Factor VIII— von Willebrand Factor

Volume I
Biochemical, Methodological, and Functional Aspects

Editors

M. J. Seghatchian, B.Sc., Ph.D.
Principal Biochemist and Head of Department
North London Blood Transfusion Centre
and
Honorary Lecturer, Department of Pharmacology
Guy's Hospital Medical School
London, England

and

G. F. Savidge, M.A., M.D.
Senior Lecturer and Honorary Consultant
Department of Haematology
United Medical and Dental Schools
of Guy's and St. Thomas' Hospital
and
Director of the Haemophilia Reference Centre
at St. Thomas' Hospital
London, England

CRC Press, Inc.
Boca Raton, Florida

Library of Congress Cataloging-in-Publication Data

Factor VIII-von Willebrand factor/editors, M. J. Seghatchian and G. F.
  Savidge.
    p. cm.
  Includes bibliographies and index.
  Contents: v. 1. Biochemical, methodological, and functional
aspects -- v. 2. Clinical aspects of deficiency states.
  ISBN 0-8493-6828-6 (v. 1). ISBN 0-8493-6829-4 (v. 2)
  1. Hemophilia. 2. Blood coagulation factor VIII. 3. Von
Willebrand factor. I. Seghatchian, M. J. II. Savidge, G. F.
(Geoffrey F.) III. Title: Factor 8-von Willebrand factor.
    [DNLM: 1. Factor VIII. 2. Hemophilia. 3. Von Willebrand's
Disease. 4. Von Willebrand Factor. WH 310 F14243]
RC642.F34 1989
616.1'572--ds19
DNLM/DLC   88-26288
for Library of Congress   CIP

This book represents information obtained from authentic and highly regarded sources. Reprinted material is
quoted with permission, and sources are indicated. A wide variety of references are listed. Every reasonable effort
has been made to give reliable data and information, but the author and the publisher cannot assume responsibility
for the validity of all materials or for the consequences of their use.

Direct all inquiries to CRC Press, Inc., 2000 Corporate Blvd., N.W., Boca Raton, Florida, 33431.

International Standard Book Number 0-8493-6828-6
International Standard Book Number 0-8493-6829-4

Library of Congress Card Number 88-26288
Printed in the United States

FOREWORD

Despite intensive research over two decades, the nature of factor VIII and von Willebrand factor in plasma has yet to be fully elucidated. This is due, in part, to the fact that VIII itself circulates as a trace protein in nanogram concentrations per milliliter of plasma, and although its site of synthesis has now been identified, the mechanism of its release has yet to be established. The elusive nature of factor VIII is well known, as it is characteristically labile and susceptible to proteolysis with the formation of activated and inactivated intermediate forms. Both factor VIII and von Willebrand factor, furthermore, demonstrate a propensity to form circulating complexes with other plasmatic and cellular components of the blood. Difficulties encountered in the characterization of these proteins are further compounded by the nature of the anticoagulants used for the collection of blood and also by the diverse methodologies that have been adopted for their purification. It is, thus, not surprising that in purification procedures using citrated plasma, purified VIII is identified as a series of polypeptides ranging from 90 to 210 kDa, while with heparin anticoagulation the major polypeptide appears to have an apparent molecular weight of 260 kDa. It follows that the constraints of the various methodologies are such that even with the most stringent purification methods with the inclusion of enzyme inhibitors, one cannot relate with certainty in vitro data to the true nature of circulating factor VIII in vivo. A further complicating issue has become apparent from recent evidence, which suggests that there is a difference between free factor VIII and complexed factor VIII with respect to synthesis, release and catabolism which may be related to pathophysiological states. Despite these seemingly insurmountable problems, the development of elegant biochemical and physiocochemical techniques over the last 10 years have led to greater insight into the structure/function relationships of VIII/vWf in both the normal condition and in the deficiency disorders of Hemophilia A and von Willebrand's Disease. Many of the previously held concepts as to the nature of the biological role of these proteins, which were often open to speculation and empiricism, have been subjected to substantial reappraisal in the light of new findings, if only to reveal an increasing degree of complexity.

A number of issues have been resolved through advances in monoclonal antibody and other technologies, and through their application to the purification of VIII and vWf, leading to the molecular cloning of the relevant genes. The derivation of the primary nucleotide sequences of these proteins from the cDNA sequences, and the elucidation of molecular events occurring during proteolytic processing are of considerable scientific and practical importance.

During the same period of time, we have witnessed unprecedented advances in the clinical and diagnostic approach to patients with VIII/vWf deficiency states and with factor VIII inhibitors. These dramatic changes have naturally led to a greater increase in patient expectation, often exceeding available medical resources. To some extent, new approaches have evolved as a consequence of the application of newer technology and to the adoption of more rational and cost-effective medical and surgical care programs.

The most significant impact on current clinical concepts, however, is attributable to the emergence of HIV related disease and an increasing awareness of the morbidity induced by other transmissible viral agents in therapeutic products. Inevitably the issues of product safety, efficacy, and purity have attained maximum priority in the face of increasing clinical demands for improved therapeutic materials at a time of financial constraint. In order to achieve these objectives, greater collaboration and cooperation between clinical and scientific disciplines have become mandatory, as has the application of more advanced manufacturing technologies and quality control.

On the basis of these recent advances, it seems most timely that a state-of-the-art review should be produced to place into perspective the many and diverse developments in the field. We have attempted to collect the most significant advances into the two volumes on Factor VIII/von Willebrand factor for this express purpose, and have invited contributions from both well-established investigators and clinicians and from a number of younger researchers of high caliber about to make their mark in VIII/vWf research. For clarity and conciseness, the two volumes have been allocated to cover scientific and methodological aspects and clinical aspects of the relevant factor deficiency states.

In volume I, the purification and structure/function relationships of VIII and vWf have been extensively reviewed, as has the relevance of advances in these areas to improved methodology and biotechnology. Emphasis has been stressed on the importance of VIII/vWf interactions with plasmatic and cellular components which inevitably will provide greater insight into the physiological role of these proteins. The issues of plasma procurement and advances in the production of therapeutic products have been included in this volume to illustrate the importance of the application of scientific advancement to the solution of practical problems.

An extensive update of progress in the clinical aspects of VIII and vWf deficiency states is presented in Volume II, where the critical issues of scientific advancement and achievement attain fruition through their relevance in improved patient diagnosis and care.

In any state-of-the-art publication, it would seem mandatory to speculate on likely future trends within the subject, although clearly this is no easy task in the rapidly changing scientific and clinical arena of factor VIII/vWf. The significant impact of the application of molecular biology in our understanding of factor VIII/vWf from both scientific and potential therapeutic aspects will obviously be sustained and enhanced with further developments in cell biology. Gene expression and regulation in both normal and pathological states will be areas of intensive interest in physiological and diagnostic terms. Information on genes encoding specific protein domains and site-directed mutagenesis may provide greater insight into the solution of practical issues such as carrier detection and inhibitor patient management. The expanding field of cell biology should provide rewarding data on processes involving post-translational modification, regulation, storage, and release of gene products. Thus, contentious issues of the role of prosequence, carbohydrate, sulfation, and phosphorylation in the expression of functional vWf may be logically explained, and an interpretation of dimerization and polymerization of vWf with respect to intracellular and membrane enzymes and receptors made possible. Although such information would appear superficially only to be of academic interest, it could potentially provide the basis of a scientific classification of vWD and possibly indicate alternative therapeutic approaches. In terms of understanding the role of vWf in primary hemostasis, myeloproliferative states, and thrombotic disease such data could be invaluable.

It can be envisaged that many analytical procedures now accepted as 'gold standard' diagnostic tests will be superseded by more specific assays requiring less technical expertise or by assays based upon *ex vivo* concepts (e.g., systems containing endothelial cell coated particles) or by the release of tritiated activation peptides. In the areas of chromogenic and fluorometric methodology designed for the more precise quantitation of factor VIII and its various forms of activation, the introduction of novel substrates or enzyme inhibitors will enhance assay specificity and sensitivity to levels currently anticipated with methods based upon antigen-antibody interactions. Developments in methodology will complement molecular and cellular biological principles for the intensive study of interactions between components of VIII/vWf and other proteins and in particular cellular structures. We would envisage that rapid advances in our knowledge of such interactions will be the major area of advance over the next decade, and will directly influence the choice of therapeutic options available for patient management.

Of grave concern at the present time are the anticipated consequences of HIV and other viral infections in both high-risk groups and in the general population, and the impact that projected developments may have upon blood banking practice and the production of co-agulation factor concentrates. In terms of HIV alone, the identification of supplementary genes and their respective functions has been a significant achievement and may result in the development of analytical procedures (e.g., NEF antibody) for improved screening purposes. Gene amplication methodology (polymerase chain reaction PCR) merits particular reference as this may provide a fundamental analytical procedure for the detection of latent HIV and other viruses in asymptomatic individuals. Once this method is fully developed it may become an obligatory test, as HTLV I, in blood donors. In a similar vein, the recent isolation of the genome of one of the strains of Non-A, Non-B hepatitis is an exciting development, and tests based upon gene analysis or antibodies to the gene products obtained may be available for blood donor screening. Of particular importance in the hemophilia patient is the elucidation of the interplay between viral cofactors which can transactivate HIV and lead to the transition between an asymptomatic state to ARC and AIDS. Although future developments in the virology, molecular and cell biology, and immunology of HIV and other viruses are well beyond the scope of these volumes, any advances will have a major impact on blood product development, manufacture, and regulatory control.

Due to the emergence of HIV and the increasing awareness of the significance of other viral contaminants in blood products, patients and physicians alike have demanded greater guarantees of blood product safety and purity from plasma procurers and blood product fractionators. Through a process of fairly rapid evolution of numerous viral inactivation procedures and a gradual but significant departure from conventional fractionation principles to high-tech chromatography procedures, this has been achieved. However, the price has been high, not only in pure monetaristic terms but also in yield from plasma starting material, leading to the current global situation of poor availability of therapeutic materials. Although the commercial development of monoclonal antibody purified virus inactivated factor con-centrates is now a reality, the long-term viability of such products derived from plasma source material must be precarious, and logically these procedures at their inception were ultimately aimed at the purification of recombinant material. It is envisaged that the inherent drawbacks in such methods will be overcome by the application of general ligand systems involving highly specific affinity peptides bound to inert matrices which can be easy re-generated and sterilized.

In the final analysis, the availability of blood products will be critically influenced by socio-economic factors, and a balance has to be struck between the realistic demands of patients and physicians and the prevailing resources at the levels of plasma procurement and manufacturing. Clearly, the generally accepted concern for safety will be reinforced in future years but constrained by the cost implications of expanding screening programs for donors. It is hoped that these problems will be resolved when recombinant products established to be safe, efficacious, and free from potential inhibitor induction through clinical trials, attain adequate availability and commercial viability.

As the scope of these volumes is wide, it is hoped that they will present modern views of various approaches and opinions to readers with both scientific and clinical interests at all levels, and stimulate new ideas and concepts in this rapidly developing subject.

NOTE

Please see Appendix for nomenclature and abbreviations used in this book.

THE EDITORS

Dr. M. J. Seghatchian is Principle Biochemist in charge of Blood Product Quality Control at the North London Blood Transfusion Centre, and he is also Honorary Lecturer in the Department of Pharmacology at Guy's Hospital Medical School. His basic training is in chemistry, specializing in Radio/Radiation Chemistry in various Nuclear Research Centers in France, obtaining in 1964 his doctorate in Physical Chemistry from the University of Paris. Subsequent to further postdoctoral studies in the practical application of radioisotopes in medicine and spectroscopic techniques in the investigation of drug enzyme interactions, he also obtained a Ph.D. in Medical Biochemistry from the University of London in 1972. Since 1973 Dr. Seghatchian's interests have been focused in the field of hemostasis, initially as a visiting scientist for a number of years at the National Institute of Biological Standards and Control in Hampstead, North London and the MRC Epidemiology and Medical Care Unit at Northwick Park Hospital, Harrow. During this time he worked on the standardization/automation of coagulation assays, the activation/fragmentation/VIII/vWf in clinical concentrates, and the interaction of VIII/vWf with other plasma proteins and polyanions. In the capacity of visiting scientist he has also collaborated with several leading scientists and clinicians in Sweden, France, Italy, the U.S., Canada, and South America on the molecular abnormalities and activation states of hemostatic proteins including inhibitors of proteolytic enzymes, substances responsible for the thrombogenicity of Vitamin K-dependent coagulation concentrates and the application of chromogenic substrates and other molecular markers in general hemostasis. More recently, he has become involved in the development of methods for the evaluation of the nature of low molecular weight and standard heparin-induced thrombocytopenia.

Dr. Seghatchian's current research interests include the characterization of the activity state of coagulation factors implicated in aphoresis procedures, hypercoagulability and thrombogenicity, with particular reference to clinical and methodological aspects of VIII/VIIIa/vWf fragments, VIIa/VII, Protein C/Ca, release of activation peptides, and the formation of circulating tenase and prothrombinase complexes in various pathophysiologic states. He has pioneered the chromogenic assay of VIII and the development of methodologies for the characterization of native and altered forms of VIII/vWf complexes in clinical concentrates and specific disorders.

Dr. Seghatchian is a founder member of both the British Society of Blood Transfusion and the British Society of Haemostasis and Thrombosis, an active member of the Working Party on VIII:C standardization and an ordinary member of several International Societies. He has recently contributed to two CRC Press books on thrombin and chromogenic substrates and acts as an advisory member for CRC Press. Dr. Seghatchian is currently an editor of the *Thrombosis Research Journal* and has previously acted as a WHO Consultant Coagulation expert for the Mediterranean countries.

Dr. G. F. Savidge is currently Senior Lecturer and Honorary Consultant in the Department of Haematology, United Medical and Dental Schools of Guy's and St. Thomas' Hospital in London, U.K. and Director of the Haemophilia Reference Centre at St. Thomas' Hospital. After Matriculation in 1959 he gained an Honours Degree in Natural Sciences from Queens' College, Cambridge in 1962, and upon completion of clinical studies at St. Bartholomew's Hospital, degrees in Medicine and Surgery and subsequently Master of Arts degree from the same University. After three years hospital practice in London, he continued his postgraduate studies in General Medicine and Pathology in Scandinavia, obtaining further medical qualifications and specialist accreditation in Stockholm. During this time his interests in thrombosis and hemostasis were actively encouraged and skillfully focused under the scientific expertise of Professor Birger Blömback at the Institute of Coagulation Research and as a Physician under Professor Margaretha Blömback in the Department of Coagulation Disorders at the Karolinska Institute in Stockholm.

Upon completion of his doctoral thesis on the study of the Biological Effects of Chemical and Physiological Reducing Agents on VIII/vWf, he returned to London to take up his present position. As part of his commitment as Reference Centre Director, he is Chairman of Working Parties involved in the National Reorganisation of Haemophilia Care, and in the Surveillence of von Willebrand's Disease. Dr. Savidge is also Haematology Representative on the WFH Orthopaedic Advisory Committee and Adviser in General Haematology and Coagulation to IHG, which provides postgraduate medical education links between the United Kingdom and Saudi Arabia. His particular clinical interests include the management of factor VIII inhibitor patients and studies of the long-term cost effectiveness of early orthopedic intervention and associated rehabilitation programs in hemophilia.

His academic interests have centered on the application of general ligand matrices for the purification of VIII/vWf, the interaction of VIII/vWf with other biological components, the biosynthesis of vWf, ultrastructural studies of platelet/vWf, erythrocyte modification of fibrin structure, and the study of coagulation changes induced by extracorporeal circulation.

He is a member of a number of National and International Scientific Societies and a founder member of the British Society of Thrombosis and Haemostasis.

CONTRIBUTORS, VOLUME I

D. L. Aronson
Research Professor of Medicine
George Washington University
 Medical Center
Washington, D.C.

Stephen I. Chavin, M.D.
Associate Professor
Departments of Medicine and
 Biochemistry
School of Medicine & Dentistry
University of Rochester
Rochester, New York

Elisabeth M. Cramer, M.D.
Associate Professor
Department of Hematology
CHU Xavier Bichat
Paris, France

R. G. Dalton
Department of Hematology
St. Thomas' Hopsital
London, England

Susan Elödi, Ph.D.
Professor and Deputy Director
National Institute of Haematology
 and Blood Transfusion
Budapest, Hungary

Thomas Exner, Ph.D.
Principal Scientific Officer
Department of Hematology
Westmead Hospital
Sydney, New South Wales, Australia

Philip J. Fay, Ph.D.
Assistant Professor
Department of Medicine and Hematology
School of Medicine & Dentistry
University of Rochester
Rochester, New York

Alison Helena Goodall, Ph.D.
Lecturer in Immunology
Haemophilia Centre and
 Haemostasis Unit
Royal Free Hospital School of Medicine
London, England

R. M. Hardisty, M.D.
Emeritus Professor
Hemophilia Center and
 Hemostasis Unit
Royal Free Hospital
London, England

Paul Harrison, Ph.D.
Research Scientist
Coagulation Research Unit
Rayne Institute
St. Thomas' Hospital
London, England

Margaret A. Howard, Ph.D.
Research Fellow
Department of Medicine
Monash University
Melbourne, Victoria, Australia

Jerry Koutts, M.D.
Head, Clinical Haematology Unit
Department of Medicine
Sydney University
Westmead Hospital
Sydney, New South Wales, Australia

R. S. Lane, M.D.
Director
Blood Products Laboratory
Elstree, Hertfordshire, England

Claudine Mazurier, Ph.D.
Head, Hemostasis Research Laboratory
Centre Regional de Transfusion Sanguine
Lille, France

Pierre Meulien, Ph.D.
Research Scientist
Division of Molecular and Cellular
  Biology
Transgene S.A.
Strasbourg, France

Hans Pannekoek, Ph.D.
Head of Department of Molecular
  Biology
Blood Transfusion Service
The Netherlands Red Cross
Amsterdam, Netherlands

Andrea Pavirani, Ph.D.
Research Scientist
Division of Molecular and Cellular
  Biology
Transgene S.A.
Strasbourg, France

J. H. Reinders, Ph.D.
Cell Biologist
Department of Pharmacology
Duphar b.v.
Weesp, Netherlands

Richard Howard Saundry, Ph.D.
Senior Biochemist
Department of Hematology
St. Thomas' Hospital
London, England

Geoffrey F. Savidge, M.A., M.D.
Director
Hemophilia Center
St. Thomas' Hospital
London, England

M. J. Seghatchian, B.Sc., Ph.D.
Principal Biochemist and Head
Blood Products Quality Control
  and Research Development
North London Blood Transfusion
Edgware, England

Cees Th. Smit Sibinga, M.D., Ph.D.
Medical Director
Red Cross Blood Bank Groningen-
  Drenthe
Groningen, Netherlands

T. J. Snape, Ph.D.
Manufacturing Manager
Blood Products Laboratory
Elstree, Hertfordshire, England

James K. Smith, Ph.D.
Chief Project Scientist
Plasma Fractionation Laboratory
Churchill Hospital
Oxford, England

J. A. van Mourik, Ph.D.
Head, Department of Blood Coagulation
Central Laboratory of the Netherlands
  Red Cross
Blood Transfusion Service
Amsterdam, Netherlands

Cornelis L. Verweij
Department of Molecular Biology
Central Laboratory of the Netherlands
  Red Cross
Blood Transfusion Service
Amsterdam, Netherlands

CONTRIBUTORS, VOLUME II

Judy Beard, M.B.
Senior Registrar
Department of Hematology
St. Thomas' Hospital
London, England

Donna C. Boone, M.S.
Statistician
Clinical Laboratory
University of Southern California
Los Angeles, California

Shelby L. Dietrich, M.D.
Director
Southern California Hemophilia Center
Huntington Orthopedic Hospital
Pasadena, California

Elizabeth Fischer
Department of Pediatrics
Cornell University Medical Center
New York, New York

John B. Graham, M.D.
Distinguished Professor
Department of Pathology
University of North Carolina
Chapel Hill, North Carolina

Margaret W. Hilgartner, M.D.
Harold Weil Professor and Vice
  Chairman
Department of Pediatrics
Chief, Pediatric Hematology/Oncology
New York Hospital
Cornell Medical Center
New York, New York

Robert Hill, F.R.C.S.
Department of Orthopedics
St. Thomas' Hospital
London, England

Martin J. Inwood, M.D.
Professor
Department of Medicine
University of Western Ontario
London, Ontario, Canada

Peter M. Jones, M.D.
Director
Newcastle Hemophilia Center
Royal Victoria Infirmary
Newcastle Upon Tyne, England

Peter B. A. Kernoff, M.D.
Director
Hemophilia Center and Hemostasis Unit
Royal Free Hospital
London, England

Kathryn Siena Kirwin, M.D.
Instructor
Department of Hematology/Oncology
George Washington University Medical
  Center
Washington, D.C.

Christine A. Lee, M.D.
Consultant
Hemophilia Center and Hemostasis Unit
Royal Free Hospital
London, England

Peter H. Levine, M.D.
Chairman and Director
Department of Medicine
Comprehensive Hemophilia Center
Worcester Memorial Hospital
Worcester, Massachusetts

C. A. Ludlam, M.B., Ch.B.
Consultant
Department of Hematology
Royal Infirmary
Edinburgh, Scotland

Reuben S. Mibashan, M.D.
Reader
Department of Hematology
School of Medicine and Dentistry
King's College
London, England

Inga M. Nilsson, M.D.
Department of Coagulation Disorders
University of Lund
Lund, Sweden

Michael J. O'Doherty, M.R.C.P.
Consultant Physician
Haemophilia Center
St. Thomas' Hospital
London, England

Marcus E. Pembrey, M.D.
Professor
Mothercare Department of Pediatric
  Genetics
Institute of Child Health
London, England

Holger Pettersson, M.D.
Professor and Chairman
Department of Radiology
University Hospital
Lund, Sweden

Laura E. Pickard, M.A.
Research Coordinator
Department of Clinical Epidemiology
  and Biostatistics
McMaster University
Hamilton, Ontario, Canada

Christopher V. Prowse, D.Phil.
Top Grade Scientist
Blood Transfusion Service
Royal Infirmary
Edinburgh, Scotland

Harold R. Roberts, M.D.
Professor
Department of Medicine
University of North Carolina
Chapel Hill, North Carolina

G. F. Savidge, M.D.
Hemophilia Center
St. Thomas' Hospital
London, England

M. J. Seghatchian, Ph.D.
Principal Biochemist and Head
Blood Products Quality Control
  and Research Development
North London Blood Transfusion
Edgware, England

Uri Seligsohn, M.D.
Professor, Institute of Hematology
Tel Aviv Medical Center
Ichilov Hospital
Sackler School of Medicine
Tel Aviv University
Tel Aviv, Israel

Michael A. Smith, M.A.
Consultant Orthopedic Surgeon
Department of Orthopedics
St. Thomas' Hospital Medical School
London, England

TABLE OF CONTENTS, VOLUME I

Chapter 1
The Purification, Structure, and Function of Factor VIII 1
S. I. Chavin and P. J. Fay

Chapter 2
Advances in Biotechnology of Factor VIII 25
A. Pavirani and P. Meulien

Chapter 3
Purification, Biochemistry, and Structure/Function Relationships of vWf 41
C. Mazurier

Chapter 4
Molecular Cloning of Genetic Material Encoding vWf 83
C. L. Verweij and H. Pannekoek

Chapter 5
Advances in Amidolytic Assay of Factor VIII: Variables Affecting the Rate of Xa
Generation 97
M. Seghatchian

Chapter 6
Progress in vWf Methodology and Its Relevance in vWD 129
R. G. Dalton and G. F. Savidge

Chapter 7
Advances in Immunochemical Aspects of vWD 147
A. H. Goodall

Chapter 8
vWf and the Vessel Wall 173
J. A. van Mourik and J. H. Reinders

Chapter 9
vWf, Platelets, and Megakaryocytes 187
R. M. Hardisty

Chapter 10
Electron Microscopic Studies of vWf in Platelets and Megakaryocytes 201
E. M. Cramer

Chapter 11
Interaction of Surface-Bound Factor VIII with Other Coagulation Factors 215
S. Elodi

Chapter 12
Interaction of Factor VIII with vWf in Mixed Immunoradiometric Assay Systems 227
T. Exner and J. Koutts

Chapter 13
Interaction of Cell Proteases with Factor VIII and vWf 237
M. A. Howard

Chapter 14
Interaction of Factor VIII/vWf with Solid Matrices and Matrix-Bound Ligands........257
R. H. Saundy and P. Harrison

Chapter 15
Factor VIII in Regional Blood Banking Practice 279
C. Th. Smit Sibinga

Chapter 16
Advances in Plasma Fractionation and in the Production of Factor VIII Concentrates..289
J. K. Smith, T. J. Snape, and R. S. Lane

Chapter 17
Virus Transmission by Factor VIII Products...301
D. L. Aronson

Appendix — Nomenclature and Abbreviations 325

Index 327

TABLE OF CONTENTS, VOLUME II

Chapter 1
Phenotypic and Genotypic Carrier Detection in Hemophilia..............................1
J. B. Graham

Chapter 2
Prenatal Diagnosis of Hemophilia A 17
M. E. Pembrey and R. S. Mibashan

Chapter 3
Clinical and Laboratory Assessment of Patients with Hemophilia 33
J. Beard and G. F. Savidge

Chapter 4
Diagnostic Imaging in Hemophilia 49
H. Pettersson

Chapter 5
Orthopedic Assessment of the Hemophilic Patient......................................65
R. A. Hill and M. A. Smith

Chapter 6
Combined Factor V and VIII Deficiency 89
U. Seligsohn

Chapter 7
Progress in von Willebrand's Disease: Diagnosis, Classification, and Management 101
I. M. Nilsson

Chapter 8
Mechanism of Action and Clinical Use of DDAVP 119
C. V. Prowse and C. A. Ludlam

Chapter 9
Comprehensive Care in Hemophilia 135
P. Jones

Chapter 10
Current Therapy in Hemophilia 145
M. Hilgartner and E. Fischer

Chapter 11
Current Concepts on the Management of Inhibitors to Factor VIII 157
K. S. Kirwin and H. R. Roberts

Chapter 12
Orthopedic Management of Hemophilia 183
M. A. Smith

Chapter 13
Regulatory Control, Standardization, and Characterization of Clinical Concentrates....223
M. J. Seghatchian

Chapter 14
Liver Disease in Hemophilia 255
C. A. Lee and P. B. A. Kernoff

Chapter 15
Non-Viral Complications of Factor Replacement in Hemophilia and von Willebrand's
Disease 269
J. Beard, G. F. Savidge, and M. J. Seghatchian

Chapter 16
ARC and AIDS in Hemophilia 281
S. L. Dietrich and D. C. Boone

Chapter 17
Clinical Manifestations of Aids and Their Management 297
M. J. O'Doherty and G. F. Savidge

Chapter 18
The Implications of Acquired Immunodeficiency Syndrome for the Management of
Hemophilia 321
P. H. Levine

Chapter 19
Socio-Economic Aspects of Modern Hemophilia Care 329
M. J. Inwood and L. E. Pickard

Appendix — Nomenclature and Abbreviations 343

Index 345

Chapter 1

THE PURIFICATION, STRUCTURE, AND FUNCTION OF FACTOR VIII

Stephen I. Chavin and Philip J. Fay

TABLE OF CONTENTS

I.   Introduction 2

II.   Procedures for the Purification of VIII 2
        A.   Cryoprecipitation 2
        B.   Separation of VIII from Fibrinogen 3
        C.   Selective Precipitation of VIII Using Polyelectrolytes 3
        D.   Dissociation of VIII from its Complex with vWf 3
        E.   The Use of Antibodies to Purify VIII 3
                1.   Antibodies to vWf 3
                2.   Antibodies to VIII 4
        F.   Affinity Chromatography 4
        G.   High Performance Liquid Chromatography (HPLC) 4
        H.   Purification Schemes 4

III.   Structure and Biochemical Characterization of VIII 5
        A.   The Precursor Form of VIII 5
        B.   Polypeptide Composition of VIII 5
                1.   Human VIII 5
                2.   Animal VIII 6
        C.   Size of Native VIII in Plasma 6
        D.   Domains of VIII 6
        E.   Factor VIII and Ceruloplasmin: is VIII a Copper Binding
                Protein? 9
        F.   Sulfhydryl Groups and Disulfide Bridges in VIII 10
        G.   Role of Carbohydrate in VIII 10

IV.   Regulation of VIII:C 11
        A.   Activators of VIII 11
                1.   Thrombin 11
                2.   Factor X_a 13
                3.   Factor IX_a 14
                4.   What is the "Physiological" Activator of VIII? 15
                5.   Does Nonactivated VIII Possess Significant Clotting
                        Activity? 16
        B.   Inactivation of VIII 16
                1.   Inactivation of VIII_a 16
                2.   Inactivation by Activated Protein C 16
        C.   The Role of VIII in Blood Clotting 17

References 19

I. INTRODUCTION

Biochemical characterization of factor VIII (VIII) was an elusive goal until around 1980. Prior to that time, investigations on VIII used plasma or partially purified preparations in which VIII was merely a trace contaminant (often accounting for less than 1% of the total protein). Many of these early studies focused upon the gel filtration properties, the effects of ionic strength, and divalent cations (mostly calcium) and measured only the procoagulant activity (VIII:C) and not VIII protein. The results from different laboratories often were contradictory and were additionally confusing because of the failure of investigators to distinguish between VIII (previously called the antihemophilic factor) and von Willebrand factor (vWf). It is likely that many of the properties of VIII revealed in these earlier experiments reflected its interactions with different populations of vWf multimers and perhaps with other plasma proteins as well.

These earlier studies have been reviewed extensively[1-7] and therefore will not be covered in the present chapter.

The major biochemical advances in our understanding of VIII are the result of the development and application of a variety of purification techniques. The dramatic achievements in protein purification finally were crowned by the successful molecular cloning of the entire gene for VIII. The combination of data about VIII in plasma plus the size and structure of its gene and mRNA have given us a much clearer picture of the structure of this protein, although our knowledge of its function remains incomplete. This chapter will concentrate upon the structure and function of VIII based primarily upon these recent data and will utilize earlier results when appropriate.

Attempts to purify VIII have been plagued by a number of difficult problems: (1) low concentrations in plasma of the protein, (2) loss of activity during purification, making it difficult to keep track of the protein, and (3) association of VIII with a variety of other plasma proteins, e.g., fibrinogen and/or vWf, either because of physical association or similar physicochemical properties. During the past 5 years, these problems have been circumvented, and several research groups have been able to isolate very highly purified preparations of VIII.

Although a variety of different procedures and combinations of procedures have been used, most of these are based upon a small number of basic procedures. These common features will be discussed first, followed by the details of several representative purification schemes.

II. PROCEDURES FOR THE PURIFICATION OF VIII

A. Cryoprecipitation

This phenomenon was first recognized by Pool et al.[8] Certain proteins, predominantly fibrinogen, precipitate and fail to redissolve when the frozen plasma is thawed. Many proteins, including VIII, fibronectin, and vWf, also are found in this precipitate. Fibrinogen plays a central role in this phenomenon, as shown by the absence of cryoprecipitation in patients who lack fibrinogen. Between 50 and 80% of the original VIII is recovered in the cryoprecipitate. The reason for the co-precipitation of VIII is not known although it is likely to be related to its physical association in plasma with vWf.

Virtually all purifications, in their early stages, take advantage of cryoprecipitation. In those which start from plasma, the initial step is cryoprecipitation. In those which utilize commercial concentrates, the cryoprecipitation was carried out earlier in the production of the concentrates. The procedure itself involves freezing citrated plasma to $-20°C$, leaving it for 12 to 24 h, and then thawing it without disturbing the layer near the bottom of the container; this layer is enriched in protein and salt. The use of rapid freezing and rapid thawing appears to result in higher yields of VIII.[9] The physical basis for cryoprecipitation probably is at least in part a low temperature salting out of a mixture of sparingly soluble proteins.

B. Separation of VIII from Fibrinogen

This can be accomplished by immunochemical means or by utilizing the differences in size between VIII and fibrinogen. VIII in plasma circulates in a complex with vWf and perhaps other proteins, the apparent molecular weight of this complex varying between 1 to 2×10^6 and 20×10^6 Da or higher. The majority of fibrinogen circulates as molecules of 340,000 Da. Thus gel filtration chromatography using low percentage agarose resin will allow separation of the majority of fibrinogen from the VIII/vWf complex. The void volume fraction is predominantly vWf, with the VIII comprising between 0.1 and 1.0% of total protein. In addition, there are usually small amounts of fibrinogen, fibronectin, and other proteins of high molecular weight and low solubility.

C. Selective Precipitation of VIII Using Polyelectrolytes

Some of the earliest attempts to purify VIII (especially for therapeutic purposes) utilized organic solvents such as ethanol or ether, which were already being used in more general schemes of plasma fractionation.[10] VIII usually was recovered in the early (less soluble) fractions. More recently, polyethylene glycol has been used with some success. The most successful innovation was the use by Johnson and collaborators[11] of co-polymers composed of ethylene and maleic anhydride cross-linked with dimethylaminopropylamide. Low charge and high charge (designated E5 and E100, respectively) have been utilized. The low charge polyelectrolyte was used by Rotblat et al.[12] to purify VIII 112,000-fold over plasma.

D. Dissociation of VIII from its Complex with vWf

In the 1960s, it was realized that the physical properties of VIII were highly influenced by its ionic conditions. In addition to the effects of high concentration of a variety of divalent cations,[13] high concentration of sodium chloride,[14,15] increasing pH,[13] or very low ionic strength also affected such properties as sedimentation rates and gel filtration.[16-18] The major effect of these treatments probably is to cause the dissociation of VIII from vWf. The condition most efficient in dissociating VIII from vWf while preserving VIII:C is 250 mM Ca^{++}.[13] This dissociating effect of Ca^{++} is surprising inasmuch as the constituent polypeptide chains of VIII itself may be held together in part by calcium and/or other divalent cations.

When the plasma form of VIII is subjected to high concentration of Ca^{++}, its sedimentation rate becomes much slower and its relative molecular weight decreases considerably.[18] By passing the VIII through a gel filtration column in the presence of high Ca^{++}, the lower relative molecular weight VIII may be partially separated from many of the contaminating proteins, whose molecular properties are not affected by high Ca^{++}. In some procedures, the calcium dissociation step is carried out in conjunction with an anti-vWf antibody to immobilize the vWf.

E. The Use of Antibodies to Purify VIII

1. Antibodies to vWf

This approach utilizes the association between VIII and vWf. Polyclonal or monoclonal antibody to vWf is coupled to an insoluble column support such as sepharose.[19-22] The vWf plus its associated VIII are retained on the column. The VIII then can be selectively eluted using buffers containing 250 mM Ca^{++} which weakens interaction between VIII and vWf, but does not disrupt the binding between vWf and its antibody. Using this method VIII may be obtained in high yield and relatively high purity.

Table 1
PURIFICATION SCHEMES FOR VIII

Starting material	Technique	Final specific activity U/mg	Comments	Ref.
Bovine plasma	Ammonium sulfate precipitation Glycine precipitation DEAE sephadex Sulfate sepharose Sephadex G200 Factor X-sepharose	4,500	Reduction of disulfide bonds with 2-mercaptoethanol	29
Porcine plasma	Aluminum hydroxide adsorption PEG 5000 precipitation QAE cellulose Dextran sulfate agarose Anti-VIII monoclonal antibody column	6,000	Elution of VIII from antibody column required 50% ethylene glycol	19,24
Human therapeutic concentrate	Anti-vWf monoclonal antibody column Amino hexylsepharose	2,300	Final product contaminated with vWf and fibrinogen	31
Human cryoprecipitate	Polyelectrolyte 5 Anti-vWf monoclonal antibody column Anti-VIII monoclonal antibody column	4,700	Elution of VIII from column with 20% ethylene glycol	28
Human therapeutic concentrate	Biogel A15M gel filtration Aminohexyl sepharose adsorption chromatography Sephacryl S400 gel filtration HPLC anion exchange chromatography	20,000	Resolved several distinct forms of active VIII	30

2. Antibodies to VIII

Earlier investigations used (polyclonal) human antibodies, usually from hemophilic patients with acquired inhibitors to VIII.[22] One problem with these reagents is that VIII may be destroyed irreversibly after association with them, thereby making it difficult to isolate VIII which retains clotting activity. A more satisfactory approach uses monoclonal antibodies to VIII.[24-28] These need to be carefully selected for optimal affinity for VIII; if the affinity is too low, the VIII will be bound inefficiently, whereas if it is too high, elution will require severe conditions which may result in loss of VIII:C.

F. Affinity Chromatography

VIII interacts during clotting with a number of other clotting proteins, especially factors IX and X. Vehar and Davie[29] utilized a column with covalently attached factor X to selectively absorb VIII and were able to achieve a tenfold increase in the specific activity of the VIII.

G. High Performance Liquid Chromatography (HPLC)

High resolution anion exchange chromatography was used by Fay et al.[30] as a final purification step for human VIII. This technique allowed the partial separation of different active forms of VIII.

H. Purification Schemes

Several purification schemes which have yielded highly purified VIII are summarized in Table 1. Although a great variety of steps are used, most of the procedures give final products with specific activities in the range of 2000 to 20,000 U/mg protein. This wide range may be the result of varying degrees of activation of the final products or may reflect differences in methods used to determine clotting activity and/or protein concentration. Some of the preparations may also contain partially inactive VIII peptides. Fay et al.[30] observed that some VIII polypeptides eluted from an HPLC anion exchange resin in a region lacking VIII:C clotting activity, the overall yields varying between 1 and 20% of the initial activity. Nevertheless, the similarities among the final products are more striking than the differences, especially considering the different starting materials and different techniques.

III. STRUCTURE AND BIOCHEMICAL CHARACTERIZATION OF VIII

A. The Precursor Form of VIII

Based upon the composition of the cDNA from molecular clones of VIII, VIII is synthesized as a single polypeptide chain containing either 2332[32,33] or 2351[34] amino acid residues and has a 267,039 M_r.[34] These estimates do not include carbohydrate, of which VIII possesses an unknown amount.

Assuming a sugar content of 10%, the precursor molecule would have about 300,000 M_r.[32,34] Attempts to isolate significant amounts of precursor have included the use of an impressive variety of enzyme inhibitors to prevent proteolysis,[38] the analysis of plasma samples as quickly and with as little manipulation as possible, and the use of rapid immunoadsorbent procedures.[12] Rotblat et al.[28] and Fulcher et al.[39,40] succeeded in demonstrating small amounts of a single polypeptide in the 300- to 360-kDa range, but this high molecular weight form was a minor constituent compared with the predominant smaller molecules. It would seem that VIII undergoes rapid proteolysis before or very soon after secretion into plasma.

B. Polypeptide Composition of VIII

1. Human VIII

When analyzed by sodium-dodecyl sulfate (SDS) polyacrylamide gel electrophoresis (PAGE) after reduction of disulfide bonds, all of the VIII preparations consist of multiple polypeptides which belong to one of two groups: a family of heavy chains from around 90 up to 210 kDa and a light chain which consists of a closely spaced doublet of 79 to 83 kDa[24,28-31,33] as seen in Table 2.

The heavy chains share the same N-terminal sequences and appear to be the products of proteolytic cleavage at a number of sites in their carboxy terminal portions.[35] This group of chains is derived from the N-terminal portion of the precursor VIII polypeptide as shown in Figure 1. The largest member of this group (albeit not the predominant one) is 210 kDa (measured by SDS PAGE). It consists of between 1155 and 1194 residues and, therefore, has a polypeptide weight of approximately 135,000 Da. There are 14 potential asparagine-linked glycosylation sites,[18,19] starting at residue 757 and extending C-terminally to residue 1512; thus, some of the unaccounted-for mass may be carbohydrate. In most preparations, the predominant heavy chains are in the range of 90 to 120 kDa, but all share a common N-terminus; the C-terminal end of the heavy chain seems to be especially susceptible to proteolytic cleavage.

The light chain doublet is derived from the C-terminal third of the precursor. The N-terminal of the light chain corresponds to residue 1649 of the mature protein, and the C-terminal of the isolated light chain corresponds to that predicted from the cDNA sequence.[33-35] Thus, the light chain of VIII appears to be relatively more resistant to proteolysis.

None of the preparations of purified VIII contains significant amounts of the single chain precursor of VIII. Furthermore, significant amounts of the middle portion of the molecule,

Table 2

**OLIGOMERIC MOLECULAR WEIGHTS AND POLYPEPTIDE
COMPOSITION OF PURIFIED VIII**

| Species | Oligomer molecular weight | | Constituent polypeptides (kDa)[a] | | Ref. |
	Method	M_r, (kDa)	Heavy chains	Light chains	
Bovine	Gel filtration	250	93, 88, 85[b]		29
Porcine	—	Not reported	166, 130, 82	76	19,24
Human	—	Not reported	188—92[c]	80/79	31
Human	Polyacrylamide gel electrophoresis, with protein denatured but unreduced	360	210—110[c]	80/79	28
Human	—	Not reported	210—90[c]	80	35
Human	Sucrose density gradient centrifugation and gel filtration	237	170, 155, 146	83/81	30
		201	146, 120, 110	83/81	
		141	93	83/81	

a M_r determined by polyacrylamide gel electrophoresis, under reducing and denaturing conditions.
b   The bovine polypeptides were not designated as heavy or light chains.
c   Multiple chains, in varying amounts, in these preparations.

with most of the potential glycosylation sites, residues 1155 to 1649, have not yet been isolated.[28,35] Once this region of the precursor molecule has been cleaved, it appears to dissociate from the active VIII, although its destination and function are not known.

2. Animal VIII

Vehar and Davie[29] isolated bovine VIII consisting of three polypeptides of 93, 88, and 85 kDa. The polypeptide pattern was unchanged by reduction (although the protein earlier had been subjected to disulfide bond cleavage in the course of its purification). This form of bovine VIII may correspond to the low relative molecular weight human heterodimer isolated by Fay et al.[30] consisting of a 93-kDa heavy chain plus the 83/81-kDa light chain. Porcine VIII, isolated by Knutson and Fass[19] and Fass and colleagues,[24] consists primarily of 82- and 72-kDa polypeptides with smaller amounts of 166- and 133-kDa polypeptides. The 166-, 130-, and 82-kDa polypeptides all share the same N-terminal sequence and appear to represent the heavy chain family in this species. The 76-kDa polypeptide represents the light chain. The relative simplicity of the polypeptide composition of both animal species is in contrast to the heterogeneity in humans.

C. Size of Native VIII in Plasma

One of the earliest estimates of the size of bovine VIII by Vehar and Davie[29] based upon gel filtration analysis was about 250,000 Da. Fay and colleagues[30] were able to partially separate, by HPLC anion exchange, active forms of VIII with different polypeptide compositions as shown in Figure 2A and B. Each form contained different predominant heavy chains plus the same light chain doublet. One form consisted of heavy chains of 155 or 146 kDa. A second fraction contained a heavy chain of either 120 or 110 kDa. The third fraction contained only a 93-kDa heavy chain. All of the fractions contained the light chain doublet (83/81 kDa). The average molecular weights for each of these forms, calculated from the Stokes radii and sedimentation coefficients, were 237,500, 201,000, and 141,000 Da, respectively. Thus, purified VIII appears to be a heterodimeric molecule consisting of one heavy and one light chain, as suggested earlier for porcine VIII by Fass et al.[24]

These recent estimates of molecular weight, using purified VIII, may be compared with

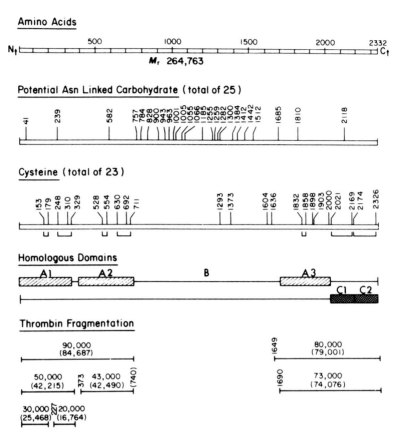

FIGURE 1. Schematic representation of the single chain precursor of VIII. Locations of asparagine and cysteine residues are shown to illustrate potential, but not proven, sites of carbohydrate additions and disulfide pairing, respectively. Domain structures are shown as boxes which indicate the triplicated "A" domain and the duplicated "C" domain. The M_r of the thrombin-derived fragments were determined by SDS PAGE; values shown in parenthesis represent the M_r calculated from amino acid composition. The position of cleavage of the 90-kD polypeptide has not been determined. (From Vehar, G. A., Keyt, B., Eaton, D., et al., *Nature (London)*, 312, 337, 1984, Macmillan Journals Ltd. With permission.)

earlier ones utilizing different techniques and VIII preparations of lower purity as presented in Table 3. Hoyer and Trabold[36] measured the sedimentation coefficient and Stokes radius of partially purified VIII:C and calculated a relative molecular weight of approximately 285,000. Harman et al.,[37] using irradiation inactivation, calculated a relative molecular weight of about 140,000. In this latter paper, however, it should be noted that the molecular weight of vWf was underestimated to a significant degree. Weinstein et al.[38] used an immunochemical procedure combined with nonreducing SDS gel electrophoresis to estimate the relative molecular weight of plasma VIII of around 240,000.

Most of the above results suggest that the circulating form of VIII has a molecular weight of around 200,000 Da and consists of two different polypeptide chains. There appears to be little of the uncleaved single chain precursor molecule in circulation. Much of the size heterogeneity is the result of proteolytic processing of the larger species of VIII.

The heterodimer appears to be held together by noncovalent bonds. The electrophoretic pattern in an SDS gel is the same before and after reduction.[24,29-31] Thus, the constituent polypeptides are not held together by disulfide bonds. They can be dissociated from one another by treatment with ethylene diamine tetraacetic acid (EDTA), a chelator of Ca^{++}

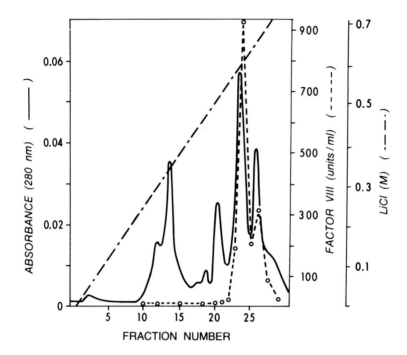

FIGURE 2A.   High performance anion exchange chromatography on a Mono-Q column to purify different forms of active VIII. The profiles of absorbance and VIII activity are slightly out of phase because the absorption was monitored continuously, whereas the activity was assayed in individual functions; the lag is due to the dead space in the collection system. An elution gradient of lithium chloride (LiCl) was used.

and other divalent cations. The divalent cation involved is presumed to be Ca^{++}, although there is no direct evidence for this. The dissociated chains are inactive, and attempts to restore activity by remixing the chains in the presence of Ca^{++} have been unsuccessful.[24,30]

D. Domains of VIII

Protein chains often consist of localized regions called domains which may subserve a particular function of a protein or may correspond approximately to an exon of DNA. Domains often comprise regions of the polypeptide chain which are relatively compact and physically distinguishable from neighboring regions.[41]

Analysis of the amino acid sequence of VIII suggested the presence of six domains which could be grouped into three categories on the basis of internal sequence homology.[33] The A-domains are represented by three regions: residues 1 to 329, 389 to 711, and 1649 to 2019, with 30% amino acid homology to one another as shown in Figure 1. These domains also have a pairwise homology of 30% when compared with the copper binding protein ceruloplasmin. The long sequence (about 900 amino acids) between the second and third A-domains constitutes the C-terminal region of the heavy chain and has been designated as the B-domain, which is susceptible to proteolytic cleavage and contains most of the potential glycosylation sites. The third type, the C-domain, consists of a pair of sequences adjacent to one another and constituting the C-terminal portion of the precursor molecule. The C-domains have a 20% homology with a family of lectins from the slime mold Dictyostelium. Thus the domain structure of VIII is represented by NH_2-A1-A2-B-A3-C1-C2-COOH. The heavy chain corresponds to the A1-A2-B-domains (variability in its size results from proteolysis within the B-region), whereas the light chain corresponds to the A3-C1-C2-domains.

Very little is known about the functions of the different domains. There has been a direct

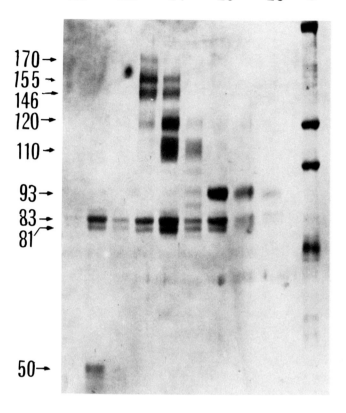

FIGURE 2B. Polypeptide composition of the various forms of VIII eluted from the column shown in Figure 2A. The polypeptides were analyzed by SDS polyacrylamide gel electrophoresis, after reduction. The numbers across the top of the figure indicate the column fractions. The column "S" contains molecular weight standards. The numbers along the left edge are the molecular radii, in kiloDaltons, of the various polypeptides described in the text. The bulk of the eluted VIII activity was found in fractions 23 to 27. Fractions 21 and 22, with virtually no VIII activity, appear to contain only the 83/81 light chain doublet. (Figures 2A and 2B from Fay, P. J., Anderson, M., Chavin, S. I., and Marder, V. J., *Biochim. Biophys. Acta*, 871, 268, 1986. With permission.)

demonstration of binding of the 80-kDa light chain to vWf.[42] None of the other known functional sites on VIII, e.g., those which bind either to phospholipid, factor IX_a or factor X, can at this time be related to any of these regions of the molecule.

E. Factor VIII and Ceruloplasmin: Is VIII a Copper Binding Protein?

The homology between VIII and ceruloplasmin[32,34] was totally unexpected. The amino acid residues which are thought to be involved in one of the three types of copper coordination complexes in ceruloplasmin are found in the first and the third of the A-domains, suggesting a possible role for copper in the structure of VIII.[33,43,44] The well-known structural and functional similarities between VIII and factor V have recently been extended to at least limited sequence homology.[43] Furthermore, factor V has been shown by atomic absorption spectroscopy to have one tightly bound copper atom per mole of protein;[45] similar findings have not yet been reported for VIII. Although it is possible that the inhibitor effect of EDTA on VIII is by means of chelation of Cu^{++}, it is likely that calcium or other divalent cations may also play a critical role in the integrity of VIII.

Table 3
MOLECULAR WEIGHTS OF "NATIVE" HUMAN VIII ACTIVITY
DEVOID OF vWf

M$_r$ (kDa)	Method of analysis	Comments	Ref.
285	Sucrose density centrifugation	Partially purified VIII separated from vWf and measured as clotting activity	36
240	Electrophoresis of immune complex unreduced in presence of SDS	VIII in plasma, measured as VIII coagulant antigen (VIII:Ag)	38
140	Electron inactivation	VIII in plasma, measured as clotting activity	37

F. Sulfhydryl Groups and Disulfide Bridges in VIII

Many earlier studies using plasma or partially purified VIII indicated that VIII either was unaffected or minimally affected by agents which react with free sulfhydryl groups.[47-51] For example, Kirby and Mills[47] showed a 5 to 10% prolongation in clotting time of VIII:C assay after prolonged incubation of bovine VIII/vWf with *p*-hydroxymercuribenzene sulfonic acid or *N*-ethylmaleimide. Counts et al.[48] reported no significant loss of VIII:C after reduction with 2-mercaptoethanol. Fukui et al.[51] similarly saw no effects with DTT. Vehar and Davie[29] and Eaton and colleagues[35] have incorporated into their purification schemes a reduction step, with either dithiothreitol or B-mercaptoethanol, which had no effect on VIII:C.

In contrast, several studies have indicated sensitivity of VIII to reducing agents. Austen[52] reported between 25 and 50% reductions in VIII:C following reaction with a range of concentrations of *p*-chloromercuribenzoic acid; this loss of activity could be reversed by subsequent treatment with a reducing agent, suggesting that it was specifically due to a reaction with free sulfhydryl groups. With the exception of mercurials, none of the other reagents is specific for sulfhydryls, but can react with a variety of nucleophilic side chains in proteins. Using VIII in plasma, Blömback et al.[53] found that reduction with dithiothreitol at 1.3, 2.5, and 3.9 m*M*, followed by alkylation with iodoacetate, caused reductions of VIII:C by 14, 48, and 73%, respectively. Savidge and colleagues,[54] using the thioredoxin system (a physiological reduction-oxidation system) at concentrations up to 10 μM, showed no effects on VIII:C.

Although the above results are somewhat contradictory, most studies indicate little or no role for easily reducible disulfide bridges or free sulfhydryl groups in the structure and function of VIII. In addition, there probably are no disulfide bridges between the light and heavy chains of VIII. It is not possible to exclude the existence of intrachain bridges, which are reduced only by higher concentrations of reducing agents.

The actual number of cysteine residues in VIII has been calculated to be 23, based on the cDNA sequence as seen in Figure 1.[33] They tend to be clustered into several regions, particularly in the three A-domains. Vehar et al.[33] have assigned disulfide pairing in the A-domains based on the analogous bonds in ceruloplasmin[44] and keeping the linkages within each respective domain. A similar rationale was used for assigning the two pairs of disulfide bonds in the two C-domains. These hypothetical assignments do not include any disulfide bridges between the light and heavy chains, because biochemical data described above suggest the absence of interchain bridges. Nine sulfhydryl groups were left unpaired; four of these are located in the carboxyl terminal region of the B-domain. No information is available to indicate whether they are free (unlikely in a plasma protein) or involved in mixed thiols or disulfide bridges.

G. Role of Carbohydrate in VIII

Early investigations by Sodetz et al.,[55,56] using impure VIII preparations, showed that removal of 100% of the terminal sialic acid and 62% of penultimate galactose residues had no effect on VIII (the remaining 38% of galactose was resistant to enzymatic cleavage).

An earlier study by Austen and Bidwell[57] showed loss of VIII:C following treatment with poorly characterized and probably impure sugar oxidases; this loss could blocked partially by inclusion of the appropriate sugars during incubation with the enzyme.

Fukui et al.[51] also showed no loss of VIII:C after reaction with neuraminidase and β-galactosidase. On the other hand, they demonstrated significant reductions in activity after incubation with galactose oxidase; it is not clear why removal of galactose has no effect, whereas oxidation leads to inhibition. Finally, there was a marked loss of activity following use of mannosidase.

Oxidation of impure VIII with sodium periodate has given contradictory results. Fukui et al.[51] saw a marked and rapid loss of VIII:C whereas Kaelin[58] noted a moderate increase in VIII:C. Using an impure preparation of human VIII with a high specific activity (2500 U/mg), Fay et al.[59] showed that treatment with a mixture of exo- and endoglycosidases had no significant effect on VIII:C or on its potentiation by thrombin.

In summary, the studies on impure VIII suggest that removal of sialic acid and galactose does not effect VIII:C. Disruption of the sugar chain closer to the polypeptide attachment site (by mannosidase) appears to be more harmful. In none of these studies was it possible to monitor structural changes in VIII or to show directly that the carbohydrate was removed from the VIII polypeptide, because the VIII was not available as a purified protein.

Recent studies have provided more direct evidence that VIII is a glycoprotein. Several studies have shown that VIII:C can be absorbed onto an insolubilized lectin column.[29] Fulcher and Zimmerman[31] showed that at least some of the VIII polypeptides can be stained for carbohydrate. There are a total of 25 asparagine residues which potentially could participate in N-linked carbohydrate sites[33] as shown in Figure 3.

All but 6 of these 25 sites are located in the B-domain, which is largely absent from most of the circulating VIII molecules. Thus, even if all of the potential sites are in fact glycosylated, most of the carbohydrate is likely to be cleaved during the processing steps which remove the B-domain. The relative molecular weight of the predominant heavy chain (with carbohydrate) is estimated at 90,000 by SDS gel; the relative molecular weight as calculated from the amino acid composition is about 83,000. The missing 7000 Da could be carbohydrate, giving an approximate upper limit of 8% carbohydrate for this chain. The approximate relative molecular weight for the light chain is 80,000 by SDS gel and 79,000 by amino acid composition, suggesting that the light chain contains very little or no sugar.

IV. REGULATION OF VIII:C

VIII circulates in plasma in a form which is relatively inactive. This form is susceptible to limited proteolytic cleavage by several enzymes of the clotting system. Several of these cleavages result in an increase in clotting activity; cleavage at other sites leads to inactivation. This balance between activation and inactivation constitutes a means for fine regulation of VIII:C.

A. Activators of VIII
1. Thrombin
The effects of thrombin on VIII have long been appreciated.[60-68] In general, treatment of plasma or purified VIII with thrombin leads to a rapid potentiation of VIII:C, followed by a slower loss of activity, and eventually its complete disappearance. The time course of this biphasic reaction is dependent upon the ratio of thrombin to VIII, as well as upon the calcium and phospholipid concentrations.[65,66] A recent report by Hultin[66] also suggests that washed human platelets potentiate VIII activation by thrombin and that platelet stimulation is a prerequisite for this effect.

Although the activation of VIII by thrombin can be demonstrated with enzyme:substrate

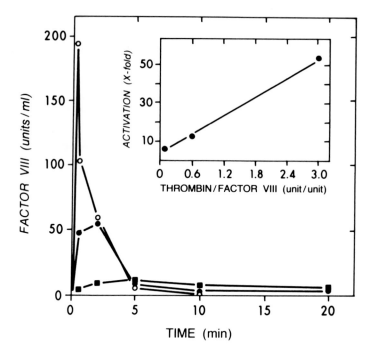

FIGURE 3.   Activation and subsequent inactivation of VIII after incubation with thrombin. Highly purified VIII and thrombin were used in these experiments. The samples were removed from the incubation mixture and assayed immediately at the times indicated. The inset shows the linear relationship between the extent of activation and the ratio of thrombin:VIII in the incubation mixture. The values of "activation" are the ratios of VIII activity at a maximum activation relative to the activity prior to thrombin activation. (From Fay, P. J., Chavin, S. I., Meyer, D., and Marder, V. J., in *Blood Coagulation,* Hemker, H. C. and Zwaal, R., Eds., Elsevier Biomedical, Amsterdam, 1986, 35. With permission.)

ratios as low as 1:50,[33,35] a number of studies[60,67,68] have shown that the extent of activation of VIII increases with increasing ratios of thrombin:VIII. For example, a thrombin:VIII ratio of 1:10 (unit:unit) gave a peak potentiation of fivefold, whereas higher ratios of enzyme:substrate gave as much as 50-fold potentiation and resulted in a more rapid rate of inactivation as demonstrated in Figure 3. Thus it appears that the activity measured may represent a balance between activation of VIII and inactivation of the activated form. Lollar et al.[69] have presented a detailed analysis showing that the K_{cat}/K_m for the activation of VIII by thrombin is $5 \times 10^6 \ M^{-1}s^{-1}$ and that the catalytic efficiency for the activation is comparable to that of other coagulation enzyme catalyzed reactions.

Whatever the exact mechanism of the activation of VIII by thrombin, it is well established that both heavy and light chains of VIII are proteolytically cleaved by thrombin.[28,31,60,70,71] Thrombin cleaves between Arg 372 and Ser 373 in the heavy chain; and between Arg 1689 and Ser 1690 in the light chain, as shown in Figure 1, Figure 4, and Table 4. All of the heavy chain classes also are cleaved by thrombin, this overall reaction proceeding slightly more slowly than the light chain cleavage. There is some evidence that the 90-kDa heavy chain may be an intermediate product common to cleavage of several of the heavy chains, but this has not been demonstrated rigorously. The end products of heavy chain cleavage are a pair of chains, 50 and 40 kDa. Although one group[70,71] has reported further breakdown of these two chains after prolonged incubation with thrombin, other workers[29,30,35,69] have been unable to confirm this. The cleavage of the 80-kDa light chain doublet occurs very quickly and results in conversion to a 72-kDa doublet.

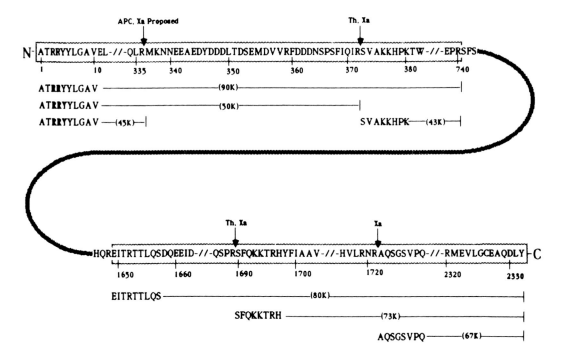

FIGURE 4. Diagrammatic representation of the single chain precursor VIII to show the locations and amino acid sequences around various enzymatic cleavage sites. The cleavage site after arginine 337 has not been identified directly. APC and Th stand for activated protein C and thrombin, respectively. The conventional one letter code is as follows: A, Ala; R, Arg; N, Asn; D, Asp; C, Cys; Q, Gln; E, Glu; G, Gly; H, His; I, Ile; L, Leu; K, Lys; M, Met; F, Phe; P, Pro; S, Ser; T, Thr; W, Trp; Y, Tyr; and V, Val. (From Eaton, D., Rodriguez, H., and Vehar, G. A., *Biochemistry*, 25, 505, 1986. Copyright 1986, American Chemical Society. With permission.)

It still is unclear exactly which of the cleavages is responsible for the activation. Fay et al.[30] have presented data which suggest that cleavage of the light chain is completed early in the course of activation, well before the peak of activation. In most preparations of human VIII, the heterogeneity of the heavy chains makes it difficult to correlate cleavage of a particular chain with activation. However, Fay et al.[30] showed that an VIII protein with only a 93-kDa heavy chain plus the light chain was fully activatable and suggested that a major portion of the activation can be attributed to the cleavage of the 93-kDa polypeptide to the 51- and 43-kDa fragments. It was not possible to assess whether any additional activation might result from conversion of the higher relative molecular weight heavy chains to the 93-kDa intermediate. Based on the above data, we suggest that the most likely polypeptide composition of VIII$_a$ is represented by the cleaved doublet plus the 51- and 43-kDa polypeptides derived from the heavy chains as demonstrated in Figure 5. However, it is not known if VIII$_a$ exists as a 73/51/43-kDa trimer or as a dimer consisting of the 73-kDa light chain plus either the 51- or the 43-kDa heavy chain derivative (with one of the heavy chain derivatives dissociating from the remaining two polypeptides).

The cleavage which separates the 80-kDa doublet light chain from the middle (B) domain is between Arg 1648 and Glu 1649. Since the sites cleaved by thrombin are Arg-Ser bonds, and those cleaved by factor X$_a$ are Arg-Ser or Arg-Ala, Vehar et al.[33] and Eaton et al.[35] suggested that a protease other than thrombin may be responsible for this cleavage. Fay et al.,[30] using a different argument based on the stability of the activities of the various forms, suggested that some of the heterogeneity of the VIII heavy chain may also be due to an enzyme other than thrombin.

2. Factor X$_a$

By analogy with the prothrombinase complex, in which thrombin is the activator of factor

Table 4
THE EFFECTS OF THROMBIN ON THE POLYPEPTIDES OF VIII

Species		Polypeptide M_r (kDa)		Comments	Ref.
		Before thrombin	After thrombin		
Bovine		93, 88, 85	75 (doublet), 38	No distinction made between heavy and light chains; only 93 kD$_a$ is cleaved by activated protein C, suggesting that this chain is the bovine equivalent of the heavy chain	29
Porcine	Heavy	166, 130, 82	69, 44, 25		19, 24
	Light	76	76		
Human	Heavy	188—92	92, 54, 44	Activation correlated with generation of 92-kDa chain; inactivation was related to further cleavage of this chain to 50 and 40 kDa	70
	Light	80/79	72/71		
Human	Heavy	210—110	55/40		28
	Light	80/79	70/69		
Human	Heavy	210—90	50, 43		35
	Light	80	73		
Human	Heavy	170, 155, 146	93, 51, 43	See text for details of the three different forms of VIII	30
	Light	83/81	73/71		
Human	Heavy	146, 120, 110	93, 51, 43	Activation appeared to be correlated with production of 51- and 43-kDa chains from larger heavy chain precursor; 93-kDa chain appears to be only a transient intermediate; inactivation not related to additional proteolytic cleavages	
	Light	83/81	73/71		
	Heavy	93	51, 43		
	Light	83/81	73/71		

V, one might expect factor X_a to be an important activator of VIII. Factor X_a is indeed capable, *in vitro,* of activating VIII.[29,33,69,73] Eaton et al.[35] have shown clearly a total of four cleavage sites cleaved by factor X_a, involving both heavy and light chains. Two of these (on the carboxyl-terminal side of residues 372, 1689) are identical to the thrombin sites. One site (following residue 1721) is unique to factor X_a. The fourth site, which they propose but have not proven, follows residue 336 and is shared by activated protein C as shown in Figure 4. Lollar et al.[69] and Mertens and Bertina[73] have shown that thrombin-activated VIII$_a$ is more potent than factor X_a activated VIII$_a$. Lollar et al.[69] and Eaton et al.,[35] using polyacrylamide gel analysis, have noted at least one additional cleavage site by factor X_a, compared to those produced by thrombin.

3. Factor IX$_a$

In the original formulations of the clotting cascade,[74,75] VIII was proposed as the substrate for factor IX$_a$. Lundblad and Davie[76] reported that factor IX$_a$ appeared to convert VIII into an activated product which accelerated clotting. Vehar and Davie[29] were the first to show activation of purified VIII by factor IX$_a$. In these experiments, they were unable to demonstrate proteolytic cleavage of the VIII polypeptides and therefore concluded that some unknown mechanism was involved. More recently, Rick[77] showed that very high concen-

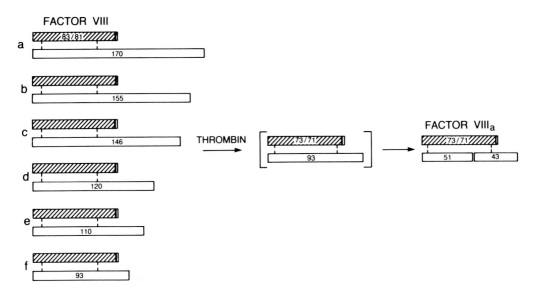

FIGURE 5. Schematic representation of the several proposed heterodimeric forms of VIII and of the proteolytic cleavages which are associated with activation by thrombin. Each heterodimer consists of a heavy chain of differing size plus the light chain doublet 83/81 kD. Type c M_r (237,500) was the major component of fraction 23 in Figure 2. Types d and e M_r (201,000) predominated in fraction 24. Type f M_r (141,000) was the only constituent in fraction 26. Cleavage by thrombin initially results in the generation of a 73/71-kD doublet from the original light chains, and the production of a 93-kD heavy chain is cleaved to give polypeptides of 51 and 43 kD. See text for further details. (From Fay, P. J., Anderson, M., Chavin, S. I., and Marder, V. J., *Biochim. Biophys. Acta,* 871, 268, 1986. With permission.)

trations of factor IX_a produced modest activation of VIII:C contained in the VIII/vWf complex. We have confirmed this finding using highly purified factor IX_a and IX_a/VIII complex (unpublished results). A 50:1 molar ratio (IX_a:VIII) was required to obtain a fivefold activation of VIII. Although this is an unusually high enzyme:substrate ratio, it might easily be attained *in vivo*, given the large excess of factor IX over VIII in plasma. Lower levels of factor IX_a had no apparent effect. SDS PAGE of VIII_a activated by factor IX_a showed proteolysis of both chains of the VIII heterodimer. Lollar et al.[69] using a lower concentration of factor IX_a, as well as a lower ratio of factors IX_a:VIII were unable to demonstrate activation.

4. What is the "Physiological" Activator of VIII?

VIII clearly can be activated by at least three clotting proteases, thrombin, factor X_a and factor IX_a. The nonactivated precursors of these proteases are present at relatively high concentrations: factor II, 1 μM; factor X, 0.1 μM; and factor IX, 0.05 μM. VIII exists in plasma at approximately 1 nM. Therefore, even if as little as 1% of these proenzymes were activated, it would be nearly equimolar to VIII itself. Thus, any one, or a combination, of these factors would be capable of activating VIII. Earlier work by Neal and Chavin,[78] showing that VIII:C could be expressed in the presence of a high concentration of hirudin (a potent and specific inhibitor of thrombin), suggested that activation of VIII by thrombin is not necessary, although it is likely to occur under normal circumstances.

The K_{cat}/K_m for the activation of VIII by factor X_a was shown to be 10^6 $M^{-1}s^{-1}$,[71] or about fivefold lower than the comparable value for thrombin; thus activation of VIII by thrombin was about five times more efficient. It appears that VIII_a generated by thrombin was about threefold more active than that generated by factor X_a.[69,73]

According to the currently accepted formulation of the clotting cascade, significant amounts of either factors IX_a or X_a will be present at an earlier stage than will similar amounts of thrombin. Therefore, VIII might well be activated under physiological conditions by either of these active enzymes. The available experimental data do not permit an unambiguous choice of any one enzyme as the most important activator of VIII; it even is possible that more than one enzyme is important *in vivo*.

5. Does Nonactivated VIII Possess Significant Clotting Activity?

Preparations of factor V containing only a single polypeptide chain have little or no clotting activity until they have been proteolytically activated by thrombin.[79-81] It has not been possible to study this question for VIII because of the difficulty of isolating significant amounts of a single chain form of VIII.[28,40] One possible explanation for the absence of an intact VIII precursor is that activation already has occurred during the long and complicated purification procedures. There are several arguments against this possibility. Knutson and Fass[19] and Fass and colleagues[24] showed that there were no systematic or progressive changes in the degree of thrombin activatability of the VIII in the starting material (plasma) compared with each of the stages of purification. Switzer et al.[82] found only a two- to threefold difference in specific activity with thrombin activatability of partially purified VIII when the initial blood samples were collected directly into a mixture of proteolytic inhibitors compared to collection without such inhibitors. The predominant mixture of smaller heterodimers may be the result of processing within the cell or very shortly after secretion. Thus, the heterodimers may already be partially activated, albeit to stable intermediate forms. If single chain VIII could be isolated it might prove to be virtually devoid of clotting activity, but it is not yet possible to give a definitive answer to this question.

B. Inactivation of VIII

1. Inactivation of VIII_a

Several reports[29,30,35,67,69,83,84] show that VIII_a produced by thrombin undergoes inactivation in the absence of additional proteolytic cleavages other than those which are responsible for activation. Switzer and McKee[67] using dansyl-arginine-4-ethylpiperidine amide (DAPA) to competitively inhibit further action by thrombin, failed to see a reduction in the rate of inactivation of thrombin-enhanced VIII:C. Furthermore, rapid separation of VIII_a from a thrombin-agarose resin did not alter the rate of decay of activity compared with the rate seen with continued exposure to thrombin. Hultin and Jesty[83] reported studies on the effects of thrombin inhibitors on potentiation and inactivation of VIII. They noted that thrombin-potentiated VIII:C decreased in the presence of either DAPA (a competitive inhibitor), or diisopropylfluorophosphate (DFP) or hirudin (irreversible inhibitors), and that the initial period of decay was even more rapid than in the absence of the inhibitors. They concluded that only the initial potentiation step depends upon the concentration of thrombin, whereas inactivation was the result of a first-order decay reaction, perhaps because VIII_a is intrinsically unstable. Furthermore, Lollar et al.[69] showed that the half-life of VIII_a could be prolonged significantly by inclusion of factor IX_a, phospholipid, and Ca^{++}; when inactivation did occur, it was not correlated with the appearance of new degradation products. These authors postulated that the interaction of VIII_a with factor IX_a, Ca^{++}, and phospholipid maintained the VIII_a in its active conformaton. In contrast, Fulcher et al.[70] and Zimmerman and Fulcher[71] have shown that inactivation of VIII_a after prolonged incubation with thrombin is accompanied by the appearance of smaller degradation products. We conclude that most of the data available currently favors the hypothesis that VIII_a is intrinsically unstable and becomes inactivated without further proteolytic cleavages.[61,69]

2. Inactivation by Activated Protein C

Protein C is a vitamin K dependent serine protease precursor.[85] The activated form of protein C causes rapid inactivation of factors VIII and V, in addition to activation of the fibrinolytic system.[85-88] The proteolytic activity of activated protein C is directed entirely at the heavy chains in human VIII[33,35,86,89] and at the presumed bovine counterpart, 93 kDa.[29] The light chain appears to be unaffected. Fulcher et al.[86] and Eaton et al.[35] noted a predominant degradation product of 45 kDa. This site of cleavage by activated protein C is near the middle of the heavy chain (following Arg 336); this same site is believed to be cleaved as well by factor X_a.[35] Inasmuch as activated protein C appears to cause only inactivation of VIII, whereas the cleavages at the other locations by thrombin and factor X_a result in activation first, and inactivation subsequently, Eaton et al.[35] suggested that the cleavage after Arg 336 is responsible solely for inactivation. More recently, Walker et al.[89] showed that activated protein C cleaved the 170- to 110-kDa heavy chains in at least four sites. The initial cleavage, which appeared to be correlated with the onset of inactivation, resulted in the formation of 93- and 53-kDa polypeptides. Further proteolysis converted the 93 kDa to a 68-kDa polypeptide which in turn was cleaved to fragments of 48 and 23 kDa. Cleavage products from the 53-kDa polypeptide have not been identified, but the progressive appearance of low relative molecular weight peptides in the dye front suggested that this fragment may have undergone extensive proteolysis. Polypeptide composition analysis following interaction of activated protein C with a purified 93/83-kDa VIII heterodimer[30] also showed the generation of a transient 68-kDa polypeptide which was converted to the 48- and 23-kDa fragments. No fragment of 53-kDa was observed, suggesting that this polypeptide was derived from a segment of the VIII molecule (perhaps representing a portion of the B-domain) that is different from the 93-kDa polypeptide.

Walker[90,91] has demonstrated that another vitamin K dependent protein, protein S, is a nonenzymic co-factor for activated protein C which increases the rate at which activated protein C cleaves factor V_a. This enhancement may be due to increased binding of activated protein C to negatively charged phospholipids.[92] Lawrence et al.[93] and Walker et al.[89] have demonstrated a similar enhancement of cleavage of VIII by activated protein C/protein S complex with no change in the pattern of the final polypeptides.

Thus, in some respects the inactivation of activated VIII by protein C was similar to that of factor V_a. The main cleavage of factor V_a appeared to be in the 94-kDa heavy chain.[88] One difference was that VIII per se is a substrate and prior activation of VIII is not required for inactivation, although some evidence has been presented that the activated co-factor is inactivated more rapidly than the non-activated co-factor.[87] This difference between factors VIII and V may be related to the fact that VIII can exist as a two-chain molecule prior to activation by thrombin or factor X_a, whereas nonactivated factor V is a single chain polypeptide.[79]

C. The Role of VIII in Blood Clotting

The majority of plasma clotting factors are serine proteases whose mechanism of action is the limited proteolytic activation and/or inactivation of other clotting factors. In recent years, several nonenzymatic proteins have been described which can affect the properties of various clotting factors. These modifying proteins include high molecular weight kininogen, protein S, thrombomodulin, VIII, and factor V. Although Vehar and Davie[94] earlier raised the possibility that VIII_a might be a serine protease, these results have been neither confirmed nor extended, and the consensus is that factors VIII and V are co-factors with no intrinsic enzymatic activities.

Early experiments by Østerud and Rapaport,[95] using polyclonal antisera to either VIII or factor IX, showed that both components needed to be active and present simultaneously in order to achieve maximum shortening of the clotting time. These workers proposed the occurrence of a bimolecular complex between factors IX_a and VIII. More direct evidence for such a complex has been presented recently by Bajaj et al.[96] using a monoclonal antibody which interfered with binding between VIII_a and factor IX_a. Because the epitope against which the antibody was directed was in the C-terminal portion of factor IX_a, they suggested that interaction with VIII involved the C-terminal region. The stabilizing effect of factor IX_a on VIII[69] and protection of VIII by factor IX from degradation by activated protein C[89] also are consistent with the occurrence of a complex between VIII and factors IX or IX_a. Mertens et al.[97] recently described a genetically defective VIII which could be activated normally by factor X_a and thrombin, but kinetically appeared to have a reduced affinity for phospholipid-bound factor IX_a. Therefore, even though a complex of factor IX and VIII has not been isolated, there are strong kinetic and immunological data supporting its existence.

Factor IX_a alone is sufficient to convert factor X to X_a, although in the absence of VIII relatively high concentrations of factor IX_a are required and the reaction proceeds very slowly.[78,98-100] The addition of VIII causes the reaction to proceed more rapidly and more completely.[99,101] While it generally is agreed that the major effect of VIII_a is to increase the maximum velocity of the reaction, the experimental values from different laboratories varied widely between 54-fold[100] and 2×10^5-fold.[101] The K_m is only minimally affected by the presence of VIII, with a two- to threefold reduction when VIII_a is present, compared to when it is absent.[98,100-102] All of the above studies utilized VIII which had been activated to VIII_a by prior incubation with thrombin. In contrast, Neal and Esnouf[103] showed that prior activation of VIII was not required, and that in the presence of apparently nonactivated VIII there was a 170-fold increase in the V_{max} for activation of factor X. These results with VIII are analogous to the effect of factor V upon the rate of prothrombin activation.[105-107]

In a recent paper, van Dieijen and colleagues[104] showed that the presence of VIII reduces the dissociation constant (K_D) of factor IX_a for phospholipid from 10^{-6} to $10^{-8} M$, suggesting an increased binding affinity. These workers postulated that the activator of factor X is a stoichiometric (1:1) complex of factor IXa and VIII bound to phospholipid. Similarly, Mertens et al.[108] suggested that VIII forms a complex with phospholipid-bound factor IX_a and that in this ternary complex the turnover rate (catalytic efficiency) of factor IX_a is increased 500-fold.

The exact mechanism(s) by which VIII and factor V effect their respective mechanisms are subject to speculation. Mertens et al.[108] suggest that the co-factors provide high affinity binding sites for the active enzyme and its substrate. Nesheim et al.[109] demonstrated that most of prothrombin activation (and presumably factor X activation) occurs within a very small volume (interface shell) at the surface of phospholipid or all membrane bilayers, and that the volume of this region is about 1/10,000 the volume of the bulk solution. If most of the available clotting proteins are confined to this small interface shell, their concentrations may be increased by three to four orders of magnitude. A schematic representation incorporating some of these ideas is shown in Figure 6. The increased concentration plus the high affinity interactions between the proteins and phospholipids may account for most of the observed rate increases which are so characteristic of these complex systems.

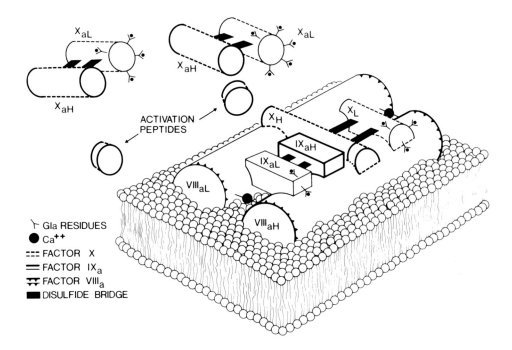

FIGURE 6. Schematic representation of the multimolecular complex responsible for the activation of factor X via the intrinsic pathway. This "tenase complex" consists of factors IX_a, VIII_a, calcium, and phospholipid, with factor X as its substrate. The phospholipid is shown as a typical lipid bilayer with the polar head groups (small open spheres) oriented towards the solvent and the aliphatic fatty acid chains oriented inwards. VIII_a is shown as two polypeptides which are linked by two divalent calcium bridges. The number, nature, and location of these interchain bridges have not yet been demonstrated and the exact number of polypeptide chains in VIII_a has not been shown. The relative sizes of the different proteins have not been drawn to scale. (From Fay, P. J., Chavin, S. I., Meyer, D., and Marder, V. J., in *Blood Coagulation*, Hemker, H. C. and Zwaal, R., Eds., Elsevier Biomedical, Amsterdam, 1986, 35. With permission.)

REFERENCES

1. **Barrow, E. M. and Graham, J. B.,** Blood coagulation factor VIII (anti-hemophilic factor) with comments on von Willebrand's disease and Christmas disease, *Physiol. Rev.*, 54, 23, 1974.
2. **Hershgold, E. J.,** Properties of factor VIII (antihemophilic factor), *Progr. Hemostasis Thromb.*, 2, 99, 1974.
3. **Hoyer, L. W.,** Immunological properties of antihemophilic factor, *Progr. Hematol.*, 8, 191, 1973.
4. **Bouma, B. N. and Van Mourik, J. A.,** The biochemistry of factors VIII and IX, in *Haemostasis: Biochemistry, Physiology and Pathology.*, Bennett, B. and Ogston, D., Eds., John Wiley & Sons, London 1977, 56.
5. **Davie, E. W. and Fujikawa, K.,** Basic mechanisms in blood coagulation, *Ann. Rev. Biochem.*, 44, 799, 1975.
6. **Hoyer, L. W.,** The factor VIII complex: structure and function, *Blood*, 58, 1, 1981.
7. **Hoyer, L. W.,** Biochemistry of factor VIII, in *Hemostasis and Thrombosis: Basic Principles and Clinical Practice*, Colman, R. W., Hirsh, J., Marder, V. J., and Salzman, E. W., Eds., Lippincott, Philadelphia, 1982, 39.
8. **Pool, J. G., Hershgold, E. J., and Pappenhagen, A. R.,** High potency anti-hemophilic factor concentrate prepared from cryoglobulin in precipitate, *Nature (London)*, 203, 312, 1964.
9. **Prowse, C. V. and McGill, A.,** Evaluation of the "Mason" (continuous-thaw-siphon) method for cryoprecipitate production, *Vox Sang.*, 37, 235, 1979.
10. **Bidwell, E., Dike, G. W. R., and Snape, T. J.,** Therapeutic materials, in *Human Blood Coagulation, Haemostasis and Thrombosis*, Biggs, R., Ed., Blackwell Scientific, Oxford, 1976, 249.

11. **Johnson, A. J., MacDonald, V. E., Semar, M., Fields, J. E., Shuck, L. C., and Brind, J.,** Preparation of the major plasma fractions by solid phase polyelectrolytes, *J. Lab. Clin. Med.,* 92, 194, 1978.
12. **Rotblat, F., Goodall, A. H., O'Brien, D. P., Rawlings, E., Middleton, S., and Tuddenham, E. G. D.,** Monoclonal antibodies to human procoagulant factor VIII, *J. Lab. Clin. Med.,* 101, 736, 1983.
13. **Owen, W. G. and Wagner, R. H.,** Anti-hemophilic factor: separation of an active fragment following dissociation by salts or detergent, *Thromb. Diath. Haemorrh.,* 27, 502, 1972.
14. **Austen, D. E. G.,** Factor VIII of small molecular weight and its aggregation, *Br. J. Haematol.,* 27, 89, 1974.
15. **Sussman, I. I., Rosner, W., and Weiss, H. J.,** Concentration dependent dissociation of factor VIII in 1M NaCl, *Am. J. Physiol.,* 230, 434, 1976.
16. **Vermylen, J.,** Physical and chemical properties of normal and haemophilic factor VIII, *Pathol. Biol.,* Suppl. 23, 5, 1975.
17. **Bouma, B. N., Van Mourik, J. A., De Graaf, S., Hordyk-Hos, J. A., and Sixma, J. J.,** Immunologic studies on human factor VIII (antihemophilic factor A, AHF) components produced by low ionic strength dialysis, *Blood,* 47, 253, 1976.
18. **Weiss, H. J. and Kochwa, S.,** Molecular forms of antihaemophilic globulin in plasma, cryoprecipitate and after thrombin activation, *Br. J. Haematol.,* 18, 89, 1970.
19. **Knutson, G. J. and Fass, D. N.,** Porcine factor VIII C prepared by affinity interaction with von Willebrand factor and heterologous antibodies: sodium dodecyl sulfate polyacrylamide gel analysis, *Blood,* 59, 615, 1982.
20. **Holmberg, K. L. and Ljung, R.,** Purification of factor VIII C by antigen-antibody chromatography, *Thromb. Res.,* 12, 667, 1978.
21. **Tuddenham, E. G. D., Trabold, N. C., Collins, J. A., and Hoyer, L. W.,** The properties of factor VIII coagulant activity prepared by immunoadsorbent chromatography, *J. Lab. Clin. Med.,* 93, 40, 1979.
22. **Horowitz, B., Lippin, A., and Woods, K. R.,** Purification of low molecular weight factor VIII by affinity chromatography using factor VIII sepharose, *Thromb. Res.,* 14, 463, 1979.
23. **Zimmerman, T. S., De La Pointe, L., and Edgington, T. S.,** Interaction of factor VIII antigen in hemophilic plasmas with human antibodies to factor VIII, *J. Clin. Invest.,* 59, 984, 1977.
24. **Fass, D. N., Knutson, G. J., and Katzmann, J. A.,** Monoclonal antibodies to porcine factor VIII coagulant and their use in the isolation of active coagulant protein, *Blood,* 59, 594, 1985.
25. **Nordfang, O., Ezban, M., Favaloro, J. M., Dahl, H. H. M., and Hansen, J. J.,** Specificity of monoclonal antibodies to factor VIII, *Thromb. Haemost.,* 54, 586, 1985.
26. **Rotblat, F., Goodall, A. H., O'Brien, D. P., Rawlings, E., Middleton, S., and Tuddenham, E. G. D.,** Monoclonal antibodies to human procoagulant factor VIII, *J. Lab. Clin. Med.,* 101, 736, 1983.
27. **Muller, H. P., Van Tilburg, H. J., Derles, J., Klein-Berteler, E., and Bertina, R. M.,** Monoclonal antibody to VIII:C produced by a mouse hybridoma, *Blood,* 58, 1000, 1981.
28. **Rotblat, F., O'Brien, D. P., O'Brien, F. J., Goodall, A. H., and Tuddenham, E. G. D.,** Purification of human factor VIII C and its characterization by Western blotting using monoclonal antibodies, *Biochemistry,* 24, 4294, 1985.
29. **Vehar, G. A. and Davie, E. W.,** Preparation and purification of bovine factor VIII (antihemophilic factor), *Biochemistry,* 19, 401, 1980.
30. **Fay, P. J., Anderson, M., Chavin, S. I., and Marder, V. J.,** The size and heterodimeric structure of human factor VIII and the effects produced by thrombin, *Biochim. Biophys. Acta,* 871, 268, 1986.
31. **Fulcher, C. A. and Zimmerman, T. S.,** Characterization of the human factor VIII procoagulant protein with a heterologous precipitating antibody, *Proc. Nat. Acad. Sci. U.S.A.,* 79, 1648, 1982.
32. **Gitschier, J., Wood, W. I., Goralka, T. M., et al.,** Characterization of the human factor VIII gene, *Nature (London),* 312, 326, 1984.
33. **Vehar, G. A., Keyt, B., Eaton, D., et al.,** Structure of human factor VIII, *Nature (London),* 312, 337, 1984.
34. **Toole, J. J., Knopf, J. L., Wozney, J. M., et al.,** Molecular cloning of a cDNA encoding human antihaemophilic factor, *Nature (London),* 312, 342, 1984.
35. **Eaton, D., Rodriguez, H., and Vehar, G. A.,** Proteolytic processing of human factor VIII, *Biochemistry,* 25, 505, 1986.
36. **Hoyer, L. A. and Trabold, N. C.,** The effect of thrombin on human factor VIII. Cleavage of the protein during activation, *J. Lab. Clin. Med.,* 97, 50, 1981.
37. **Harmon, J. T., Jamieson, G. A., and Rock, G. A.,** The functional molecular weights of factor VIII activities in whole plasma as determined by electron irradiation, *J. Biol. Chem.,* 257, 14245, 1982.
38. **Weinstein, M., Chute, L., and Deykin, D.,** Analysis of factor VIII coagulant antigens in normal, thrombin treated, and hemophilic plasma, *Proc. Natl. Acad. Sci. U.S.A.,* 78, 5137, 1981.
39. **Fulcher, C. A., Roberts, J. R., Holland, L. Z., and Zimmerman, T. S.,** Human factor VIII protein: monoclonal antibodies define precursor-product relationships and functional epitopes, *J. Clin. Invest.,* 76, 117, 1985.

40. **Fulcher, C. A., Mahoney, S. de G., Roberts, J. R., Kasper, C. K., and Zimmerman, T. S.,** Localization of human factor VIII inhibitor epitopes to two polypeptide fragments, *Proc. Natl. Acad. Sci. U.S.A.,* 82, 7728, 1985.

41. **Wodak, S. J. and Janin, J.,** Location of structural domains in proteins, *Biochemistry,* 20, 6544, 1981.

42. **Hamer, R. J., Koedam, J. A., Besser-Visser, N. H., and Sixma, J. J.,** Factor VIII binds to the von Willebrand factor (vWD) through its M_r 80 kDa light chain, *Thromb. Haemost.,* 54 (Abstr.), 251, 1985.

43. **Church, W. R., Jernigan, R. L., Toole, J., et al.,** Coagulation factors V and VIII and ceruloplasmin constitute a family of structurally related protens, *Proc. Natl. Acad. Sci. U.S.A.,* 81, 6934, 1984.

44. **Bauman, R. A., Dwulet, F. E., and Wang, C.-C.,** Internal triplication in the structure of ceruloplasmin, *Proc. Natl. Acad. Sci. U.S.A.,* 80, 115, 1983.

45. **Mann, K. G., Lawler, C. M., Vehar, G. A., and Church, W. R.,** Coagulation factor V contains cooper ion, *J. Biol. Chem.,* 259, 12949, 1984.

46. **Weiss, H. J.,** A study of the cation and pH-dependent stability of factors V and VIII in plasma, *Thromb. Diath. Haemorrh.,* 14, 32, 1965.

47. **Kirby, E. P. and Mills, D. C. B.,** The interaction of bovine factor VIII with human platelets, *J. Clin. Invest.,* 56, 491, 1975.

48. **Counts, R. B., Paskell, S. L., and Elgee, S. K.,** Disulfide bonds and the quaternary structure of factor VIII/von Willebrand factor, *J. Clin. Invest.,* 62, 702, 1978.

49. **Peake, I. R. and Bloom, A. L.,** The dissociation of factor VIII by reducing agents, high salt concentration and affinity chromatography, *Thromb. Haemost.,* 35, 191, 1976.

50. **Harris, R. B., Newman, J., and Johnson, A. J.,** Partial purification of biologically active low molecular weight human antihemophilic factor free of von Willebrand factor I, *Biochim. Biophys. Acta,* 668, 456, 1981.

51. **Fukui, H., Mikami, S., Okuda, T., et al.,** Studies of the von Willebrand factor: effects of different kinds of carbohydrate oxidases, SH inhibitors, and some other chemical reagents, *Br. J. Haematol.,* 36, 259, 1970.

52. **Austen, D. E. G.,** Thiol groups in the blood clotting action of factor VIII, *Br. J. Haematol.,* 19, 472, 1970.

53. **Blombäck, B., Hessel, B., Savidge, G., Wikstrom, L., and Blombäck, M.,** The effect of reducing agents on factor VIII and other coagulation factors, *Thromb. Res.,* 12, 1177, 1978.

54. **Savidge, G., Carlebjork, L., Thorell, L., Hessel, B., Holmgren, A., and Blombäck, B.,** Reduction of factor VIII and other coagulation factors by the thioredoxin system, *Thromb. Res.,* 16, 587, 1979.

55. **Sodetz, J. M., Pizzo, S. V., and McKee, P. A.,** Relationship of sialic acid to function and in vivo survival of human factor VIII/von Willebrand factor protein, *J. Biol. Chem.,* 252, 5539, 1977.

56. **Sodetz, J. M., Paulson, J. C., Pizzo, S. V., and McKee, P. A.,** Carbohydrate on human factor VIII/ von Willebrand factor, *J. Biol. Chem.,* 253, 7202, 1978.

57. **Austen, D. E. G. and Bidwell, E.,** Carbohydrate structure in factor VIII, *Thromb. Diath. Haemorrh.,* 28, 464, 1972.

58. **Kaelin, A. C.,** Sodium periodate modification of factor VIII procoagulant activity, *Br. J. Haematol.,* 31, 349, 1971.

59. **Fay, P. J., Chavin, S. I., Malone, J. E., Schroeder, D., Young, F. E., and Marder, V. J.,** The effect of carbohydrate depletion on procoagulant activity and in vivo survival of highly purified human factor VIII, *Biochim. Biophys. Acta,* 800, 152, 1984.

60. **Chavin, S. I.,** Factor VIII: structure and function, *Am. J. Hematol.,* 16, 297, 1984.

61. **Fay, P. J., Chavin, S. I., Meyer, D., and Marder, V. J.,** Factor VIII, in *Blood Coagulation,* Hemker, H. C. and Zwaal, R., Eds., Elsevier Biomedical, Amsterdam, 1986, 35.

62. **Langdell, R. D., Wagner, R. H., and Brinkhous, K. M.,** Effect of antihemophilic factor on one-stage clotting tests, *J. Lab. Clin. Med.,* 41, 637, 1953.

63. **Rapaport, S. I., Schiffman, S., Patch, M. J., and Ames, S. B.,** The importance of activation of antihemophilic globulin, and proaccelerin by traces of thrombin in the generation of intrinsic prothrombinase activity, *Blood,* 21, 221, 1963.

64. **Biggs, R., MacFarlane, R. G., Denson, K. W. E., and Ash, B. J.,** Thrombin and the interaction of factors VIII and IX, *Br. J. Haematol.,* 11, 276, 1965.

65. **Østerud, B., Rapaport, S. I., Schiffman, S., and Chong, M. N. Y.,** Formation of intrinsic factor X activator activity with special reference to the role of thrombin, *Br. J. Haematol.,* 21, 643, 1971.

66. **Hultin, M. B.,** Modulation of thrombin-mediated activation of factor VIII:C by calcium ions, phospholipid, and platelets, *Blood,* 66, 53, 1985.

67. **Switzer, M. P. and McKee, P. A.,** Reactions of thrombin with factor VIII/von Willebrand factor protein, *J. Biol. Chem.,* 255, 10606, 1981.

68. **Fay, P. J., Chavin, S. I., Schroeder, D., Young, F. E., and Marder, V. J.,** Purification and characterization of a highly purified human factor VIII consisting of a single type of polypeptide chain, *Proc. Natl. Acad. Sci. U.S.A.,* 79, 7200, 1982.

69. **Lollar, P., Knutson, G. J., and Fass, D. N.,** Activation of porcine factor VIII:C by thrombin and factor Xa, *Biochemistry,* 24, 8056, 1985.
70. **Fulcher, C. A., Roberts, J. R., and Zimmerman, T. S.,** Thrombin proteolysis of purified factor VIII procoagulant protein, *Blood,* 61, 807, 1983.
71. **Zimmerman, T. S. and Fulcher, C. A.,** Factor VIII procoagulant protein, *Clin. Haematol.,* 14, 343, 1985.
72. **Davie, E. W., Fujikawa, K., Legaz, M. E., and Kato, H.,** Role of proteases in blood coagulation, in *Proteases and Biological Control,* Reich, E., Rifkin, D. B., and Shaw, E., Eds., Cold Spring Harbor Laboratory, Cold Spring Harbor, N.Y., 1975, 65.
73. **Mertens, K. and Bertina, R. M.,** Activation of human coagulation factor VIII by activated factor X, the common product of the intrinsic and extrinsic pathway of blood coagulation, *Thromb. Haemost.,* 47, 96, 1982.
74. **MacFarlane, R. G.,** An enzyme cascade in the blood clotting mechanism and its function as a biochemical amplifier, *Nature (London),* 202, 498, 1964.
75. **Davie, E. W. and Ratnoff, O. D.,** Waterfall sequence for intrinsic blood clotting, *Science,* 145, 1310, 1964.
76. **Lundblad, R. L. and Davie, E. W.,** The activation of antihemophilic factor (factor VIII) by activated Christmas factor (activated factor IX), *Biochemistry,* 3, 1720, 1964.
77. **Rick, M. E.,** Activation of factor VIII by factor IXa, *Blood,* 60, 744, 1982.
78. **Neal, G. G. and Chavin, S. I.,** The role of factors VIII and IX in the activation of bovine coagulation factor X, *Thromb. Res.,* 16, 473, 1979.
79. **Nesheim, M. E., Myrmel, K. H., Hibbard, L., and Mann, K. G.,** Isolation and characterization of single chain bovine factor V, *J. Biol. Chem.,* 254, 508, 1979.
80. **Mann, K. G., Nesheim, M. E., and Tracy, P. B.,** Molecular weight of undegraded plasma factor V, *Biochemistry,* 20, 28, 1981.
81. **Suzuki, K., Dahlback, B., and Stenflo, J.,** Thrombin-catalyzed activation of human coagulation factor V, *J. Biol. Chem.,* 257, 6556, 1982.
82. **Switzer, M. E., Pizzo, S. V., and McKee, P. A.,** Immunologic studies of native and modified human factor VIII/von Willebrand factor, *Blood,* 54, 310, 1979.
83. **Hultin, M. B. and Jesty, J.,** The activation and inactivation of human factor VIII by thrombin. Effect of inhibition of thrombin, *Blood,* 57, 476, 1981.
84. **Rick, M. E. and Hoyer, L. W.,** Thrombin activation of factor VIII. The effect of inhibitors, *Br. J. Haematol.,* 36, 585, 1977.
85. **Stenflo, J.,** Structure and function of protein C, *Semin. Thromb. Hemost.,* 10, 109, 1984.
86. **Fulcher, C. A., Gardiner, J. E., Griffin, J., and Zimmerman, T. S.,** Proteolytic inactivation of human factor VIII procoagulant protein by activated protein C and its analogy with factor V, *Blood,* 63, 486, 1984.
87. **Marler, R. A., Kleiss, A. J., and Griffin, J. H.,** Mechanism of action of human activated protein C, a thrombin dependent anticoagulant enzyme, *Blood,* 59, 1067, 1982.
88. **Walker, F. J., Sexton, P. W., and Esmon, C. T.,** The inhibition of blood coagulation by activated protein C through the selected inactivation of activated factor V, *Biochim. Biophys. Acta,* 571, 333, 1979.
89. **Walker, F., Chavin, S. I., and Fay, P. J.,** Inactivation of factor VIII by activated protein C and proteins, *Arch. Biochem. Biophys.,* 252, 322, 1987.
90. **Walker, F. J.,** The regulation of activated protein C by a new protein, a possible function for bovine protein S, *J. Biol. Chem.,* 255, 5521, 1980.
91. **Walker, F. J.,** Protein S and the regulation of activated protein C, *Semin. Thromb. Hemost.,* 10, 131, 1984.
92. **Walker, F. J.,** Regulation of activated protein C by protein S, *J. Biol. Chem.,* 256, 11128, 1981.
93. **Lawrence, J. E., Batard, M. A., Berridge, C. W., and Fulcher, C. A.,** Protein S enhances protein C, *Thromb. Haemost.,* 54, 83, 1985.
94. **Vehar, G. A. and Davie, E. W.,** Formation of a serine enzyme in the presence of bovine factor VIII (antihemophilic factor) and thrombin, *Science,* 197, 374, 1977.
95. **Østerud, B. and Rapaport, S. I.,** Synthesis of intrinsic factor X activator. Inhibition of function of formed activator by antibodies to factor VIII and to factor IX, *Biochemistry,* 9, 1854, 1970.
96. **Bajaj, S. P., Rapaport, S. I., and Maki, S. L.,** A monoclonal antibody to factor IX that inhibits the factor VIII:C$_a$ potentiation of factor X activation, *J. Biol. Chem.,* 260, 11574, 1985.
97. **Mertens, K., Ven Wijngaarden, A., Bertina, R. M., and Veltkamp, J. J.,** The functional defect of factor VIII Leiden, a genetic variant of coagulation factor VIII, *Thromb. Haemost.,* 54, 650, 1985.
98. **Brown, J. E., Baugh, R. F., and Hougie, C.,** Substrate inhibition of the intrinsic generation of activated factor X (Stuart factor), *Thromb. Res.,* 13, 893, 1978.
99. **Hultin, M. B. and Nemerson, Y.,** Activation of factor X by factors IXa and factor VIII. A specific assay for factor IXa in the presence of thrombin activated factor VIII, *Blood,* 52, 928, 1978.

100. **Hultin, M. B.,** Role of human factor VIII in factor X activation, *J. Clin. Invest.,* 69, 950, 1982.
101. **Van Dieijen, G., Tans, G., Rosing, J., and Hemker, H. C.,** The role of phospholipid and factor VIIIa in the activation of bovine factor X, *J. Biol. Chem.,* 256, 3433, 1981.
102. **Kosow, D. P.,** Purification and activation of human factor X: cooperative effects of Ca^{++} on the activation reaction, *Thromb. Res.,* 9, 565, 1976.
103. **Neal, G. G. and Esnouf, M. P.,** Kinetic studies of the activation of factor X by factors IXa and VIII:C in the absence of thrombin, *Br. J. Haematol.,* 57, 123, 1984.
104. **Van Dieijen, G., Van Rijn, J. L. M., Govers-Riemslag, J. W. P., Hemker, H., Coenrad, and Rosing, J.,** Assembly of the intrinsic factor X_a activating complex-interaction between factor IX_a, factor VIII_a, and phospholipid. *Thromb. Haemost.,* 53, 396, 1985.
105. **Jackson, C. M.,** The biochemistry of prothrombin activation, *Br. J. Haematol.,* 39, 1, 1978.
106. **Rosing, J., Tans, G., Govers-Riemsing, J. W. P., and Hemker, H. C.,** The role of phospholipids and factor V_a in the prothrombinase complex, *J. Biol. Chem.,* 255, 274, 1980.
107. **Esmon, C. T., Owen, W. G., and Jackson, C. M.,** A plausible mechanism for prothrombin activation by factor X_a, factor V_a, phospholipid, and calcium ions, *J. Biol. Chem.,* 249, 8045, 1974.
108. **Mertens, K., Van Wijngarrden, and Bertina, R. M.,** The role of factor VIII in the activation of human blood coagulation factor X by activated factor IX, *Thromb. Haemost.,* 54, 654, 1985.
109. **Nesheim, M. E., Tracy, R. B., and Mann, K. G.,** "Clotspeed", a mathematical simulation of the functional properties of prothrombinase, *J. Biol. Chem.,* 259, 1447, 1984.

Chapter 2

ADVANCES IN BIOTECHNOLOGY OF FACTOR VIII

Andrea Pavirani and Pierre Meulien

TABLE OF CONTENTS

I.   Introduction 26

II.   Basic Principles of Biotechnology 26
        A.   Cloning 26
        B.   Expression 27

III.   Recombinant VIII 28
        A.   The Cloning of VIII cDNA 28
        B.   Expression of rVIII 29
        C.   Properties of rVIII 29

IV.   Novel Procoagulant Polypeptides Based on VIII 32

V.   Concluding Remarks 35

Acknowledgments 36

References 36

INTRODUCTION

Present day therapy for hemophilia A is associated with well-known and documented clinical, social, and economic problems which are directly related to the quality of factor VIII (VIII) preparations available, these being obtained from the only possible source of VIII which has existed until now, human plasma. The recent cloning and expression of the VIII gene[1-4] have thus brought new hope to hemophiliacs of a safer therapeutic preparation. Many scientific disciplines participate in the field of biotechnology, and for the first time, molecular and cellular biologists, protein chemists, and fermentation scientists within many biotechnology companies are close to producing large quantities of highly purified recombinant VIII (rVIII) free from the contaminants usually associated with many blood products. This new preparation will, therefore, constitute a revolution in the presently problematic treatment of hemophilia A.

In this chapter we shall describe the cloning and expression of the VIII gene, which has been acclaimed as one of the most important technical achievements of the decade, and the important aspects of expressing such a large and complex molecule[5] which need to be considered when large scale production is in mind.

Another important area of development to be discussed stems from the deduction (from the cDNA sequence) of the primary structure of the VIII molecule[1-3] which along with the elucidation of the proteolytic processing of VIII during its activation[2,5-12] has led molecular biologists to manipulate the cDNA sequence with the aim of producing new VIII derivatives. These engineered molecules may have beneficial properties which would overcome undesirable characteristics of VIII such as its extreme lability and its susceptibility to proteolytic attack. This "fine tuning" of the VIII molecule has to be performed with care in order neither to destroy or diminish its procoagulant activity nor to prolong its stability in an active form which could lead to thrombotic complications. One other major consideration concerns the possible problematic immunogenicity of these "new molecules", and because of the necessary and time consuming antigenicity testing required, their therapeutic potential will not be known for some time.

II. BASIC PRINCIPLES OF BIOTECHNOLOGY

While it is not our purpose to explain the fundamentals of molecular biology or to write a laboratory manual (interested readers are referred to References 13 and 14), we feel it necessary to describe, in outline, the theoretical and practical steps involved when confronted with the cloning and expression of a given gene.

A. Cloning

Cloning a specific DNA sequence requires two essential steps: first the construction of a library of DNA sequences complementary to the messenger RNA present in a given tissue/organ and second the isolation of the specific cDNA of interest. The major problem encountered in the first step is to ensure that the sequence of interest is present in the library, this being directly associated with the abundance of the mRNA in the tissue. If one compares levels of mRNA encoding albumin, for example, with those for VIII (both expressed in the liver), one will find a ratio of at least 500:1, respectively. Therefore, in order to ensure that VIII mRNA is present in the library, the number of individual clones required will need to be large.[15]

There exist three basic methods for isolating the cDNA sequence of interest. These rely on:

1. The ability of the cDNA to hybridize to a synthetic oligonucleotide probe deduced from back-translating a portion of amino acid sequence of the natural molecule

2. The ability of the protein encoded by the cDNA expressed in *Escherichia coli* to be recognized by a specific antibody made against the natural molecule
3. The ability of the cDNA to encode a specific biological function when expressed in a suitable host (normally mammalian cells)

When designing oligonucleotide probes from amino acid sequences, many alternatives are possible due to the degeneracy of the genetic code.[16] It is, therefore, desirable, when possible, to choose stretches of amino acid sequence containing methionine or tryptophan residues as both have unique codons. The choice is then made for using either a mixture of short oligonucleotides covering all possibilities — the disadvantage here is that one lowers the specific activity of the correctly matching probe — or a long oligonucleotide containing a unique sequence which is hybridized in conditions of low stringency[17] which can result in many false positives. While each route has its disadvantages, both have been used successfully.[16]

When screening clones using antibodies specific for the natural protein, several points should be born in mind. The cDNA is expressed in bacteria usually as a fusion protein, i.e., fused to the product of another gene (β-galactosidase, for example[18]). This protein is not glycosylated and will certainly not have the conformation of the natural molecule. Polyclonal rather than monoclonal antibodies should, therefore, be used, and by preference these antibodies should give a signal in a "Western" blot demonstrating that the denatured protein is recognized.[18] In some cases it is advisable to use the denatured protein for making the antibodies to be utilized in screening.

In cases when neither antibody nor amino acid sequence exists but a specific biological function is known for the gene of interest, the possibility of screening by biological activity is feasable. In this method, normally used in conjunction with a mammalian cell expression system,[19] complete cDNA sequences are cloned into a plasmid capable of expressing heterologous genes in mammalian cells. After construction of the cDNA bank, pools of clones are screened for the required biological function. Subsequent subcloning allows the isolation of the expressing clone and the rescue of the gene.

B. Expression

The goal of the molecular and cellular biologists is to produce a cell secreting respectable amounts of biologically active product in a stable fashion. While bacteria and yeasts have been the preferred hosts for the production of various molecules, including insulin[20] and the hepatitis B surface antigen (HBsAg),[21] little success has been achieved when complex proteins have been expressed in these systems. This is mainly due to the inability of these cells to perform the posttranslational modifications (glycosylation and γ-carboxylation in the case if IX[22-24], for example) necessary to guarantee a fully active product. For the coagulation factors, mammalian cells alone have been exploited with success.

Many strategies exist in order to establish permanent mammalian cell lines secreting a given protein.[25,26] In the first instance it is important to ensure that in a particular cell line the protein in question will be correctly processed giving full biological activity. A procedure is therefore desirable which allows the screening of many cell lines in order to find the best performing host. These so-called transient expression assays consist either of (1) testing a mixed population of transfected cells for production shortly after the introduction of the foreign gene or (2) the use of a recombinant vaccinia virus[27-29] carrying the gene of interest which can infect a large range of host cell types and has been shown to produce large amounts of recombinant protein shortly after infection.[30,31]

Having chosen a suitable host, permanent cell lines can be obtained. In this case the gene will be placed downstream of promoter/enhancer sequences (often of viral origin) and will be either integrated along with a marker gene needed to select the clones or be maintained as an autonomously replicating element within the nucleus, in which case the vector will be based on a viral genome such as bovine papilloma virus (BPV). Many markers are available for selection and are based either on mutant cell lines (dihydrofolate reductase gene [DHFR] for chinese hamster ovary: CHO DHFR⁻ cells) or are dominant in nature (adenosine deaminase [ADA],[32] xanthine-guanine phosphoribosyltransferase [XGPRT], and G418 resistance gene, for example), having a wider application.[25,26]

III. RECOMBINANT VIII

A. The Cloning of VIII cDNA

For decades the purification of VIII eluded biochemists, and in fact it is only relatively recently that VIII has been separated into its two components:[33] the VIII antihemophilic factor and the von Willebrand factor (vWf), a large glycoprotein involved in platelet adhesion to damaged subendothelium and the carrier molecule for VIII.[34] The characterization of monoclonal antibodies specific for either component of the complex[35] resulted in substantial progress being made in purification techniques,[5,36] culminating in the determination by microsequencing of several stretches of amino acids on peptides generated by proteolytic cleavage.[2,3,5] The protein sequence was the first essential tool required for the successful isolation of the DNA coding sequence of VIII; the second would be the discovery of the site of synthesis of the messenger RNA.

Three groups independently cloned a complete VIII cDNA using different variations on the same theme. Toole et al.[2] used protein sequence data from porcine VIII (used in some cases to replace human VIII *in vivo*) to make synthetic oligonucleotide probes enabling the isolation of a porcine genomic clone which was in turn used to isolate a human genomic sequence. This allowed the synthesis of homologous probes to be used in the screening for sites of synthesis of VIII mRNA, the resulting cDNA clones being isolated from human liver. Wood et al.[1] used a more direct approach using amino acid sequence from highly purified human VIII to design oligonucleotide probes allowing the isolation of human genomic sequences. This group then looked at 80 different cell lines and tissue samples to find a suitable source of VIII mRNA, opting ultimately for the T-cell hybridoma line AL-7. A similar strategy was taken by Truett et al.,[3] however, in this case the cDNA was cloned from a human kidney library.

One point worth noting is that all three groups chose for indirect approach passing by a genomic cloning step. This was necessary due to the uncertainty of the source of the mRNA and because of its extremely low abundance (1 out of 200 to 300 × 10³ mRNA molecules in the liver) which made it too risky to screen cDNA banks directly using partially homologous probes.

Another major problem to be overcome was the isolation of cDNAs spanning the complete length (~9000 ntd) of the VIII mRNA which at that time was the longest nonviral message known. This was achieved by priming the mRNA internally with synthetic oligonucleotides designed from 5′ portions of the initially isolated cDNA clones. cDNAs were cloned using either λgt10-like vector systems[18] or a primer-adapter technique using the plasmid pUC9,[3] both methods giving a large number of recombinants per nanogram of cDNA.

The information obtained from the analysis of the cDNA sequence has been enormous. The primary translation product of VIII is 2351 residues including a 19-amino acid signal peptide. Internal homologies were found which predicted a domain structure for the VIII protein consisting of a triplicated A-domain, a unique B-domain, and a duplicated C-domain arranged as follows: A1-A2-B-A3-C1-C2. The unique B-domain encoded by a large 3.1-Kbp exon (exon 14 of the VIII gene[4]) contains 19 of the 25 potential asparagine linked glycosylation sites and corresponds to the portion of VIII which is lost during thrombin activation. Homologies among VIII and two other plasma proteins, factor V and ceruloplasmin, have also been documented.[37,38]

One group isolated and characterized the complete VIII gene which consists of ~200 kbp representing 0.1% of the X-chromosome.[4] As already mentioned the largest exon is 3.1 kbp in length while the smallest is 69 bp. It has been suggested[4] that the origin of the unusually large exon 14 derives from the insertion of a processed gene (cDNA) into a sequence encoding the A2-A3 junction.

Comparison of cDNA sequences from different laboratories reveals surprisingly few nucleotide differences considering the size of the message and the variety of sources used in its isolation. The ~9000-ntd message is organized as 170 ntd of 5' untranslated sequence, an open reading frame of 7053 ntd, and 1806 ntd corresponding to the 3' noncoding region. Our goup at Transgene S.A., Strasbourg, may have found a true polymorphism present in the B-domain encoding portion (position 3564, A to C: silent)[39] as this region of the completed VIII cDNA was derived from a genomic clone and thus this base change cannot be due to a reverse transcriptase error. The distribution of this polymorphism (if it is such) in the population has not yet been determined.

B. Expression of rVIII

The capability of the rVIII cDNA to encode a protein which reduces the coagulation time of hemophilic plasma has been reported by several groups.[1-3,39] The cDNA was placed in an expression vector downstream of a suitable promoter sequence used usually in conjunction with viral enhancer sequences which are known to increase transcription. This vector was then transfected into either BHK 21[1] or COS-7[2,3] cells and levels of between 0.01 to 0.10 U ml^{-1} of VIII:C were detected. More recently we have screened various mammalian cell lines for their ability to express VIII using recombinant vaccinia virus.[39] One advantage of this system is that many cell lines can be tested due to the wide host range of VV, and normally reasonable yields of recombinant protein are produced enabling preliminary characterization of the recombinant product from a given cell line. This strategy has been successfully used for rIX,[31] and outlines of the experimental procedure using VIII are described below and also shown in Figure 1.

The VIII cDNA from nucleotides -64 to 8235 was inserted into a vector such that expression is driven from the VV 7.5K promoter.[27,28,30] Viral TK gene sequences are situated 5' and 3' to the VIII expression block allowing the *in vivo* recombination with the vaccinia virus genome to take place. Several cell lines were infected with recombinant virus (VV.TG. VIII 10.2-1)[39] selected with 5-bromodeoxyuridine, and after 24 h supernatants were assayed for VIII:Ag levels.[40]

As shown in Table 1 variable levels of VIII:Ag were detected in the supernatants of the different cell lines tested. When identical samples were analyzed for VIII:C (APTT assay[41]) the importance of the negative controls became clear as supernatants from Vero (monkey kidney), HeLa, or MDCK (canine kidney) cells infected with WT VV gave high background values. This could be due to the release of proteases following cell lysis which interfere with this test. Supernatants from infected HepG2 (human hepatoma G2) cells, on the other hand, contained no VIII:C, a result in direct contrast with the VIII:Ag determination suggesting that while VIII is produced in these cells it is either inactive or inactivated after secretion. It should be noted that HepG2 cells are known to produce both protein C and factor X, the activated forms of which are involved in the inactivation of VIII.

Baby hamster kidney cells (BHK 21) produced the highest values of both VIII:C and VIII:Ag (~0.10 U ml^{-1} of VIII:C). This activity was demonstrated to be VIII derived as monoclonal antibody CAG-1 175A7[42] or serum from a hemophilia A-inhibitor patient completely abolished the procoagulant activity. An interesting point was that after 24 h the VIII:C decreased rapidly demonstrating the fragility of the molecule (either due to proteolytic attack or thermolability at 37°C).[43] In attempts to stabilize the rVIII within the context of the VV system, the natural carrier molecule of VIII, vWf, was used. On supplementing cell

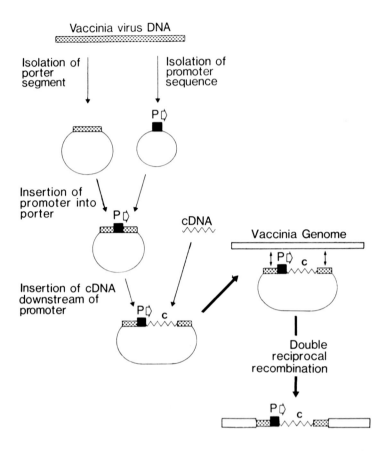

FIGURE 1.   Schematic representation of the different steps involved in the introduction of a foreign cDNA sequence into the VV genome. The *in vitro* manipulations consist of the construction of a recombinant plasmid containing a porter segment (usually the TK gene), whose DNA sequence is interrupted by a VV promoter, e.g., the 7.5 K, which drives the expression of the inserted cDNA. On the transfection of this plasmid into a suitable host infected with WT VV, the DNA homology between the porter sequence and the corresponding VV gene allows a double reciprocal recombination event (*in vivo* step) resulting in a recombinant VV expressing the heterologous cDNA but defective in the function carried by the porter (TK deficiency in the case of the TK porter). Subsequent rounds of selection for the TK⁻ virus lead to the isolation of the recombinant VV. (By courtesy of Kieny, M. P., Lathe, R., and Lecocq, J.-P., Transgene, S. A., Strasbourg. With permission.)

culture medium with preparations of vWf (0.5 U ml^{-1}) an almost linear increase in VIII:C was observed after 24 h, the usual decline being noted when vWf was absent from the medium as seen in Figure 2. Moreover it was established that 0.1 U ml^{-1} vWf was sufficient to stabilize rVIII as depicted in Figure 3.

This demonstrates that vWf recognizes and protects rVIII which may be an important point if vWf is to be used either in a production or purification step on an industrial scale. If so, it is obvious that recombinant vWf (rvWf) may well be required for such a process.

C. Properties of rVIII

Recently the biochemical characterization of rVIII produced in a permanent BHK 21 cell line has been performed by Eaton et al.[44] This study showed that purified VIII consists of

Table 1
VIII:Ag LEVELS (U ml⁻¹) IN THE SUPERNATANTS OF
DIFFERENT CELL LINES

	Cell line				
	BHK21	**Vero**	**HeLa**	**HepG2**	**MDCK**
VV.TG. VIII 10.2-1	0.120	0.049	0.035	0.028	0.025

Note: 2×10^6 cells were infected (1 pfu/cell) for 1 h with recombinant VV expressing the complete VIII sequence (VV.TG. VIII 10.2-1). After several washes of the cells, serum-free medium supplemented with 4% bovine serum albumin (BSA) and 1 mM CaCl$_2$ was added. The immunoradiometric assay (IRMA)[40] was performed at 24 h post-infection on solid phase using purified immunoglobulin G from hemophilic inhibitor patient serum as the first antibody and secondly an anti-VIII monoclonal antibody.

From Pavirani et al., *Bio/Technology,* 5(4), 389, 1987. With permission.

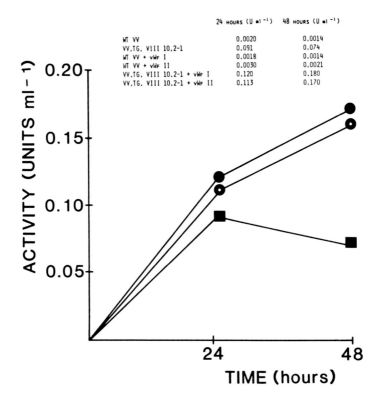

FIGURE 2. VIII:C (U ml⁻¹) levels in the supernatant of BHK 21 cells at 24 and 48 h after infection with VV.TG. VIII 10.2-1 or WT VV. At time 0 medium containing 4% BSA + 1 mM CaCl$_2$ + 0.5 U ml⁻¹ of vWf preparation I (●——●), preparation II (○——○), or lacking vWf (■——■) was added. (From Pavirani et al., *Bio/Technology,* 5(4), 389, 1987. With permission.)

multiple polypeptides exhibiting the same pattern on sodium dodecyl sulfate-polyacrylamide gels as plasma derived VIII, that these polypeptides are recognized in a "Western" blot by antibodies to human VIII, and that both proteins display the same banding pattern in iso-electric focusing experiments.

Functional aspects of VIII were also studied.[44] Thrombin, X$_a$, and activated protein C

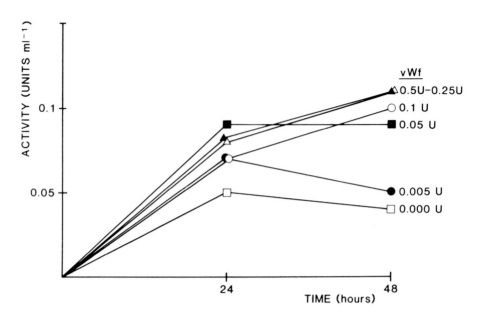

FIGURE 3.   Dose response of vWf concentrations (U ml^{-1}) on the VIII:C (U ml^{-1}) at 24 and 48 h post-infection. Recombinant VV is VV.TG.VIII 10.2-1. See Figure 2 for technical details.

were shown to process rVIII in the same manner they do the native molecule. Animal trials have also started using hemophilic dogs, and it has been shown that rVIII can shorten the cuticle bleeding time and that the half-life of the recombinant molecule is similar to that of plasma derived VIII.[45,46] These studies have produced promising results and lead the way to clinical trials.

IV. NOVEL PROCOAGULANT POLYPEPTIDES BASED ON VIII

One of the most recent and powerful developments in recombinant DNA technology is the ability to modify the primary structure of a protein by changing the corresponding DNA sequence in order to obtain information regarding the functional importance of distinct regions of amino acid sequences.[47] For example, these changes can be single base mutations altering a processing site, changes in several amino acids to determine antigenic sites (high resolution epitope mapping), or more dramatic changes such as specific deletions. The primary structure of the VIII protein together with the knowledge of the proteolytic processing known to modulate its activity has led several investigators to engineer novel VIII derived polypeptides with the aim of avoiding problems linked to the inherent instability of VIII which is associated with its susceptibility to proteolytic attack.

The role of the B-domain in this regard has attracted much attention. Figure 4 shows a representation of the current model of the processing of VIII.[2,5-12] In this model the initial activation event consists of a cleavage of the VIII primary translation product at the Arg 1648-Glu 1649 bond producing a light chain precursor (80 kDa) and a heavy chain precursor (>200 kDa). Presumably the two chains are already associated before this cleavage occurs. The subsequent degradation of the B-domain by successive proteolytic cleavages is followed by a thrombin activation step cleaving at Arg 739-Ser 740 and Arg 1689-Ser 1690 which results in a 90-kDa heavy chain and a 73-kDa light chain. Whether a further cleavage by thrombin at Arg 371-Ser 372 is necessary for maximal activity or whether this cleavage destabilizes the complex is a controversial point at present.[6,9] It is generally accepted, however, that prolonged incubation with thrombin leads to a rapid decline in activity. Other factors which are known to inactivate VIII are activated protein C and X$_a$ cleaving the protein at several positions, one of which is Arg 336/ Met 337.

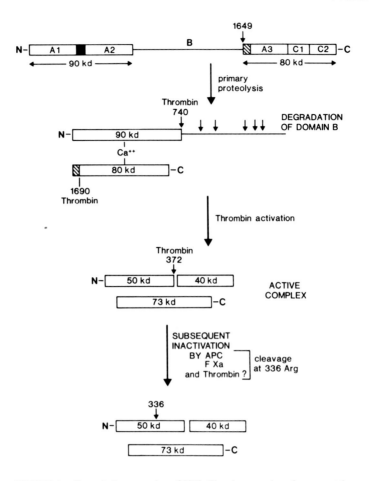

FIGURE 4.   Proteolytic processing of VIII. The cleavage sites shown are taken from Vehar et al.[5] Toole et al.,[2] and Eaton et al.[9] The primary cleavage at aa 1649 is produced by an unknown protease. The activated protein C cleavage site at aa 336 is thought to be associated with the inactivation of VIII.[9] The association of the two chains is thought to be dependent on the presence of Ca,[++] but other cations may be implicated.

One striking feature in this process is that the B-domain does not seem to play a role in the active complex as it is lost after thrombin cleavage. Furthermore, Toole et al.[48] have compared nucleotide sequences from human and porcine VIII, and, while the respective DNA sequences encoding the heavy and light chains are highly conserved, the two B-domains show surprising divergence. This suggested to Toole et al.[48] and subsequently to others[49-51] that the B-domain could be dispensed without losing procoagulant function.

Two approaches have been used to test this hypothesis. Either large sections of the DNA encoding the B-region were deleted from the complete cDNA resulting in shorter VIII derivatives[48,49] or DNA fragments corresponding to the heavy and light chains have been co-expressed in mammalian cells.[50,51] It has thus been demonstrated that a molecule lacking domain-B, but retaining the processing sites at aa positions 740, 1649, and 1690 necessary for activation, displays procoagulant activity and has the added advantage of being ten times more efficiently expressed in mammalian cells.[48] This molecule can be activated by thrombin in a similar manner to the complete VIII molecule. Eaton et al.[49] have demonstrated that similar molecules bind vWf efficiently and therefore would presumably have a reasonable half-life in plasma.

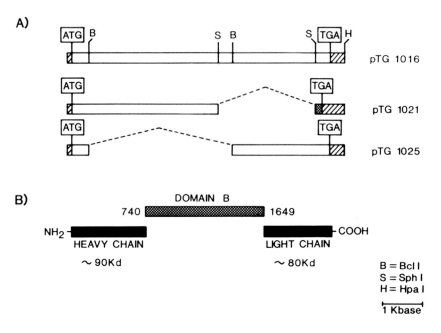

FIGURE 5.   (A) Schematic representation of the construction of two separate plasmids containing either the heavy chain (pTG1021)[51] or the light chain (pTG1025)[51] VIII cDNA sequence. At the top the complete VIII cDNA sequence in pTG1016[39] is shown. 5′ and 3′ untranslated regions are hatched. The start (ATG) and stop (TGA) codons are indicated. The restriction endonuclease sites used for the assembly of the two sequences are shown. pTG1016[39] which carries the entire VIII coding sequence was modified by deleting DNA between ntd 3936 and 6585 cleaving with SphI and subsequent religation. This heavy chain construct (pTG1021) contains sequences encoding aa 1-1293 of the VIII molecule followed by 46 aa plus stop codon resulting from the frameshift due to the position of the 3′ SphI site (dotted portion). A similar light chain construct (pTG1025) was made by deleting the DNA between the two BclI sites at ntd 403 and ntd 4419. This construction encodes the VIII signal peptide (19 aa), aa 1 to aa 115 (heavy chain), aa 1455 to 2232, and the natural VIII stop codon. Both pTG1021 and pTG1025 were recombined *in vivo* with wild type VV (Copenhagen ts 26)[30] thus creating VV.TG. VIII HC-1 and VV.TG. VIII LC-1, respectively. (B) Primary (preactivation) proteolytic products of the VIII protein are shown. The size of the peptides are in scale with that of the cDNA. Note that the excision of the central domain-B is achieved by progressive proteolytical degradation starting from its own COOH terminus. Numbers indicate the aa at which cleavage occurs (see Figure 4). (From Pavirani, A., *Biochem. Biophys. Res. Commun.*, 145(1), 234, 1987. With permission.)

Others[50,51] have studied the possibility of expressing the amino terminal 90 and the carboxy terminal 80 chains as separate proteins. When co-expressed in the same cell these two chains associate to form an active VIII molecule. There follows a brief description of a study[51] using the vaccinia virus derived vectors described above. Figure 5 shows the constructs enabling the expression of either the heavy or light chains. When BHK 21 cells were co-infected with both recombinant viruses, significant VIII:C was detected after a 24-h period, albeit lower than that found when the entire molecule is expressed as shown in Table 2. Since FVIII:Ag data revealed larger quantities of the individual chains when compared to the full molecule, the lower VIII:C levels observed must be due to the association kinetics of the two chains. The failure to reconstitute VIII:C by mixing supernatants of cells expressing either the light or heavy chains would indicate that either their concentration is prohibitively low for the formation of the two-chain complex or that their association demands specific conditions which as yet remain elusive. Similar results have been reported by Burke et al.[50] using a COS-7 cell transient system. Antigenicity tests will need to be performed on such molecules as new antigenic sites may be created when alterations in the primary structure of protein are performed.

Epitope mapping studies show that many inhibitor patients make anti-VIII antibodies

Table 2
VIII:C AND VIII:Ag LEVELS (U ml⁻¹) IN THE SUPERNATANTS OF BHK21 CELLS INFECTED WITH EITHER RECOMBINANT VVs OR WT VV

	24 h		48 h	
	VIII:C	**VIII:Ag**	**VIII:C**	**VIII:Ag**
VV.TG. VIII 10.2-1	0.140	0.412	0.235	0.412
VV.TG. VIII HC-1 + VV.TG. VIII LC-1	0.010	0.195	BDL[a]	0.095
VV.TG. VIII HC-1	BDL[a]	D[b]	BDL[a]	D[b]
VV.TG.VIII LC-1	BDL[a]	0.407	BDL[a]	0.247
WT VV	BDL[a]	BDL[a]	BDL[a]	BDL[a]

Note: 2×10^6 BHK21 cells were infected at 1 pfu/cell for 1 h. Time 0 represents the time when serum-free medium containing 4% BSA + 1 mM $CaCl_2$ was added.

[a]   Below detection limits (detection limit = 0.001 U ml⁻¹).
[b]   VIII:Ag was indeed detected using an anti-VIII heavy chain monoclonal antibody (CAG-1 72A3) but, due to the different assay system used (liquid phase), these values are not comparable with those obtained using the anti-light chain antibody presented above.

From Pavirani, A., *Biochem. Biophys. Res. Commun.*, 145(1), 234, 1987. With permission.

directed against the light chain only.[52,53] While the availability of rVIII will not directly solve the problems of inhibitor patients, a therapy using preparations of purified light chain administered before the VIII preparation[53] (to trap excess anti-light chain antibodies) suggests a possible application for a gene construction expressing the light chain alone.

V. CONCLUDING REMARKS

The aim of this chapter has been to summarize the recent achievements in the biotechnology of VIII. We have focused on the wealth of scientific information which has accumulated as a direct consequence of the cloning and expression of rVIII. This has enabled the construction of a new generation of VIII derived molecules which may have therapeutic potential. There is no doubt that these developments are extremely promising and will ultimately result in the availability of an improved therapy for hemophilia A patients. We would, however, like to emphasize that before rVIII takes its place on the market the preparation will have to be submitted to stringent clinical safety and efficacy standards as is the practice for any pharmaceutical product. These lengthy preclinical and clinical tests may prevent rVIII being routinely available before 1990, but the importance of these quality controls cannot be overemphasized as VIII replacement is a life-long therapy, and therefore all the consequences due to the nature of the rVIII preparations (which will in any case differ in some degree from those containing plasma derived VIII) will need careful evaluation. This overt caution needs to be balanced with the urgency of a rVIII product when considering the increasing cost of plasma derived VIII (due in part, to the supplementary treatments now necessary to insure against human immunodeficiency virus [HIV] contamination); the inadequacy of the present preparation; and the estimated 98% probability[54] that the rVIII will work. This together with the intense competition among industrialists for a share in the market ($155 million for U.S. alone[54]) ensures that rVIII will become a reality within the shortest feasible delay. It is obvious that this will have enormous consequences for the biotechnology of other blood products and will probably lead to considerable restructuring of the blood fraction market.

Two important subjects linked to the biotechnology of VIII have not been dealt with above, these are

1.   The use of DNA probes in the diagnosis of hemophilia A
2.   Gene therapy

The former technique has become the preferred method for the diagnosis of hemophilia and is used routinely in many laboratories. Readers are referred to several articles which cover this subject.[55-57]

Gene therapy is a futuristic technology whereby a defective gene is replaced by a functional one[58] using, for example, tissue grafts or bone marrow transplants (using ideally cells from the patient himself), these tissues having been transfected *in vitro* with a functional gene. In this regard initial experimentations injecting transfected cells into mice look promising.[59]

ACKNOWLEDGMENTS

We thank Jean-Pierre Lecocq for stimulating discussions, encouragement, and critical reading of the manuscript. We would like to thank H. Harrer, F. Mischler, and K. Dott for technical assistance; M.-L. Wiesel for the FVIII:C tests; C. Mazurier for the IRMA assays; H. Van de Pol for providing the CAG-1 175A7 and CAG-1 72A3 monoclonal antibodies; P. Chambon, P. Kourilsky, E. Eisenmann, and M. Courtney for continued interest in our research; M. Garretta, M. Goudemand, G. Jacquin, J.-P. Cazenave, and D. Meyer for helpful discussions; and M. De Bazouges and N. Monfrini for excellent secretarial assistance. The experiments using the vaccinia virus system carried out at Transgene S.A. have been made possible by the support of the Centres de Transfusion Sanguine Française (C.T.S.).

REFERENCES

1. **Wood, W. I., Capon, D. J., Simonsen, C. C., Eaton, D. L., Gitschier, J., Keyt, B., Seeburg, P. H., Smith, D. H., Hollingshead, P., Wion, K. L., Delwart, E., Tuddenham, E. G. D., Vehar, G. A., and Lawn, R. M.,** Expression of active human factor VIII from recombinant DNA clones, *Nature,* 312, 330, 1984.

2. **Toole, J. J., Knopf, J. L., Wozney, J. M., Sultzman, L. A., Buecker, J. L., Pittman, D. D., Kaufman, R. J., Brown, E., Shoemaker, C., Orr, E. C., Amphlett, G. W., Foster, B. W., Coe, M. L., Knuston, G. J., Fass, D. N., and Hewick, R. M.,** Molecular cloning of a cDNA encoding human antihaemophilic factor, *Nature,* 312, 342, 1984.

3. **Truett, M. A., Blacher, R., Burke, R. L., Caput, D., Chu, C., Dina, D., Hartog, K., Kuo, C. H., Masiarz, F. R., Merryweather, J. P., Najarian, R., Pachl, C., Potter, S. J., Puma, J., Quiroga, M., Rall, L. B., Randolph, A., Urdea, M. S., Valenzuela, P., Dahl, H. H., Favalaro, J., Hansen, J., Nordfang, O., and Ezban, M.,** Characterization of the polypeptide composition of human factor VIII:C and the nucleotide sequence and expression of the human kidney cDNA, *DNA,* 4, 333, 1985.

4. **Gitschier, J., Wood, W. I., Goralka, T. M., Wion, K. L., Chen, E. Y., Eaton, D. H., Vehar, G. A., Capon, D. J., and Lawn, R. M.,** Characterization of the human factor VIII gene, *Nature,* 312, 326, 1984.

5. **Vehar, G. A., Keyt, B., Eaton, D., Rodriguez, H., O'Brien, D. P., Rotblat, F., Oppermann, H., Keck, R., Wood, W. I., Harkins, R. N., Tuddenham, E. G. D., Lawn, R. M., and Capon, D. J.,** Structure of human factor VIII, *Nature,* 312, 337, 1984.

6. **Fulcher, C. A., Roberts, J. R., and Zimmerman, T. S.,** Thrombin proteolysis of purified factor VIII procoagulant protein: correlation of activation with generation of a specific polypeptide, *Blood,* 61, 807, 1983.

7. **Fulcher, C. A., Roberts, J. A., Holland, L. Z., and Zimmerman, T. S.,** Human factor VIII procoagulant protein. Monoclonal antibodies define precursor-product relationships and functional epitops, *J. Clin. Invest.,* 76, 117, 1985.

8. **Rotblat, F., O'Brien, D. P., O'Brien, F. J., Goodall, A. H., and Tuddenham, E.,** Purification of human factor VIII:C and its characterization by western blotting using monoclonal antibodies, *Biochemistry,* 24, 4294, 1985.

9. **Eaton, D., Rodriguez, H., and Vehar, G. A.,** Proteolytic processing of human factor VIII. Correlation of specific cleavages by thrombin, factor Xa, and activated protein C with activation and inactivation of factor VIII coagulant activity, *Biochemistry,* 25, 505, 1986.

10. **Andersson, L.-O., Forsman, N., Huang, K., Larsen, K., Lundin, A., Pavlu, B., Sandberg, H., Sewerin, K., and Smart, J.,** Isolation and characterization of human factor FVIII: molecular forms in commercial factor VIII concentrate, cryoprecipitate, and plasma, *Proc. Natl. Acad. Sci. U.S.A.,* 83, 2979, 1986.

11. **Fay, P. J., Anderson, M. T., Chavin, S. I., and Marder, V. J.,** The size of human factor VIII heterodimers and the effects produced by thrombin, *Biochim. Biophys. Acta,* 871, 268, 1986.

12. **Hamer, R. J., Koedam, J. A., Beeser-Visser, N. H., and Sixma, J. J.,** Human factor VIII: purification from commercial factor VIII concentrate, characterization, identification and radiolabeling, *Biochim. Biophys. Acta,* 873, 356, 1986.

13. **Maniatis, T., Fritsch, E. F., and Sambrook, J.,** *Molecular Cloning: A Laboratory Manual,* Cold Spring Harbor Laboratory, Cold Spring Harbor, N.Y., 1982.

14. **Lathe, R. F., Lecocq, J.-P., and Everett, R.,** DNA engineering, in *Genetic Engineering,* Vol. 4, Williamson, R., Ed., Academic Press, London, 1983, 1.

15. **Williams, J. G.,** The preparation and screening of a cDNA clone bank, in *Genetic Engineering,* Vol. 1, Williamson, R., Ed., Academic Press, London, 1981, 1.

16. **Lathe, R.,** Synthetic oligonucleotide probes deduced from amino acid sequence data — theoretical and practical considerations, *J. Mol. Biol.,* 183, 1, 1985.

17. **Jaye, M., De La Salle, H., Schamber, F., Balland, A., Kohli, V., Findeli, A., Tolstoshev, P., and Lecocq, J.-P.,** Isolation of a human antihaemophilic factor IX cDNA clone using a unique 52-base synthetic oligonucleotide probe deduced from the amino acid sequence of bovine factor IX, *Nucleic Acids Res.,* 11, 2325, 1983.

18. **Huynh, T. V., Young, R. A., and Davis, R. W.,** Constructing and screening cDNA libraries in λgt10 ahd λgt11, in *DNA Cloning. A Practical Approach,* Vol. 1, Glover, D. M., Ed., IRL Press, Oxford, 1985, 49.

19. **Wong, G. G., Witek, J. S., Temple, P. A., Wilkens, K. M., Leary, A. C., Luxenberg, D. P., Jones, S. S., Brown, E. L., Kay, R. M., Orr, E. C., Shoemaker, C., Golde, D. W., Kaufman, R. J., Hewick, R. M., Wang, E. A., and Clark, S. C.,** Human GM-CSF: molecular cloning of the complementary DNA and purification of the natural and recombinant proteins, *Science,* 228, 810, 1985.

20. **Riggs, A. D., Itakura, K., and Boyer, H. W.,** From somatostatin to human insulin, in *Recombinant DNA Products: Insulin, Interferon and Growth Hormones,* Bollon, A. P., Ed., CRC Press, Boca Raton, FL, 1984, 37.

21. **Valenzuela, P., Medina, A., and Rutter, W. J., Ammerer, G., and Hall, B. D.,** Synthesis and assembly of hepatitis B virus surface antigen particles in yeast, *Nature,* 298, 347, 1982.

22. **Chavin, S. I. and Weidner, S. M.,** Blood clotting factor IX, *J. Biol. Chem.,* 259, 3387, 1984.

23. **Friedman, P. A.,** Vitamin K-dependent proteins, *N. Engl. J. Med.,* 310, 1458, 1984.

24. **Jorgensen, M. J., Cantor, A. B., Furie, B. A., Brown, C. L., Shoemaker, C. B., and Furie, B.,** Recognition site directing vitamin K-dependent γ-carboxylation resides on the propeptide of factor IX, *Cell,* 48, 185, 1987.

25. **Rigby, P. W. J.,** Expression of cloned genes in eukaryotic cells using vector systems derived from viral replicons, in *Genetic Engineering,* Vol. 3, Williamson, R., Ed., Academic Press, London, 1982, 84.

26. **Strauss, M., Kiessling, U., and Platzer, M.,** Gene transfer in animal cells, *Biol. Zentralbl.,* 105, 209, 1986.

27. **Smith, G. L., Mackett, M., and Moss, B.,** Infectious vaccinia virus recombinants that express hepatitis B virus surface antigen, *Nature,* 302, 490, 1983.

28. **Panicali, D., Davis, S. W., Weinberg, R. L., and Paoletti, E.,** Construction of live vaccines by using genetically engineered poxviruses: biological activity of recombinant vaccinia virus expressing influenza virus hemagglutinin, *Proc. Natl. Acad. Sci. U.S.A.,* 80, 5364, 1983.

29. **Mackett, M. and Smith, G. L.,** Vaccinia virus expression vectors, *J. Gen. Virol.,* 67, 2067, 1986.

30. **Kieny, M. P., Lathe, R., Drillien, R., Spehner, D., Skory, S., Schmitt, D., Wiktor, T., Koprowski, H., and Lecocq, J.-P.,** Expression of rabies virus glycoprotein from a recombinant vaccinia virus, *Nature,* 312, 163, 1984.

31. **De La Salle, H., Altenburger, W., Elkaim, R., Dott, K., Dieterlé, A., Drillien, R., Cazenave, J.-P., Tolstoshev, P., and Lecocq, J.-P.,** Active γ-carboxylated human factor IX expressed using recombinant DNA techniques, *Nature,* 316, 268, 1985.

32. **Kaufman, R. J., Murtha, P., Ingolia, D. E., Yeung, C. Y., and Kellems, R. E.,** Selection and amplification of heterologous genes encoding adenosine deaminase in mammalian cells, *Proc. Natl. Acad. Sci. U.S.A.,* 83, 3136, 1986.

33. **Hoyer, L. W.,** The factor VIII complex: structure and function, *Blood,* 58, 1, 1981.

34. **Zimmermann, T. S. and Meyer, D.**, Factor VIII-von Willebrand factor and the molecular basis of von Willebrand's disease, in *Hemostasis and Thrombosis: Basic Principles and Clinical Practice*, Colman, R. W., Hirsch, J., Marder, V. J., and Salzman, E. W., Eds., Lippincott, Philadelphia, 1982, 54.

35. **Goodall, A. H. and Meyer, D.**, Registry of monoclonal antibodies to factor VIII and von Willebrand factor, *Thromb. Haemost.*, 54, 878, 1985.

36. **Fass, D. N., Knutson, G. J., and Katzmann, J. A.**, Monoclonal antibodies to porcine factor VIII coagulant and their use in the isolation of active coagulant protein, *Blood*, 59, 594, 1982.

37. **Church, W. R., Jernigan, R. L., Toole, J., Hewick, R. M., Knopf, J., Knutson, G. J., Nesheim, M. E., Mann, K. G., and Fass, D. N.**, Coagulation factors V and VIII and ceruloplasmin constitute a family of structurally related proteins, *Proc. Natl. Acad. Sci. U.S.A.*, 81, 6934, 1984.

38. **Fass, D. N., Hewick, R. M., Knutson, G. J., Nesheim, M. E., and Mann, K. G.**, Internal duplication and sequence homology in factors V and VIII, *Proc. Natl. Acad. Sci. U.S.A.*, 82, 1688, 1985.

39. **Pavirani, A., Meulien, P., Harrer, H., Schamber, F., Dott, K., Villeval, D., Cordier, Y., Wiesel, M.-L., Mazurier, C., Van de Pol, H., Piquet, Y., Cazenave, J.-P., and Lecocq, J.-P.**, Choosing a host cell for active recombinant factor VIII production using vaccina virus, *Bio/Technology*, 5, 389, 1987.

40. **Girma, J.-P., Lavergne, J.-M., Meyer, D., and Larrieu, M.-J.**, Immunoradiometric assay of factor VIII: coagulant antigen using four human antibodies. Study of 27 cases of haemophilia A, *Br. J. Haemotol.*, 47, 269, 1981.

41. **Soulier, J. P. and Larrieu, M. J.**, Nouvelle méthode de diagnostic de l'hémophile. Dosage des facteurs antihemophiliques A et B, *Sang*, 14, 205, 1953.

42. **Croissant, M.-P., Van de Pol, H., Lee, H. H., and Allain, J.-P.**, Characterization of four monoclonal antibodies to factor VIII coagulant protein and their use in immunopurification of factor VIII, *Thromb. Haemost.*, 56, 271, 1986.

43. **Rock, G. A., Cruickshank, W. H., Tackaberry, E. S., Ganz, P. R., and Palmer, D. S.**, Stability of FVIII:C in plasma: the dependence on protease activity and calcium, *Thromb. Res.*, 29, 521, 1983.

44. **Eaton, D. L., Hass, P. E., Riddle, L., Mather, J., Wiebe, M., Gregory, T., and Vehar, G. A.**, Characterization of recombinant human factor VIII, *J. Biol. Chem.*, 262, 3285, 1987.

45. **Giles, A. R., Bowie, E. J. W., Fournel, M. A., and Pancham, N.**, Evaluation of recombinant factor VIII (rFVIII) kinetics and functional activity in a canine model of hemophilia A, *Ric. Clin. Lab.*, 16, 201, 1986.

46. **Amphlett, G.**, Advances in gene technology of factor VIII:C, in *Recent Advances and New Developments in Hemostaseology*, Breddin, H. K., Bender, N., and Scharf, R. E., Eds., S. Karger, Basel, Switzerland, 1986, 4.

47. **Leatherbarrow, R. J. and Fersht, A. R.**, Protein engineering, *Protein Eng.*, 1, 7, 1986.

48. **Toole, J. J., Pittman, D. D., Orr, E. C., Murtha, P., Wasley, L. C., and Kaufman, R. J.**, A large region ($\approx$ 95 kDa) of human factor VIII is dispensable for in vitro procoagulant activity, *Proc. Natl. Acad. Sci. U.S.A.*, 83, 5939, 1986.

49. **Eaton, D. L., Wood, W. I., Eaton, D., Haas, P. E., Hollingshead, P., Wion, K., Mather, J., Lawn, R. M., Vehar, G. A., and Gorman, C.**, Construction and characterization of an active factor VIII variant lacking the central one-third of the molecule, *Biochemistry*, 25, 8343, 1986.

50. **Burke, R. L., Pachl, C., Quiroga, M., Rosenberg, S., Haigwood, N., Nordfang, O., and Ezban, M.**, The functional domains of coagulation factor VIII:C, *J. Biol. Chem.*, 261, 12574, 1986.

51. **Pavirani, A., Meulien, P., Harrer, H., Dott, K., Mischler, F., Wiesel, M.-L., Mazurier, C., Cazenave, J.-P., and Lecocq, J.-P.**, Two independent domains of FVIII co-expressed using recombinant vaccinia virus have procoagulant activity, *Biochem. Biophys. Res. Commun.*, 145, 234, 1987.

52. **Fulcher, C. A., De Graaf Mahoney, S., Roberts, J. R., Kasper, C. K., and Zimmerman, T. S.**, Localization of human factor FVIII inhibitor epitopes to two polypeptide fragments, *Proc. Natl. Acad. Sci. U.S.A.*, 82, 7728, 1985.

53. **Knudsen, B. J., Scheibel, E., Nordfang, O., and Ezban, M.**, Effect of a novel FVIII:CAg preparation in a high-responder inhibitor patient, *Ric. Clin. Lab.*, 16, 103, 1986.

54. **Klausner, A.**, Handicapping pharmaceuticals' prospects, *Bio/Technology*, 5, 116, 1987.

55. **Graham, J. B., Green, P. P., McGraw, R. A., and Davis, L. M.**, Application of molecular genetics to prenatal diagnosis and carrier detection in the hemophilics: some limitations, *Blood*, 66, 759, 1985.

56. **Gitschier, J., Wood, W. I., Shuman, M. A., and Lawn, R. M.**, Identification of a missense mutation in the factor VIII gene of a mild hemophiliac, *Science*, 232, 1415, 1986.

57. **Youssoufian, H., Kazazian, H. H., Jr., Philips, D. G., Aronis, S., Tsiftis, G., Brown, V. A., and Antonarakis, S. E.**, Recurrent mutations in haemophilia A give evidence for CpG mutation hotspots, *Nature*, 324, 380, 1986.

58. **Williams, D. A. and Orkin, S. H.**, Somatic gene therapy. Current status and future prospects, *J. Clin. Invest.*, 77, 1053, 1986.

59. **Garver, R. I., Jr., Chytil, A., Courtney, M., and Crystal, R. G.**, Clonal gene therapy: transplanted mouse fibroblast clones express human α_1-antitrypsin gene *in vivo*, *Science*, 237, 762, 1987.

60. **Foster P. A., Fulcher, C. A., Houghton, R. A., and Zimmerman, T. S.,** An immunogenic region within residues val1670-Glu1684 of the factor VIII light chain induces antibodies which inhibit binding of FVIII to von Willebrand Factor, *J. Biol. Chem.,* 263, 5230, 1988.

61. **Hamer, R. J., Koedam, J. A., Beeser-Visser, N. H., Bertina, R. M., Van Mourik, J. A., and Sixma, J. J.,** Factor VIII binds to von Willebrand factor via its Mr-80,000 light chain, *Eur. J. Biochem.,* 166, 37, 1987.

62. **Meulien, P., Faure, T., Mischler, F., Harrer, H., Ulrich, P., Bouderbala, B., Dott, K., Sainte-Marie, M., Mazurier, C., Wiesel, M-L., Van de Pol, H., Cazenave, J-P., Courtney, M., and Pavirani, A.,** A new recombinant procoagulant protein derived from the cDNA encoding human factor VIII, *Protein Engienering,* 2, in press.

63. **Nordfang, O. and Ezban, M.,** Generation of active coagulation factor VIII from isolated subunits, *J. Biol. Chem.,* 263, 1115, 1988.

64. **Pittman, D. D. and Kaufman, R. J.,** Proteolytic requirements for thrombin activation of anti-hemophilia factor (factor VIII), *Proc. Natl. Acad. Sci. U.S.A.,* 85, 2429, 1988.

65. **Roberts, H., McMillan, C. W., High, K., and White II, G. C.,** Preliminary experience with factor VIII prepared by recombinant DNA techniques for the treatment of hemophilia. Abstract SYM-TY-3-4 at 12th congr. Int. Soc. Haematology, August 23 to September 2, 1988, Milan, Italy.

65. **Sarver, N., Ricca, G. A., Link, J., Nathan, M. H., Newman, J., and Drohan, W. N.,** Stable expression of recombinant factor VIII molecules using a bovine papillomavirus vector, *DNA,* 6, 553, 1987.

Chapter 3

PURIFICATION, BIOCHEMISTRY, AND STRUCTURE/FUNCTION RELATIONSHIPS OF vWf

Claudine Mazurier

TABLE OF CONTENTS

I.   Introduction 42

II.   Purification of vWf 42
        A.   Preparation of Fractions Enriched with VIII/vWf 42
        B.   Purification of VIII/vWf 43
        C.   Dissociation of VIII from vWf 44

III.   Biochemistry of vWf 45
        A.   Earlier Characterization 45
                1.   Chemical Composition 45
                2.   Physical Properties 45
                        a.   Molecular Weight 45
                        b.   Electrophoretic Mobility 49
                3.   Subunits 49
        B.   Primary Structure of vWf 50
                1.   Peptide Chain 50
                        a.   Strategic Approach 50
                        b.   Experimental Results 51
                2.   Glycans 51
        C.   Three Dimensional Structure vWf 53
                1.   Secondary Structure 53
                2.   Domains 54
                3.   Protomer 57
                4.   Polymers 59
        D.   Particular Features of the Platelet vWf 60
        E.   Von Willebrand Antigen II 60

IV.   Structure/Function Relationships of vWf 61
        A.   The Role of vWf Multimeric Structure 62
                1.   Clinical Data 62
                2.   Experimental Data 62
                        a.   vWf/Platelet Interaction 62
                        b.   vWf/Subendothelium Interaction 63
                        c.   vWf Involvement in Platelet Adhesion 63
        B.   The Role of vWf Organization in Domains 64
                1.   Ristocetin-Induced vWf Binding to Platelets 64
                2.   vWf Binding to Gp IIb/IIIa Platelet Receptor 66
                3.   vWf Binding to Collagen 67
                4.   Ristocetin-Induced Platelet Agglutination 67
                5.   Platelet Adhesion 68
        C.   The Role of vWf Carbohydrate Moiety 68

1.   Studies of vWf from vWD Patients 68
2.   Studies of Carbohydrate-Modified vWf 69
      a.   Effects of Lectins 69
      b.   Effects of Galactose Oxidase Treatment 69
      c.   Effects of Neuraminidase Treatment 70
      d.   Effects of β-Galactosidase Treatment 70
      e.   Effects of Endoglycosidase Treatment 71

V.   Concluding Remarks 71

Acknowledgments 72

Addendum 72

References 73

I. INTRODUCTION

The major part of human von Willebrand factor (vWf) synthesized and secreted by endothelial cells[1,2] circulates in plasma at a concentration of about 8 $\mu g/m\ell$.[3,4] Plasma vWf is associated noncovalently with the antihemophilic factor (VIII) as a complex VIII/vWf. As most of this complex ($\cong 98\%$) consists of vWf, its physical properties are essentially those of vWf. Another part of the total vWf, representing approximately 20% of its circulating pool,[5-7] is synthesized by megakaryocytes[8] and is found in platelet α granules.[9] This platelet vWf is difficult to purify, and its biochemistry, like its function, has still to be clearly defined.

In this chapter, purification procedures for VIII/vWf and the methods of separating vWf from VIII will be presented, and an update on the biochemical and structural features, in particular of plasma vWf, will be covered. In conclusion, the relationships between the structure and the different functions of vWf will be discussed.

II. PURIFICATION OF vWf

Factor VIII/vWf may be purified from either plasma or from different kinds of therapeutic preparations used for the treatment of patients with hemophilia A or von Willebrand's disease (vWD), as shown in Figure 1. Purified factor VIII/vWf complex can be further dissociated in order to obtain vWf devoid of VIII.

A. Preparation of Fractions Enriched with VIII/vWf

In the initial ethanol fractionation procedures as described by Cohn et al.,[10] fraction I was found to contain the highest concentrations of plasma VIII/vWf and fibrinogen. Separation of part of the contaminating proteins in fraction I was achieved using glycine,ethanol, and citrate buffer.[11] This led to the production of the therapeutic fraction F 1-0 which has been further purified by the elimination of fibrinogen with tannic acid producing F 1-0-Ta.[12]

However, the easiest and simplest way of obtaining fractions five to ten times enriched with VIII/vWf is cryoprecipitation. Cryoprecipitation, the therapeutic usefulness of which was shown by Pool and Shannon,[13] consists of thawing fresh frozen plasma at $4 \pm 2°C$ and, after centrifugation, harvesting the insoluble part, the so-called cryoprecipitate. Cryo-

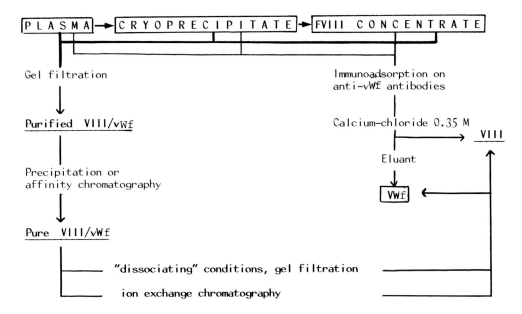

FIGURE 1.   Schematic presentation of the different means of purifying plasma vWf.

precipitation of VIII/vWf which may be caused in part by a salting-out effect, requires the presence in the plasma of both fibrinogen[14] and fibronectin.[15] Under the best conditions, almost all vWf:Ag is recovered in cryoprecipitate whereas 20 to 40% of VIII:C is lost in the supernatant. However, even on a small scale, VIII/vWf does not represent more than 0.5% of proteins in the cryoprecipitate.

Various procedures have been developed in order to further enrich VIII/vWf from cryoprecipitate by eliminating some of the contaminants, particularly fibrinogen and fibronectin. Such methods include adsorption on aluminium hydroxide or bentonite; precipitation with polyethylene glycol, either alone or associated with glycine or ethanol;[16-18] and/or cold precipitation at low ionic strength,[19] acidic pH,[20] or using heparin.[14] However, these precipitation steps, which are often applied for the preparation of therapeutic factor VIII concentrates used in hemophilia A treatment, may induce a loss of the larger molecular weight (MW) forms of VIII/vWf. In fact commercial factor VIII concentrates, except those specially prepared to retain all vWf forms,[21,22] have a limited efficacy in the treatment of vWD and are not the ideal means of purifying vWf with a view to undertaking structure/function studies. Nevertheless, as these concentrates contain 1 to 5% vWf of the total protein, they are a useful starting material for the purification and chemical analysis of vWf.

B. Purification of VIII/vWf

The most usual and efficient method of purifying VIII/vWf from cryoprecipitate or factor VIII concentrates has been shown to be gel filtration using large pore beads such as Sepharose 6B, 4B, and 2B.[23-25] Due to its particularly high MW, VIII/vWf is recovered in void volume fractions (Vo). In these Vo fractions, which may be contaminated with chylomicrons, VIII/vWf represents at least 90% of the total protein. Precipitation with agents such as β-alanine, concanavalin A, ammonium sulfate, polyethylene glycol, etc. is generally used to eliminate most of the contaminants remaining in the supernatant and thus concentrate VIII/vWf. Although VIII/vWf obtained in this way is in some cases immunologically pure, it is generally still contaminated with plasma proteins. Contaminants may be eliminated by affinity chromatography on insolubilized antibodies directed against all plasma proteins except vWf[26] or on heparin-Sepharose.[27]

Most purification procedures reported above were described during the 1970s. Few methods have been published more recently. Affinity chromatography on agmatine- and gelatin-Sepharose succeeds in removing most of the contaminants from void fractions obtained from size exclusion chromatography of VIII/vWf concentrates.[28] Dextran-sulfate agarose[29] and a molecular sieving agent with a high flow rate[30] enable enrichment of VIII/vWf from plasma in a single step. Theoretically some immobilized monoclonal antibodies directed against vWf can be used for the purification of plasma vWf. Nevertheless, whereas many antibodies have been reported to be suitable for immunopurification,[31] we are not aware of published data concerning the purity and physico-chemical properties of vWf obtained in this way. In our laboratory, we have tested ten monoclonal antibodies for this purpose. Though most of them bind plasma VIII/vWf and may be used to purify VIII, they do not easily release vWf. Eluants containing chaotropic agents or sodium-dodecyl sulfate (SDS) are generally required for this purpose. Nevertheless, in one case, vWf is eluted with a pH shift permitting immunoisolation of either VIII/vWf complex[32] or VIII and vWf separately.[33]

C. Dissociation of VIII from vWf

The simplest way of obtaining vWf totally devoid of VIII is to apply one of the purification procedures described above to a starting material consisting of plasma from a hemophilia A CRM$^-$ patient. The amount of vWf obtained by this way is, of course, limited.[34]

Other procedures are based on the dissociation of VIII from purified VIII/vWf complex. High ionic strength buffers, containing either 1 M sodium chloride[35,36] or 0.25 M calcium chloride,[37,38] have often been used to separate VIII from vWf. Dissociation also occurs under other conditions.[35,39-46] Some of these conditions are based on the use of chemical agents or proteolytic enzymes which are liable to modify the structure of dissociated proteins and consequently do not seem suitable for purification and subsequent functional analysis of vWf. After dissociation, vWf is generally separated from VIII by gel filtration. Factor VIII and vWf may also be obtained separately by chromatography on aminohexyl-Sepharose,[47,48] quaternary amino ethyl-Sepharose,[49] and diaminoalkane- and alkane-derivatized Sepharose[48] and by adsorption using polyelectrolytes.[50] In point of fact, as changes in ionic strength and pH could modify conformation and aggregation states of some proteins[51] and assuming the trace concentrations of VIII in the VIII/vWf complex in these preparations, most biochemical studies of vWf have been made on purified vWf not totally devoid of VIII.

Thus, it appears that gel filtration is the basic essential step in the purification of vWf. Depending on the amount of vWf required and on the purpose of the subsequent use of the purified vWf, different starting materials may be selected. If relatively high concentrations (>50 mg of vWf) are required, commercial factor VIII concentrates with a specific activity higher than 1 vWf unit/mg protein are of value as starting material, but it must be stressed that they generally do not contain all the multimeric forms of plasma vWf. From 750 ml of this material (35,000 vWf units), it is possible to obtain in 2 dℓ 300 mg of VIII/vWf complex suitable for some vWf chemical analyses.[62] Nevertheless, if subsequent dissociation of VIII is required, the overall yield is decreased, and only 100 mg of vWf with a purity in excess of 95% is obtained.[28] If all the molecular forms of plasma vWf are required, cryoprecipitate may be used. In our laboratory, using a two-step procedure involving precipitation of a great part of contaminants and gel filtration, we obtain from 600 ml cryoprecipitate ($\cong$6000 vWf units, specific activity $\cong$ 0.25 vWf units/mg protein) 7 to 10 mg of VIII/vWf of more than 95% purity.[22,26] In order to avoid possible denaturation or proteolysis of vWf which can occur during cryoprecipitation, plasma must be used as starting material. For example, when less than 1 mg is needed, vWf may be prepared from fresh plasma within 12 h after blood collection with a purification protocol involving only two steps.[30]

III. BIOCHEMISTRY OF vWf

A. Earlier Characterization

Previous reviews on vWD or on VIII/vWf complex have broached the major physico-chemical properties and structural features of plasma vWf.[52-56]

1. Chemical Composition

Although its low absorption at 280 nm led to early doubts regarding its protein nature,[57] it is now well known that a major part of vWf is composed of amino acids. Several amino acid analyses of human VIII/vWf have been published since 1971. At that time, scientists were already aware of the low levels of methionine, tyrosine, and tryptophan;[3,4] the high half-cysteine content;[58] and the absence of free sulfhydryl groups.[3,58,59] These characteristics were later confirmed by analyzing vWf devoid of VIII[28,60,61] and more recently in publications dealing with the amino acid sequence of vWf.[62] The percentages of amino acid residues recalculated on the basis of the different compositions published are reported in Table 1. A comparison of these data with those recently obtained on the basis of cDNA sequencing shows good consistency except for the number of glycine, cysteine, and, above all, tryptophan residues.

Since vWf is stained by periodic acid Schiff stain[67] and reacts with concavalin A,[68] it was previously considered that vWf might contain a carbohydrate moiety. Although the glyco-protein nature of vWf is now accepted, there is still no general agreement as to the percentage carbohydrate composition and relative percentage carbohydrate content of the protein as shown in Table 2.[3,28,58,59,65,69-83] Nevertheless, the simultaneous presence of mannose and N-acetylgalactosamine residues suggesting the presence of both O- and N-glycosidically linked glycans has been remarked upon in several publications.[65,74,80]

The presence of lipids in highly purified VIII/vWf preparations was first reported in 1971.[58] As the percentage of lipid in different VIII/vWf preparations was reproducible and as contamination did not seem to be a likely problem,[60] some authors have considered that the vWf molecule itself contains a lipid moiety. However, it appears that both the percentage of lipids and their nature (the proportion between phospholipids and neutral groups of lipids) differ according to the starting material and purification procedures used.[58-60,65,84] Further-more, it has been demonstrated that VIII/vWf may be associated with chylomicrons and binds various sulfated glycolipids.[85] As lipid transfer from the very low density lipoproteins (VLDL) to VIII/vWf may also occur,[86] it now seems likely that lipids represent a contam-ination of vWf preparations.

2. Physical Properties

a. Molecular Weight

Much of the early work was directed at using gel filtration, ultracentrifugation, and electron microscopy to characterize the molecular weight (MW) of vWf. Different teams[5,17,23,24,58,69,87,88] successively showed that VIII/vWf was excluded from Sephadex G 200; Sepharose 6B, 4B, and 2B; and Biogel A-5M and A-1.5M, but the only conclusion drawn was that the apparent MW of vWf was greater than 0.5 or 1.5×10^6 Da. Due to the fact that VIII/vWf was included in a 2.5% agarose gel, and on the basis of its partial specific volume (0.77 ml/g) and sedimentation coefficient (18 S), Hershgold et al.[67] estimated the MW of vWf as 2.8×10^6 Da. Later Hershgold[89] reported that vWf demonstrated a molecular weight of 4.5×10^6 Da, calculated on the basis of a 26.1 S value, and that its Stokes radius was 39 nm and frictional ratio 3.43, indicating a high degree of asymmetry.

Initially, ultracentrifugation in saccharose gradients showed that the sedimentation constant of VIII/vWf was greater than that of fibrinogen.[17] Values of 18, 40, 26, 26.1, 30, and 21 S were successively reported.[23,58,67,89-91] Few analytical ultracentrifugations were performed.

Table 1

PERCENTAGES OF AMINO ACID RESIDUES RECALCULATED ON THE BASIS OF DIFFERENT COMPOSITIONS

	Herhsgold et al. 1971[58]	Marchesi et al. 1972[59]	Shapiro et al. 1973[4]	Legaz et al. 1973[3]	Holmberg et al. 1975[63]	Casillas et al. 1976[64]	Olson et al. 1977[60a]
Lys	6.2	5.6	5.4	4.4	5.3	4.8	5.2
His	2.1	—	3.0	2.5	2.4	2.2	2.9
Arg	5.3	4.6	5.3	4.4	4.2	5.1	3.7
AsX	9.6	13.1	9.1	9.5	8.3	7.6	10.0
Thr	6.2	5.9	5.6	6.7	5.3	5.1	5.8
Ser	7.7	8.9	7.3	7.9	9.5	9.2	9.3
GlX	12.5	12.0	12.6	10.0	12.2	12.3	14.4
Pro	6.3	8.2	6.6	6.8	5.8	7.1	4.6
Gly	8.0	9.8	7.4	7.0	9.4	8.5	13.4
Ala	6.6	6.4	5.4	4.9	5.7	5.4	7.9
Cys	2.9	—	6.8	7.3	6.5	6.3	—
Val	7.2	8.1	8.5	8.5	7.5	7.4	6.8
Met	1.2	1.1	1.4	0.9	1.4	2.7	1.3
Ile	3.9	4.4	3.5	3.8	3.4	3.4	3.6
Leu	8.3	6.2	7.5	7.3	6.8	7.8	6.7
Tyr	2.8	2.5	1.9	2.3	1.9	2.4	2.2
Phe	3.2	3.2	2.8	3.0	2.6	2.7	2.2
Trp	—	—	—	2.8	1.8	—	

	Mazurier et al. 1976[65]	Hessel et al. 1984[61a]		Hamilton et al. 1985[66]	Chopek et al. 1986[28a]	Titani et al. 1986[62]	Mean ± SD	Titani et al. 1986[62b]
Lys	4.2	4.3	4.5	4.5	4.3	4.4	4.85 ± 0.6	4.3 (88)
His	2.5	2.5	2.9	2.5	2.7	2.4	2.55 ± 0.28	2.5 (52)
Arg	4.8	4.2	5.9	4.7	4.7	5.0	4.76 ± 0.57	4.9 (101)
AsX	10.3	9.1	9.9	9.2	9.3	9.0	9.54 ± 1.28	9.1 (187)
Thr	5.7	5.3	5.3	5.7	5.6	5.3	5.65 ± 0.48	5.6 (116)
Ser	7.6	8.3	6.5	7.0	6.5	6.9	7.89 ± 1.06	5.6 (116)
GlX	12.2	11.6	12.7	11.6	12.7	12.6	12.26 ± 0.97	11.6 (237)
Pro	7.9	6.8	7.2	6.6	6.5	6.5	6.68 ± 0.89	6.6 (136)

Gly	7.6	10.1	9.6	7.0	6.8	7.7	8.64 ± 1.83	6.7 (137)
Ala	5.4	5.4	5.5	5.3	5.2	5.4	5.73 ± 0.80	5.4 (104)
Cys	6.8	—	3.8	7.0	7.2	7.9	6.25 ± 1.60	8.2 (169)
Val	6.4	9.1	7.5	8.9	7.6	8.0	7.83 ± 0.84	9.0 (184)
Met	1.7	1.9	1.2	1.4	1.9	1.8	1.53 ± 0.47	2.0 (41)
Ile	3.0	3.0	3.1	3.7	3.5	3.6	3.53 ± 0.38	3.8 (78)
Leu	7.6	7.0	7.7	7.6	7.5	7.8	7.37 ± 0.56	7.6 (156)
Tyr	2.9	1.9	1.7	2.6	2.7	2.7	2.35 ± 0.40	2.4 (49)
Phe	3.2	2.6	2.5	2.7	3.0	2.9	2.81 ± 0.30	2.7 (56)
Trp	—	1.7	1.5	2.0	2.1	—	1.98 ± 0.45	0.9 (18)

a   Data obtained on vWf devoid of VIII.

b   Data obtained from amino acid sequence, with the number of residues per mature vWf subunit expressed in parenthesis.

Table 2
PERCENTAGE CARBOHYDRATE COMPOSITION AND RELATIVE PERCENTAGE CARBOHYDRATE CONTENT OF HUMAN vWf [a]

Ref.	Total carbohydrate	Osamines			N-acetyl neuraminic acid	Neutral hexoses			
		Total	GlcNAc[b]	GalNAc[c]		Total	Fuc[d]	Man[e]	Gal[f]
McKee 1970[69]									
Hershgold et al., 1971[58]	11					5			
Marchesi et al., 1972[59]		2.87	2.7	0.17	0.98	1 — 2			
Legaz et al., 1973[3]	6	2.7			0.9 — 1.2	2.2			
Paulssen et al., 1974[70]	20 — 30	3 — 5			0 — 1		1 — 2		
Gralnick et al., 1977[71]					1.18				
Sodetz et al., 1977[72]					4.74, 4.93				
Gralnick et al., 1978[73]					3.33, 3.48				
Sodetz et al., 1979[74]	15	4.07	4	0.7	3.7	6.6	1.0	3.2	2.4
Rosenfeld and Kirby, 1979[75]					4.0				
Mazurier et al., 1980[65]	14.5	4.25	3.25	1.0	3.8	6.5	0.9	2.4	3.2
Kao et al., 1980[76]					3.56				2.97
Morisato and Gralnick, 1980[77]					3.38				3.11
De Marco and Shapiro, 1981[78]					4.03				
Gralnick et al., 1982[79]	14.4	4.16	3.60		4.68 — 5.02	6.32	0.89		2.6, 2.9
Samor et al., 1982[80]			3.4	0.76	3.9		0.85	2.4	3.07
Gralnick et al., 1983[81]					4.48				3.69
Federici et al., 1984[82]			5.7		4.08		1.15		
Gralnick and Williams, 1985[83]					4.35				3.26
Chopek et al., 1986[28]	18.7	8.7			3.5	6.5			

[a] Results are expressed in percentages (w/w) related to glycoprotein.
[b] N-acetyl glucosamine.
[c] N-acetyl galactosamine.
[d] Fucose.
[e] Mannose.
[f] Galactose.

The sedimentation constant and corresponding MW values were 16.3 S,[58] 23.7 ± 0.5 S (MW = 1.12 ± 0.098 × 10^6 Da),[3] 20.5 S,[92] 27 S,[93] and 29 S (MW = 2.2 × 10^6 Da).[94] These results on the VIII/vWf complex obtained by gel filtration and ultracentrifugation were confirmed using vWf devoid of VIII isolated from hemophilic plasma.[90]

Hershgold[89] was the first to observe filaments of variable length in a VIII/vWf preparation dried and shadowed with carbon-platinum. On the other hand, globular particles 20 to 50 nm in size,[95] rod shaped particles measuring 22 by 42 nm with or without bends at approximately 90 and 120° angles,[96] or irregularly branched thick fibrils rarely exceeding 120 nm in length[97] were demonstrated by other authors observing both dried and freeze-etched specimens of VIII/vWf preparations. Their respective deduced MW values were approximately 3 × 10^6, 8.5 × $10,^6$ and 0.6 to 6 × 10^6 Da. Recent data obtained in two laboratories[30,99,100] will be discussed below as they represent an essential contribution to current knowledge of the three dimensional structure of vWf.

b. Electrophoretic Mobility

The electrophoretic mobility of VIII/vWf has remained a mystery for a long time. Discrepant results reporting that VIII/vWf migrates from a zone between albumin and α_1 components[101] to γ components[70] have been obtained. The techniques used at this time resulted in fact in erroneous results attributable to the high MW, to the tendency of vWf to aggregate with itself and other proteins or lipids, and to the methods used to detect the VIII/vWf complex after electrophoresis. It is now evident that vWf, due to its large size, does not enter into conventional gels such as 7.5 and 5% polyacrylamide. In fact, Van Mourik et al.[39] were the first to succeed in making purified factor VIII/vWf migrate into 4.35% acrylamide gel with a low degree of cross-linkage. After staining with Coomassie blue, they obtained a series of bands demonstrating the polydispersity of vWf. Many authors, using various agarose gels or composite gels made of acrylamide- or glycoxyl-agarose confirmed this polydispersity of purified VIII/vWf as illustrated in Figure 2 and drew conclusions as to its MW.[97,102-106] Gralnick et al.[103] reported that 47% of a purified VIII/vWf preparation had a MW between 4.2 and 5.6 × 10^6 Da while 34 and 19% corresponded to lower and higher MW forms ranging from 1.6 to 2.8 × 10^6 Da and from 6.8 to 10.2 × 10^6 Da, respectively. These results obtained on possibly denatured purified VIII/vWf preparations were later confirmed by electrophoresing plasma and revealing vWf bands with radiolabeled anti-vWf antibodies.[104,106,107] Thus, this polydispersity which was observed in the presence of SDS and urea did not seem to be an artifact and was thought to be related to the existence of variable MW forms of vWf. This polydispersity accounts for the breadth of VIII/vWf peaks obtained on different molecular sieving columns, for the variability of sedimentation constants previously reported, and also for the asymmetric pattern of vWf observed previously when plasma was submitted to crossed immunoelectrophoresis.[108]

3. Subunits

As early as in 1970,[69] disc-electrophoresis showed that VIII/vWf reduced with β-mercaptoethanol (β-Me) entered 5% acrylamide gels and gave a major band estimated at 260 kDa. Many reports confirmed that complete reduction of vWf was achieved with either 0.1 M β-Me or 5 mM dithiothreitol (DTT) giving rise to a single major band in disc-electrophoresis (Figure 2) with a MW estimate between 195[4] and 280 kDa.[107] These results were in agreement with those obtained by ultracentrifugation[4] and gel filtration.[110] When very high concentrations of reducing agents (0.4 M β-Me or 90 mM DTT) were used, even in the presence of dissociating agents (8 M urea or 6 M guanidine-HCl), no further decrease in subunit MW was observed. In contrast, conditions of limited reduction produced vWf forms with MW intermediate components between native vWf and the vWf subunit, and in particular a dimeric form of this subunit.[102] Furthermore, it was proved[97] that the different vWf forms present in both purified preparations and plasma were mainly composed of the same MW subunit.

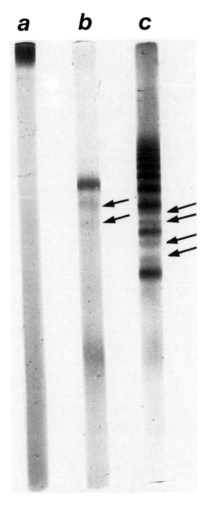

FIGURE 2.   Disc-electrophoreses stained with Coomassie blue of a preparation of purified vWf. In lane a (nonreduced) and b (reduced), the gel is in 5% acrylamide; in lane c, the gel is 4.35%. acrylamide and 0.25%. agarose. The arrows indicate the minor forms of vWf distinguishable either in the vWf subunits (b) or in native vWf (c).

Thus, it appeared that vWf was a very large polydisperse molecule comprised of multiple covalently linked major 250-kDa subunits. Recent studies have attempted to establish a more precise definition of the nature of vWf subunits and their relationship in native vWf.

B.Primary Structure of vWf

1. Peptide Chain

a. Strategic Approach

Direct determination of the sequence of amino acids in a single polypeptide chain of ≅250 kDa MW present in trace concentrations in plasma is a real challenge. The first attempts were made by Titani et al.[111] and Hessel et al.[61] who determined by Edman degradation the amino terminal sequence (15 residues) of reduced and alkylated vWf. One peptide obtained by plasmin proteolysis[66] was also sequenced for its 33 N-terminal residues and was assigned to be the N-terminus of plasma vWf because its sequence matched the 15 residues previously reported.[61] Recently, Titani et al.[62] established a large-scale and fast purification procedure[28] and developed the methods necessary to cleave reduced and carboxymethylated vWf. After cyanogen bromide treatment they isolated and characterized 41 resultant peptides which were partially sequenced. A major contribution was the observation of Girma et al.[112] that *Staphylococcus aureus* V8 protease (SpV8) hydrolyses one Glu-Glu peptide bond between residues 1365 and 1366, giving two complementary fragments named SpII and SpIII with respective MWs of 110 and 170 kDa. Methionyl fragments and subpeptides obtained by cleaving lysyl or arginyl bonds in SpII and SpIII were then isolated, sequenced, and aligned.[62]

b. Experimental Results

The sequenator analyses succeeded in placing about 80% of the 2050 amino acid residues proven, by cDNA sequencing,[113-114] to represent the entire circulating peptide chain.[62] The information not available by direct analysis of the protein sequence was provided by the nucleotide sequence of the cDNA clone λHvWf 3.[115] This sequence together with the designation of some residues of interest is shown in Figure 3. The composition derived from this sequence is Asp: 113, Asn: 74, Thr: 116, Ser: 141, Glu: 137, Gln: 100, Pro: 136, Gly: 137, Ala: 104, CySH: 169, Val: 184, Met: 41, Ile: 78, Leu: 156, Tyr: 49, Phe: 56, Trp: 18, His: 52, Lys: 88, Arg: 101. The calculated MW of the polypeptide moiety is 225,843 Da. The distribution of charged groups in the sequence is rather balanced: 55% basic amino acids to 45% amino acids with acidic side chains. The half-cystinyl residues are clustered principally in three segments: they constitute 14% of the 685 carboxy terminal residues, 11% of the 510 amino terminal residues, and 11% of the segment from residue 1109 to residue 1238. This last segment is on the fragment Sp I obtained by secondary cleavage of SpV8 between Glu (910) and Gly (911), as shown in Figures 3 and 4.

Research on internal homologies of amino acid sequence in the vWf subunit revealed five[115,116] or four[113] unrelated repeated sequences (these duplicated or triplicated domains are described in a later chapter dealing with vWf cDNA). Furthermore, the amino acid sequence of vWf was compared to NBRF Protein Sequence Database. It appeared that a domain triplicated in vWf is homologous to a portion of complement factor B and to a short sequence of complement component C2a.[116] No apparent homology with any other protein was shown.

2. Glycans

In collaboration with Montreuil's laboratory we have studied the carbohydrate moiety of vWf. In preliminary experiments,[65,80] delipidated purified VIII/vWf was treated either with mild alkaline-borohydride (β-elimination) or with anhydrous hydrazine (hydrazinolysis). Mild alkaline treatment led to a mixture of reduced oligosaccharides, derived from O-glycosidically linked glycans, and glycopeptides with N-glycosidically linked glycans. On the other hand, hydrazinolysis specifically released N-deacetylated glycans which were N-glycosidically linked and destroyed O-linked glycans. Analysis by gas-liquid chromatography of monosaccharides from the oligosaccharides or glycopeptides thus obtained demonstrated the coexistence of approximately 30% O- and 70% N-glycosidically linked glycans. Furthermore, results obtained by thin layer chromatography provided evidence of the high degree of heterogeneity of these glycans: at least ten O-linked oligosaccharides and three N-linked glycans were characterized. One of them was a major glycan representing about 60% of the N-glycans and belonging to the N-acetyl lactosaminic type. Later it was isolated from vWf hydrazinolysate by high voltage electrophoresis, as shown in Figure 5, and its complete structure demonstrated in Figure 6A was determined by a combination of methylation, mass spectrometry, and nuclear magnetic resonance spectroscopy.[117] Recently N-glycosidically linked glycopeptides obtained by β-elimination were fractionated by serial affinity chromatography on immobilized lectins (Figure 5). Both the major and a pure minor glycopeptide were thus isolated. The structure of this minor N-glycosidically linked glycan was established.[118] It is a monosialylated monofucosylated tetraantennary structure of the N-acetyl lactosaminic type which has not previously been described in human glycoproteins (Figure 6B).

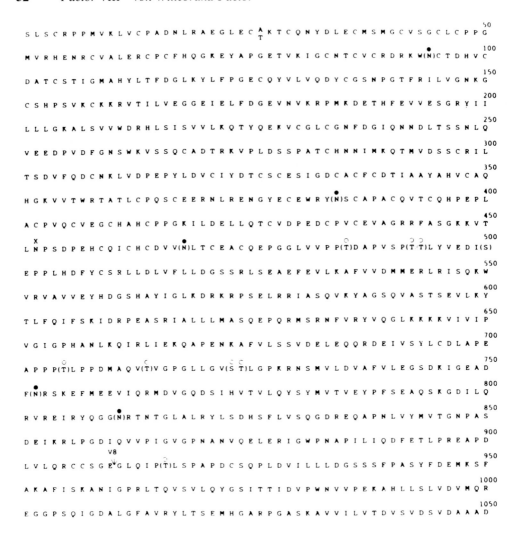

```
                                                                        50
S L S C R P P M V K L V C P A D N L R A E G L E C A K T C Q N Y D L E C M S M G C V S G C L C P P G
                                                  T
                                                                        100
M V R H E N R C V A L E R C P C F H Q G K E Y A P G E T V K I G C N T C V C R D R K W(N)C T D H V C
                                                                        150
D A T C S T I G M A H Y L T F D G L K Y L F P G E C Q Y V L V Q D Y C G S N P G T F R I L V G N K G
                                                                        200
C S H P S V K C K K R V T I L V E G G E I E L F D G E V N V K R P M K D E T H F E V V E S G R Y I I
                                                                        250
L L L G K A L S V V W D R H L S I S V V L K Q T Y Q E K V C G L C G N F D G I Q N N D L T S S N L Q
                                                                        300
V E E D P V D F G N S W K V S S Q C A D T R K V P L D S S P A T C H N N I M K Q T M V D S S C R I L
                                                                        350
T S D V F Q D C N K L V D P E P Y L D V C I Y D T C S C E S I G D C A C F C D T I A A Y A H V C A Q
                                                                        400
H G K V V T W R T A T L C P Q S C E E R N L R E N G Y E C E W R Y(N)S C A P A C Q V T C Q H P E P L
                                                                        450
A C P V Q C V E G C H A H C P P G K I L D E L L Q T C V D P E D C P V C E V A G R R F A S G K K V T
    X                                                                   500
L N P S D P E H C Q I C H C D V V(N)L T C E A C Q E P G G L V V P P(T)D A P V S P(T T)L Y V E D I(S)
                                                                        550
E P P L H D F Y C S R L L D L V F L L D G S S R L S E A E F E V L K A F V V D M M E R L R I S Q K W
                                                                        600
V R V A V V E Y H D G S H A Y I G L K D R K R P S E L R R I A S Q V K Y A G S Q V A S T S E V L K Y
                                                                        650
T L F Q I F S K I D R P E A S R I A L L L M A S Q E P Q R M S R N F V R Y V Q G L K K K K V I V I P
                                                                        700
V G I G P H A N L K Q I R L I E K Q A P E N K A F V L S S V D E L E Q Q R D E I V S Y L C D L A P E
                                                                        750
A P P P(T)L P P D M A Q V(T)V G P G L L G V(S T)L G P K R N S M V L D V A F V L E G S D K I G E A D
                                                                        800
F(N)R S K E F M E E V I Q R M D V G Q D S I H V T V L Q Y S Y M V T V E Y P F S E A Q S K G D I L Q
                                                                        850
R V R E I R Y Q G G(N)R T N T G L A L R Y L S D H S F L V S Q G D R E Q A P N L V Y M V T G N P A S
                                                                        900
D E I K R L P G D I Q V V P I G V G P N A N V Q E L E R I G W P N A P I L I Q D F E T L P R E A P D
        V8                                                              950
L V L Q R C C S G E G L Q I P(T)L S P A P D C S Q P L D V I L L L D G S S S F P A S Y F D E M K S F
                                                                        1000
A K A F I S K A N I G P R L T Q V S V L Q Y G S I T T I D V P W N V V P E K A H L L S L V D V M Q R
                                                                        1050
E G G P S Q I G D A L G F A V R Y L T S E M H G A R P G A S K A V V I L V T D V S V D S V D A A A D
```

FIGURE 3.   Amino acid sequence of human vWf. ● and ○ denote sites of N- and O-glycosylation, and X denotes two potential glycosylation sites that are not glycosylated. Vertical arrows indicate major (⇒) and minor (→) sites of limited proteolysis by *S. aureus* V8 protease. The RGDS sequence is enclosed in a rectangle. (From Titani, K., Kumar, S., Takio, K., Ericsson, L. H., Wade, R. D., Ashida, K., Walsh, K. A., Chopek, J. E., and Fujikawa, F., *Biochemistry*, 25, 3171, 1986. Copyright, American Chemical Society. With permission.)

It is well known that most of the glycans with an N-acetyl glucosamine residue at their reducing end are linked to an Asn residue occurring in the characteristic sequence: Asn-X-Thr/Ser. Owing to cDNA sequencing, 13 of such potential N-glycosylation sites have been located on the mature vWf subunit in position 94, 452, 468, 752, 811, 1460, 1527, 1594, 1637, 1783, 1822, 1872, and 2027.[113,114] By direct amino acid sequencing, Titani et al.[62] identified 22 probable glycosylation sites corresponding to the lack of identifiable phenyl-thiohydantoins. Of them, 11 appeared to belong to the potential glycosylation sites described above, 2 Asn (in position 452 and 1872) being unglycosylated and 1 additional Asn (residue 384), in the sequence Asn-X-Cys, being glycosylated. The last ten probable glycosylation sites corresponded to eight threonyl and two seryl residues. As shown in Figures 3 and 4, the glycosylation sites are distributed between the amino-terminal (Sp III) and the carboxy-terminal (Sp II) fragment of mature vWf, most (eight of ten) of O-glycosylation sites being clustered in two narrow segments of Sp III.

The structures of the glycans corresponding to more than 50% of the monosaccharides of vWf remain to be identified as does the exact location of each glycan on the peptide chain.

```
                                                                    1100
A A R S N R V T V F P I G I G D R Y D A A Q L R I L A G P A G D S N V V K L Q R I E D L P T M V T L
                                                                    1150
G N S F L H K L C S G F V R I C M D E D G N E K R P G D V W T L P D Q C H T V T C Q P D G Q T L L K
                                                                    1200
S H R V N C D R G L R P S C P N S Q S P V K V E E T C G C R W T C P C V C T G S S T R H I V T F D G
                                                                    1250
Q N F K L T G S C S Y V L F Q N K E Q D L E V I L H N G A C S P G A R Q G C M K S I E V K H S A L S
                                                                    1300
V E L H S D M E V T V N G R L V S V P Y V G G N M E V N V Y G A I M H E V R F N H L G H I F T F T P
                                                                    1350
Q N N E F Q L Q L S P K T F A S K T Y G L C G I C D E N G A N D F M L R D G T V T T D W K T L V Q E
                                  V8
                                  ( )                               1400
W T V Q R P G Q T C Q P I L E E Q C L V P D S S H C Q V L L L P L F A E C H K V L A P A T F Y A I C
                                                                    1450
Q Q D S C H Q E Q V C E V I A S Y A H L C R T N G V C V D W R T P D F C A M S C P P S L V Y N H C E
                       •                                            1500
H G C P R H C D G (N) V S S C G D H P S E G C F C P P D K V M L E G S C V P E E A C T Q C I G E D G V
                                                                    1550
Q H Q F L E A W V P D H Q P C Q I C T C L S G R K V (N) C T T Q P C P (T) A K A P T C G L C E V A R L R
                                                           •        1600
Q N A D Q C C P E Y E C V C D P V S C D L P P V P H C E R G L Q P T L T N P G E C R P (N) F T C A C R
                                                 •                  1650
K E E C K R V S P P S C P P H R L P T L R K T Q C C D E Y E C A C N C V (N) S T V S C P L G Y L A S T
                                                                    1700
A T N D C G C T T T T C L P D K V C V H R S T I Y P V G Q F W E E G C D V C T C T D M E D A V M G L
                                                            1750
R V A Q C S Q K P C E D S C R S G F T Y V L H E G E C C G R C L P S A C E V V T G S P [R G D S] Q S S
                                          •                         1800
W K S V G S Q W A S P E N P C L I N E C V R V K E E V F I Q Q R (N) V S C P Q L E V P V C P S G F Q L
                                  •                                 1850
S C K T S A C C P S C R C E R M E A C M L (N) G T V I G P G K T V M I D V C T T C R C M V Q V G V I S
                          X                                         1900
G F K L E C R K T T C N P C P L G Y K E E N N T G E C C G R C L P T A C T I Q L R G G Q I M T L K R
                                                                    1950
D E T L Q D G C D T H F C K V N E R G E Y F W E K R V T G C P P F D E H K C L A E G G K I M K I P G
                                                                    2000
T C C D T C E E P E C N D I T A R L Q Y V K V G S C K S E V E V D I H Y C Q G K C A S K A M Y S I D
                                         •                          2050
I N D V Q D Q C S C C S P T R T E P M Q V A L H C T (N) G S V V Y H E V L N A M E C K C S P R K C S K
```

FIGURE 3 (continued)

C. Three Dimensional Structure of vWf

The sequence of the side chains of amino acids determines all that is unique in glyco-proteins, including conformational and biological function. Although all the information required for the folding of a protein is contained in its amino acid sequence, no prediction of a detailed three dimensional structure is possible on the basis of this sequence. Furthermore, as vWf has not as yet been analyzed by X-ray diffraction, a detailed picture of this molecule is not available. Nevertheless, an attempt will be made to report recent data on the conformation of vWf in the context of the different hierarchical levels of protein structure.

1. Secondary Structure

The first level of folding by hydrogen bond interactions within continuous stretches of the vWf polypeptide chain is not known. Whereas the knowledge of the distribution and pattern of α helices and β sheets is dependent upon X-ray diffraction analysis, circular dichroism spectra have provided some information about their relative percentages: vWf appeared to have 24% α helix and 18% β sheet structure in its native state, while reduction with 50 mM βMe and alkylation decreased β sheet content by 50% without affecting α helix.[119]

We examined the available amino acid sequence[62] to predict the secondary structure of

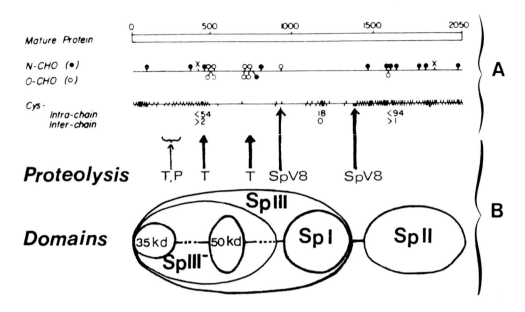

FIGURE 4. Schematic views of structural features of mature vWf. (A) The N- (●) and O- (○) glycosidically linked oligosaccharides and cystine residues are located. X indicates unglycosylated potential sites of glycosylation. (Part A from Titani, K., Kumar, S., Takio, K., Ericsson, L. H., Wade, R. D., Ashida, K., Walsh, K. A., Chopek, J. E., and Fujikawa, F., *Biochemistry*, 25, 3171, 1986. Copyright, American Chemical Society. With permission.) (B) A tentative diagram of some vWf domains based on the location of the sites of proteolysis with either *S. aureus* V8 protease (Sp V8),[112] trypsin (T),[121,172] or plasmin (P).[66]

mature vWf. Using the prediction method of Garnier et al.[120] we obtained the following information: mature vWf polypeptide chain contained 22.3% α helix, 23.8% β sheet, and 39.2% β turn. Thus, it is probably a very structured molecule in which five different regions may be distinguished. This takes into account both the cysteine content and the distribution of α helix and β turn conformational states, as shown in Table 3. The N-terminal region extending from N-terminal Ser to Ser (510), the central region between CySH residues (1109) and (1238), and the region containing the 685 carboxy-terminal residues are all rich in cysteine and contain 46.2, 59.9, and 53% β turn type of conformation, respectively. In contrast, the internal regions extending from Arg (511) to Leu (1108) and from Met (1239) to Glu (1365) are very poor in cysteine and contain 31.5 and 34.3% helical structures, respectively.

Disulfide bridges which have already been considered as part of the primary structure are normally not required for protein folding. However, S-S links appear to influence the secondary structure of proteins by providing local stabilization. In vWf, all 169 CySH are involved in either intrachain or interchain disulfide bridges. By cleaving native vWf with SpV8, Girma et al.[112] obtained dimers of fragments Sp II and Sp III and monomers of fragment Sp I. This indicates that S-S links probably connect two carboxy-terminal regions and two amino-terminal regions together as depicted in Figure 9. This also provides evidence that CySHs localized on fragment Sp I are not involved in interchain bridges and that amino- and carboxy-terminal parts of the vWf subunit are not linked together by S-S. It is thus likely that many disulfide loops exist on terminal parts of the vWf subunit and in the central part of the segment corresponding to Sp I. However, the disulfide connections have not yet been identified.

2. Domains

Within a single subunit, contiguous portions of the polypeptide chain frequently fold into

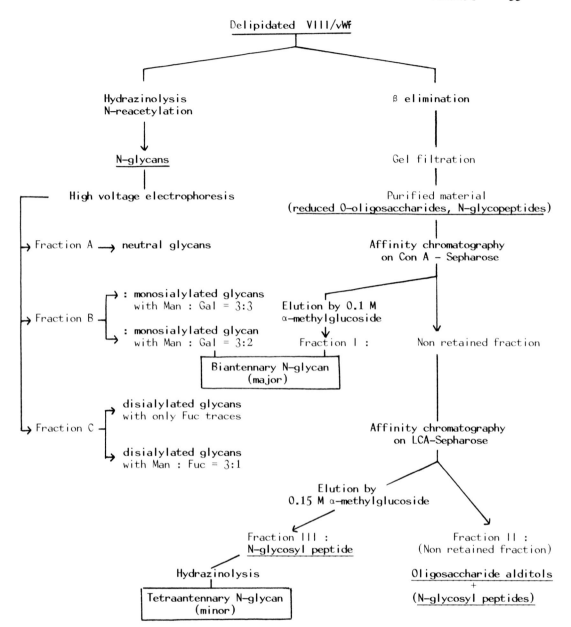

FIGURE 5. Diagrammatic representation of the protocols used to obtain the two N-linked glycans of human vWf of which the structure was established.[118,119] Con A = concanavalin A; LCA = lens culinaris agglutinin.

compact, local, and semiindependent units called domains. Domains have proved fruitful in explaining both the structure and the function of some proteins.

Recently a combination of spectroscopic techniques[119] showed that vWf may contain discrete ordered conformational domains linked by coil regions. Nevertheless, these structural domains have not as yet been characterized. In order to attempt to locate some domains, we have included in Figure 4B the few precise data available on the peptides obtained after limited proteolysis of vWf with different enzymes. Sites of proteolysis were then assumed to be located in the relatively open lengths of polypeptide chain usually stringing contiguous domains. Consequently, the last line of Figure 4 is only a preliminary and tentative scheme

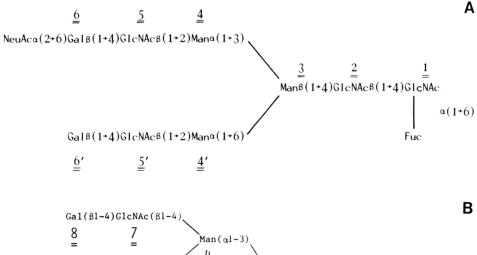

FIGURE 6.   (A) Primary structure of the major N-glycosidically linked glycan of human vWf. (From Debeire, P., Montreuil, J., Samor, B., Mazurier, C., Goudemand, M., Van Halbeck, H., and Vliegenthart, J. F. G., *FEBS Lett.*, 1983. With permission.) (B) Primary structure of a minor N-glycosidically linked glycan of human vWf. (From Samor, B., Michalski, J. C., Debray, H., Mazurier, C., Goudemand, M., Van Halbeek, H., Vliegenthart, J. F. G., and Montreuil, J., *Eur. J. Biochem.*, 158, 295, 1986. With permission.)

Table 3
SECONDARY STRUCTURE PREDICTION OF HUMAN vWf [a]

	Region[b]					Total polypeptide chain
	I	II	III	IV	V	
Extending from amino acid:	1	511	1109	1239	1365	1
to amino acid:	510	1108	1238	1364	2050	2050
Percentage of α helix	16.9	31.5	7.8	34.3	19.7	22.3
Percentage of β sheet	23.7	35.2	12.4	19.4	16.7	23.8
Percentage of β turn	46.2	8.9	59.9	24.6	53.5	39.2
Percentage of cysteine	11[c]	0.7	11[c]	2.5	14[c]	8.2[c]

[a]   According to amino acid sequence reported by Titani et al.[62] and the method of Garnier et al.[120]

[b]   The distinction between five regions of vWf polypeptide chain is based on both cysteine content and the distribution of the different conformational states.

[c]   Results reported by Titani et al.[62]

of some of the probable domains of the vWf subunit. In fact, it is tempting to speculate that vWf is composed of two large regions connected by a coil easily accessible to SpV8. The C-terminal region, named Sp II, is rich in CySH and probably contains seven N- but only one O-glycan. The N-terminal region extending from N-terminal amino acid of mature vWf protein to residue 1364 may be further divided in two different substructures probably connected by a coil around the sequence Glu-Gly accessible to SpV8. The central substructure, Sp I, contains only one O-glycan and its CySH residues are clustered in its central part. In the amino-terminal substructure, designated Sp III $^-$ in Figure 4, we can distinguish at least two domains. One is the N-terminus of the vWf subunit which contains one N-glycan and is probably connected by a coil extending around amino acids 310—330 which is easily accessible to both trypsin[121] and plasmin.[66] The second probable domain extends from Val (449) to Tyr (729)[62,121] and corresponds to a tryptic fragment probably containing one N-glycan and eight O-glycans clustered four by four in two narrow segments located at either end of the domain.

3. Protomer

The protomeric form of vWf may be considered either from the quaternary or tertiary structural level. From the quaternary standpoint, the vWf protomer is the smallest circulating multimer in human plasma. From the tertiary standpoint, it is an association of different polypeptide chains referred to as subunits.

The protomeric form of plasma vWf was first visualized by disc-electrophoresis analysis. It was found to be the fastest migrating specific intense band, generally named band 1, revealed by radiolabeled anti-vWf antibodies after electrophoresing plasma in SDS through a large pore gel, as shown in Figure 7. Different results for the MW of the protomer have been obtained. Some[103,105] are in agreement with a protomer composed of two subunits (dimer). On the other hand, other results[106,107,122,123] suggest that the smallest multimer has an apparent MW of between 850 and 860 kDa and appears to be a tetramer of the basic polypeptidic subunit. Nevertheless, there is general agreement that the protomer is a disulfide-bonded poly(di- or tetra-)mer of only one $\cong$ 250-kDa subunit.

Recent observations[30,99,100] made by electron microscopy have also contributed to the characterization of the vWf protomer. It is the shortest distinguishable organized form of plasma vWf (100 to 120 nm in length $\times$ 1.5 to 2 nm) constituting the basic unit of chains up to 2 μm. Some authors[80] observed a protomeric structure composed of two large globular end domains (G) symmetrically connected to a small central node (n) by two flexible rod domains (R), as depicted in Figure 8. The size of these different parts (G $=$ 22 $\times$ 6.5 nm, R $=$ 34 $\times$ 2 nm, n $=$ 6.4 $\times$ 3.4 nm) was consistent with the following values for their MW: G $\cong$ 150 kDa, R $\cong$ 106 kDa, n $=$ 35 kDa. These calculations gave a MW estimate of $\cong$540 kDa for the vWf protomer, thus assuming it to be comprised of a dimer of $\cong$250-kDa vWf subunits.[30] Further observations after fragmentation with plasmin and SpV8 suggested that the rod domain R can probably be assigned to the carboxy-terminal part of vWf subunit and the globular domain G to its amino-terminal part.[124] Other authors,[99,100] using dark field photographs, provided evidence that each symmetrical half of a protomer contains a linear tail and a binodular head possibly corresponding to the domains R and G, respectively, as described above. As each head is probably the terminus of a single polypeptide chain the vWf protomer could be a tetramer of the vWf subunit. Nevertheless, recent data obtained by quasi-elastic light scattering lend greater support to the dimer model.[125]

Discontinuous SDS gel electrophoresis in high resolution conditions[123,126-129] has provided evidence that plasma vWf is not a simple series of polymers of the protomer described above. As shown in Figure 7, each multimeric unit may appear to be comprised of either three (triplet pattern)[123] or, at least, five bands[126-129] with the major band situated in the central position. The presence of these satellite bands is explained on the basis of the possible heterogeneity of the vWf protomer. This is concordant with the fact that purified vWf,

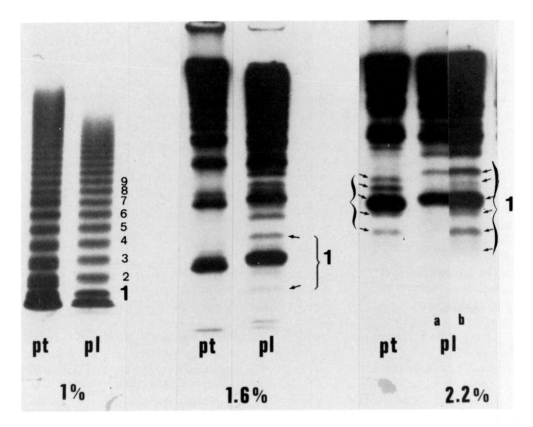

FIGURE 7. Multimeric patterns of vWf from platelet lysate (pt) and plasma (pl) of a normal individual. Auto-radiographs obtained after SDS discontinuous electrophoresis in different gels with increasing agarose concentration and overlay with ^{125}I-labeled anti-vWf antibodies. In low resolution gel (agarose 1%), vWf is resolved in a series of bands numbered one to nine corresponding to the protomer (1) and related polymers; larger multimers are seen in platelets than in plasma. In intermediate resolution gel (agarose 1.6%), protomeric form (1) and oligomers of plasma vWf show a triplet pattern whereas vWf platelet protomer has a predominant band flanked by fainter bands. In high resolution gel (agarose 2.2%), plasma vWf protomer (1) appears to be composed of at least six bands (a and b are two different exposure times of the same gel lane), and vWf platelet protomer also shows a complex pattern composed by a central predominant band and some additional fainter bands having a different rate of movement compared with the corresponding bands from plasma. (From Lopez-Fernandez, M. F., Lopez-Berges, C., Nieto, J., Martin, R., and Batlle, J., *Thromb. Res.*, 44, 125, 1986. Pergamon Journals Ltd. With Permission.)

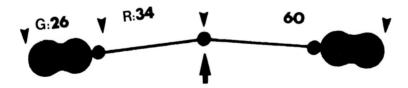

FIGURE 8. Schematic representation of human plasma vWf protomer observed in electron microscopy, showing the two subunits joined at central twofold symmetry axis (large arrow). Maximum dimensions in nanometers, uncorrected for replica thickness, of the rod (R) and globular domains (G) are indicated within the smaller arrows. (From Fowler, W. E., Fretto, L. J., Hamilton, K. K., Erikson, H. P., and McKee, P. A., *J. Clin. Invest.*, 76, 1491, 1985. Copyright American Society for Clinical Investigation, with permission.)

prepared in the presence of protease inhibitors[28,130] and subsequently completely reduced, produces not only a major band of ≅250 kDa MW on electrophoresis, but also one or more minor bands migrating ahead of the subunit position (Figure 2). Recently, after reduction of vWf rapidly purified from plasma in the presence of a variety of protease inhibitors, Zimmerman et al.[131] obtained a major 225-kDa subunit and additional minor components of 189-, 176-, and 140-kDa values as revealed by anti-vWf antibodies. These results suggest that the subunit composition of plasma vWf is not quite homogeneous, and that minor subunits and satellite bands are probably, at least in part, the result of *in vivo* proteolysis of the major plasma form of vWf. Such an explanation is in agreement with the observations of Fowler et al.[30] who noticed morphological differences at the globular end domain of vWf multimers and suggested that proteolytic cleavage was the most likely explanation of their presence. This also correlates well with recent results[28] demonstrating that the smallest protomer of vWf contains equimolar ratios of 270-, 140-, and 120-kDa subunits, the latter two subunits probably produced by limited proteolysis of the 270-kDa subunit. One other explanation of the heterogeneity of vWf comes from the study of vWf biosynthesis in endothelial cells.[2,132,133] In fact, vWF from both cell lysates and culture media gave several bands in SDS-acrylamide after reduction. The elution of the major and satellite bands of multimers separated by SDS-agarose and their subsequent analysis in SDS-acrylamide after reduction[133] enabled different subunits of vWf to be characterized. Their apparent molecular weights of ≅225, 250, and 270 kDa were considered sufficient to explain the appearance of two satellite bands to the major protomer. Thus, the heterogeneity of the plasma vWf protomer may also be due to differential posttranslational modifications of vWf. This heterogeneity probably accounts for the results obtained by isoelectric focusing of plasma in agarose-ampholytes in the presence of urea, in which a discrete series of bands may be observed with corrected isoelectric point estimates between pH 5.03 and 5.43.[109]

4. Polymers

SDS electrophoresis in discontinuous gel systems was the first technique to demonstrate that vWf consists of a series of multimers of increasing MW derived from mainly one protomeric form. The MW of the larger multimeric form is difficult to assign since these forms are not well distinguished from one another, as seen in Figure 7. As 15 to 20 multimers can be identified under optimal experimental conditions, the largest multimers may have an MW of approximately 10 to 20 × 10^6 kDa.[107] Furthermore, it has been shown that multimers, which progressively decrease in size[102] and increase in electrophoretic mobility on SDS-agarose gels[98] under reducing conditions, contain an even number of the 250-kDa subunits.[28,102] The heterogeneity of the vWf protomer also induces heterogeneity in vWf multimers. The major bands, generally numbered 2, 3, 4, obtained by SDS-agarose gel electrophoresis, correspond to 2-, 3-, 4-, . . . mers, respectively, of the major protomer. These bands, like the protomer, may be flanked by at least two satellite bands (Figure 7) which are generally assumed to be the multimers of the minor forms of the vWf protomer. Nevertheless, recent data[28] show that each isolated vWf multimer is composed of a variable percentage of the different subunits (270, 140, and 120 kDa) of vWf.

Recent sedimentation analyses using partition cells[134] in the analytical ultracentrifuge confirmed that vWf is highly asymmetric and behaves as a heterogeneous population of molecules. Furthermore, these investigators indicated that the sedimentation coefficient and the Stokes radius of vWf fractions separated by gel filtration on Sepharose CL2B ranged between 23 and 13 S and 15.3 and 8.1 nm, respectively.

Electron microscopy has also provided evidence of very large molecular forms of vWf. Either very flexible filaments up to 1.15 μm in length and containing irregularly spaced small nodules,[98] flexible strands up to 2 μm consisting of a chain of a basic unit assumed to be vWf protomer,[30] or both linear flexible polymers up to 1.3 μm and "ball of yarn" elliptic structures due to considerable folding of filaments[99,100] were observed. These latter mentioned globular structures could be an artifact since Furlan et al.[135] using an alternative technique of surface labeling permitting the examination of vWf multimers in solution, indicated that the accessible surface of each vWf protomeric form is only very slightly affected by polymerization. This is in agreement with the existence of elongated filaments. Nevertheless, other data obtained in solution by quasi-elastic light scattering showed that the average vWf polymers, with 83- $\pm$ 37-nm radius of gyration and 59- $\pm$ 25-nm Stoke radius, are not fully extended but rather assumed to have a shape between that of a rigid rod and an oblate ellipsoid.[100,125]

Recent data have defined the mode of connection between protomers. In vWf preparations further purified by gel filtration, Fowler et al.[30] clearly distinguished structures corresponding to the association of 2, 3, 4 . . . protomeric basic units GRnRG. Their observations provided evidence that vWf protomers are linked within multimers by their globular domain G, corresponding to the amino-terminal part of the vWf subunit in the following fashion: —GRnRG-GRnRG— . . . It seems that this link does not involve a CySH residue localized in the extreme N-terminus of vWf. In fact plasmin cleavage induced the release of a monomeric 34-kDa fragment (Figure 4B), the sequence of which matched the amino-terminal sequence of the intact vWf subunit.[66] On the other hand, one disulfide bridge at least was localized on a segment extending from residue 449 to residue 729 of the vWf subunit (Figure 4B). Indeed the $\cong$50-kDa tryptic fragment corresponding to this sequence[121] is a dimer in its native form.[62]

Recently, Loscalzo et al.[125] investigated the reversible association of vWf protomers using quasi-elastic light scattering and gel filtration techniques. Their data demonstrated that, in appropriate conditions, the vWf multimers persist after disulfide reduction due to hydrophobic interaction.[100,125] The fact that this and previous data demonstrate that vWf multimers may be dissociated in nonreducing conditions (low pH and high ionic strength,[39] storage in 1% SDS,[102] sonication,[136,137] and penultimate galactose removal[81,138]) emphasizes the importance of the possible role of noncovalent forces in maintaining the quaternary structure of vWf.

D. Particular Features of Platelet vWf

There are little available data on the biochemistry of platelet vWf. Platelet vWf appears to be immunologically similar to plasma vWf and originates as the result of biosynthesis processes in the megakaryocytes which closely resemble those of vWf in endothelial cells.[3] Furthermore, before and after reduction, platelet and plasma vWf behave similarly in SDS-polyacrylamide gel electrophoresis.[139] Nevertheless, platelet vWf exhibits some differences when compared with plasma vWf. First, it is not associated with VIII. Secondly, it appears that the tryptic peptide maps of plasma and platelet vWf are not quite identical in that 7 of the 41 peptides observed from plasma vWf are not detected in platelet vWf.[139] Last, as illustrated in Figure 7, plasma and platelet vWf show differing patterns on SDS electrophoresis when high resolution techniques are used, in that

1. Platelet vWf contains slower migrating (i.e., larger) multimers than those seen in plasma[107,140-142]
2. The mobility of the two smaller multimers (bands 1 and 2) is greater in platelets than in plasma, i.e., the opposite to larger multimers[141,142]
3. Each multimeric unit of platelet vWf is composed of bands having a different electrophoretic mobility compared with the corresponding bands from plasma[142]

E. Von Willebrand Antigen II

Recent data,[113,114] presented in the later chapter dealing with vWf cDNA have provided evidence that vWf cDNA encodes a 2813-amino acids polypeptide denoted pre-pro vWf.

This polypeptide, after sequential cleavage of an N-terminal signal peptide (22 amino acid residues) and a polypeptide of 741 amino acid residues, results in a 2050-amino acids polypeptide corresponding to the major plasma vWf subunit described above. The N-terminal sequence of the polypeptide corresponding to the prosequence of vWf deduced from the 5' end of vWf cDNA has recently proved to be identical to the N-terminal sequence of a protein denoted von Willebrand antigen II (vW:Ag II) which, like vWf, is present in plasma and platelets of normal individuals and absent from those with severe vWD. This sequence also matched the N-terminal sequence of a plasma glycoprotein with a MW $\cong$ 100 kDa which was initially believed to be VIII.[144] Thus, our present knowledge of vW:Ag II biochemistry comes from the direct study of both vW:Ag II, the plasma 100-kDa glycoprotein, and from the data derived from vWf cDNA.

Montgomery and Zimmerman,[91] who discovered vW:Ag II in 1978, showed that this antigen was distinct from vWf by demonstrating immunologic nonidentity. Furthermore, plasma and platelet vW:Ag II, isolated by gel filtration from cryoprecipitate or platelet lysates, shared similar electrophoretic mobility (between α_1 and α_2 components), sedimentation velocity (4.8 S), and behavior on gel filtration (elution in fractions corresponding to $2.5 \times$ Vo in Biogel A-15 M) which clearly distinguished this protein from vWf.[91]

The plasma glycoprotein isolated by Fay et al.,[143] which could exist as a noncovalent complex of two or four 100-kDa subunits, was shown to be converted into 75- and 26-kDa MW peptides[143,144] by thrombin cleavage. Furthermore, as the vW:Ag II migrated faster in its nonreduced form, it very likely contains intrachain disulfide bonds.[144] The 781-amino acid residues sequence derived from cDNA has indicated that vW:Ag II is composed of two homologous domains (two copies of this domain are also present in native plasma vWf) and contains four potential sites of N-glycosylation.[113]

IV. STRUCTURE/FUNCTION RELATIONSHIPS OF vWf

vWf has a dual biological function. Indeed, the pathology associated with the absence of vWf and observed in the severe forms of vWd is linked to abnormalities in both the coagulation cascade and in primary hemostasis. It has been established that vWf is the carrier protein of VIII, and thus the function of vWf in the cascade is dependent on its interaction with this factor. Nevertheless, the structural requirements for the binding of vWf to VIII are as yet unknown. Furthermore, vWf plays a key role in platelet adhesion to subendothelium. This mechanism, which is difficult to reproduce *in vitro*, apparently involves various steps requiring vWf. Most of these steps are related to the binding of vWf to both platelets and subendothelial components. These various binding properties of vWf are functions which are easier to study as well as the ability of vWf to induce platelet agglutination in the presence of ristocetin. Whereas the physiological relevance of the functions of vWf measured *in vitro* may not be understood comprehensively, binding and ristocetin cofactor activities of vWf represent, however, essential tools for the study of the relationships between its structure and functions.

Information pertaining to relevant structure/function relationships of vWf can be derived from three types of studies:

1. Studies involving analysis of pathological vWf samples; biochemical and functional studies of abnormal vWf molecules present in the variant forms of vWD contribute valuable insight into those components of the vWf structure which may be of functional significance
2. Data obtained from functional studies using purified vWf modified by either chemical or enzymatic agents
3. Data obtained from topographical studies involving epitope mapping of anti-vWf monoclonal antibodies inhibiting a given vWf function

These numerous sources of information have provided evidence that various levels of conformation of the vWf molecule are involved in its functions.

A. The Role of vWf Multimeric Structure

There is convincing evidence that the hemostatic efficacy of vWf resides in its higher molecular weight (HMW) forms. Such evidence is provided by clinical observations supporting the importance of HMW vWf multimers in its biological activity and also by experimental data demonstrating the role of vWf multimeric structure in vWf/platelet, vWf/subendothelium interactions, and vWf involvement in platelet adhesion.

1. Clinical Data

The biological function of vWf is defined as that activity that corrects the bleeding time in patients with vWD. A number of studies have shown that the bleeding time is prolonged in patients lacking HMW plasma vWf.[145-147] Furthermore, cryoprecipitate which contains all the HMW vWf plasma forms has proved to be hemostatically effective, whereas most commercial factor VIII concentrates deficient in HMW vWf forms are less efficacious in stopping hemorrhagic symptoms in vWD.[148-150] All these *in vivo* observations support the concept that the function of vWf in the primary phase of hemostasis is significantly governed by its multimeric size. The *in vitro* experimental data reported below will distinguish those vWf functions which are also linked to the same structural requirement.

2. Experimental Data
a. vWf/Platelet Interaction

Preliminary work on VIII/vWf[102,151] showed that, under conditions of chemical reduction, VIII:C levels remained essentially unaltered, whereas vWf ristocetin cofactor (vWf:RCo) activity decreased progressively. Furthermore, it had been previously shown that the HMW forms of plasma vWf had a higher affinity to formalin-fixed platelets in the presence of ristocetin.[152] Subsequent publications, particularly those dealing with the different MW forms of purified vWf obtained either by mild reduction or separation by gel filtration, have reported that some vWf functions reside preferentially in the HMW.

Forms of HMW vWf present in cryoprecipitate but not in cryosupernatant[153] were identified as the only vWf components possessing the ability to agglutinate platelets in the presence of ristocetin.[152,153] Using gel filtration or gradient ultracentrifugation, Martin et al.[105] isolated vWf forms with different MWs and measured their vWf:RCo activity. These investigators showed that vWf forms with MWs greater than 10×10^6 Da demonstrated 12 to 28 times more vWf:RCo activity than vWf forms below 4.6×10^6 Da, measured either relative to protein concentration or vWf antigen levels. Furthermore, they reported that all the different MW polymeric forms studied exhibited the same carbohydrate content and the same pattern of tryptic degradation. These results emphasizing the role of MW or size of vWf in the expression of its vWf:RCo activity were confirmed in other studies.[61,98,100,101,137,150,154] The reduction of half of the disulfide bonds of a vWf preparation by NADPH, thioredoxin reductase, and thioredoxin was shown to decrease vWf:RCo activity to about 20% of the original activity, without production of the protomeric form.[61] Also, among vWf forms synthesized by endothelial cells, only those greater than 3.76×10^6 Da possessed vWf:RCo activity.[137] Furthermore, not only reduction of disulfide bonds but also sonication, which induces a decrease in size of vWf multimers, resulted in decreased vWf:RCo activity.[137] Subsequent adsorption on gold granules of small MW forms of vWf obtained by partial reduction was shown to enhance the vWf:RCo activity.[155] Finally, quasi-elastic light scattering showed that ristocetin-dependent platelet agglutination depends directly on vWf polymer size as a function of both gyration and Stokes radii of vWf.[100] Nevertheless, molecular size is seemingly not the only requirement since Martin et al.[105] showed that low MW forms of vWf obtained after partial reduction of large multimers expressed more vWf:RCo activity than natural vWf forms of similar size.

One report[103] showed that HMW vWf bound preferentially with high affinity to low capacity sites on human platelets in the presence of ristocetin and that, as their MW decreased, the affinity of the smaller vWf multimers for the platelet receptors decreased while the binding capacity increased. Another report[98] added that vWf function most sensitive to structural alteration induced by reduction involved the binding to Gp Ib platelet receptors. However, like native vWf, reduced and alkylated vWf showed a good correlation between binding and the rate of platelet agglutination induced by ristocetin.[92] These reports[98,103] and recent ones[28,112] have stated that the dimer of vWf had a lower binding constant for ristocetin-stimulated platelets than native vWf. In contrast, other authors have indicated that vWf binding to platelets in the presence of ristocetin is preserved after intensive reduction.[156-158] Nevertheless, it has been shown that, in the presence of divalent cations, it is the HMW forms of radiolabeled purified vWf which are associated with thrombin-stimulated platelets.[140]

Thus, controversy is still abundant with respect to the role of the vWf quaternary structure as to its binding properties to platelets. Nevertheless, there are a number of experiments proving that optimal vWf:RCo activity of vWf is dictated mainly by its size and by implication is thus related to its multimeric structure. Furthermore, a recent paper reported that the initiation of shear-induced platelet aggregation, which did not require exogenous agents such as ristocetin and was inhibited by both anti-GP Ib and anti-GP IIa/IIIa monoclonal antibodies, was dependent on large vWf multimeric forms.[158a]

b. vWf/Subendothelium Interaction

Santoro[159] showed that rapid anodic migrating forms of vWf, presumed to have lower MW, were not readily adsorbed by collagen. Later he[160] and others,[161] using intact physiological monomeric type I collagen, confirmed this result in observing that collagen fibers preferentially removed HMW vWf from plasma. Recently it has been reported that reduction of radiolabeled purified vWf with 0.01, 0.1, and 1% β-Me decreased the binding to type I collagen fibers by 25, 50, and more than 90%, respectively.[162] Furthermore, the isolated dimeric form of vWf was shown to be unable to compete with polymeric vWf in binding to soluble acid collagen.[158] All these results have provided evidence that the multimeric state of vWf is important for its binding to different types of collagen. On the other hand, it is not yet known whether the quaternary structure is required for its binding to noncollageneous components of endothelium since vWf multimers of different size bind equally to subendothelium in a perfusion system.[150] However, Wagner et al.[163] recently observed that the small multimers synthesized by endothelial cells in the presence of monensin were not stored in these cells nor were they incorporated in the extracellular matrix.

c. vWf Involvement in Platelet Adhesion

Sixma et al.[150] studied the effect of three different fractions of vWf multimers with apparent MW of 6.5 to 14, 4.0 to 9.0, and 2.0 to 7.5 $\times$ 10^6 Da and of different therapeutic concentrates on platelet adhesion. They showed that concentrates lacking vWf multimers with MWs greater than 5.5 $\times$ 10^6 Da did not support platelet adhesion. However, they noticed no evident differences in platelet adhesion to subendothelium mediated by the three fractions of the purified vWf preparation. Other experiments performed with partially reduced vWf indicated that the ability of vWf to bind to subendothelium was not significantly changed even after treatment with 50 m*M* dithiothreitol. However, ability of vWf to support adhesion was decreased when dithiothreitol at concentrations exceeding 3 m*M* was used, but the effect was less apparent than in systems assessing vWf:RCo activity.[150] Furthermore, Sakariassen et al.[164] recently showed that the dimeric fragment Sp III obtained by Sp V8 protease was able to promote the same extent of platelet adhesion to collagen as multimeric vWf. These authors concluded that the multimeric structure of vWf was not required for platelet adhesion to collagen. In order to reconcile this conclusion with the importance of the multimeric structure of vWf in the requisite preliminary step of vWf binding to collagen, one must consider that, under these conditions, the Sp III fragments bound to collagen may mimic the quaternary conformation of native vWf.

Although most of the above data provide convincing evidence that the role of the molecular size of vWf, governed by its multimeric state, exerts critical influence on some of its characteristics or functional properties which seem to be directly involved in its biological activity, on the other hand, some data indicate that HMW forms of vWf are not always required even for platelet adhesion. Furthermore, there is some suggestion that other structural features of vWf apart from its multimeric size are probably important in determining its biological efficacy. The importance of the structural organization at a level below the multimeric structure is emphasized in the data reported below.

B. The Role of vWf Organization in Domains

The knowledge of the requirements related to the primary, secondary, or tertiary structure of vWf in the context of its different functional properties necessitates prior location of vWf substructures involved in various functional attributes. These substructures, named functional domains, have been studied in recent years in two main ways. The first is by characterizing proteolytic fragment of vWf maintaining a given function and localizing each of them in the vWf subunit. The second is by identifying the epitopes of monoclonal antibodies (MAb) to vWf which inhibit some of the functional activities. Since most of the vWf functions are dependent on its multimeric state and on its size, only low residual functional activity is usually demonstrated by cleavage products of the vWf molecule. Furthermore, as MAbs may change the conformation state of the whole molecule, the fact that a MAb inhibits a specific function does not necessarily imply that its epitope is directly involved in the corresponding functional site. In spite of these difficulties, some information concerning vWf domains required for a number of functional properties is now available. As the subject of MAbs against vWf is discussed elsewhere, we will mainly focus on the data obtained after mild proteolysis of vWf in the context of the various functions of vWf as measured *in vitro*.

1. Ristocetin-Induced vWf Binding to Platelets

There is little information derived from the characterization of MAbs directly inhibiting vWf binding to ristocetin-stimulated platelets. Most of such MAbs (RFF VIII:R1 and RFF VIII:R2,[165,166] CLB RAg:35,[167,168] and 211-A6[169]) not only inhibited this binding but also affected ristocetin-induced aggregation and platelet adhesion to the same extent. In contrast, RFF VIII:R1 and VIII:R2,[166] H9,[140] CLBRAg:35,[169] and 211 A6[169] did not inhibit vWf binding to thrombin-stimulated platelets. These data indicate that ristocetin-induced vWf binding and platelet adhesion share at least one structural requirement of vWf. This differential property of these MAbs enabled the nonidentical nature of the vWf domains involved in ristocetin- and thrombin-induced binding of vWf to platelets to be substantiated. Complementary studies on different proteolytic digests of vWf underscore the remoteness of these separate domains from one another.

Mild proteolysis of vWf by Sp V8, trypsin, thermolysin, α-chymotrypsin, and elastase was shown to induce a 53 to 77% decrease in ristocetin-induced vWf binding to platelets.[28] Proteolysis of vWf by Sp V8 exhibited the particularity of generating two major fragments, Sp II and Sp III (Figure 4). First, it was shown that Sp III, but not Sp II, is a potent inhibitor of ^{125}I-vWf binding to ristocetin-stimulated platelets, as demonstrated in Table 4,[112,170] and the Sp III fragment was found to bind to platelets. At ligand saturation levels, this binding was even higher than observed for native vWf (16 compared to 12 μg per 10^8 platelets).[112] Furthermore, this binding was completely inhibited by both a MAb to the GP Ib platelets

Table 4
**RECEPTOR BINDING AFFINITY OF NATIVE, REDUCED, AND
PROTEOLYSED HUMAN vWf [a]**

	Girma et al.[112]	Bockenstedt et al.[158]	Fujimura et al.[121]
Native vWf	9.4 μg/ml (7.8 nM)[b]		9 μg/ml (7.5 nM)[b]
vWf dimer	76 μg/ml (170 nM)[b]	100 μg/ml[b] (227 nM)	
vWf subunit			1.4 mg/ml (6.5 μM)
Sp III fragment[d]	76 μg/ml (241 nM)[b]		
Fragment 2[d]		22 μg/ml[b] (77 nM)	
52/48-kDa fragment[c]			26 μg/ml[b] (520 nM)

[a] Affinity is shown by the concentration necessary to achieve 50% inhibition (IC$_{50}$) of the binding of ^{125}I-native vWf to platelets in the presence of ristocetin.
[b] Results calculated on the basis of following MW: native vWf: 1.2×10^6 Da, vWf dimer: 440×10^3 Da, vWf subunit: 220×10^3 Da, Sp III: 315×10^3 Da, fragment 2: 285×10^3 Da, 52/58-kDa fragment: 50×10^3 Da.
[c] Fragment isolated from reduced and alkylated tryptic digest.[121]
[d] Proteolytic fragments isolated after proteolysis with *S. aureus* V8 protease.[112,158]

receptor and by an anti-vWf MAb (H9) inhibiting more than 90% ristocetin-induced vWf binding to the platelets (Figure 9).[170,171] Complementary experiments showed that the MAb H9 bound not only to Sp III but also to the 33- and 28-kDa monomeric fragments obtained by subtilisin cleavage.[171] Bockenstedt et al.[158] identified a 285-kDa Sp V8 fragment of vWf, composed of two disulfide-linked 175- and 115-kDa polypeptides, which competed with ^{125}I-vWf for binding to GP Ib as seen in Table 4. Furthermore, this fragment, named fragment 2, exhibited the property of binding to insolubilized heparin. These studies indicate that the vWf binding site for the platelet receptor GP Ib is contained in the dimeric fragments Sp III or fragment 2, composed of two disulfide-bound polypeptide chains probably corresponding to either 1365 or 910 amino acid residues from the amino-terminal part of mature vWf and able to bind to heparin. Furthermore, this site is modified by the interaction with the MAb H9, the epitope of which extends on relatively small monomeric segments, the location of which remain to be precisely determined.

Sixma et al.[172] isolated a 116-kDa MW fragment from trypsin-digested vWf by using immunoprecipitation with CLB-RAg 35. After disulfide-bond reduction and electrophoresis, this fragment could be visualized as two bands of 52/56 and 14 kDa. Using a vWf tryptic digest, Fujimira et al.[121] isolated a reduced and alkylated fragment migrating in SDS-polyacrylamide gels as a 52/48-kDa doublet. This doublet was recognized by three MAbs (RG21, RG42, and RG46) which were able to inhibit ristocetin-induced platelet aggregation, vWf binding to platelets, and the binding of native vWf to ristocetin-stimulated platelets (Table 4). The amino acid sequence of this fragment permitted the localization of its N-terminal amino acid residue at position 449 on the native vWf polypeptide chain[121] and subsequently the characterization of its C-terminal end at position 729.[62] Houdijk et al.[173] demonstrated the direct binding of a single 50-kDa fragment by incubating the tryptic digest of radiolabeled vWf with platelets and analyzing radioactive material bound to platelets. When this incubation was performed in the presence of *N*-ethylmaleimide (an agent blocking sulfydryl groups), a predominant 116-kDa fragment was obtained which immunoprecipitated with the MAb CLB RAg 35 and also bound to platelets. It is thus likely that identical tryptic fragments have been isolated by both groups.

Thus a vWf binding site for the platelet receptor GP Ib was localized on a peptide segment from residue 449 to residue 729 containing at least one interchain disulfide bond and requiring either a linear amino acid sequence or a conformation modified by the interaction of vWf with some MAbs (such as H9, CLB RAg 35, RG 21 . . .).

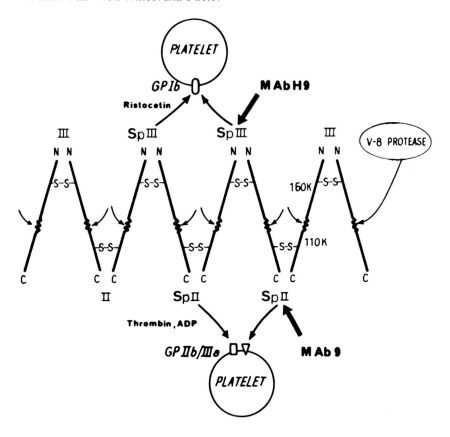

FIGURE 9.   Model for the structure of vWf multimer. Schematic representation of the fragments SpII and III obtained by limited proteolysis by *S. aureus* V8 protease, their binding to platelet receptors (GP Ib and GPIIb/IIIa), and the inhibition of these binding sites by two anti-vWf monoclonal antibodies (MAbs 9 and H9). (From Girma, J. P., Kalafatis, M., and Meyer, D., in *Factor VIII-von Willebrand Factor*, Ciavarella, N. L., Ruggeri, Z. M., and Zimmerman, T. S., Eds., Wichtig Editore, Milan, 1986, 137. With permission.)

2. vWf Binding to Gp IIb/IIIa Platelet Receptor

At this time of writing, only one MAb (9) has been reported to inhibit vWf binding to thrombin-stimulated platelets.[166] Using a proteolytic digestion procedure of vWf with Sp V8, Girma et al.[112] isolated a homodimeric fragment with a MW of 215 kDa. Each polypeptide of this homodimeric fragment corresponded to the 685 C-terminal amino acid residues of the vWf subunit (Figure 4). Contrary to fragment Sp III, this fragment, named Sp II, inhibited the binding of vWf multimers to thrombin-stimulated platelets.[170] A saturable binding of Sp II to thrombin-stimulated platelets was observed and was found to be inhibited by both MAb 9 and by a MAb to the platelet receptor Gp IIb/IIIa (Figure 9).[171] In addition, MAb 9 also reacted with a dimeric 86-kDa fragment obtained by thermolysin proteolysis of Sp II. Nevertheless, the exact location of this fragment giving rise to the two bands of 42 and 23 kDa after reduction remains to be elucidated. Recent observations with tryptic digests show that the epitope of MAb 9 is also present on a 116-kDa fragment. However, this fragment composed of 54-, 43-, 30-, and 21-kDa MW fragments[69] is different from the one precipitated by MAb CLB RAg 35.

There is evidence that the amino acid triplet RGD (Arg-Gly-Asp) which is shared by several adhesive proteins, i.e., fibrinogen, fibronectin, and vitronectin, interacts with different cellular receptors.[174,175] As this amino acid triplet also occurs in Sp II (Figure 4), and RGD-containing peptides inhibit vWf binding to GP IIb/IIIa,[176] it is likely that the GP IIb/IIIa binding domain of vWf contains this triplet sequence.

3. vWf Binding to Collagen

Two groups have characterized MAbs (CLB RAg 201 and B 200 through B 205) to vWf which inhibit its binding to collagen.[171,172] The first group showed that a vWf tryptic fragment of 48 kDa contained not only the epitope of CLB RAg 201[172] but also bound to collagen fibrils of type III.[173] The second group has reported that Sp III as well as subtilisin fragments of 26 and 33 kDa contain the epitope of the MAb B 203.[171] Using immunoprecipitation techniques on trypsin-digested vWf, these two groups[169a] have demonstrated that the collagen binding domain of the vWf subunit is localized between GP Ib- and GP IIb/IIIa-binding domains, approximately coinciding with the Sp I fragment extending from Gly (911) to Glu (1365) on the vWf subunit (Figure 4). Sakariassen et al.[164] recently showed that Sp III incubated with collagen coated on glass cover slips promoted platelet adhesion. They concluded that Sp III was able to bind to collagen and thus possessed a binding site for collagen. This binding site was assumed to be located on a part of the N-terminal portion of vWf different from the one required for the binding of vWf to GP Ib, as it interacted with MAbs different from those inhibiting ristocetin-induced vWf binding. This conclusion is in agreement with the recent data of Pareti et al.[177] This group showed that out of the 15 antibodies directed against the 52/48-kDa fragment previously found to mediate vWf interaction with GP Ib, 7 inhibited both collagen and GP Ib binding activities. The remaining eight antibodies inhibited vWf/collagen interaction without affecting GP Ib binding ability. The reduced and alkylated 52/48-kDa fragment was shown to inhibit the binding of native vWf to collagen type I with an IC_{50} (concentration necessary to achieve 50% inhibition) of approximately 0.4 μM. This fragment extended from Val (449) to Lys (728) and was different from the 48-kDa (unreduced) and 58-kDa (reduced) MW fragments previously mentioned.[172,173] Thus, at present, we cannot rule out that the vWf subunit has more than one collagen binding site.

4. Ristocetin-Induced Platelet Agglutination

Andersen et al.[178] have shown that vWf:RCo activity of purified VIII/vWf submitted to thrombin or plasmin proteolysis was unchanged or reduced to 70%, respectively. Terminal plasmin fragments, still supporting vWf:RCo activity, were identified as fragments of MW 103 kDa or less. On the other hand, N-terminal Sp III fragments obtained after vWf proteolysis by Sp V8 were shown to contain 11% of the original specific vWf:RCo activity of the purified native vWf.[112]

By submitting vWf to trypsin, Martin et al.[130] noticed a decrease of up to 90% in the starting ristocetin activity after 20 min coinciding with a quantitative decrease in the 250-kDa vWf subunit and the appearance of 154- and 116-kDa fragments. The fact that vWf:RCo activity was dramatically decreased by tryptic digestion was subsequently confirmed by others,[179] but the digestion procedure did not influence the subsequent isolation of tryptic fragments supporting significant vWf:RCo activity. A 116-kDa fragment, composed of two disulfide bond chains of MW 73 and 43 (or 46) kDa, isolated in nonreducing conditions, was able to induce platelet aggregation in the presence of ristocetin.[130] Furthermore, the previously mentioned reduced 52/48-kDa fragment, at a concentration of 500 μg/ml (10 μM) completely inhibited the aggregation of washed platelets induced by the addition of both ristocetin and purified native vWf.[121]

Results from all these experiments indicate that the structure and conformation of native vWf and the intact vWf subunit are not necessary to inhibit vWf-induced platelet agglutination in the presence of ristocetin. The proteolytic fragments which were previously reported to support vWf binding to ristocetin-stimulated platelets are able to inhibit vWf:RCo activity of native vWf and are recognized by MAbs inhibiting both ristocetin-induced functions of vWf. However, ristocetin-induced platelet aggregation may require some structural features in addition to the vWf binding capacity since two MAbs (ES vWf 3 and ES vWf 5) exhibiting no effect on vWf binding to fixed platelets were shown to enhance the rate of platelet agglutination in the presence of ristocetin.[180] In this context, it would be of interest to ascertain whether some of the anti-vWf MAbs, inhibiting vWf:RCo activity, could fail to inhibit ristocetin-induced vWf binding.

5. Platelet Adhesion

Recently, Sakariassen et al.[164] have shown that fragment Sp III, but not Sp II, could perform the same role as purified native vWf in supporting platelet adhesion to collagen. Stel et al.[167] have characterized 2 of 19 MAbs to vWf which completely inhibit platelet adhesion to human arterial subendothelium. As these two antibodies (CLB RAg 34 and CLB RAg 35) also inhibited vWf:RCo activity, it was suggested that a vWf domain was associated both with ristocetin-induced aggregation and the ability of vWf to support platelet adhesion. This hypothesis is in agreement with the data of Sakariassen et al.[164] but at variance with the conclusion drawn by Meyer et al.[181] Indeed of four MAbs to vWf inhibiting platelet adhesion on rabbit aortic endothelium, only one also attenuated vWf:RCo activity. On the other hand, a MAb inhibiting vWf:RCo activity had no effect on adhesion. The observation that several antibodies inhibit both vWf:RCo activity and platelet adhesion[166,167,169] does not disprove the hypothesis that two different molecular loci of vWf are involved in vWf:RCo activity and platelet adhesion.[181] However, it does at least raise questions as to their exact location and the mechanism of their interaction. Finally, it must be emphasized that platelet adhesion is likely to require several vWf functional domains as some MAb interacting with collagen binding domains also inhibit platelet adhesion in a perfusion system.[172]

In conclusion, all the above results provide evidence that at least three distinct sites on the vWf molecule are involved in some of its functions. The first site involved in vWf binding to the platelet in the presence of ristocetin was localized on a segment from Val (449) to Arg (729) contained on the N-terminal part of the vWf subunit. The second site involved in vWf binding to collagen was also localized on the amino-terminal half of vWf, but either on the segment 449-729 or on the Sp I fragment extending from Gly (911) to Glu (1365). Thus, the occurrence of two distinct vWf binding sites for collagen must be considered. The third site involved in vWf binding to the Gp IIb/IIIa complex was localized on the C-terminal part of the vWf subunit and was thought to require the presence of the RGD sequence occurring at position 1744-1746 on the vWf subunit. Nevertheless, the existence of additional vWf binding sites, involved either in the binding to collagen or in functions not yet identified, cannot be excluded. The understanding of the structural requirements for the expression of the biological activity of vWf necessitates prior determination of the exact locations of all of the different functional domains. Indeed, it is likely that multiple sites in the vWf molecule are involved in its biological activity.

C. The Role of the vWf Carbohydrate Moiety

vWf is a glycoprotein, and, as with other glycoproteins, there is continuing debate as to the role of the carbohydrate moiety. Elucidation of the functional importance of such structures can be gained through investigations either of the carbohydrate moiety of functionally abnormal vWf isolated from the plasma of vWd patients, or by study of the functional properties of carbohydrate-modified vWf.

1. Studies of vWf from vWD Patients

The first indication of an abnormality in the vWf carbohydrate moiety in vWD came from a study of periodic acid-Schiff (PAS) staining of bands obtained after electrophoresis of reduced purified vWf. Indeed, an absence of PAS coloration was noticed by Gralnick et al.[182] in three patients with a variant form of vWD (probably type IIA). The frequency of such abnormalities in vWD was challenged by Zimmerman et al.[183] who found a normal Coomassie/PAS staining ratio in 15 of 16 patients with either type I or IIA vWD. It must be stressed that this approach lacked methodological sensitivity since a 50% reduction in the carbohydrate moiety will not modify the ratio.[184] Another method based on isoelectric focusing failed to provide evidence of a sialic acid deficiency in several vWD patients.[109] An indirect method which has been used to detect vWf carbohydrate abnormalities involved affinity studies with lectins. Initially concanavalin A, a lectin specific for α-mannose and α-glucose residues was used. In the presence of this lectin both a decrease in vWF precipitation[185-187] and an abnormality in the electrophoretic pattern[188] of vWF were characterized in several vWD patients. The affinity of vWf for a lectin from *Ricinis communis*, specific to galactose residues, also was shown to be decreased in three patients with type IIA vWD, but was normal in six patients with type I vWD.[189] In fact, only few direct analyses of the carbohydrate composition of vWf purified from vWD plasma have been performed. Although the sialic acid levels were initially found to be dramatically decreased in three patients[71,78] more precise analysis performed on vWf isolated from 2.5 l of plasma from a patient with vWD showed a deficiency not only in sialic acid but also in galactose and *N*-acetyl glucosamine residues.[79] These data emphasize the need for more extensive evaluation of the carbohydrate moiety of vWf in vWD, but such studies are restricted by plasma availability.

2. Studies of Carbohydrate-Modified vWf
a. Effects of Lectins

Fluorescein isothiocyanate labeled concanavalin A has been shown to give a similar intensity of staining on the different forms of vWf separated by SDS-agarose electrophoresis.[190] With this observation and the fact that all vWf forms stain with a constant dansyl hydrazine/Coomassie blue ratio, Furlan et al.[190] concluded that neither size distribution nor vWf:RCo activity of vWf were related to carbohydrate content. Nevertheless, they later reported that reduced chains derived from HMW vWf multimers exhibited stronger affinity for two *R. communis* lectins, both specific of galactose residues, than those obtained from smaller multimers.[191] Howard et al.[188] showed that vWf from cryoprecipitate bound three times more to concanavalin A than vWf from cryosupernatant. Additionally, Furlan et al.[190] reported that vWf:RCo activity of purified vWf was inhibited by both *Ricinus* lectins and concanavalin A and was restored by further incubation with D-galactose and α-methyl-D mannoside, respectively. As high concentrations of these two sugars produced only 20% inhibition in vWf:RCo activity, these authors concluded that vWf binding to the platelet membrane receptors did not involve sugar/lectin interaction.[191]

b. Effects of Galactose Oxidase Treatment

Fukui et al.[192] were the only authors who directly treated native purified VIII/vWf with galactose oxidase, an enzyme which is known to oxidise the C-6 hydroxymethyl group of galactose to an aldehyde group. They reported dramatic decrease in both vWf:RCo activity and the apparent MW of the protein as deduced from molecular sieving experiments. Later some investigators took advantage of the reversibility of this treatment in the presence of reducing agents, such as potassium borohydride (KBH_4), to demonstrate the specificity of the modification of galactose residues which can be oxidized after prior removal of ultimate sialic acid by neuraminidase. Although removal of more than 95% sialic acid did not affect vWf activity, Gralnick[73] reported that oxidation of asialo-vWf resulted in a progressive loss of up to 45% of the initial vWf:RCo activity. Subsequent reduction with KBH_4 resulted in a 6-aldehydo group of galactoses and concomitant regeneration of vWf:vWf:RCo activity. These results were later confirmed in part by Kao et al.[76] After removal of sialic acid they observed a decrease in vWf:RCo activity to 39%. A further decrease to 19% occurred after oxidation of 39% of the galactose residues of asialo-vWf by galactose oxidase. Subsequent reduction of galactose oxidized, asialo-vWf restored vWf:RCo activity to 33%. The IC_{50}

for ^{125}I-vWf binding to platelets in the presence of ristocetin for native vWf was 2.0 μg/ml (1.1 nM); for asialo-vWf, 14.8 μg/ml (12.5 nM); for galactose oxidized, asialo-vWf, 66 μg/ml (53.8 nM); and 30 μg/ml (18.9 nM) for KBH4-reduced galactose-oxidized asialo-vWf. Later Gralnick et al.[81] reported that the modification of penultimate galactose residues by the treatment of asialo-vWf with galactose oxidase resulted in the loss of HMW multimers with an increase in intermediate and small multimers.[81] This treatment was reported to markedly reduce vWf adsorption to fibrillar collagen[193] and the residual vWf:RCo activity of a 116-kDa tryptic fragment of vWf.[179] These results indicate the importance of the penultimate galactose residue in both multimeric integrity and functional activity of vWf.

c. Effects of Neuraminidase Treatment

Neuraminidases from two different sources, *Clostridium perfringens* or *Vibrio cholerae*, are generally used at values approximately pH 5 and 7, respectively. These agents have been shown to be able to remove more than 90% vWf sialic acid in 2 to 6 h. The properties of so-called asialo-vWf thus obtained have been extensively studied. Sodetz et al.[72] showed that the half-life of human asialo-vWf in rabbits was dramatically decreased (5 min as opposed to 240 min for native vWf). Indeed, consistent with other asialoglycoproteins, asialo-vWf, but not native vWf, binds to a rabbit liver lectin.[194] Some investigators have found that desialylation reduces the ability of vWf either to bind to the GP Ib receptor or to induce platelet aggregation in the presence of ristocetin.[72,75,76] There is, however, general agreement that asialo-vWf retains these two ristocetin-induced activities.[72,77,78,81,138,192,195] Recently, we[138] demonstrated that vWf binding to thrombin-stimulated platelets was not impaired following more than 90% desialylation and confirmed that the multimeric pattern of asialo-vWf is similar to that of the native molecule.[81,82] As asialo-vWf was reported to be adsorbed on type I collagen to a similar degree as native vWf,[193] it thus seems that the removal of sialic acid does not affect the majority of the *in vitro* properties of native vWf. However, in the absence of any agonist, asialo-vWf has been found to bind significantly more to normal and thrombasthenic platelets than unmodified vWf[78,138,196,197] and induced platelet aggregation in platelet rich plasma.[78,194,196,198] The mechanism of this aggregation was studied using MAbs specific for GP Ib and the GP IIb/IIIa complex in a system with plasma containing variable concentrations of fibrinogen, and platelets from patients with either Glanzmann's thrombasthenia or Bernard-Soulier syndrome. Asialo-vWf bound to the GP Ib receptor was shown to render additional GP IIb/IIIa receptors available on the platelet surface and consequently induce aggregation in the presence of fibrinogen.[78,196,197] This calcium-dependent mechanism is analogous to the recently reported observation[199] involving platelet aggregation induced by abnormal vWf isolated from the plasma of a patient with type IIB vWD.

d. Effects of β-Galactosidase Treatment

Few investigators have studied the direct effects of β-galactosidase on native vWf. This treatment, which only removes the nonreducing terminal β1-4 linked galactose residues of glycanic chains, was found to induce a release of about 20% galactose residues.[81,138] On the one hand, galactosidase was found to induce no loss in vWf:RCo activity[81,192] and no changes in the multimeric structure in spite of a 19% decrease in galactose.[81] On the other hand, using galactosidase from two different sources, Goudemand et al.[138] have shown that a removal of 20% galactose was associated with a loss of HMW forms of vWf and with a decrease in the vWf binding to ristocetin-, but not to thrombin-, stimulated platelets.

Many investigators have assessed the effects of β-galactosidase on previously desialylated vWf. This treatment is expected to release both terminal and penultimate β1-4 linked galactose residues from glycanic chains. Whereas the extent of galactose removal reported by several groups was variable (from 39[76] to 83%[81]), general agreement has been reached as to its dramatic effect on several vWf functions. The treatment of asialo-vWf with β-galactosidase was first shown to induce a decrease in the vWf:RCo activity proportional to the amount of galactose released.[73,76,77,81,194] This decrease of up to 90% is probably related to a decrease in vWf binding to ristocetin-stimulated platelets[76,77,79,138] and to an eightfold increase in its dissociation constant.[79] Furthermore, the treatment of asialo-vWf with β-galactosidase was reported to markedly reduce vWf adsorption on fibrillar collagen[193] and to result in a dramatic change in vWf multimeric structure.[81,138] In contrast, Federici et al.[82] found no change in either the vWf:RCo activity or the multimeric structure of purified vWf after sequential neuraminidase and galactosidase treatment when protease inhibitors were present throughout the enzyme incubation period. These authors also showed that vWf:RCo activity was reduced to 62% of the initial value in the absence of protease inhibitors, and that carbohydrate-modified vWf lost its HMW forms in the presence of traces of plasmin.[82]

e. Effects of Endoglycosidase Treatment

Endoglycosidases are enzymes which are able to cleave N-glycosidically linked glycans in hydrolysing β1-4 linkage between the two *N*-acetyl glucosamine residues close to the peptide chain. The recent availability of endoglycosidase F which cleaves both high mannose and complex type N-glycans[200] enabled Federici et al. to study the effect of the removal of N-glycans on vWf. In spite of a release of 69% of total hexoses and galactose and of 71% sialic acid, they reported no loss in HMW multimers nor any alteration in the "triplet" pattern, with only 11% decrease in vWf:RCo activity. In this system purified native vWf was treated with a high concentration of the enzyme (50 U endoglycosidase per milligram of vWf).[82] Using the same enzyme on the 52/48-kDa vWf tryptic fragment, retaining vWf ability to bind to the GP Ib platelet receptor in the presence of ristocetin, Fujimura et al.[121] removed 70% of the total hexoses and obtained a 46-kDa fragment equally effective in blocking ristocetin-induced platelet binding of ¹²⁵I-native vWf.

The available data suggest that the carbohydrate moiety of vWf plays an important role principally in the multimeric organization and in the interaction of vWf with platelets in the presence of ristocetin. The biological importance of the vWf carbohydrate moiety is still a subject of controversy. As the multimeric state of vWf has been shown to influence some of its essential properties, it is possible that vWf carbohydrates act indirectly in maintaining vWf multimeric conformation. However, this hypothesis and the possible direct action of the vWf carbohydrate moiety have been refuted by several investigators. An alternative explanation is that carbohydrate may simply protect vWf against proteases, which could account for the previously observed depolymerization of vWf subjected to exoglycosidase treatment.[82] Recently Wagner et al.[201] emphasized the importance of initial N-glycosylation in the essential events for vWf processing in human endothelial cells and once more raised the possibility of a glycosylation defect operative in Type IIA vWD. In our opinion, a more precise analysis of the glycans, both from native and carbohydrate-modified normal vWf and from abnormal vWf occurring in variants of vWD, is essential before any valid conclusions can be reached.

V. CONCLUDING REMARKS

Our understanding of the biochemistry of vWf has advanced considerably during the 1980s. Both high resolution electrophoretic and electron microscopic procedures have contributed to a greater degree of characterization of the polydispersity and heterogeneity of vWf, which have hampered physiochemical studies for more than a decade. These new techniques combined with other physicochemical methodologies permitting the study of vWf in solution, have contributed significantly in the elucidation of the morphological features of the predominant forms of plasma vWf and the existence of minor forms. Aided by methodological advances in the preparation of large amounts of highly purified VIII/vWf and by the new technology of vWf and VIII cDNA cloning, the particular identity of vWf has been established and its amino acid sequence demonstrated. We now know that the predominant forms of plasma vWf consist of a series of multimers composed of a variable number of protomers associated by disulfide bonds located on amino-terminal parts of peptide chains. Furthermore, each protomer includes two or four glycopeptidic subunits linked by disulfide bonds located on their carboxy-terminal parts. Their polypeptide moiety with a MW of 225, 843 Da contains approximately 15% carbohydrates distributed among 12 N-glycosidically linked oligosaccharides and probably 10 O-glycosidically linked chains.

Nevertheless, full knowledge of the primary structure of plasma vWf still depends upon identification of the glycanic structure of half of the monosaccharides in vWf, the location of each glycan on polypeptide chains, the characterization of the sites of sulfatation (the occurrence of which was recently reported[202]), and the biochemical characterization of vWf heterogeneity. Furthermore, only few data are available on the three dimensional conformation of vWf which may be important in the context of structural and functional correlations within this molecule. It is, however, noteworthy that we already know that both the multimeric state and specific regions of the glycoprotein chain involved in several ligand binding sites for platelet receptors and collagen are required for vWf biological activity. However, the relative importance of these two requirements is not as yet understood, as no information is available concerning the possible abnormalities of receptor binding sites in vWf from vWD patients. Furthermore, it is still not clear whether vWf carbohydrate has an indirect role or a direct role in vWf activity. If vWf glycans, like glycans from other glycoproteins, are involved in the stabilization of protein conformation and in the recognition of receptors, irrefutable proof of this is still needed as are the exact nature and structural requirements of the various vWf functional domains.

It is likely that answers to these questions will be forthcoming and will contribute to an increase in our understanding of molecular events involved in platelet adhesion. However, the mechanism of association between vWf and VIII, and the particular features of platelet vWf remain to be elucidated if we are to fully comprehend all the molecular aspects of the complex physiological function of vWf.

ACKNOWLEDGMENTS

I thank Prof. M. Goudemand for critical reading of the manuscript and for his stimulation. Many thanks are due to Dr. J. Mazurier and to C. Taillefer for their help with the computer analysis used in the section on predictive secondary structure. I am also grateful to my co-workers, B. Samor, C. De Romeuf, and S. Jorieux, for their support and comments during the preparation of this manuscript. I am indebted to B. Wittouck for her excellent secretarial assistance.

ADDENDUM

Since the writing of this chapter, knowledge of the localization of plasma vWf domains involved in its binding to factor VIII,[203-205] heparin,[206] platelet receptors,[207,208] and subendothelium components,[209-211] has significantly improved. Furthermore, recent progress in expression of recombinant vWf has opened new horizons in the understanding of structure-function relationships of this molecule.

REFERENCES

1. **Jaffe, E. A., Hoyer, L. W., and Nachman, R. L.,** Synthesis of antihemophilic factor antigen by cultured human endothelial cells, *Proc. Natl. Acad. Sci. U.S.A.,* 71, 1966, 1974.
2. **Wagner, D. D. and Marder, V. J.,** Biosynthesis of von Willebrand protein by human endothelial cells: processing steps and their intracellular localization, *J. Cell Biol.,* 99, 2123, 1984.
3. **Legaz, M. E., Schmer, G., Counts, R., and Davie, E.,** Isolation and characterization of human factor VIII (antihemophilic factor), *J. Biol. Chem.,* 248, 3946, 1973.
4. **Shapiro, G. A., Andersen, J. C., Pizzo, S. V., and McKee, P. A.,** The subunit structure of normal and hemophilic factor VIII, *J. Clin. Invest.,* 52, 2198, 1973.
5. **Howard, M. A., Montgomery, D. C., and Hardisty, R. M.,** Factor VIII-related antigen in platelets, *Thromb Res.,* 4, 617, 1974.
6. **Nachman, R. L. and Jaffe, E. A.,** Subcellular platelet factor VIII antigen and von Willebrand factor, *J. Exp. Med.,* 141, 1101, 1975.
7. **Zucker, M. B., Broekman, M. J., and Kaplan, K. L.,** Factor VIII-related antigen in human blood platelets. Localization and release by thrombin and collagen, *J. Lab. Clin. Med.,* 94, 675, 1979.
8. **Sporn, L. A., Chavin, S. I., Marder, V. J., and Wagner, D. D.,** Biosynthesis of von Willebrand protein by human megakaryocytes, *J. Clin. Invest.,* 76, 1102, 1985.
9. **Slot, J. W., Bouma, B. N., Montgomery, R. M., and Zimmerman, T. S.,** Platelet factor VIII-related antigen: immunofluorescent localization, *Thromb. Res.,* 13, 871, 1978.
10. **Cohn, E. J., Strong, L. E., Hughes, W. L., Mulford, D. J., Asworth, J. N., Melin, M., and Taylor, H. L.,** Preparation and properties of serum and plasma proteins. IV. A system for the separation into fractions of proteins and lipoprotein components of biological tissues and fluids, *J. Am. Chem. Soc.,* 68, 459, 1946.
11. **Blomback, M.,** Purification of antihemophilic globulin, *Arch. Kemi,* 12, 387, 1958.
12. **Simonetti, C., Casillas, G., and Pavlovsky, A.,** Tannic acid purification of factor VIII, in *The Hemophilia,* Brinkhous, K. M., Ed., University of North Carolina Press, Chapel Hill, 1964, 100.
13. **Pool, J. G. and Shannon, A. E.,** Production of high potency concentrates of anti-hemophilic globulin in a closed bag system, *N. Engl. J. Med.,* 273, 1443, 1965.
14. **Amrani, D. L., Mosesson, M. W., and Hoyer, L. W.,** Distribution of plasma fibronectin (CIG) and components of the factor VIII complex after heparin-induced precipitation of plasma, *Blood,* 59, 657, 1982.
15. **Mazurier, C., Samor, B., De Romeuf, C., and Goudemand, M.,** The role of fibronectin in factor VIII/von Willebrand factor cryoprecipitation, *Thromb. Res.,* 37, 651, 1985.
16. **Webster, W. P., Roberts, H. R., Thelin, G. M., Wagner, R. H., and Brinkhous, K. M.,** Clinical use of a new glycine-precipitated antihemophilic fraction, *Am. H. Med. Sci.,* 250, 643, 1965.
17. **Johnson, A. J., Newman, J. J., Howell, M. B., and Puszkin, S.,** Purification of antihemophilic factor (AHF) for clinical and experimental use, *Thromb. Diath. Haemorrh.,* 26, 377, 1967.
18. **Newman, J., Johnson, A. J., Karpatkin, M. H., and Puszkin, S.,** Methods for the production of clinically intermediate and high purity factor VIII concentrates, *Br. J. Haematol.,* 21, 1, 1971.
19. **Hershgold, E. J., Pool, J. G., and Pappenhagen, A. R.,** The potent antihemophilic globulin concentrate derived from a cold-insoluble fraction of human plasma, *J. Lab. Med.,* 67, 23, 1966.
20. **Smith, J. K., Evans, D. R., Stone, V., and Snape, T. J.,** A factor VIII concentrate of intermediate purity and higher potency, *Transfusion,* 19, 299, 1979.
21. **Thorell, L. and Blomback, B.,** Purification of the factor VIII complex, *Thromb. Res.,* 35, 431, 1984.
22. **Mazurier, C., Maillard, J., Parquet-Gernez, A., and Goudemand, M.,** Etude d'un concentré thérapeutique de facteur VIII/vWF préparé en circuit clos, *Rev. Fr. Transfus. Immunohematol.,* 25, 25, 1982.
23. **Ratnoff, O. D., Kass, L., and Lang, P. D.,** Studies on the purification of antihemophilic factor (factor VIII). II. Separation of partially purified antihemophilic factor by gel filtration on plasma, *J. Clin. Invest.,* 48, 957, 1969.
24. **Paulssen, M. M., Wouterlood, A. C., and Scheffers, H. L.,** Purification of the antihemophilic factor by gel filtration on agarose, *Thromb. Diath. Haemorrh.,* 22, 577, 1969.
25. **Van Mourik, J. A. and Mochtar, I. A.,** Purification of human antihemophilic factor (factor VIII) by gel chromatography, *Biochim. Biophys. Acta,* 221, 677, 1970.
26. **Mazurier, C., Parquet-Gernez, A., Samor, B., Goudemand, M., and Montreuil, J.,** Etude de l'antigène lié au facteur VIII (VIIIR:Ag). Purification par chromatographie d'immunoaffinité, *C.R. Acad. Sci. (Paris),* 288, 1431, 1979.
27. **Madaras, F., Bell, W. R., and Castaldi, P. A.,** Isolation and insolubilization of human factor VIII by affinity chromatography, *Haemostasis,* 7, 321, 1978.
28. **Chopek, M. W., Girma, J. P., Fujikawa, K., Davie, E. W., and Titani, K.,** Human von Willebrand factor: a multivalent protein composed of identical subunits, *Biochemistry,* 25, 3171, 1986.
29. **Saundry, R. H., Harrison, P., and Savidge, G. F.,** The purification of factor VIII using dextran sulphate-agarose chromatography, *Thromb. Haemost.,* 54 (Abstr.), 79, 1985.

30. **Fowler, W. E., Fretto, L. J., Hamilton, K. K., Erikson, H. P., and McKee, P. A.,** Substructure of human von Willebrand factor, *J. Clin. Invest.,* 76, 1491, 1985.
31. **Goodall, A. H. and Meyer, D.,** Registry of monoclonal antibodies to factor VIII and von Willebrand factor, *Thromb. Haemost.,* 54, 878, 1985.
32. **Mejan, O., Delezay, M., Fert, V., Cheballah, R., and Bourgois, A.,** Immunopurification of FVIII/vWF complex from plasma, presented at Int. Conf. on FVIII/vWF, Bari, June 10 to 15, 1985, 26.
33. **Jorieux, S., Mazurier, C., De Romeuf, C., and Goudemand, M.,** Properties and interests of a monoclonal antibody to human von Willebrand factor, presented at Int. Conf. on FVIII/vWF, Bari, June 10 to 15, 1985, 14.
34. **Bouma, B. N., Wiegernick, Y., Sixma, J. J., Van Mourik, J. A., and Mochtar, I. A.,** Immunochemical characterization of purified anti-haemophilic factor A which corrects abnormal platelet retention in vWD, *Nature (London) New Biol.,* 236, 104, 1972.
35. **Weiss, H. J. and Kochwa, S.,** Molecular forms of antihaemophilic globulin in plasma, cryoprecipitate and after thrombin activation, *Br. J. Haematol.,* 18, 89, 1970.
36. **Weiss, H. J. and Hoyer, L. W.,** Von Willebrand factor: dissociation from antihemophilic factor procoagulant activity, *Science,* 182, 1149, 1973.
37. **Rick, M. E. and Hoyer, L. W.,** Immunologic studies of antihemophilic factor VIII. Immunologic properties of AHF subunits produced by salt dissociation, *Blood,* 42, 737, 1973.
38. **Owen, W. G. and Wagner, R. H.,** Antihemophilic factor: separation of an active fragment following dissociation by salts or detergents, *Thromb. Diath. Haemorrh.,* 27, 502, 1972.
39. **Van Mourik, J. A., Bouma, B. N., La Bruyere, W. T., De Graaf, S., and Mochtar, I. A.,** Factor VIII a series of homologous oligomers and a complex of two proteins, *Thromb. Res.,* 4, 155, 1974.
40. **Barrow, E. M. and Graham, J. B.,** Factor VIII (AHF) activity of small size produced by succinylating plasma, *Am. J. Physiol.,* 222, 134, 1972.
41. **Kaelin, A. C.,** Sodium periodate modification of factor VIII procoagulant activity, *Br. J. Haematol.,* 31, 349, 1975.
42. **Anderson, J. C. and McKee, P. A.,** The effects of proteolytic enzymes on the coagulant properties and molecular structure of human factor VIII, *Circulation,* 46(Suppl. 2), 52(Abstr.), 1972.
43. **Cooper, H. A., Reisner, F. F., Hall, M., and Wagner, R. H.,** Effects of thrombin treatment on preparations of factor VIII on the Ca^{2+}-dissociated small active fragment, *J. Clin. Invest.,* 56, 751, 1975.
44. **Austen, D. E. G.,** Factor VIII of small molecular weight and its aggregation, *Br. J. Haematol.,* 27, 89, 1974.
45. **Mikaelsson, M. E., Forsman, N., and Oswaldsson, U. M.,** Human factor VIII: a calcium linked protein complex, *Blood,* 62, 1006, 1983.
46. **Tran, T. H. and Duckert, F.,** Dissociation of factor VIII:CAg and FVIII:RAg by EDTA. Influence of divalent cation on the binding of VIII:CAg and VIII:RAg, *Thromb. Haemost.,* 50, 547, 1983.
47. **Austen, D. E. G.,** The chromatographic separation of factor VIII on aminohexyl Sepharose, *Br. J. Haematol.,* 43, 669, 1979.
48. **Morgenthaler, J. J.,** Chromatography of antihemophilic factor on diaminoalkane and aminoalkanes derivatized Sepharose, *Thromb. Haemost.,* 47, 124, 1982.
49. **Baugh, R., Brown, J., Sargeant, R., and Hougie, C.,** Separation of human factor VIII activity from the von Willebrand's antigen and ristocetin platelet aggregation activity, *Biochim. Biophys. Acta,* 371, 360, 1974.
50. **Johnson, A. J., McDonald, V. E., Semar, M., Fields, J. E., Schuck, J., Lewis, C., and Brind, J.,** Preparation of the major plasma fractions by solid phase polyelectrolytes, *J. Lab. Clin. Med.,* 92, 194, 1978.
51. **Shaltield, S.,** Hydrophobic chromatography, in *Methods in Enzymology,* Vol. 34, Colowick, F. P. and Kaplan, N. O., Eds., Academic Press, New York, 1974, 126.
52. **Hershgold, E. J.,** Properties of factor VIII, in *Progress in Hemostasis and Thrombosis,* Vol. 2, Spaet, T. H., Ed., Grune & Stratton, New York, 1974, 99.
53. **Hoyer, M. D.,** Von Willebrand's disease, in *Progress in Hemostasis and Thrombosis,* Vol. 3, Spaet, T. H., Ed., Grune & Stratton, New York, 1976, 231.
54. **Hoyer, L. W.,** The factor VIII complex: structure and function, *Blood,* 58, 1, 1981.
55. **Zimmerman, T. S. and Meyer, D.,** Structure and function of factor VIII/von Willebrand factor, in *Haemostasis and Thrombosis,* Bloom, A. L. and Thomas, D. P., Eds., Churchill Livingstone, London 1981, 111.
56. **Zimmerman, T. S. and Meyer, D.,** Factor VIII-von Willebrand factor and the molecular basis of von Willebrand's disease, in *Haemostasis and Thrombosis,* Colman, R. W., Hirsh, J., Marder, V. J., and Salzman, E. W., Eds., Lippincott, Philadelphia, 1982, 54.
57. **Barrow, E. S. and Graham, J. B.,** Blood coagulation factor VIII (antihemophilic factor) — with comments on von Willebrand's disease and Christmas disease, *Physiol. Rev.,* 54, 23, 1974.

58. **Hershgold, E. J., Davison, A. M., and Janszen, M. E.,** Isolation and some chemical properties of human factor VIII (antihemophilic factor), *J. Lab. Clin. Med.,* 77, 185, 1971.
59. **Marchesi, S. L., Shulman, N. R., and Gralnick, H. R.,** Studies on the purification and characterization of human factor VIII, *J. Clin. Invest.,* 51, 2151, 1972.
60. **Olson, J. D., Brockway, W. J., Fass, D. N., Bowie, E. J., and Mann, K. G.,** Purification of porcine and human ristocetin — Willebrand factor, *J. Lab. Clin. Med.,* 89, 1278, 1977.
61. **Hessel, B., Jornvall, H., Thorell, L., Soderman, S., Larsson, U., Egberg, N., Blomback, B., and Holmgren, A.,** Structure-function relationships of human factor VIII complex studied by thioredoxin dependent disulfide reduction, *Thromb. Res.,* 35, 637, 1984.
62. **Titani, K., Kumar, S., Takio, K., Ericsson, L. H., Wade, R. D., Ashida, K., Walsh, K. A., Chopek, J. E., and Fujikawa, F.,** Amino acid sequence of human von Willebrand factor, *Biochemistry,* 25, 3171, 1986.
63. **Holmberg, L., Jeppson, J. O., Nilsson, I. M., and Stenflo, J.,** Cyanogen bromide and tryptic fragments of normal and haemophilic factor VIII, *Thromb. Res.,* 6, 523, 1975.
64. **Casillas, G., Simonetti, C., Vasquez, C., and Pavlovsky, A.,** Physical and immunological studies on bovine factor VIII, *Haemostasis,* 5, 1, 1976.
65. **Mazurier, C., Samor, B., Parquet-Gernez, A., Fournet, B., Goudemand, M., and Montreuil, J.,** Chemical composition of factor VIII, in *Protides of Biological fluids,* Peeters, H., Ed., Pergamon Press, Oxford, 1980, 299.
66. **Hamilton, K. K., Fretto, L. J., Grierson, D. S., and McKee, P. A.,** Effects of plasmin on von Willebrand factor multimers. Degradation in vitro and stimulation of release in vivo, *J. Clin. Invest.,* 76, 261, 1985.
67. **Hershgold, E. J., Silverman, L., Davison, A. M., and Janszen, M.,** Native and purified factor VIII: molecular and electron microscopical properties and a comparison with hemophilic plasma, *Fed. Proc. Fed. Am. Soc. Exp. Biol.,* 26 (Abstr.), 488, 1967.
68. **Kass, L., Ratnoff, O. D., and Leon, M. A.,** Studies on the purification of antihemophilic factor (factor VIII). I. Precipitation of antihemophilic factor by concanavalin A, *J. Clin. Invest.,* 48, 351, 1969.
69. **McKee, P. A.,** Purification and electrophoretic analysis of human antihemophilic factor (factor VIII), *Fed. Proc. Fed. Am. Soc. Exp. Biol.,* 29 (Abstr.), 647, 1970.
70. **Paulssen, M. M. P., Vandenbussche-Scheffers, H. L., Spaan, P. B., De Jong, T., and Planje, M. C.,** Studies on the characterization of factor VIII and a cofactor VIII, *Thromb. Diath. Haemorrh.,* 31, 328, 1974.
71. **Gralnick, H. R., Sultan, Y., and Coller, B.,** Von Willebrand's disease. Combined qualitative and quantitative abnormalities, *N. Engl. J. Med.,* 296, 1024, 1977.
72. **Sodetz, J. M., Pizzo, S. V., and McKee, P.,** Relationship of sialic acid to function and in vivo survival of human factor VIII/von Willebrand factor protein, *J. Biol. Chem.,* 252, 5538, 1977.
73. **Gralnick, H.,** Factor VIII/von Willebrand factor protein: galactose, a cryptic determinant of von Willebrand factor activity, *J. Clin. Invest.,* 62, 496, 1978.
74. **Sodetz, J. M., Paulson, J. C., and McKee, P. A.,** Carbohydrate composition and identification of blood group A, B and H oligosaccharide structures on human factor VIII/von Willebrand factor, *J. Biol. Chem.,* 254, 10754, 1979.
75. **Rosenfeld, L. and Kirby, E. P.,** The effect of neuraminidase treatment on the biological activities of factor VIII, *Thromb. Res.,* 15, 255, 1979.
76. **Kao, K. J., Pizzo, S. V., and McKee, P. A.,** Factor VIII/von Willebrand and protein. Modification of its carbohydrate causes reduced binding to platelets, *J. Biol. Chem.,* 255, 10134, 1980.
77. **Morisato, D. K. and Gralnick, H. R.,** Selective binding of the FVIII/vWf protein to human platelets, *Blood,* 55, 9, 1980.
78. **De Marco, L. and Shapiro, S. S.,** Properties of human asialo-factor VIII. A ristocetin-independent platelet-aggregating agent, *J. Clin. Invest.,* 68, 321, 1981.
79. **Gralnick, H. R., Cregger, M. C., and Williams, S. B.,** Characterization of the defect of the factor VIII/von Willebrand factor protein in von Willebrand's disease, *Blood,* 59, 542, 1982.
80. **Samor, B., Mazurier, C., Goudemand, M., Debeire, P., Fournet, B., and Montreuil, J.,** Preliminary results on the carbohydrate moiety of factor VIII/von Willebrand factor (FVIII/vWF), *Thromb. Res.,* 25, 81, 1982.
81. **Gralnick, H. R., Williams, S. B., and Rick, M. E.,** Role of carbohydrate in multimeric structure of factor VIII/von Willebrand factor protein, *Proc. Natl. Acad. Sci. U.S.A.,* 80, 2771, 1983.
82. **Federici, A. B., Elder, J. H., De Marco, L., Ruggeri, Z. M., and Zimmerman, T. S.,** Carbohydrate moiety of von Willebrand factor is not necessary for maintaining multimeric structure and ristocetin cofactor activity but protects from proteolytic degradation, *J. Clin. Invest.,* 74, 2049, 1984.
83. **Gralnick, H. R. and Williams, S. B.,** Asialo von Willebrand factor interactions with platelets. Interdependence of glycoproteins Ib and IIb/IIIa for binding and aggregation, *J. Clin. Invest.,* 75, 19, 1985.
84. **Green, D.,** A simple method for the purification of factor VIII (antihemophilic factor) employing snake venom, *J. Lab. Clin. Med.,* 77, 153, 1971.

85. **Roberts, D. D., Rao, N., Liotta, L. A., Gralnick, H. R., and Ginsburg, V.,** Comparison of the specificities of laminin, thrombospondin, and von Willebrand factor for binding to sulfated glycolipids, *J. Biol. Chem.,* 261, 6872, 1986.

86. **Vukovich, T., Marktl, M., and Nemeth, G.,** Heterogeneity of human factor VIII/vWF in lipaemic plasma, *Thromb. Res.,* 38, 215, 1985.

87. **Casillas, G., Simonetti, C., and Pavlosky, A.,** Molecular sieving experiments on human factor VIII, *Coagulation,* 3, 123, 1970.

88. **Weiss, H. J., Phillips, L. L., and Rosner, W.,** Separation of subunits of antihemophilic factor by agarose gel chromatography, *Thromb. Diath. Haemorrh.,* 27, 212, 1971.

89. **Hershgold, E. J.,** Discussion paper: factor VIII, *Ann. N.Y. Acad. Sci.,* 240, 70, 1975.

90. **Bennett, B., Forman, W. B., and Ratnoff, O. D.,** Studies on the nature of antihemophilic factor (factor VIII). Further evidence relating the AHF-like antigens in normal and hemophilic plasmas, *J. Clin. Invest.,* 52, 2191, 1973.

91. **Montgomery, R. R. and Zimmerman, T.,** Von Willebrand's disease antigen II (a new plasma and platelet antigen deficient in severe von Willebrand's disease), *J. Clin. Invest.,* 61, 1498, 1978.

92. **Mazurier, C., Parquet-Gernez, A., Goudemand, M., and Montreuil, J.,** Contribution à l'isolement et à l'étude de la masse moléculaire du facteur VIII humain, *Pathol. Biol.,* 23(Suppl.), 11, 1975.

93. **Bouma, B. N., Dodds, W. J., Van Mourik, J. A., Sixma, J. J., and Webster, W. P.,** Infusion of human and canine factor VIII in dogs with von Willebrand's disease: studies of the von Willebrand and Factor VIII synthesis stimulating factors, *Scand. J. Haematol.,* 17, 263, 1976.

94. **Bolhuis, P. A., Besser-Visser, N. H., and Sixma, J. J.,** Molecular weight of human plasma factor VIII, *Thromb. Res.,* 16, 497, 1979.

95. **Marder, U. J., Tranqui-Pouit, L., Hudry-Clergeon, G., Atichartakarn, V., and Suscillon, M.,** Electron microscopic studies of the factor VIII-von Willebrand factor protein, *Thromb. Haemost.,* 38(Abstr.), 88, 1977.

96. **Tan, H. K. and Andersen, J. C.,** Human factor VIII. Morphometric analysis of purified material in solution, *Science,* 198, 932, 1977.

97. **Beck, E. A., Tranqui-Pouit, L., Chapel, A., Perret, B. A., Furlan, M., Hudry-Clergeon, G., and Suscillon, G.,** Studies on factor VIII-related protein. I. Ultra-structural and electrophoretic heterogeneity of human factor VIII related protein, *Biochim. Biophys. Acta,* 578, 155, 1979.

98. **Ohmori, K., Fretto, L. J., Harrison, R. L., Switzer, M. E. P., Erikson, H. P., and McKee, P. A.,** Electron microscopy of human factor VIII/von Willebrand glycoprotein: effect of reducing agents on structure and function, *J. Cell Biol.,* 95, 632, 1982.

99. **Slayter, H., Loscalzo, J., Bockenstedt, P., and Handin, R. I.,** Native conformation of human von Willebrand protein. Analysis by electron microscopy and quasi-elastic light scattering, *J. Biol. Chem.,* 260, 8559, 1985.

100. **Loscalzo, J., Slayter, H., Handin, R. I., and Farber, D.,** Subunit structure and assembly of von Willebrand factor polymer: complementary analysis by electron microscopy and quasi elastic light scattering, *Biophys. J.,* 49, 49, 1986.

101. **Bidwell, E., Dike, G. W., and Denson, D. W.,** Experiments with factor VIII separated from fibrinogen by electrophoresis in free buffer film, *Br. J. Haematol.,* 12, 583, 1966.

102. **Counts, R. B., Paskell, S. L., and Elgee, S. K.,** Disulfide bonds and the quaternary structure of factor VIII/von Willebrand factor, *J. Clin. Invest.,* 62, 702, 1978.

103. **Gralnick, H. R., Williams, S. B., and Morisato, D. K.,** Effect of multimeric structure of the factor VIII/vWF protein on binding to platelets, *Blood,* 58, 387, 1981.

104. **Perret, B. A., Furlan, M., and Beck, E. A.,** Studies on factor VIII-related protein. II. Estimation of molecular size differences between factor VIII oligomers, *Biochim. Biophys. Acta,* 578, 164, 1979.

105. **Martin, S. E., Marder, V. J., Francis, C. W., and Barlow, G. H.,** Structural studies on the functional heterogeneity of von Willebrand protein polymers, *Blood,* 57, 313, 1981.

106. **Hoyer, L. W. and Shainoff, J. R.,** Factor VIII-related protein circulates in normal human plasma as high molecular weight multimers, *Blood,* 55, 1056, 1980.

107. **Ruggeri, Z. M. and Zimmerman, T. S.,** Variant von Willebrand's disease. Characterization of two subtypes by analysis of multimeric composition of factor VIII/von Willebrand factor in plasma and platelets, *J. Clin. Invest.,* 65, 1318, 1980.

108. **Zimmerman, T. S., Roberts, J., and Edgington, T. S.,** Factor VIII-related antigen: multiple molecular forms in human plasma, *Proc. Natl. Acad. Sci. U.S.A.,* 72, 5121, 1975.

109. **Fulcher, C. A., Ruggeri, Z. M., and Zimmerman, T. S.,** Isoelectric focusing of human von Willebrand factor in urea-agarose gels, *Blood,* 61, 304, 1983.

110. **Austen, D. E., Carey, M., and Howard, M. A.,** Dissociation of factor VIII-related antigen into subunits, *Nature,* 53, 55, 1975.

111. **Titani, K., Ericsson, L. H., Kumar, S., Dorsam, H., Chopek, M. W., and Fujikawa, K.,** Chemical characterization of human von Willebrand factor, *Circulation,* 70-II(Abstr.), 210, 1984.

112. **Girma, J. P., Chopek, M. W., Titani, K., and Davie, E. W.,** Limited proteolysis of human von Willebrand factor by Staphylococcus aureus V-8 protease: isolation and partial characterization of a platelet-binding domain, *Biochemistry,* 25, 3156, 1986.

113. **Verweij, C. L., Diergaarde, P. J., Hart, M., and Pannekoek, H.,** Full-length von Willebrand factor (vWF) cDNA encodes a highly repetitive protein considerably larger than mature vWF subunit, *EMBO J.,* 5, 1839, 1986.

114. **Bonthron, D., Orr, E. C., Mitsock, L. M., Ginsburg, D., Handin, R. I., and Orkin, S. H.,** Nucleotide sequence of pre-pro von Willebrand factor cDNA, *Nucleic Acids Res.,* 14, 7125, 1986.

115. **Sadler, J. E., Shelton-Inloes, B. B., Sorace, J. M., Harlan, J. M., Titani, K., and Davie, E. W.,** Cloning and characterization of two cDNAs coding for human von Willebrand factor, *Proc. Natl. Acad. Sci. U.S.A.,* 82, 6394, 1985.

116. **Shelton-Inloes, B. B., Titani, K., and Sadler, J. E.,** cDNA sequences for human von Willebrand factor reveal five types of repeated domains and five possible protein sequence polymorphisms, *Biochemistry,* 25, 3164, 1986.

117. **Debeire, P., Montreuil, J., Samor, B., Mazurier, C., Goudemand, M., Van Halbeek, H., and Vliegenthart, J. F. G.,** Structure determination of the major asparagine-linked sugar chain of human factor VIII/von Willebrand factor, *FEBS Lett.,* 151, 22, 1983.

118. **Samor, B., Michalski, J. C., Debray, H., Mazurier, C., Goudemand, M., van Halbeek, H., Vliegenthart, J. F. G., and Montreuil, J.,** Primary structure of a new tetraantennary glycan of the N-acetyl lactosaminic type isolated from human factor VIII/von Willebrand factor, *Eur. J. Biochem.,* 158, 295, 1986.

119. **Loscalzo, J. and Handin, R. I.,** Conformational domains and structural transitions of human von Willebrand protein, *Biochemistry,* 23, 3880, 1984.

120. **Garnier, J., Osguthorpe, D. J., and Robson, B.,** Analysis of the accuracy and implications of simple methods for predicting the secondary structure of globular proteins, *J. Mol. Biol.,* 120, 97, 1978.

121. **Fujimura, Y., Titani, K., Holland, L., Russell, S., Roberts, J. T., Elder, J. H., Ruggeri, Z., and Zimmerman, T. S.,** von Willebrand factor. A reduced and alkylaled 52/48 kDa fragment beginning at amino acid residue 449 contains the domain interacting with platelet glycoprotein Ib, *J. Biol. Chem.,* 261, 381, 1986.

122. **Meyer, D., Obert, B., Pietu, G., Lavergne, J. M., and Zimmerman, T. S.,** Multimeric structure of factor VIII/von Willebrand factor in von Willebrand's disease, *J. Lab. Clin. Med.,* 95, 590, 1980.

123. **Ruggeri, Z. M. and Zimmerman, T. S.,** The complex multimeric composition of factor VIII/von Willebrand factor, *Blood,* 57, 1140, 1981.

124. **Fretto, L. T., Fowler, W. E., Hamilton, K. K., and McKee, P. A.,** Substructure of human von Willebrand factor (vWF) protomer: fragmentation by plasmin and S. aureus V8 protease (V8), *Thromb. Haemost.,* 54(Abstr. 348), 59, 1985.

125. **Loscalzo, J., Fish, M., and Handin, R. I.,** Solution studies of the quaternary structure and assembly of human von Willebrand factor, *Biochemistry,* 24, 4468, 1985.

126. **Kinoshita, S., Harrison, J., Lazerson, J., and Abildgaard, C. F.,** A new variant of dominant type II von Willebrand's disease with aberrant multimeric pattern of factor VIII related antigen (type II D), *Blood,* 63, 1369, 1984.

127. **Ciavarella, G., Ciavarella, N., Antoncecchi, S., De Mattia, D., Ranieri, P., Dent, J., Zimmerman, T. S., and Ruggeri, Z. M.,** High resolution analysis of von Willebrand factor multimeric composition defines a new variant of type I von Willebrand disease with aberrant structure but presence of all size multimers (type I C), *Blood,* 66, 1423, 1985.

128. **Tuddenham, E. G. D.,** The varieties of von Willebrand's disease, *Clin. Lab. Haematol.,* 6, 307, 1984.

129. **Mazurier, C., Samor, B., and Goudemand, M.,** Improved characterization of plasma von Willebrand factor heterogeneity when using 2.5% agarose gel electrophoresis, *Thromb. Haemost.,* 55, 61, 1986.

130. **Martin, S. E., Marder, V. J., Francis, C. W., Loftus, L. S., and Barlow, G. H.,** Enzymatic degradation of the factor VIII-von Willebrand protein: a unique tryptic fragment with ristocetin cofactor activity, *Blood,* 55, 848, 1980.

131. **Zimmerman, T. S., Dent, J. A., Ruggeri, Z. M., and Nannini, L. H.,** Subunit composition of plasma von Willebrand factor, *J. Clin. Invest.,* 77, 947, 1986.

132. **Wagner, D. D. and Marder, V. J.,** Biosynthesis of von Willebrand protein by human endothelial cells: identification of a large precursor polypeptide chain, *J. Biol. Chem.,* 258, 2065, 1983.

133. **Lynch, D. C., Zimmerman, T. S., Ling, E. H., and Browning, P. J.,** An explanation for minor multimer species in endothelial cell-synthesized von Willebrand factor, *J. Clin. Invest.,* 77, 2084, 1986.

134. **Barlow, G. H., Martin, S. E., and Marder, V. J.,** Sedimentation analysis of von Willebrand and factor VIII:C protein using partition cells in the analytical ultracentrifuge, *Blood,* 63, 940, 1984.

135. **Furlan, M., Stalder, M., Perret, B. A., and Beck, E. A.,** Surface of factor VIII/von Willebrand factor in solution: studies with dye-sensitized photochemical labelling, *Thromb. Res.,* 323, 343, 1983.

136. **Casillas, G., Simonetti, C., Lazzari, M., and Kempfer, A.,** Effects of ultrasonication on factor VIII, *Thromb. Haemost.,* 43, 68, 1980.

137. **Chan, V. and Chan, T. K.,** Characterization of factor VIII related protein synthesized by human endothelial cell: a study of structure and function, *Thromb. Haemost.,* 48, 177, 1982.

138. **Goudemand, J., Mazurier, C., Samor, B., Bouquelet, S., Montreuil, J., and Goudemand, M.,** Effect of carbohydrate modification of factor VIII/von Willebrand factor on binding to platelets, *Thromb. Haemost.,* 53, 390, 1985.

139. **Nachman, R. L., Jaffe, E. A., and Ferris, B.,** Peptide mape analysis of normal plasma and platelet factor VIII antigen, *Biochem. Biophys. Res. Commun.,* 92, 1208, 1980.

140. **Lopez-Fernandez, M. F., Ginsberg, M. H., Ruggeri, Z. M., Batlle, P. J., and Zimmerman, T. S.,** Multimeric structure of platelet factor VIII/von Willebrand factor: the presence of larger multimers and their reassociation with thrombin-stimulated platelets, *Blood,* 60, 1132, 1982.

141. **Gralnick, H. R., Williams, S. B., McKeown, L. P., Krizek, D. M., Shafer, B. C., and Rick, M. E.,** Platelet von Willebrand factor: comparison with plasma vWF, *Thromb. Res.,* 38, 623, 1985.

142. **Lopez-Fernandez, M. F., Lopez-Berges, C., Nieto, J., Martin, R., and Batlle, J.,** Platelet and plasma vWF: structural differences, *Thromb. Res.,* 44, 125, 1986.

143. **Fay, P. J., Kawai, Y., Wagner, D. D., Ginsburl, D., Bonthron, D., Ohlsson-Wilhelm, B. M., Chavin, S. I., Abraham, G. N., Handin, R. I., Ordin, S. H., Montgomery, R. R., and Marder, V. J.,** Propolypeptide of von Willebrand factor circulates in blood and is identical to von Willebrand antigen II, *Science,* 232, 995, 1986.

144. **Fay, P. J., Chavin, S. I., Schroeder, D., Young, F. E., and Marder, V. J.,** Purification and characterization of a highly purified human factor VIII consisting of a single type of polypeptide chain, *Proc. Natl. Acad. Sci. U.S.A.,* 79, 7200, 1982.

145. Italian Working Group, Spectrum of von Willebrand's disease: a study of 100 cases, *Br. J. Haematol.,* 35, 101, 1977.

146. **Shoa'i, I., Lavergne, J. M., Ardaillou, N., Obert, T., Ala, F., and Meyer, D.,** Heterogeneity of von Willebrand's disease: study of 40 Iranian cases, *Br. J. Haematol.,* 37, 67, 1977.

147. **Ruggeri, Z. M., Mannucci, P. M., Lombardi, R., Federici, A. B., and Zimmerman, T. S.,** Multimeric composition of factor VIII/von Willebrand factor following administration of DDAVP: implications for pathophysiology and therapy of von Willebrand's disease subtypes, *Blood,* 59, 1272, 1982.

148. **Blatt, P. M., Brinkhous, K. M., Culp, H. R., Krauss, J. S., and Robert, H. R.,** Antihemophilic factor concentrate therapy in von Willebrand disease. Dissociation of bleeding-time factor and ristocetin-cofactor activities, *JAMA,* 236, 2770, 1976.

149. **Green, D. and Potter, E. V.,** Platelet bound ristocetin aggregation factor in normal subjects and patients with von Willebrand's disease, *J. Lab. Clin. Med.,* 87, 976, 1976.

150. **Sixma, J., Sakariassen, K. S., Beeser-Visser, N. H., Ottenhof-Rovers, M., and Bolhuis, P. A.,** Adhesion of platelets to human artery subendothelium: effect of factor VIII-von Willebrand factor of various multimeric composition, *Blood,* 63, 128, 1984.

151. **Blomback, B., Hessel, B., Savidge, G., Wikstrom, L., and Blomback, M.,** The effect of reducing agents on factor VIII and other coagulation factors, *Thromb. Res.,* 12, 1177, 1978.

152. **Doucet-De-Bruine, M. H., Sixma, J. J., Over, J., and Beeser-Visser, N. H.,** Heterogeneity of human factor VIII. II. Characterization of forms of factor VIII binding to platelets in the presence of ristocetin, *J. Lab. Clin. Med.,* 92, 96, 1978.

153. **Over, J., Bouma, B. N., Van Mourik, J. A., Sixma, J. J., Vlooswijk, R., and Bakker-Woudenberg, I.,** Heterogeneity of human factor VIII. I. Characterization of the factor VIII present in the supernatant of cryoprecipitate, *J. Lab. Clin. Med.,* 91, 32, 1978.

154. **Pietu, G., Obert, B., Larrieu, M. J., and Meyer, D.,** Structure-function relationship of factor VIII/von Willebrand factor. Application to the study of variant von Willebrand's disease and cryosupernatant prepared from normal plasma, *Thromb. Res.,* 19, 671, 1980.

155. **Furlan, M., Perret, B. A., and Beck, E. A.,** Von Willebrand activity of low molecular weight human factor VIII increases by binding to gold granules, *Thromb. Haemost.,* 46, 242, 1981.

156. **Suzuki, K., Nishioka, J., and Hashimoto, S.,** The influence of 2 mercapto ethanol on von Willebrand factor and bovine aggregating factor, *Thromb. Res.,* 17, 443, 1980.

157. **Loscalzo, J. and Handin, R. I.,** Preservation of the polymeric structure and biologic activity of von Willebrand's protein after extensive disulfide reduction, *Clin. Res.,* 31(Abstr.), 318, 1983.

158. **Bockenstedt, P., Greenberg, J., and Handin, R. I.,** Structural basis of vWF binding to platelet glycoprotein Ib and collagen. Effects of disulfide reduction and limited proteolysis of polymeric vWF, *J. Clin. Invest.,* 77, 743, 1986.

158a. **Moake, J. L., Turner, N. A., Stathopoulos, N. A., Nolasco, L. H., and Hellums, J. D.,** Involvement of large plasma von Willebrand factor (vWF) multimers and unusually large vWF forms derived from endothelial cells in shear stress-induced platelet aggregation, *J. Clin. Invest.,* 78, 1456, 1986.

159. **Santoro, S. A.,** Adsorption of von Willebrand factor/factor VIII by the genetically distinct interstitial collagens, *Thromb. Res.,* 21, 689, 1981.

160. **Santoro, S. A.,** Preferential binding of high molecular weight forms of von Willebrand factor to fibrillar collagen, *Biochim. Biophys. Acta,* 756, 123, 1983.

161. **Kessler, C. M., Floyd, C. M., Rick, M. E., Krizek, D. M., Lee, S. L., and Gralnick, H. R.,** Collagen — factor VIII/von Willebrand factor protein interaction, *Blood,* 63, 1291, 1984.

162. **Morton, L. F., Griffin, B., Pepper, D. S., and Barnes, M. J.,** The interaction between collagens and factor VIII/von Willebrand factor: investigation of the structural requirement for interaction, *Thromb. Res.,* 32, 545, 1983.

163. **Wagner, D. D., Mayadas, T., Urban-Pickering, M., Lewis, B., and Marder, V. J.,** Inhibition of disulfide bonding of von Willebrand protein by monensin results in small, functionally defective multimers, *J. Cell Biol.,* 101, 112, 1985.

164. **Sakariassen, K. S., Fressinaud, E., Girma, J. P., Baumgartner, H. S., and Meyer, D.,** Mediation of platelet adhesion to fibrillar collagen in flowing blood by a proteolytic fragment of human von Willebrand factor, *Blood,* 67, 1515, 1986.

165. **Goodall, A. H., Jarvis, J., Chand, S., Rawlings, E., O'Brien, D. P., McGraw, A., Hutton, R., and Tuddenham, E. G. D.,** An immunoradiometric assay for human factor VIII/von Willebrand factor (VIII:vWf) using a monoclonal antibody that defines a functional epitope, *Br. J. Haematol.,* 59, 565, 1985.

166. **Nokes, T. J. C., Mahmoud, N. A., Savidge, G. F., Goodall, A. H., Meyer, D., Edington, T. S., and Hardisty, R. M.,** Von Willebrand factor has more than one binding site for platelets, *Thromb. Res.,* 34, 361, 1984.

167. **Stel, H. V., Sakariassen, K. S., Scholte, B. J., Veerman, E. C., Van Der Kwast, T. H., De Groot, P., Sixma, J. J., and Van Mourik, J. A.,** Characterization of 25 monoclonal antibodies to factor VIII — von Willebrand factor: relationship between ristocetin induced platelet aggregation and platelet adherence to subendothelium, *Blood,* 63, 1408, 1984.

168. **Stel, H. V., Sakariassen, K. S., De Groot, P. G., Van Mourik, J. A., and Sixma, J. J.,** Von Willebrand factor in the vessel wall mediates platelet adherence, *Blood,* 65, 85, 1985.

169. **Jorieux, S., De Romeuf, C., Samor, B., Goudemand, M., and Mazurier, C.,** Characterisation of a monoclonal antibody to von Willebrand factor as a potent inhibitor of ristocetin-mediated platelet interaction and platelet adhesion, *Thromb. Haemost.,* 57, 278, 1987.

169a. **Houdijk, W. P. M., Girma, J. P., Van Mourik, J. A., Sixma, J. J., and Meyer, D.,** Comparison of tryptic fragments of von Willebrand factor involved in binding to thrombin-activated platelets with fragments involved in ristocetin-induced binding and binding to collagen, *Thromb. Haemost.,* 56, 391, 1986.

170. **Girma, J. P., Kalafatis, M., and Meyer, D.,** Mapping of von Willebrand factor functional domains with monoclonal antibodies, in *Factor VIII-von Willebrand Factor,* Ciavarella, N. L., Ruggeri, Z. M., and Zimmerman, T. S., Eds., Wichtig Editore, Milan, 1986, 137.

171. **Girma, J. P., Kalafatis, M., Pietu, G., Lavergne, J. M., Chopek, M. W., Edgington, T. S., and Meyer, D.,** Mapping of distinct von Willebrand factor domains interacting with platelet GP Ib and GP IIb/IIIa and with collagen using monoclonal antibodies, *Blood,* 67, 1356, 1986.

172. **Sixma, J. J., Sakariassen, K. S., Stel, H. V., Houdijk, W. P. M., In Der Maur, D. W., Hamer, R. J., De Groot, P. G., and Van Mourik, J. A.,** Functional domains of von Willebrand factor. Recognition of discrete tryptic fragments by monoclonal antibodies that inhibit interaction of von Willebrand factor with platelets and with collagen, *J. Clin. Invest.,* 74, 736, 1984.

173. **Houdijk, W. P. M., Schiphorst, M. E., and Sixma, J. J.,** Identification of functional domains on von Willebrand factor by binding of tryptic fragments to collagen and to platelets in the presence of ristocetin, *Blood,* 67, 1498, 1986.

174. **Ruoslahti, E. and Pierschbacher, M. D.,** Arg-Gly-Asp: a versatile cell recognition signal, *Cell,* 44, 517, 1986.

175. **Pytela, R., Pierschbacher, M. D., Ginsberg, M. H., Plow, E. F., and Ruoslahti, E.,** Platelet membrane glycoprotein IIb/IIIa: member of a family of Arg-Gly-Asp-specific adhesion receptors, *Science,* 231, 1559, 1986.

176. **Plow, E. F., Pierschbacher, M. D., Ruoslahti, E., Marguerie, G. A., and Ginsberg, M. H.,** The effect of Arg-Gly-Asp-containing peptides on fibrinogen and von Willebrand factor binding to platelets, *Proc. Natl. Acad. Sci. U.S.A.,* 82, 8057, 1985.

177. **Pareti, F. I., Fujimura, Y., Dent, J. A., Holland, L. Z., Zimmerman, T. S., and Ruggeri, Z. H.,** Isolation and characterization of a collagen binding domain in human vWF, *J. Biol. Chem.,* 261, 15310, 1986.

178. **Andersen, J. C., Switzer, M. E. P., and McKee, P. A.,** Support of ristocetin-induced platelet aggregation by procoagulant-inactive and plasmin-cleaved forms of human factor VIII/von Willebrand factor, *Blood,* 55, 101, 1980.

179. **Martin, S. E., Francis, C. W., and Marder, V. J.,** Potentiation of wheat germ agglutinin aggregation of platelets by von Willebrand protein and by a 116 000 molecular weight tryptic fragment, *Thromb. Res.,* 31, 437, 1983.

180. **Hornsey, V., Micklem, L. R., McCann, M. C., James, K., Dawes, J., McClelland, D. B. L., and Prowse, C. V.,** Enhancement of factor VIII-von Willebrand factor ristocetin activity by monoclonal antibodies, *Thromb. Haemost.,* 54, 510, 1985.

181. **Meyer, D., Baumgartner, H. R., and Edgington, T. S.,** Hybridoma antibodies to human von Willebrand factor II. Relative role of intramolecular loci in mediation of platelet adhesion to the subendothelium, *Br. J. Haematol.,* 57, 609, 1984.

182. **Gralnick, H. R., Coller, B. S., and Sultan, Y.,** Carbohydrate deficiency of the factor VIII/von Willebrand factor protein in von Willebrand's disease variants, *Science,* 192, 56, 1976.

183. **Zimmerman, T. S., Voss, R., and Edgington, T. S.,** Carbohydrate of the factor VIII/von Willebrand factor in von Willebrand's disease, *J. Clin. Invest.,* 64, 1298, 1979.

184. **Gralnick, H. R., Jackson, G. M., Williams, S. B., and Cregger, M. C.,** Factor VIII/von Willebrand factor protein: sensitivity of periodic acid Schiff stain to carbohydrate deficiency, *Blood,* 59, 1310, 1982.

185. **Peake, I. R. and Bloom, A. L.,** Abnormal factor VIII related antigen (FVIIIR:Ag) in von Willebrand's disease (vWD): decreased precipitation by concanavalin A, *Thromb. Haemost.,* 37, 361, 1977.

186. **Takahashi, H., Sakuragawa, N., and Shibata, A.,** Decreased precipitation of factor VIIIR:Ag with concanavalin A in patients with a variant of vWD and disseminated intravascular coagulation, *Tohoku J. Exp. Med.,* 132, 141, 1980.

187. **Howard, M. A., Hendrix, L., and Firkin, B. G.,** Further studies on the factor VIII of a patient with a variant form of von Willebrand's disease, *Thromb. Res.,* 14, 609, 1979.

188. **Howard, M. A., Perkin, J., Koutts, J., and Firkin, B. G.,** Quantitation of binding of factor VIII antigen to concanavalin A, *Br. J. Haematol.,* 47, 607, 1981.

189. **Mikami, S., Veda, M., Yasvi, M., Takahashi, Y., Nishino, M., and Fukui, H.,** Heterogeneity of sugar composition of factor VIII/von Willebrand factor in von Willebrand's disease. Analysis by crossed affino-immunoelectrophoresis using lectin (Ricinus communis agglutinin 120), *Thromb. Haemost.,* 49, 87, 1983.

190. **Furlan, M., Perret, B. A., and Beck, E. A.,** Studies on factor VIII-related protein III. Size distribution and carbohydrate content of human and bovine factor VIII, *Biochem. Biophys. Acta.,* 579, 325, 1979.

191. **Furlan, M., Perret, B. A., and Beck, E. A.,** Studies on factor VIII-related protein IV. Interaction of galactose-specific lectins with human factor VIII/von Willebrand factor, *Biochem. Biophys. Acta,* 623, 402, 1980.

192. **Fukui, H., Mikami, S., Okuda, T., Murashima, N., Takase, T., and Yoshioka, A.,** Studies on von Willebrand factor: effect of different kinds of carbohydrate oxidases, SH inhibitors and some other chemical reagents, *Br. J. Haematol.,* 36, 259, 1977.

193. **Kessler, C. M., Floyd, C. M., and Franz, S.,** Effect of carbohydrate modification on factor VIII/von Willebrand factor protein-collagen interaction, *Clin. Res.,* 31(Abstr.), 316 A, 1983.

194. **Sodetz, J. M., Paulson, J., Pizzo, S. V., and McKee, P. A.,** Carbohydrate on human factor VIII/von Willebrand factor. Impairment of function by removal of specific galactose residues, *J. Biol. Chem.,* 253, 7202, 1978.

195. **Vermylen, J., Bottechia, D., and Szpilman, H.,** Factor VIII and human platelet aggregation III. Further studies on aggregation of human platelets by neuraminidase-treated human factor VIII, *Br. J. Haematol.,* 34, 321, 1976.

196. **De Marco, L., Girolami, A., Russell, S., and Ruggeri, Z. M.,** Interaction of asialo von Willebrand factor with glycoprotein Ib induces fibrinogen binding to the glycoprotein IIb/IIIa complex and mediates platelet aggregation, *J. Clin. Invest.,* 75, 1198, 1985.

197. **Gralnick, H. R., Williams, S. B., and Coller, B. S.,** Asialo von Willebrand factor interactions with platelets. Interdependence of glycoproteins Ib and IIb/IIIa for binding and aggregation, *J. Clin. Invest.,* 75, 19, 1985.

198. **Vermylen, J., Donati, M. B., De Gaetano, G., and Verstraete, M.,** Aggregation of human platelets by bovine or human factor VIII: role of carbohydrate, *Nature,* 244, 167, 1973.

199. **De Marco, L., Girolami, A., Zimmerman, T. S., and Ruggeri, Z. M.,** Interaction of purified type IIB von Willebrand factor with the platelet membrane glycoprotein Ib induces fibrinogen binding to the glycoprotein IIb/IIIa complex and initiates aggregation, *Proc. Natl. Acad. Sci. U.S.A.,* 82, 7424, 1985.

200. **Elder, J. H. and Alexander, S.,** Endo-N-acetylglucosaminidase F from Flavobacterium meningosepticum that cleaves both high mannose and complex glycoproteins, *Proc. Natl. Acad. Sci. U.S.A.,* 79, 4540, 1982.

201. **Wagner, D. D., Mayadas, T., and Marder, V. J.,** Initial glycosylation and acidic pH in the Golgi apparatus are required for multimerization of von Willebrand factor, *J. Cell Biol.,* 102, 1320, 1986.

202. **Browning, P. J., Ling, E. H., Zimmerman, T. S., and Lynch, D. C.,** Sulfation of von Willebrand factor by human umbilical vein endothelial cells, *Blood,* 62(Suppl.), 281, 1983.

203. **Jorieux, S., Magallon, T., and Mazurier, C.,** Evidence that NH2-terminal but not COOH-terminal moiety of plasma von Willebrand factor binds to factor VIII, *Thromb. Res.,* 48, 205, 1987.

204. **Foster, P. A., Fulcher, C. A., Marti, T., Titani, K., and Zimmerman, T. S.,** A major factor VIII binding domain resides within the amino-terminal 272 amino acid residues of von Willebrand factor, *J. Biol. Chem.,* 262, 8443, 1987.

205. **Takahashi, Y., Kalafatis, M., Girma, J. P., Sewerin, K., Andersson, L. O., and Meyer, D.,** Localization of a factor VIII binding domain on a 34 kilodaltons fragment of the N-terminal portion of von Willebrand factor, *Blood,* 70, 1679, 1987.
206. **Fujimura, Y., Titani, K., Holland, L. Z., Roberts, J. R., Kostel, P., Ruggeri, Z. M., and Zimmerman, T. S.,** A heparin-binding domain of human von Willebrand factor. Characterization and localization to a tryptic fragment extending from amino acid residue Val 449 to Lys 728, *J. Biol. Chem.,* 70, 1734, 1987.
207. **Titani, K., Takio, K., Handa, M., and Ruggeri, Z. M.,** Amino acid sequence of the von Willebrand factor-binding domain of platelet membrane glycoprotein Ib, *Proc. Natl. Acad. Sci. U.S.A.,* 84, 5610, 1987.
208. **Fujimura, Y., Holland, L. Z., Ruggeri, Z. M., and Zimmerman, T. S.,** The von Willebrand factor domain mediating botrocetin-induced binding to glycoprotein Ib lies between Val 449 an Lys 728, *Blood,* 70, 985, 1987.
209. **Roth, G. J., Titani, K., Hoyer, L. W., and Hickey, M. J.,** Localization of binding sites within human von Willebrand factor for monomeric type III collagen, *Biochemistry,* 25, 8357, 1986.
210. **Kalafatis, M., Takahashi, Y., Girma, J. P., and Meyer, K.,** Localization of a collagen-interactive domain of human von Willebrand factor between amino acid resudues Gly 911 and Glu 1365, *Blood,* 70, 1577, 1987.
211. **Fitzsimmons, C. M., Cockburn, C. G., Hornsey, V., Prowse, C. V., and Barnes, M. J.,** The interaction of von Willebrand factor (vWf) with collagen: investigation of vWf-binding sites in the collagen molecule, *Thromb. Haemost.,* 59, 186, 1988.

Chapter 4

MOLECULAR CLONING OF GENETIC MATERIAL ENCODING vWf

C. J. Verweij and H. Pannekoek

TABLE OF CONTENTS

I. Introduction 84

II. Molecular Cloning of vWf:cDNA 84

III. Nucleotide Sequence of Full Length vWf:cDNA 85

IV. Repetitive Structures of the Precursor Protein 88

V. Identity the Pro-Sequence and von Willebrand Antigen II 90

VI. The Chromosomal vWf Gene 91

VII. Concluding Remarks 92

Acknowledgments 93

References 93

I. INTRODUCTION

The von Willebrand factor (vWf) is a large glycoprotein of complex multimeric structure which mediates the adhesion of platelets to subendothelium after injury.[1] The vWf protein is synthesized by endothelial cells and is believed to be produced as a 275-kDa precursor which has been subjected to glycosylation and sulfatation and subsequently proteolytically processed to the mature 220-kDa subunit. Dimers aggregate to an array of heterogeneous structures which may consist of more than 50 subunits.[2-4] The larger multimers are most essential for the hemostatic function of vWf, namely the aggregation of platelets upon injury of the vessel wall.[5] A number of observations indicate that the mature protein is stored in the Weibel-Palade bodies.[6]

In plasma, vWf is the "carrier" protein for factor VIII, a crucial co-factor in the intrinsic coagulation cascade. It has been suggested that this function may be important for the observed survival of factor VIII *in vivo*.[7] However, the mechanism of this protective effect and the nature of the interaction remain to be fully elucidated.

vWf is clearly a multifunctional glycoprotein, displaying numerous and distinct protein-protein interactions. This is exemplified by the binding of vWf to platelets as its association and interaction with glycoprotein Ib[8-10] and the glycoprotein IIb/IIIa complex.[11,13] Components within the subendothelium which have been shown to interact with vWf include type I and type III collagen.[14] Furthermore, vWf self-aggregates into specific multimers interacting with VIII representing the circulating forms of the protein in plasma.

The localization of the sites responsible for the various interactions of the vWf protein and the elucidation of the mechanisms of such interactions remain a scientific challenge. The large molecular size and heterogeneity of the vWf protein have imposed further constraints on studies of structure/function relationships. However, the application of molecular biological techniques offers a direct and precise approach for the investigation of both the structure and function of vWf. In particular, the introduction of well-defined mutations within genetic material (e.g., cDNA) encoding vWf, and the subsequent expression of the mutated vWf:cDNA in a suitable host, should permit a detailed, unambiguous analysis of the different interaction sites. In this respect, the successful construction of a full-length vWf:cDNA[15,16] is a significant initial step towards such an analysis. Moreover, if the chromosomal vWf gene is shown to consist of several structural domains ("exons") which encode separate, autonomous functions, then a logical approach would be to express defined segments of vWf:cDNA and subsequently assay for the function(s) of the peptide. A similar strategy has been employed successfully to study another multifunctional plasma protein, tissue-type plasminogen activator (t-PA), where well-defined functions have been localized to a specific exon or a set of exons.[17,18] The use of restriction endonucleases, DNA modifying enzymes, site-directed mutagenesis, and other molecular biological tools should thus provide a powerful approach to elucidate the structure and function of the vWf glycoprotein.

II. MOLECULAR CLONING OF vWf:cDNA

The choice of the strategy for cloning vWf:cDNA has been rather limited due to scanty knowledge of the primary structure of the protein. Early groups of investigators were restricted by the lack of amino acid sequence data derived from the C-terminal part of vWf. Therefore, the obvious approach to detect vWf:cDNA by colony hybridization with a radiolabeled, complementary oligonucleotide derived from an amino acid sequence could not be applied. Using an alternative approach, by the application of poly- and monoclonal anti-vWf antibodies, four groups of investigators have recently and simultaneously reported the isolation of plasmids or bacteriophages which harbor partial vWf:cDNA inserts.[19-22]

Starting with polyA$^+$-RNA preparations, isolated from cultured human endothelial cells derived from unbilical vein, double-stranded cDNA was synthesized, which was then inserted either into a plasmid[19,21] or into a bacteriophage.[20,22] The resulting expression libraries, based on plasmid pUC9[23,24] or on phase λgtll,[25] were then screened with rabbit polyclonal anti-human vWf antibodies. In some cases, further screening was performed with a radiolabeled or a peroxidase-conjugated "anti-antibody". Using an alternative strategy, Lynch et al.[19] employed polyclonal anti vWf antibodies to isolate polysomes from which an enriched vWf mRNA preparation was obtained. The mRNA was then used as substrate for the synthesis of a single-stranded DNA probe.

The main conclusions which can be drawn from these studies[19-22] concern the predicted C-terminal amino acid sequence and the 3' part of the vWf mRNA. The sequence of the 11 C-terminal amino acid residues derived from the established nucleotide sequence is fully in agreement with the sequence determined by Edman degradation of the C-terminal cyanogen-bromide fragment of mature vWf (Glu-Cys-Lys-Cys-Ser-Pro-Arg-Lys-Cys-Ser-Lys).[46] This would imply that the vWf precursor glycoprotein is not proteolytically processed at its C-terminus. Furthermore, it is of interest that cysteine (Cys) residues are relatively abundant in the C-terminal part of vWf. Since dimerization of vWf subunits involves the formation of disulfide bonds between the C-termini of two vWf molecules,[26] it is feasible that these cysteine residues may participate in such interactions.

Nucleotide sequencing has provided evidence that vWf mRNA contains a relatively short 3' untranslated region of 136 nt. A typical polyadenylation signal (AATAAA)[27] was present 18 nucleotides upstream from the polyA tail. Northern blot analysis of human endothelial polyA[+] RNA, using vWf:cDNA as a probe, revealed an unexpectedly long mRNA of approximately 9000 nt.[19-21] This result was unexpected, since the coding sequence required for the presumed precursor of the vWf glycoprotein (275 kDa)[28] would approximate to 6000 nt. If vWf mRNA resembles other mRNAs and does not contain a very extensive 5' untranslated region, then it is likely that the actual precursor form of vWf is considerably larger than 275 kDa. Perhaps in this context it is worthwhile to reemphasize that large glycoproteins frequently behave anomalously in sodium-dodecyl sulfate (SDS)-polyacrylamide gel systems whereby molecular weight estimations may lack precision. Thus, these data should be reevaluated when accurate molecular weights are established by mulecular biological procedures.

III. NUCLEOTIDE SEQUENCE OF FULL LENGTH vWf:cDNA

Two groups of investigators have pursued the construction of a recombinant DNA molecule containing a full length vWf:cDNA.[15,16] These studies have provided new insights into the structure and the biosynthesis of the vWf glycoprotein and have resolved the enigma of the molecular weight of the vWf precursor protein. The entire nucleotide sequence of the full-length vWf:cDNA is given in Figure 1. This sequence is a compilation of the work by Sadler et al.,[22] mainly on the region encoding mature vWf, and Verweij et al.[15] on the region which codes for the pre-pro sequence of vWf. The full length vWf:cDNA, constructed by Verweij et al.,[15] comprises 8803 bp excluding the polyA tail. The sequence displays an extremely long "open" translation reading frame, starting at the ATG initiation condon, denoted as positions 1—3, and terminating at a TGA nonsense codon starting at position 8440. The coding region is preceded by a 5' untranslated stretch of at least 230 bp, and as already mentioned, is followed by a 3' untranslated region of 136 bp. Hence vWf mRNA harbors a continuous translation reading frame for 2813 amino acid residues. This polypeptide constitutes the pre-pro form of vWf. A comparison of the predicted amino acid sequence of the precursor with the NIH Data Bank (Protein Sequences) did not reveal any significant homology with other proteins.[15]

The N-terminus of the 2813 amino acid residue long polypeptide contains a sequence

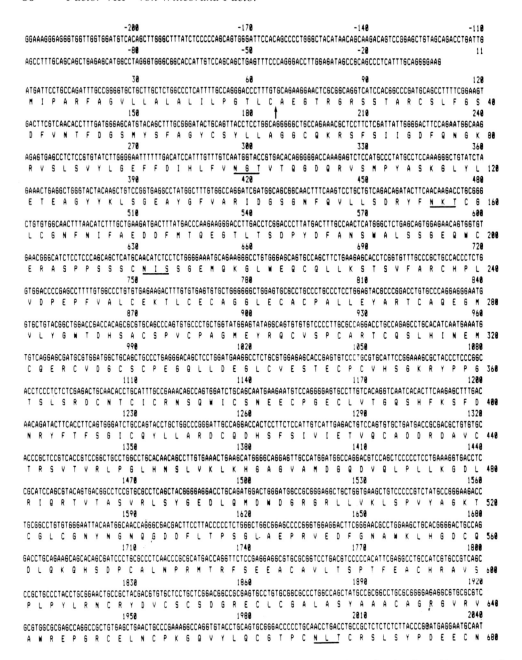

FIGURE 1. Complete nucleotide sequence of full length vWf:cDNA and the predicted amino acid sequence of pre-pro-vWf. The nucleotide sequence and the predicted amino acid sequence, which is represented by the one-letter code, are numbered separately. The arrows indicate the cleavage sites for the signal peptidase (between cysteine [C; 22] and alanine [A; 23]) and a proteinase (between arginine [R; 763] and serine [S; 764]), respectively. The pro-sequence extends from amino acid residue 23 (alanine; A) until 763 (arginine; R) and mature vWF from 764 (serine; S) until 2813 (lysine; K). The underlined sequences (N-X-S/T) represent potential asparagine (N)-linked glycosylation sites. The arginine-glycine-aspartic acid ("R-G-D") sequences, both in the pro-sequence and vWf, are boxed.

which is consistent with the consensus sequence for a signal peptide.[29] It has a core of ten consecutive hydrophobic residues, flanked by hydrophilic amino acids. The most probable cleavage site for a signal peptidase is located between the cysteine (position 22) and the alanine (position 23) residues.[29] Thus, it is likely that the N-terminus of the pro-sequence of vWf is occupied by an alanine residue. The calculated molecular weight of the precursor

```
                    2070              2100               2130              2160
GAGGCCTGCCTGGAGGGCTGCTTCTGCCCCCCAGGGCTCTACATGGATGAGAGGGGGGACTGCGTGCCCAAGGCCCAGTGCCCCTGTTACTATGACGGTGAGATCTTCCAGCCAGAAGAC
 E  A  C  L  E  G  C  F  C  P  P  G  L  Y  M  D  E [R  G  D] C  V  P  K  A  Q  C  P  C  Y  Y  D  G  E  I  F  Q  P  E  D  720
                    2190              2220               2250              2280
ATCTTCTCAGACCATCACACCATGTGCTACTGTGAGGATGGCTTCATGCACTGTACCATGAGTGGAGTCCCCGGAAGCTTGCTGCCTGACGCTGTCCTCAGCAGTCCCCTGTCTCATCGC
 I  F  S  D  H  H  T  M  C  Y  C  E  D  G  F  M  H  C  T  M  S  G  V  P  G  S  L  L  P  D  A  V  L  S  S  P  L  S  H  R  760
                    2310              2340               2370              2400
AGCAAAAGGAGCCTATCCTGTCGGCCCCCCATGGTCAAGCTGGTGTGTCCCGCTGACAACCTGCGGGCTGAAGGGCTCGAGTGTACCAAAACGTGCCAGAACTATGACCTGGAGTGCATG
 S  K  R  S  L  S  C  R  P  P  M  V  K  L  V  C  P  A  D  N  L  R  A  E  G  L  E  C  T  K  T  C  Q  N  Y  D  L  E  C  M  800
                    2430              2460               2490              2520
AGCATGGGCTGTGTCTCTGGCTGCCTCTGCCCCCCGGGCATGGTCCGGCATGAGAACAGATGTGTGGCCCTGGAAAGGTGTCCCTGCTTCCATCAGGGCAAGGAGTATGCCCCTGGAGAA
 S  M  G  C  V  S  G  C  L  C  P  P  G  M  V  R  H  E  N  R  C  V  A  L  E  R  C  P  C  F  H  Q  G  K  E  Y  A  P  G  E  840
                    2550              2580               2610              2640
ACAGTGAAGATTGGCTGCAACACTTGTGTCTGTCGGGACCGGAAGTGGAACTGCACAGACCATGTGTGTGATGCCACGTGCTCCACGATCGGCATGGCCCACTACCTCACCTTCGACGGG
 T  V  K  I  G  C  N  T  C  V  C  R  D  R  K  W  N  C  T  D  H  V  C  D  A  T  C  S  T  I  G  M  A  H  Y  L  T  F  D  G  880
                    2670              2700               2730              2760
CTCAAATACCTGTTCCCCGGGGAGTGCCAGTACGTTCTGGTGCAGGATTACTGCGGCAGTAACCCTGGGACCTTTCGGATCCTAGTGGGGAATAAGGGGATGCAGCCACCCCTCAGTGAAA
 L  K  Y  L  F  P  G  E  C  Q  Y  V  L  V  Q  D  Y  C  G  S  N  P  G  T  F  R  I  L  V  G  N  K  G  C  S  H  P  S  V  K  920
                    2790              2820               2850              2880
TGCAAGAAAACGGGTCACCATCCTGGTGGAGGGAGGAGAGATTGAGCTGTTTGACGGGGAGGTGAATGTGAAGAGGCCCATGAAGGATGAGACTCACTTTGAGGTGGTGGAGTCTGGCCGG
 C  K  K  R  V  T  I  L  V  E  G  G  E  I  E  L  F  D  G  E  V  N  V  K  R  P  M  K  D  E  T  H  F  E  V  V  E  S  G  R  960
                    2910              2940               2970              3000
TACATCATTCTGCTGCTGGGCAAAGCCCTCTCCGTGGTCTGGGACCGCCACCTGAGCATCTCCGTGGTCCTGAAGCAGACATACCAGGAGAAAGTGTGTGGCCTGTGTGGGAATTTTGAT
 Y  I  I  L  L  L  G  K  A  L  S  V  V  W  D  R  H  L  S  I  S  V  V  L  K  Q  T  Y  Q  E  K  V  C  G  L  C  G  N  F  D  1000
                    3030              3060               3090              3120
GGCATCCAGAACAATGACCTCACCAGCAGCAACCTCCAAGTGGAGGAGGACCCTGTGGACTTTGGGAAGTCCTGGGAAGTGAGCTCGCAGTGTGCTGACACCAGAAAAGTGCCTCTGGAC
 G  I  Q  N  N  D  L  T  S  S  N  L  Q  V  E  E  D  P  V  D  F  G  K  S  W  E  V  S  S  Q  C  A  D  T  R  K  V  P  L  D  1040
                    3150              3180               3210              3240
TCATCCCCTGCCACCTGCCATAACAACATCATGAAGCAGACGATGGTGGATTCCTCCTGTAGAATCCTTACCAGTGACGTCTTCCAGGACTGCAACAAGCTGGTGGACCCCGAGCCATAT
 S  S  P  A  T  C  H  N  N  I  M  K  Q  T  M  V  D  S  S  C  R  I  L  T  S  D  V  F  Q  D  C  N  K  L  V  D  P  E  P  Y  1080
                    3270              3300               3330              3360
CTGGATGTCTGCATTTACGACACCTGCTCCTGTGAGTCCATTGGGGACTGCGCCTGCTTCTGCGACACCATTGCTGCCTATGCCCACGTGTGTGCCCAGCATGGCAAGGTGGTGACCTGG
 L  D  V  C  I  Y  D  T  C  S  C  E  S  I  G  D  C  A  C  F  C  D  T  I  A  A  Y  A  H  V  C  A  Q  H  G  K  V  V  T  W  1120
                    3390              3420               3450              3480
AGGACGGCCACATTGTGCCCCCAGAGCTGCGAGGAGAGGAATCTCCGGGAGAACGGGTATGAGTGTGAGTGGCGCTATAACAGCTGTGCACCTGCCTGTCAAGTCACGTGTCAGCACCCT
 R  T  A  T  L  C  P  Q  S  C  E  E  R  N  L  R  E  N  G  Y  E  C  E  W  R  Y  N  S  C  A  P  A  C  Q  V  T  C  Q  H  P  1160
                    3510              3540               3570              3600
GAGCCACTGGCCTGCCCTGTGCAGTGTGTGGAGGGCTGCCATGCCCATTGCCCTCCAGGCAAAATCCTGGATGAGCTTTTGCAGACCTGCGTTGACCCTGAAGACTGTCCAGTGTGTGAG
 E  P  L  A  C  P  V  Q  C  V  E  G  C  H  A  H  C  P  P  G  K  I  L  D  E  L  L  Q  T  C  V  D  P  E  D  C  P  V  C  E  1200
                    3630              3660               3690              3720
GTGGCTGGCCGGCGTTTTGCCTCAGGAAAGAAAGTCACCTTGAATCCCAGTGACCCTGAGCACTGCCAGATTTGCCACTGTGATGTTGTCAACCTCACCTGTGAAGCCTGCCAGGAGCCG
 V  A  G  R  R  F  A  S  G  K  K  V  T  L  N  P  S  D  P  E  H  C  Q  I  C  H  C  D  V  V  N  L  T  C  E  A  C  Q  E  P  1240
                    3750              3780               3810              3840
GGAGGCCTGGTGGTGCCTCCACAGATGCCCCGGTGAGCCCACCACTCTGTATGTGGAGGACATCTCGGAACCGCCGTTGCACGATTTCTACTGCAGCAGGCTACTGGACCTGGTCTTC
 G  G  L  V  V  P  P  T  D  A  P  V  S  P  T  T  L  Y  V  E  D  I  S  E  P  P  L  H  D  F  Y  C  S  R  L  L  D  L  V  F  1280
                    3870              3900               3930              3960
CTGCTGGATGGCTCCTCCAGGCTGTCCGAGGCTGAGTTTGAAGTGCTGAAGGCCTTTGTGGTGGACATGATGGAGCGGCTGCGCATCTCCCAGAAGTGGGTCCGCGTGGCCGTGGTGGAG
 L  L  D  G  S  S  R  L  S  E  A  E  F  E  V  L  K  A  F  V  V  D  M  M  E  R  L  R  I  S  Q  K  W  V  R  V  A  V  V  E  1320
                    3990              4020               4050              4080
TACCACGACGGCTCCCACGCCTACATCGGGCTCAAGGACCGGAAGCGACCATCAGAGCTGCGGCGCATTGCCAGCCAGGTGAAGTATGCGGGCAGCCAGGTGGCCTCCACCAGCGAGGTC
 Y  H  D  G  S  H  A  Y  I  G  L  K  D  R  K  R  P  S  E  L  R  R  I  A  S  Q  V  K  Y  A  G  S  Q  V  A  S  T  S  E  V  1360
                    4110              4140               4170              4200
TTGAAATACACACTGTTCCAAATCTTCAGCAAGATCGACCGCCCCTGAAGCCTCCCGCATCGCCCTGCTCCTGATGGCCAGCCAGGAGCCCAACGGATGTCCCGGAACTTTGTCCGCTAC
 L  K  Y  T  L  F  Q  I  F  S  K  I  D  R  P  E  A  S  R  I  A  L  L  L  M  A  S  Q  E  P  Q  R  M  S  R  N  F  V  R  Y  1400
```

FIGURE 1 (continued).

protein of vWf, devoid of its signal peptide, is 307,029 kDa. These theoretical considerations have recently been confirmed by the demonstration that the N-terminal amino acid of the pro-sequence is alanine (position 23).[16] The entire coding sequence contains 16 potential N-linked glycosylation sites. Posttranslational modifications, such as glycosylation and sulfatation, will further increase the molecular weight. For example carbohydrate moieties contribute to about 15% by weight of the mature vWf glycoprotein.[30] Consequently, a realistic estimation of the molecular weight of the precursor of vWf is approximately 360 kDa.

The N-terminal sequence of the mature vWf subunit has been established by automated Edman degradation.[31-33] It reads Ser-Leu-Ser-Cys-Arg-Pro-Pro, and continues to align with the preducted amino acid sequence of the precursor. It was observed that this sequence

```
           4230              4260              4290              4320
GTCCAGGGCCTGAAGAAGAAGAAGGTCATTGTGATCCCGGTGGGCATTGGGCCCCATGCCAACCTCAAGCAGATCCGCCTCATCGAGAAGCAGGCCCCTGAGAACAAGGCCTTCGTGCTG
 V Q G L K K K K V I V I P V G I G P H A N L K Q I R L I E K Q A P E N K A F V L 1440
           4350              4380              4410              4440
AGCAGTGTGGATGAGCTGGAGCAGCAAAGGGACGAGATCGTTAGCTACCTCTGTGACCTTGCCCCTGAAGCCCCTCCTCCTACTCTGCCCCCCGACATGGCACAAGTCACTGTGGGCCCG
 S S V D E L E Q Q R D E I V S Y L C D L A P E A P P P T L P P D M A Q V T V G P 1480
           4470              4500              4530              4560
GGGCTCTTGGGGGTTTCGACCCTGGGGCCCAAGAGGAACTCCATGGTTCTGGATGTGGCGTTCGTCCTGGAAGGATCGGACAAAATTGGTGAAGCCGACTTCAACAGGAGCAAGGAGTTC
 G L L G V S T L G P K R N S M V L D V A F V L E G S D K I G E A D F N R S K E F 1520
           4590              4620              4650              4680
ATGGAGGAGGTGATTCAGCGGATGGATGTGGGCCAGGACAGCATCCACGTCACGGTGCTGCAGTACTCCTACATGGTGACCGTGGAGTACCCCTTCAGCGAGGCACAGTCCAAAGGGGAC
 M E E V I Q R M D V G Q D S I H V T V L Q Y S Y M V T V E Y P F S E A Q S K G D 1560
           4710              4740              4770              4800
ATCCTGCAGCGGGTGCGAGAGATCCGCTACCAGGGCGGCAACAGGACCAACACTGGGCTGGCCCTGCGGTACCTCTCTGACCACAGCTTCTTGGTCAGCCAGGGTGACCGGGAGCAGGCG
 I L Q R V R E I R Y Q G G N R T N T G L A L R Y L S D H S F L V S Q G D R E Q A 1600
           4830              4860              4890              4920
CCCAACCTGGTCTACATGGTCACCGGAAATCCTGCCTCTGATGAGATCAAGAGGCTGCCTGGAGACATCCAGGTGGTGCCCATTGGAGTGGGCCCTAATGCCAACGTGCAGGAGCTGGAG
 P N L V Y M V T G N P A S D E I K R L P G D I Q V V P I G V G P N A N V Q E L E 1640
           4950              4980              5010              5040
AGGATTGGCTGGCCCAATGCCCCTATCCTCATCCAGGACTTTGAGACGCTCCCCCGAGAGGCTCCTGACCTGGTGCTGCAGAGGTGCTGCTCCGGAGAGGGGCTGCAGATCCCCACCCTC
 R I G W P N A P I L I Q D F E T L P R E A P D L V L Q R C C S G E G L Q I P T L 1680
           5070              5100              5130              5160
TCCCCAGCACCTGACTGCAGCCAGCCCCTGGACGTGATCCTTCTCCTGGATGGCTCCTCCAGTTTCCCAGCTTCTTATTTTGATGAAATGAAGAGTTTCGCCAAGGCTTTCATTTCAAAA
 S P A P D C S Q P L D V I L L L D G S S S F P A S Y F D E M K S F A K A F I S K 1720
           5190              5220              5250              5280
GCCAATATAGGGCCTCGTCTCACTCAGGTGTCAGTGCTGCAGTATGGAAGCATCACCACCATTGACGTGCCATGGAACGTGGTCCCGGAGAAAGCCCATTTGCTGAGCCTTGTGGACGTC
 A N I G P R L T Q V S V L Q Y G S I T T I D V P W N V V P E K A H L L S L V D V 1760
           5310              5340              5370              5400
ATGCAGCGGGAGGGAGGGCCCCAGCCAAATCGGGGATGCCTTGGGCTTTGCTGTGCGATACTTGACTTCAGAAATGCATGGTGCCAGGCCGGGAGCCTCAAAGGCGGTGGTCATCCTGGTC
 M Q R E G G P S Q I G D A L G F A V R Y L T S E M H G A R P G A S K A V V I L V 1800
           5430              5460              5490              5520
ACGGACGTCTCTGTGGATTCAGTGGATGCAGCAGCTGATGCCGCCAGGTCCAACAGAGTGACAGTGTTCCCTATTGGAATTGGAGATCGCTACGATGCAGCCCAGCTACGGATCTTGGCA
 T D V S V D S V D A A A D A A R S N R V T V F P I G I G D R Y D A A Q L R I L A 1840
           5550              5580              5610              5640
GGCCCAGCAGGCGACTCCAACGTGGTGAAGCTCCAGCGAATCGAAGACCTCCCTACCATGGTCACCTTGGGCAATTCCTTCCTCCACAAACTGTGCTCTGGATTTGTTAGGATTTGCATG
 G P A G D S N V V K L Q R I E D L P T M V T L G N S F L H K L C S G F V R I C M 1880
           5670              5700              5730              5760
GATGAGGATGGGAATGAGAAGAGGCCCGGGGACGTCTGGACCTTGCCAGACCAGTGCCACACCGTGACTTGCCAGGCCAGATGGCCAGGACCTTGCTGAAGAGTCATCGGGTCAACTGTGAC
 D E D G N E K R P G D V W T L P D Q C H T V T C Q P D G Q T L L K S H R V N C D 1920
           5790              5820              5850              5880
CGGGGGGCTGAGGCCTTCGTGCCCTAACAGCCAGTCCCCTGTTAAAGTGGAAGAGACCTGTGGCTGCCGCTGGACCTGCCCCTGCGTGTGCACAGGCAGCTCCACTCGGCACATCGTGACC
 R G L R P S C P N S Q S P V K V E E T C G C R W T C P C V C T G S S T R H I V T 1960
           5910              5940              5970              6000
TTTGATGGGCAGAATTTCAAGCTGACTGGCAGCTGTTCTTATGTCCTATTTCAAAACAAGGAGCAGGACCTGGAGGTGATTCTCCATAATGGTGCCTGCAGCCCTGGAGCAAGGCAGGGC
 F D G Q N F K L T G S C S Y V L F Q N K E Q D L E V I L H N G A C S P G A R Q G 2000
           6030              6060              6090              6120
TGCATGAAATCCATCGAGGTGAAGCACAGTGCCCTCTCCGTCGAGCTGCACAGTGACATGGAGGTGACGGTGAATGGGAGACTGGTCTCTGTTCCTTACGTGGGTGGGAACATGGAGGTC
 C M K S I E V K H S A L S V E L H S D M E V T V N G R L V S V P Y V G G N M E V 2040
           6150              6180              6210              6240
AACGTTTATGGTGCCATCATGCATGAGGTCAGATTCAATCACCTTGGTCACATCTTCACATTCACTCCACAAAACAATGAGTTCCAACTGCAGCTCAGCCCCAAGACTTTTGCTTCAAAG
 N V Y G A I M H E V R F N H L G H I F T F T P Q N N E F Q L Q L S P K T F A S K 2080
           6270              6300              6330              6360
ACGTATGGTCTGTGTGGGATCTGTGATGAGAACGGAGCCAATGACTTCATGCTGAGGGATGGCACAGTCACCACAGACTGGAAAACACTTGTTCAGGAATGGACTGTGCAGCGGCCAGGA
 T Y G L C G I C D E N G A N D F M L R D G T V T T D W K T L V Q E W T V Q R P G 2120
```

FIGURE 1 (continued).

matches exactly with the residues, starting at position 764. Consequently, the mature vWf glycoprotein is preceded by a remarkably long pro-sequence of 741 amino acid residues.

IV. REPETITIVE STRUCTURES OF THE PRECURSOR PROTEIN

Sadler et al.[22] reported that about 50% of the mature vWf consists of repeated segments which display an identity ranging from 29 to 43%. Actually, these authors have observed a "head-to-tail" triplication of a domain ("A"), with the length of each repeated unit varying between 191 and 202 amino acids. Furthermore, two other duplicated domains ("B" and "C") were reported with a length of 25 to 35 amino acids and 116 to 119 amino acid residues, respectively. These findings are schematically drawn in Figure 2.

```
           6390              6420              6450              6480
CAGACGTGCCAGCCCATCCTGGAGGAGCAGTGTCTTGTCCCCGACAGCTCCCACTGCCAGGTCCTCCTCTTACCACTGTTTGCTGAATGCCACAAGGTCCTGGCTCCAGCCACATTCTAT
 Q  T  C  Q  P  I  L  E  E  Q  C  L  V  P  D  S  S  H  C  Q  V  L  L  L  P  L  F  A  E  C  H  K  V  L  A  P  A  T  F  Y    2160
           6510              6540              6570              6600
GCCATCTGCCAGCAGGACAGTTCGCACCAGGAGCAAGTGTGTGAGGTGATCGCCTCTTATGCCCACCTCTGTCGGACCAACGGGGTCTGCGTTGACTGGAGGACACCTGATTTCTGTGCT
 A  I  C  Q  Q  D  S  S  H  Q  E  Q  V  C  E  V  I  A  S  Y  A  H  L  C  R  T  N  G  V  C  V  D  W  R  T  P  D  F  C  A    2200
           6630              6660              6690              6720
ATGTCATGCCCACCATCTCTGGTCTACAACCACTGTGAGCATGGCTGTCCCCGGCACTGTGATGGCAACGTGAGCTCCTGTGGGGACCATCCCTCCGAAGGCTGTTTCTGCCCTCCAGAT
 M  S  C  P  P  S  L  V  Y  N  H  C  E  H  G  C  P  R  H  C  D  G  N  V  S  S  C  G  D  H  P  S  E  G  C  F  C  P  P  D    2240
           6750              6780              6810              6840
AAAGTCATGTTGGAAGGCAGCTGTGTCCCTGAAGAGGCCTGCACTCAGTGCATTGGTGAGGATGGAGTCCAGCACCAGTTCCTGGAAGCCTGGGTCCCGGACCACCAGCCCTGTCAGATC
 K  V  M  L  E  G  S  C  V  P  E  E  A  C  T  Q  C  I  G  E  D  G  V  Q  H  Q  F  L  E  A  W  V  P  D  H  Q  P  C  Q  I    2280
           6870              6900              6930              6960
TGCACATGCCTGAGCGGGCGGAAGGTCAACTGCACAACGCAGCCCTGCCCCACGGCCAAAGCTCCCACGTGTGGCCTGTGTGAAGTAGCCCGCCTCCGCCAGAATGCAGACCAGTGCTGC
 C  T  C  L  S  G  R  K  V  N  C  T  T  Q  P  C  P  T  A  K  A  P  T  C  G  L  C  E  V  A  R  L  R  Q  N  A  D  Q  C  C    2320
           6990              7020              7050              7080
CCCGAGTATGAGTGTGTGTGTGACCCAGTGAGCTGTGACCTGCCCCCAGTGCCTCACTGTGAACGTGGCCTCCAGCCCACACTGACCAACCCTGGCGAGTGCAGACCCAACTTCACCTGC
 P  E  Y  E  C  V  C  D  P  V  S  C  D  L  P  P  V  P  H  C  E  R  G  L  Q  P  T  L  T  N  P  G  E  C  R  P  N  F  T  C    2360
           7110              7140              7170              7200
GCCTGCAGGAAGGAGGAGTGCAAAAGAGTGTCCCCACCCTCCTGCCCCCCGCACCGTTTGCCCACCCTTCGGAAGACCCAGTGCTGTGATGAGTATGAGTGTGCCTGCAACTGTGTCAAC
 A  C  R  K  E  E  C  K  R  V  S  P  P  S  C  P  P  H  R  L  P  T  L  R  K  T  Q  C  C  D  E  Y  E  C  A  C  N  C  V  N    2400
           7230              7260              7290              7320
TCCACAGTGAGCTGTCCCCTTGGGTACTTGGCCTCAACCGCCACCAATGACTGTGGCTGTACCACCAACCACCTGCCTTCCCGACAAGGTGTGTGTCACCGAAGCACCATCTACCCTGTG
 S  T  V  S  C  P  L  G  Y  L  A  S  T  A  T  N  D  C  G  C  T  T  T  T  C  L  P  D  K  V  C  V  H  R  S  T  I  Y  P  V    2440
           7350              7380              7410              7440
GGCCAGTTCTGGGAGGAGGGCTGCGATGTGTGCACCTGCACCGACATGGAGGATGCCGTGATGGGCCTCCGCGTGGCCCAGTGCTCCCAGAAGCCCTGTGAGGACAGCTGTCGGTCGGGC
 G  Q  F  W  E  E  G  C  D  V  C  T  C  T  D  M  E  D  A  V  M  G  L  R  V  A  Q  C  S  Q  K  P  C  E  D  S  C  R  S  G    2480
           7470              7500              7530              7560
TTCACTTACGTTCTGCATGAAGGCGAGTGCTGTGGAAGGTGCCTGCCATCTGCCTGTGAGGTGGTGACTGGCTCACCGCGGGGGGACTCCCAGTCTTCCTGGAAGAGTGTCGGCTCCCAG
 F  T  Y  V  L  H  E  G  E  C  C  G  R  C  L  P  S  A  C  E  V  V  T  G  S  P [R  G  D] S  Q  S  S  W  K  S  V  G  S  Q    2520
           7590              7620              7650              7680
TGGGCCTCCCCGGAGAACCCCTGCCTCATCAATGAGTGTGTCCGAGTGAAGGAGGAGGTCTTTATACAACAAAGGAACGTCTCCTGCCCCCAGCTGGAGGTCCCTGTCTGCCCCTCGGGC
 W  A  S  P  E  N  P  C  L  I  N  E  C  V  R  V  K  E  E  V  F  I  Q  Q  R  N  V  S  C  P  Q  L  E  V  P  V  C  P  S  G    2560
           7710              7740              7770              7800
TTTCAGCTGAGCTGTAAGACCTCAGCGTGCTGCCCCAAGCTGTCGCTGTGAGCGCATGGAGGCCTGCATGCTCAATGGCACTGTCATTGGGCCCGGGAAGACTGTGATGATCGATGTGTGC
 F  Q  L  S  C  K  T  S  A  C  C  P  S  C  R  C  E  R  M  E  A  C  M  L  N  G  T  V  I  G  P  G  K  T  V  M  I  D  V  C    2600
           7830              7860              7890              7920
ACGACCTGCCGCTGCATGGTGCAGGTGGGGGTCATCTCTGGATTCAAGCTGGAGTGCAGGAAGACCACCTGCAACCCCTGCCCCCTGGGTTACAAGGAAGAAAATAACACAGGTGAATGT
 T  T  C  R  C  M  V  Q  V  G  V  I  S  G  F  K  L  E  C  R  K  T  T  C  N  P  C  P  L  G  Y  K  E  E  N  N  T  G  E  C    2640
           7950              7980              8010              8040
TGTGGGAGGATGTTTGCCTACGGCTTGCACCATTCAGCTAAGAGGAGGACAGATCATGCACACTGAAGCGTGATGAGCAGCTCCAGGATGGCTGTGATACTCACTTCTGCAAGGTCAATGAG
 C  G  R  C  L  P  T  A  C  T  I  Q  L  R  G  G  Q  I  M  T  L  K  R  D  E  T  L  Q  D  G  C  D  T  H  F  C  K  V  N  E    2680
           8070              8100              8130              8160
AGAGGAGAGTACTTCTGGGAGAAGAGGGTCACAGGCTGCCCCACCCTTTGATGAACACAAGTGTCTGGCTGAGGGAGGTAAAATTATGAAAATTCCAGGCACCTGCTGTGACACATGTGAG
 R  G  E  Y  F  W  E  K  R  V  T  G  C  P  P  F  D  E  H  K  C  L  A  E  G  G  K  I  M  K  I  P  G  T  C  C  D  T  C  E    2720
           8190              8220              8250              8280
GAGCCTGAGTCCAACGACATCHCTGCCAGTATGTCAGGACCAGTGCTGCTGCTGCTCTCCGACACGGACGGGAGCCCCATGCAGGTGGCCCTGCACTGCACCAATGGCTCTGTTGTGTACCATCAGGTTCTCAAT
 E  P  E  S  N  D  I  T  A  R  L  Q  Y  V  K  V  G  S  C  K  S  E  V  E  V  D  I  H  Y  C  Q  G  K  C  A  S  K  A  M  Y    2760
           8310              8340              8370              8400
TCCATTGACATCAACGATGTGCAGGACCAGTGCTCCTGCTGCTCTCCGACACGGACGGGAGCCCCATGCAGGTGGCCCTGCACTGCACCAATGGCTCTGTTGTGTACCATCAGGTTCTCAAT
 S  I  D  I  N  D  V  Q  D  Q  C  S  C  C  S  P  T  R  T  E  P  M  Q  V  A  L  H  C  T  N  G  S  V  V  Y  H  Q'V  L  N    2800
           8430              8460              8490              8520
GCCATGGAGTGCAAATGCTCCCCCAGGAAGTGCAGCAAGTGA
 A  M  E  C  K  C  S  P  R  K  C  S  K                                                                                    2840
```

FIGURE 1 (continued).

Besides the homologies among these domains, the distribution of the cysteine residues appears significant. The frequency of appearance and the position of cysteines are characteristic for each set of domains. The domains A1, A2, and A3 harbor relatively few of these residues (0.5 to 1.0%), whereas the domains B1, B2, and C1, C2 contain a very high percentage of cysteine residues of 20 to 24% and 13 to 15%, respectively. These observations suggest that a particular interaction of the vWf protein with another component (e.g., glycoprotein Ib, glycoprotein IIb/IIIa, collagens, or VIII) is influenced by two or three active sites (domains) on the vWf molecules. If this interpretation is valid, then it would be interesting to determine whether these sites contribute in an additive or a synergistic mode to the protein-protein interaction. In this respect, it should be noted that both collagens[34]

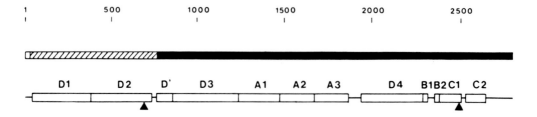

FIGURE 2..   Schematic representation of the repetitive structure of pro-vWf. The upper line in this diagram represents the vWf precursor protein (open area, signal peptide; hatched area, pro-sequence; dark area, mature vWF). Beneath this line are indicated the triplicated domain "A" (A1, A2, and A3); two duplicated domains "B" (B1 and B2) and "C" (C1 and C2), as reported by Sadler et al.;[22] the quadruplicated domain "D" (D1, D2, D3 and D4); and the partly duplicated domain D'. These repeats correspond with the following amino acid residues: A1 (1242—1480), A2 (1480—1673), A3 (1673—1875), B1 (2296—2331), B2 (2375—2400), C1 (2400—2516), C2 (2544—2663), D1 (34—387), D2 (387—746), D3 (866—1242), D4 (1947—2299) and D' (769—866). The positions of the R-G-D tripeptides are shown with a triangle.

and VIII[35,36] resemble vWf in that they also consist of repeated domains. The presence of these repeated domains could permit multiple interactions among these proteins.

The elucidation of the nucleotide sequence of the prosegment of vWf[15] revealed another domain (D') which has been quadruplicated, as seen in Figure 2. Domains D1 and D2 are present in the pro-sequence, while domains D3 and D4 are encountered on mature vWf, of which each covers 350 to 400 amino acid residues. Moreover, an incomplete D domain (D') is also found in mature vWf between the N-terminus and the domain D3. This implies that about 90% of the entire precursor protein is composed of repeated structures. In addition it has been reported[15] that both the frequency of appearance and the position of the cysteines in the various type D domains are similar, suggesting an analogous secondary structure. The observation that the pro-sequence and mature vWf each harbor two corresponding domains may imply that these polypeptides have a biological function in common, provided that the pro-sequence is a stable protein in plasma. This argument is strengthened by another common feature between these polypeptides. Sadler et al.[22] indicated that the predicted amino acid sequence of mature vWf includes an arginine-glycine-aspartic acid-(serine) stretch denoted "R-G-D-S" or "R-G-D" region. The R-G-D sequence is present in the C-terminal part of domain C1. This sequence mediates, at least in part, the cell attachment activity of fibronectin.[37,38] vWf and fibronectin compete for binding to the receptor glycoprotein IIb/IIIa on platelets, and these interactions are inhibited by R-G-D containing peptides. These results suggest that the R-G-D region on mature vWf is involved in this interaction with platelets. The pro-sequence also includes a R-G-D region which is located in the C-terminal part of domain D2. Based on the striking homology between the pro-sequence and mature vWf and the presence of a possible "cell attachment site (R-G-D)", it is tempting to speculate that the pro-sequence and mature vWf perform analogous interactions.

V. IDENTITY OF THE PRO-SEQUENCE AND VON WILLEBRAND ANTIGEN II

It has been reported that, apart from vWf, a second protein is absent in plasma from patients with severe von Willebrand's disease.[39] Analogous to vWf, this other protein, denoted von Willebrand antigen II (vW:AgII) is also synthesized in vascular endothelial cells and apparently stored in the Weibel-Palade bodies.[16,40] vW:AgII is a glycoprotein of unknown function with an apparent molecular weight of 100 kDa and is relatively stable in plasma. Both vWf and vW:AgII are released after *in vivo* stimulation with 1-desamino-8-D-arginine-vasopressin (DDAVP).[41] These observations suggest a common feature in the biosynthesis of vW and vW:AgII.

Table 1
MATCHING OF N-TERMINAL AMINO ACID SEQUENCE OF vWf:AgII AND
THAT DERIVED FROM vWf:cDNA

vWf:cDNA

5' nucleotide sequence (nucleotides 296—328):	GAC	GAA	GGA	ACT	CGC	GGC	AGG	TCA	TCC	ACG	GCC
Predicted amino acids:	Ala	Glu	Gly	Thr	Arg	Gly	Arg	Ser	Ser	Thr	Ala

Intact vWf:AgII

N-terminal sequence:	Ala	Glu	Gly	Thr	—	Gly	—	Ser	Ser	Thr	Ala
Residue position:	1	2	3	4	5	6	7	8	9	10	11

Note: The 5' nucleotide sequence has been taken from Verweij et al.[15] The numbering (296—328, see Figure 1) corresponds with nucleotides 67—99 of Fay et al.[16] The N-terminal amino acid sequence of vWf:AgII has been determined by automated Edman degradation.[16]

The molecular cloning of full length vWf:cDNA revealed an "open" reading frame of 2813 amino acids, while mature vWf comprises the C-terminal 2050 amino acid residues.[15] These data suggested that vWf mRNA may encode two distinct polypeptides, and it has been proposed that the pro-sequence may be equivalent to vW:AgII.[15] This hypothesis was recently confirmed by Fay et al.[16] who demonstrated unambiguously that the pro-sequence is identical to vW:AgII. The amino acid sequence of the N-terminus of vW:AgII, determined by automated Edman degradation, matches with the amino acid sequence predicted from a nucleotide sequence of vWf:cDNA, derived from the 5' end of vWf mRNA, as demonstrated in Table 1. Furthermore, these data are concordant to the amino acid sequence predicted from the full length vWf:cDNA nucleotide sequence of Verweij et al.[15] The observation that a monoclonal antibody, raised against vW:AgII, precipitated both vW:AgII (molecular weight approximately 100 kDa) and the precursor of vWf is consistent with this conclusion. Immunofluorescent staining of permeabilized endothelial cells with this monoclonal antibody results in the formation of specific immune complexes in the Weibel-Palade bodies, representing either free vW:AgII or the precursor of vWf. Consequently, these authors have concluded that the pro-sequence of vWf is identical to vW:AgII. The calculated molecular weight of unglycosylated vW:AgII is approximately 81 kDa,[15] a value which is consistent with the determined molecular weight of the vW:AgII glycoprotein of approximately 100 kDa.[40]

VI. THE CHROMOSOMAL vWf GENE

The chromosomal localization of the vWf gene was determined both by Southern blotting of DNA isolated from panels of somatic human-rodent cell hybrids[20,21] and by *in situ* chromosomal hybridization.[20] The results of both studies indicate that the human genome harbors a single copy of the vWf gene and that this gene is present in chromosome 12. The *in situ* hybridization experiments assigned the position to the region 12p12—12pter. It should be noted that this assignment contradicts a previous opinion based upon a more empirical immunological approach, that the vWf gene is located on chromosome 5.[42] The elucidation of the chromosomal structure of the vWf gene awaits further studies.

vWf:cDNA probes were further used to detect a restriction fragment-length polymorphism (RFLP) among normal European Caucasians.[43] The combination of blotted chromosomal DNA digested with the restriction endonuclease BgIII and a 1100-bp Pst.I vWf:cDNA fragment as a probe yielded a simple two-allele polymorphism. The hybridization reveals

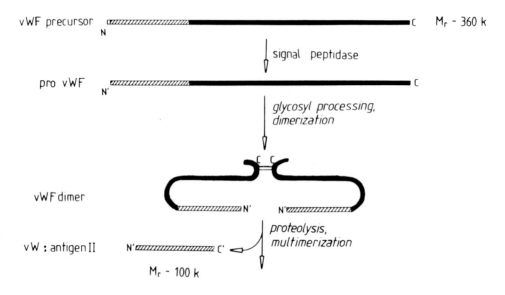

FIGURE 3. Schematic representation of the processing steps involved in the biosynthesis of mature vWf. The lines in this scheme represent the precursor vWf protein and the processing products derived from it. The open area is the signal peptide, the hatched area the pro-sequence (vWf:AgII), and the dark area the mature VWf. Pro-vWf is generated by the activity of a signal peptidase which removes 22 amino acid residues from the N-terminus of pre-pro-vWf. The pro-vWf molecules are further processed to form dimers. Multimerization of dimers is accompanied by the proteolytic cleavage of pro-vWF by a proteinase to yield both the mature vWf and vW:AgII.

two variant fragments with a length of 9 and 7.4 kb, which occur at a frequency of 69 and 31%, respectively. Recently, it has been shown that the polymorphic sequence is present in an intron which is located within the chromosomal vWf gene.[47] This observation is particularly relevant for an application of this RFLP in the genetic analysis of von Willebrand families. It indicates a close linkage between the polymorphic sequence and a possible defect within the structural gene, almost excluding crossing-over events which perturb the validity of this method. Additional RFLPs for the vWf gene are desirable to increase the reliability of diagnosis of carriers for von Willebrand's disease.

VII. CONCLUDING REMARKS

The foregoing paragraphs summarize the contribution of recent molecular biological experiments to our knowledge on the biosynthesis, the structure, and the function of the vWf glycoprotein. New data, mainly on physical parameters of the precursor and the mature vWf glycoprotein, have been generated. The finding that vWf mRNA is considerably longer than required to encode the originally presumed precursor protein has been the starting point for a new concept of the biosynthesis of vWf. It is evident that vWf mRNA codes for two distinct proteins, i.e.; the mature vWf glycoprotein and vW:AgII. The simplest scheme for the biosynthesis of mature vWf includes only two proteolytic processing steps, as shown in Figure 3. First, a signal peptidase removes the N-terminal signal peptide of 22 amino acid residues during transport of the growing polypeptide chain across the rough endoplasmatic reticulum. These pro-vWf molecules, consisting of 2791 amino acid residues will form dimers and will be subject to post translational processing (glycosylation, sulfatation), resulting in a molecular weight for each subunit of approximately 360 kDa. The discrepancy between this molecular weight for the pro-vWf glycoprotein and the value of 275 kDa reported by Wagner and Marder[28] is probably due to inaccuracy of molecular weight estimations of large glycoproteins in SDS-polyacrylamide gels. Second, a specific proteinase will cleave the pro-vWf molecular between the arginine and serine residues at positions 763 and 764, generating the two proteins vW:AgII and mature vWf. Both the proteolytic processing and multimerization of dimers may occur in the Golgi apparatus and/or within the Weibel-Palade bodies. These storage organelles may also serve for the processing of the precursor of vWf, resulting in the liberation of vWF:AgII and mature vWf. An indication that the crucial processing event may occur within the Weibel-Palade bodies can be inferred from the data of McCarroll and co-workers.[40] Using immunological methods, these investigators were able to detect a complex between vW:AgII and vWf in Weibel-Palade bodies, but only in the presence of phenyl-methyl-sulfonyl fluoride (PMSF), an inhibitor of serine proteases.

The repetitive structure of the precursor vWf protein, including two duplications, a triplication, and a quadruplication, indicates that the chromosomal gene has evolved from duplicative events of four different domains. Analogous to the mosaic gene structure of several coagulation and fibrinolysis proteins,[44,45] it is expected that separate domains are located on an exon or a set of adjacent exons. Provided that such domains display autonomous functions, similar to t-PA,[18] experiments can be devised to express selected portions of vWf:cDNA in a suitable host. The resulting mutant proteins could then be analyzed to localize a specific function and to elucidate in depth the mechanism of action of vWf with other proteins.

ACKNOWLEDGMENTS

The authors express their gratitude to Dr. D. J. Loskutoff for his critical reading of the manuscript. This study was supported by the Netherlands Organization for the Advancement of Pure Research (ZWO) (Grant no.-13/90-91).

REFERENCES

1. **Hoyer, L. W.,** The factor VIII complex: structure and function, *Blood,* 58, 1, 1981.
2. **Legaz, M. E., Schmer, G., Counts, R. B., and Davie, E. W.,** Isolation and characterization of human factor VIII (antihemophilic factor), *J. Biol. Chem.,* 248, 3946, 1973.
3. **Ruggeri, Z. M. and Zimmerman, T. S.,** Variants von Willebrand's disease: characterization of two subtypes by analysis of multimeric composition of factor VIII/von Willebrand factor in plasma and platelets, *J. Clin. Invest.,* 65, 1318, 1980.
4. **Hoyer, L. W. and Shainoff, J. R.,** Factor VIII-related protein circulates in normal human plasma as high molecular weight multimers, *Blood,* 55, 1056, 1980.
5. **Zimmerman, T. S., Ruggeri, Z. M., and Fulcher, C. A.,** Factor VIII/von Willebrand factor, in *Progress in Hematology,* Vol. 13, Brown, E. B., Ed., Grune & Stratton, New York, 1983, 279.
6. **Wagner, D. D., Olmsted, J. B., and Marder, V. J.,** Immunolocalization of von Willebrand protein in Weibel-Palade bodies of human endothelial cells, *J. Cell Biol.,* 95, 355, 1982.
7. **Tuddenham, E. G. D., Lane, R. S., Rotblat, F., Johnson, A. J., Snape, T. J., Middleton, S., and Kernoff, P. B. A.,** Response to infusions of electrolyte fractionated human factor VIII concentrate in human haemophilia A and von Willebrand's disease, *Br. J. Haematol.,* 52, 259, 1982.
8. **Jenkins, C. S. P., Phillips, D. R., Clemetson, K. J., Meyer, D., Larrieu, M.-J., and Luschen, E. F.,** Platelet membrane glycoproteins implicated in ristocetin-induced aggregation, *J. Clin. Invest.,* 57, 112, 1976.
9. **Okumura, T. and Jamieson, G. A.,** Platelet glycocalicin: a single receptor for platelet aggregation induced by thrombin or ristocetin, *Thromb. Res.,* 8, 701, 1976.
10. **Nachman, R. L., Jaffe, E. A., and Webster, B. B.,** Immuno-inhibition of ristocetin-induced platelet aggregation, *J. Clin. Invest.,* 59, 143, 1977.
11. **Fujimoto, T., Ohara, S., and Hawiger, J.,** Thrombin-induced exposure and prostacyclin inhibition of the receptor for factor VII/von Willebrand factor on human platelets, *J. Clin. Invest.,* 69, 1212, 1982.

12. **Fujimoto, T. and Hawiger, J.,** Adenosine diphosphate induces binding of von Willebrand factor to human platelets, *Nature,* 297, 154, 1982.

13. **Ruggeri, Z. M., Bader, R., and De Marco, L.,** Glanzmann thrombasthenia: deficient binding of von Willebrand factor to thrombin-stimulated platelets, *Proc. Natl. Acad. Sci. U.S.A.,* 79, 6038, 1982.

14. **Sixma, J. J., Sakariassen, K. S., Stel, H. V., Houdijk, W. P. M., In der Maur, D. W., Hamer, R., De Groot, Ph. G., and Van Mourik, J. A.,** Functional domains on von Willebrand factor: recognition of discrete tryptic fragments by monoclonal antibodies inhibiting interaction of von Willebrand with platelets and with collagen, *J. Clin. Invest.,* 74, 736, 1984.

15. **Verweij, C. L., Diergaarde, P. J., Hart, M., and Pannekoek, H.,** Full length von Willebrand factor (vWF) cDNA encodes a highly repetitive protein, considerably larger than mature vWF, *EMBO J.,* 5, 183g, 1986.

16. **Fay, P. J., Kawai, Y., Wagner, D. D., Ginsburg, D., Bonthron, D., Ohlsson-Wilhelm, B. M., Chavin, S. I., Abraham, G. N., Handin, R. I., Orkin, S. H., Montgomery, R. R., and Marder, V. J.,** The propolypeptide of von Willebrand factor circulates in blood and is identical to von Willebrand antigen II, *Science,* 232, 995, 1986.

17. **Ny, T., Elgh, F., and Lund, B.,** The structure of the human tissue-type plasminogen activator gene: correlation of intron and exon structures to functional and structural domains, *Proc. Natl. Acad. Sci. U.S.A.,* 81, 5355, 1984.

18. **Van Zonneveld, A.-J., Veerman, H., and Pannekoek, H.,** Autonomous functions of structural domains on human tissue-type plasminogen activator, *Proc. Natl. Acad. Sci. U.S.A.,* 83, 4670, 1986.

19. **Lynch, D. C., Zimmerman, T. S., Collins, C. J., Brown, M., Morin, M. J., Ling, E. H., and Livingston, D. M.,** Molecular cloning of cDNA for human von Willebrand factor: authentication by a new method, *Cell,* 41, 49, 1985.

20. **Ginsburg, D., Handin, R. I., Bonthron, D. T., Donlon, T. A., Bruns, G. A. P., Latt, S. A., and Orkin, S. H.,** Human von Willebrand (vWF): isolation of complementary DNA (cDNA) clones and chromsomal localization, *Science,* 228, 1401, 1985.

21. **Verweij, C. L., De Vries, C. J. M., Distel, B., Van Zonneveld, A.-J., Geurts van Kessel, A., Van Mourik, J. A., and Pannekoek, H.,** Construction of cDNA coding for human von Willebrand factor using antibody probes for colony screening and mapping of the chromosomal gene, *Nucleic Acids Res.,* 13, 4699, 1985.

22. **Sadler, J. E., Shelton-Inloes, B. B., Sorace, J. M., Harlan, J. M., Titani, K., and Davie, E. W.,** Cloning and characterization of two cDNAs coding for human von Willebrand factor, *Proc. Natl. Acad. Sci. U.S.A.,* 82, 6394, 1985.

23. **Vieira, J. and Messing, J.,** The UC plasmids, an M13mp7-derived system for insertion mutagenesis and sequencing with synthetic universal primers, *Gene,* 19, 259, 1982.

24. **Helfman, D. M., Feramisco, J. R., Fiddes, J. C., Thomas, G. P., and Hughes, S. H.,** Identification of clones that encode chicken tropomyosin by direct immunological screening of a cDNA expression library, *Proc. Natl. Acad. Sci. U.S.A.,* 80, 31, 1983.

25. **Young, R. A. and Davis, R. W.,** Efficient isolation of genes by using antibody probes, *Proc. Natl. Acad. Sci. U.S.A.,* 80, 1194, 1983.

26. **Fowler, W. E., Fretto, L. J., Hamilton, K. K., Erickson, H. P., and McKee, P. A.,** Substructure of human von Willebrand factor, *J. Clin. Invest.,* 76, 1491, 1985.

27. **Proudfoot, N. J. and Brownlee, G. G.,** 3′ non-coding region sequences in eukaryotic messenger RNA, *Nature,* 263, 211, 1976.

28. **Wagner, D. D. and Marder, V. J.,** Biosynthesis of von Willebrand protein by human endothelial cells: processing steps and their intracellular localization, *J. Cell Biol.,* 99, 2123, 1984.

29. **Von Heijne, G.,** Patterns of amino acids near signal-sequence cleavage sites, *Eur. J. Biochem.,* 133, 17, 1983.

30. **Sodetz, J. M., Paulson, J. C., and McKee, P. A.,** Carbohydrate composition and identification of blood group A, B and H oligosaccharide structures on human factor VIII/von Willebrand factor, *J. Biol. Chem.,* 254, 10754, 1979.

31. **Titani, K., Ericksson, L. H., Kumar, S., Dorsam, H., Chopek, M. W., and Fujikawa, K.,** Chemical characterization of the human von Willebrand factor, *Circulation,* 70 (Suppl. 2) (Abstr.), 837, 1984.

32. **Hessel, B., Jornvall, H., Thorell, L., Soderman, S., Larsson, U., Egberg, N., Blomback, B., and Holmgren, A.,** Structure-function relationships of human factor VIII complex studied by thioredoxin dependent disulfide reduction, *Thromb. Res.,* 35, 637, 1984.

33. **Hamilton, K. K., Fretto, L. J., Grierson, D. S., and McKee, P. A.,** Effects of plasmin on von Willebrand factor multimers, *J. Clin. Invest.,* 76, 261, 1985.

34. **Eyre, D. R.,** Collagen: molecular diversity in the body's protein scaffold, *Science,* 207, 1315, 1980.

35. **Gitschier, J., Wood, W. I., Goralka, T. M., Wion, K. L., Chen, E. Y., Eaton, D. H., Vehar, G. A., Capon, D. J., and Lawn, R. M.,** Characterization of the human factor VIII gene, *Nature,* 312, 326, 1984.

36. **Toole, J. J., Knopf, J. L., Wozney, J. M., Sutzman, L. A., Buecker, J. L., Pittman, D. D., Kaufman, R. J., Brown, E., Shoemaker, C., Orr, E. C., Amphlett, G. W., Foster, W. B., Coe, M. L., Knutson, G. J., Fass, D. N., and Hewick, R. M.,** Molecular cloning of a cDNA encoding human antihaemophilic factor, *Nature,* 312, 342, 1984.

37. **Pierschbacher, M. D. and Ruoslahti, E.,** Cell attachment activity of fibronectin can be duplicated by small synthetic fragments of the molecule, *Nature,* 309, 30, 1984.

38. **Pierschbacher, M. D. and Ruoslahti, E.,** Variants of the cell recognition site of fibronectin that retain attachment-promoting activity, *Proc. Nat. Acad. Sci. U.S.A.,* 81, 5985, 1984.

39. **Montgomery, R. R. and Zimmerman, T. S.,** Von Willebrand's disease antigen II: a new plasma and platelet antigen efficient in severe von Willebrand's disease, *J. Clin. Invest.,* 61, 1498, 1978.

40. **McCarroll, D. R., Levin, E. G., and Montgomery R. R.,** Endothelial cell synthesis of von Willebrand antigen II, von Willebrand factor and von Willebrand factor/von Willebrand antigen II complex, *J. Clin. Invest.,* 75, 1089, 1985.

41. **McCarroll, D. R., Ruggeri, Z. M., and Montgomery, R. R.,** The effect of DDAVP on plasma levels of von Willebrand's antigen II in normal individuals and patients with von Willebrand's disease, *Blood,* 63, 532, 1984.

42. **Kefalides, N. A.,** Expression of the gene for human factor VIII-antigen in hybrids of human endothelium and rodent fibroblasts, *Fed. Proc. Fed. Am. Soc. Exp. Biol.,* 40, 327, 1981.

43. **Verweij, C. L., Hofker, M., Quadt, R., Briet, E., and Pannekoek, H.,** RFLP for a human von Willebrand factor (vWF) cDNA clone, pvWF1100, *Nucleic Acids Res.,* 13, 8299, 1985.

44. **Doolittle, R. F.,** The genealogy of some recently evolved vertebrate proteins, *Trends Biochem. Soc.,* 10, 233, 1985.

45. **Patthy, L.,** Evolution of the proteases of blood coagulation and fibrinolysis by assembly from modules, *Cell,* 41, 657, 1985.

46. **Titani, K.,** personal communication.

47. **Verweij, C. L., Quadt, R., Briet, E., Dubbeldam, K., van Ommen, G.-J., and Pannekoek, H.,** Genetic linkage of two intragenic restriction fragment length polymorphisms with von Willebrand's disease type IIa: Evidence for a defect in the von Willebrand factor gene, *J. Clin. Invest.,* 81, 111b, 1988.

Chapter 5

ADVANCES IN AMIDOLYTIC ASSAY OF FACTOR VIII: VARIABLES AFFECTING THE RATE OF Xa GENERATION

M. J. Seghatchian

TABLE OF CONTENTS

I.   Introduction 98

II.   Basic Principles of VIII Amidolytic Assays 99
      A.   Current Concepts of Xa Generation 99
      B.   Coatest Factor VIII Kit and Modified One-Stage Procedure 100
            1.   Two-Stage VIII Amidolytic Assay (VIII:Am$_2$) 100
            2.   One-Stage VIII Amidolytic Assay (VIII:Am$_1$) 100
            3.   Working Reagents 100
            4.   Assay Procedure 101
      C.   Global Amidolytic Assays of VIII Based on APPT Principles 101

III. Variables Affecting the Amidolytic Assay of VIII 102
      A.   Calcium/Phospholipid as Variables 102
      B.   Significance of Tenase Complex(es) 104
      C.   Effect of Al(OH)$_3$ Adsorption 104
      D.   Tissue Factor or Phospholipid as Variables 104
            1.   The Influence of Tissue Factor 105
            2.   The Influence of Phospholipid(s) 105

IV.   Elevated VIII in Hypercoagulable States 108
      A.   The Nature of VIII Amidolytic Activity in Pregnancy 108
      B.   VIII Amidolytic Activity in Oral Anticoagulant Therapy 115
      C.   Possible Causes of Elevated VIII:C in Oral Anticoagulant
            Therapy 115

V.   Some Useful Applications of Coatest Factor VIII 117
      A.   Some Diagnostic Applications of Coatest Factor VIII 120
      B.   Assay Discrepancy in Potency Determination of Clinical
            Concentrates 121
      C.   Assay Discrepancies in the Evaluation of Factor VIII Inhibitors 121
      D.   VIII Amidolytic Activity Levels in Various Pathophysiological
            States 123

VI.   Future Trends/Concluding Remarks 123

Acknowledgments 124

References 124

I. INTRODUCTION

Any innovations in laboratory methodology are generally intended to improve the accuracy and/or efficacy of laboratory performance with resultant improvement in patient management. In this respect the use of chromogenic substrates for the measurement of factor VIII (VIII) potency at the level where its co-factor activity is expressed, namely factor X (X) activation by factor IXa (IXa), was greeted with interest for the following reasons.[1,2] First, such an approach would eliminate the need for clotting assays, where the distinguishing feature of abnormality is based on correction of a biologically active entity (i.e., VIII:C) with a second biological variable as substrate (fibrinogen), at the end of the clotting cascade, by a rather subjective clot end-point method. In addition, there has also been some concern over the poor accuracy of clotting methodology, and there are still some unresolved problems associated with the standardization of reagents. With the introduction of a more specific assay of VIII using standardized amounts of purified reagents, it was anticipated that VIII:C procoagulant activity could be evaluated biochemically with a greater precision and uniformity, reducing between laboratory variations.[2] Second, with the application of a more specific assay, the clinical and economic aspects of newer technologies have to be considered. VII:C assay is by far the most frequently requested clotting factor test for the investigation of deranged hemostasis and for the diagnostic and therapeutic evaluation of various deficiency states. It is obvious that inaccurate potency estimations have considerable clinical significance as well as financial consequences since the price of clinical concentrates is based upon the manufacturer's declared potency of the product. The validity of the declared potency values in terms of the consumers' methodology is still under debate.[3-5] Third, comparative analysis using different technologies will provide useful information on the activity state of VIII. In this respect further progress in the characterization of concentrates will be expected with the use of amidolytic assays, which are reportedly insensitive to traces of thrombin. Finally, with the availability of automated rate analyzers, spectrophotometric devices, and ELISA plate readers, it can be anticipated that chromogenic substrate assays of VIII will contribute to improved assay precision at a level independent of the thrombin effect and facilitate laboratory management by reducing the workload of skilled technicians.

The pioneer work[6] on the use of Xa substrates for the assessment of VIII procoagulant activity (VIII:C) potency was performed by the author in 1976 using commercially available combined reagents for the two-stage clotting assay. It was found that VIII-mediated intrinsic activation of X could be measured in the intermediate stage of the coagulation cascade by Xa-induced release of *para*-nitroaniline (pNA) from the chromogenic substrate for Xa (S2222), but long incubation times were required. Since then, several attempts have been made to improve the reaction rate by using different activators instead of serum and/or purified components of the original reagents, as described earlier.[2] Furthermore, a diazotation reaction was introduced to increase the sensitivity of the method and facilitate the application for screening purposes by using microtiter plates.[8] These innovations rendered the VIII amidolytic procedure more accessible for general nonspecialist laboratories and/or for bedside measurements. Some of the clinical applications of this methodology have been reported earlier and subsequently reviewed.[2,8,9]

Several modifications of the above basic principle for amidolytic assay of VIII have also been described by other investigators[10-15] and include the use of either human or bovine semipurified/purified coagulation factors (IXa, X); different types of phospholipid; and the use of different substrates and/or thrombin inhibitors.[13-16] It is only recently, however, with the availability of commercial reagents (Coatest Factor VIII Kabi-Vitrum) consisting of optimal concentrations of bovine IXa/X and porcine brain phospholipid that the VIII amidolytic assay has become the method of choice in many laboratories. The test is also reportedly of value in nonplasmatic environments.[16] This is currently of particular relevance since the method is applicable for the assessment of VIII in cell cultures. It has been used in the measurement of the expression of functional activity of recombinant VIII.[17] Furthermore, the species differences in the reagents have rendered the method more suitable for the accurate measurement of VIII:C potency in clinical concentrates.[18,19]

More recently, with the aim of reducing the potential interference of the plasmatic components and activated factors, the author has designed a one-stage procedure, using Coatest Factor VIII reagents. This is achieved by incorporating the synthetic substrate containing thrombin inhibitor (S2222 + I 2581) in the reaction mixture during the incubation stage. The assay was also performed on $Al(OH)_3$ adsorbed samples. This rendered the assay more specific to VIII-mediated Xa generation in the intrinsic pathway.

In this chapter, the basic principles of VIII amidolytic assays are described. The effects of variables which might influence the potency estimation are exemplified. Also, attempts have been made to define the nature of the elevated VIII:C in hypo-hypercoagulable states, using as models samples from patients receiving oral anticoagulants with variable INR values and samples during various stages of pregnancy from the same patients. Finally, the current literature on potency estimations of VIII and its inhibitors will be reviewed.

II. BASIC PRINCIPLES OF VIII AMIDOLYTIC ASSAYS

A. Current Concepts of Xa Generation

The generation of activated X by IXa is greatly stimulated by VIII. Accordingly, the extent of VIII-mediated activation of X can be evaluated by measuring amidolytic activity of Xa, through the release of PNA from the specific substrate for Xa (S2222 or S2337).[2,6-9,16]

Apart from the intrinsic pathway of Xa generation, triggered by contact activation,[20] several other mechanisms are known to contribute to Xa generation. These include the extrinsic and alternative pathways, where tissue factor (TF) VII/VIIa complexes have the major regulatory role for Xa generation.[21-28] The formation of a ternary complex between the extrinsic and intrinsic pathway (VII a-TF-IXa) makes the alternative pathway more efficient than the extrinsic pathway.[26]

Cold/surface activation,[25] as well as the exposure to extravascular surfaces or activated platelets,[29] could also lead to potent activators of IX and X, with an altered rate of Xa generation. Several other proteolytic enzymes can affect the rate of Xa generation and hence play a major role in positive and negative feedback of clotting pathways.[25-28]

More recently several investigators[30-38] have studied the role of the endothelial cell in the triggering and propagation of Xa generation. Interleukin 1-induced TF[33,34] appears to play a major role in the expression of procoagulant activity of human vascular cells. Both non-activated and activated IX and X reportedly bind to endothelial cells, and it appears that VIII in combination with X induces a high affinity binding site for IXa.[36-37]

In all above possible pathways the phospholipid moiety providing the suitable negatively charged surface is essential for optimal activation of the component of "tenase/prothrombinase" complexes. Under pathological conditions, bacterial lipopolysaccharides can serve as activated surfaces. The significance of intermediate complexes and the regulatory aspects of smaller peptides on the reaction rate are also of importance. Nawroth et al.[38] have shown that the Gla peptide derived from the amino-terminal end of IX, X, and II light chains (peptides 1—44) can inhibit Xa generation. More importantly, the decarboxylation of the peptides 1—44 rendered X inactive in all reactions necessitating surface binding, whereas the reactions involving XIa and IIa which do not need surface binding to exert their effect were not inhibited. The use of VIII-chromogenic assays in the above models would provide further insight into the mode of action and the nature of various intermediate complexes responsible for Xa generation, at a level independent of the thrombin effect.

B. Coatest Factor VIII Kit and Modified One-Stage Procedure

It is now well established that formation of "tenase complex" is essential for obtaining optimal catalytic activity of VIII.[6-16] In the purified system this is achieved by using a high concentration of the potent activator of the intrinsic pathway (IXa) and high concentrations of its substrate (X) in the presence of optimal levels of calcium and phospholipid in proportion to IXa/X. The optimal levels of these standardized reagents, warranting a reproducible assay for test samples, containing as little as 0.005 μ/ml VIII:C, are provided by the manufacturers (Coatest Factor VIII kit, Kabi). The requirement for high plasma dilutions (1:300 to 1:3000) has the additional advantage over the clotting assay, eliminating to some extent the potential interference due to activated factors (possibly present in the samples) and the inhibitory effect of proteolytic inhibitors such as antithrombin III and/or the possible formation of the fibrin clot. Nevertheless, as in clotting assays, stringent control of temperature and incubation time is essential for obtaining accurate and reproducible results. Both two-stage and one-stage procedures are applicable.

1. Two-Stage VIII Amidolytic Assay (VIII:Am$_2$)

The two-stage assay procedure is commonly employed involving an incubation stage designed to give direct proportionality between the concentration of VIII:C and the total amounts of generated Xa. A second measurement stage involves the photometric assay of Xa using the specific substrate for Xa, in the presence of a thrombin inhibitor (I-2581). The latter eliminates the contribution of thrombin, generated in the first stage, on the cleavage of S2222.

The cleavage of S2222 in this experimental condition is linearly proportional to the VIII:C content of the test samples. The pNA released can be followed by continuous recording of changes in absorbancy either at 405 nm (the initial rate method) or after stopping the reaction with acetic or citric acid (the "end point" method).

The Coatest kit for VIII:C has also been adapted to microtiter techniques either at room temperature (R.T.)[39] or at 37°C,[16] with no loss in precision or accuracy within 5 to 7%. However, in order to achieve the high level of predicted accuracy, it is crucially important to work in a carefully standardized manner throughout the procedure.

2. One-Stage VIII Amidolytic Assay (VIII:Am$_1$)

Since trace amounts of thrombin are generated during the incubation period of the conventional two-stage assay and in view of the sensitivity of various components in the reaction mixture to thrombin,[40] a one-stage assay was designed by incorporating the synthetic substrate and thrombin inhibitor mixture in the test system during the incubation period, prior to the addition of combined reagents or test plasma. In this test system, only Xa-mediated activation of the assay components was evaluated during the incubation period. The additional distinctive feature of the one-stage system, which enables one to assess progressively the pNA formation (while reactions are still in process), is that it provides further information on interfering substances (i.e., inhibitors) which may prolong the lag phase.

The time required to reach a set absorbancy value (i.e., O.D. = 0.5) in the linear regions of the curve can be used as an index of VIII:C potency. Hence an activated partial thromboplastin time (APTT)-based assay is applicable, having several additional advantages over clotting and/or global amidolytic procedures based on APTT principles requiring undiluted plasma. In the latter the presence of activated factors which may be present in trace amounts leads to substantial discrepancy in potency estimation.

3. Working Reagents

The concentration of reagents is basically the same in one-stage and two-stage procedures. The main difference is in the order of reagents applied to the microtiter plate. In order to reduce the number of pipettings while obtaining optimal catalytic activity, a combined reagent is prepared according to recommendations of the manufacturer. The working reagent consists of:

1. Five volumes of bovine IX/X mixture dissolved in 10 ml of distilled water (10 ml)
2. Two volumes of porcine phospholipid emulsion (2 ml)
3. Three volumes of 0.025-ml calcium (6 ml)

This mixture is stable for 2 to 4 h if maintained on ice to minimize the generation of Xa. For each hour of storage on ice, the formation of Xa yields approximately 0.1 unit absorbancy. Although this increase in the reagent blank activity does not affect the linearity of the method, nevertheless, the presence of the increased Xa in the reaction mixture could contribute to changes in the activation state of some components of the test system.

Standard and sample dilutions are prepared in a standard manner. In order to obtain an increased resolution at different levels of VIII:C, two working ranges for the standard are arbitrarily defined. For high ranges (VIII:C 0.2 to 1.5 U/ml), 50-μl samples are added to 300-μl buffer, and then the second solution is made by subsampling 50 μl of the prediluted sample to 2000 μl of buffer. For low ranges (VIII:C = 0.01 to 0.2 U/ml), 25 μl of samples is added to 2000 μl of buffer. Two standard curves with dilutions of 1/200 to 1/3200 (low range) and 1/50 to 1/800 (high range) are required for the respective calculations. It is advisable to perform a three-point dose response assay which will provide further information on parallelism and validity of the assay.

4. Assay Procedure

A microtitration procedure is commonly employed, allowing large-scale screening. To 25 μl of respective dilutions of standard, test samples, and blank, 75 μl of the combined reagent is added and the mixture is incubated for 20 min at 37°C (Dynatech micro-titer shaker incubator). For the room temperature assay it is essential to prewarm the reagent at 37°C for a few minutes before use. After the incubation period, 50 μl of reconstituted substrate, containing 2.7-mM S2222 and 0.06-mM I-2158 is added to the reaction mixture. This is mixed and kept for 10 to 20 min for optimal pNA production. To obtain higher resolution, the cleavage time can be increased to yield a maximal absorbancy of about 1.0. Above this value nonlinearity may arise due to substrate depletion.

In the one-stage system substrate is added at the same concentration before the addition of samples or the combined reagent to the well. pNA formation is then measured as a function of time (intervals of 5 to 10 min). In both methods the reaction can be stopped at desired intervals by 10 μl of citric acid (0.9 M) or citrated buffer pH 3.0 at R.T. Diazotation can be performed to increase the sensitivity of this procedure at least fivefold.[2]

C. Global Amidolytic Assays of VIII Based on APPT Principles

A commercial reagent (Thromboquant-APPT) for the determination of the APPT with a chromogenic substrate (Chromozyn-TH) has been designed and compared with the conventional APPT using clot and end-point techniques.[41,42] The preincubation of the activator, consisting of ellagic acid/phospholipid, with citrated plasma, followed by the addition of the starting reagent containing calcium ions leads to IIa generation which is measured by synthetic substrates. The time required for a defined amount of pNA to be cleaved from the substrate (i.e., O.D. 1.0) is recorded, and appears to be proportional to the levels of IXa and VIII in the test sample. Although the test results are independent of the fibrinogen concentration, the maximal absorbance value of the reaction can be used as an estimation of fibrinogen level. Prediluation of normal plasma in the pooled congenital VIII:C deficient plasma makes the assay rather specific for VIII:C estimation. The results obtained by the clotting method for both normal and congenitally deficient patients correlates well (r = 0.92 to 0.97) with high reproducibility (Cv. between assays = 3 to 6%). The chromogenic APPT assay appears to be a promising tool for the laboratory involved in large-scale screening of VIII potencies. Moreover, the easy adaption of this technique for biocentrifugal analyzers, allowing direct transformation absorbance to clotting times, combined with higher sensitivity and precision of photometric methods and large sample throughput (100 per hour), makes this procedure an alternative to replace the clotting APPT,[41] in the nonclinical laboratory.

The sensitivity of this method to heparin makes it valuable for the control of heparin therapy.

III. VARIABLES AFFECTING THE AMIDOLYTIC ASSAY OF VIII

In earlier investigations[6-8] using the combined reagent for the VIII:C two-stage assay, but with S2222 as an indicator of Xa generation, the system was found to be sensitive and reproducible when high concentrations of reference and test plasma were applied (1/20 to 1/100), but long incubation periods (30 to 60 min) were necessary. Furthermore, when activated factors were present in the plasma, these experimental conditions led to inaccuracy. The lag phase for X activation could be shortened by use of purified components of test reagents and through increasing the final concentration of X to the optimal level of 1.5 U/ml. In this optimized system, increasing dilutions of plasma (1/100 to 1/800) could be assayed successfully without the interference of activated factors if present in the test plasma. However, the presence of vitamin K dependent coagulation factors was found to influence both the lag phase and the reaction rate of Xa generation. This led to some difficulties in the assay of factor VIII concentrates against reference plasma and emphasized the requirement for effective $Al(OH)_3$ adsorption of plasma preparations before the assay. This procedure, however, requires stringent standardization since it can introduce further interlaboratory variations for various reasons.[43,44] The critical role of II, VII, IX, and X in increasing both the rate of Xa generation and shortening the lag phase has also been pointed out by Suomela et al.[45] in their study of the VIII amidolytic assay. The role of protein M[46,47] in enhancement of Xa and/or IIa in semipurified preparation also remains to be elucidated.

From these earlier observations,[2,7-9] it became apparent that formation of trace amounts of IIa, a potent activator of VIII, is essential for optimal catalytic efficiency of VIII. This has been confirmed with the use of S2222 by Van Dieijen et al.[11] who have investigated the effect of thrombin-activated VIII on the kinetic parameters of Xa generation, using either semipurified or purified components of the "tenase" generation system. These investigators have shown that activated VIII (and not native VIII) in the presence of optimum levels of phospholipid/calcium decreases the kinetic constant (Km) of X activation by IXa from 299 to 0.58 μM and has a potent effect on the maximum velocity. It is now established that native VIII (with reported molecular weights up to 360 kDa) has little co-factor activity while thrombin-activated VIII consisting of two chains of approximately 80 to 90 kDa is an extremely effective co-factor of IXa-induced Xa generation.[40] In terms of enhancing the activation rate of X in appropriate conditions, thrombin-activated VIII can provide a 200,000-fold increase in reaction rate. Without IXa, however, VIII does not cleave X to any measurable extent either before or after pretreatment with thrombin.[48]

The availability of the commercial kit[16] for VIII amidolytic assay, based on the Xa generation, has facilitated comparative studies among laboratories. The influence of a number of variables affecting the kinetics of Xa generation has been evaluated in the present study.

A. Calcium/Phospholipid as Variables

1. In the absence of either Ca^{++} or phospholipid, IXa has a limited capacity to generate Xa in the Coatest assay system. Furthermore, no significant shortening of the lag

Significance of Tenase in VIII:AM

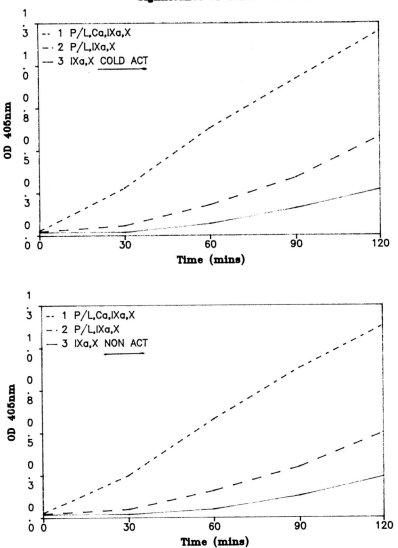

FIGURE 1.   Formation of para nitroaniline (pNA) in a system consisting of 25 μl of a 1/ 100 dilution of plasma, 50 μl of S2222 + I2581, and 75 μl of combined reagents (IXa/X/ PL/calcium) or its components, at the same final concentration. The optimal reaction rate, with optimal shortening of the lag phase, is only achieved when all components of "tenase" are present. No significant change in the reaction kinetics is observed subsequent to cold activation, (lower panel) though the lag phase is slightly shortened.

phase or increase in reaction rate was observed by prior cold activation of the reference plasma. A long lag phase and little amidolytic activity were seen in both cold activated and nonactivated samples as shown in Figure 1.

2.   Xa generation in the presence of Ca^{++} ions or phospholipid. An increase in the rate of Xa generation with a shortened lag phase was observed when either Ca^{++} or phospholipid was added to the test system. The kinetics of the reaction with Ca^{++} alone or with phospholipid alone were essentially identical. The addition of combined reagents (IXa/X, PL, Ca^{++}) greatly enhanced the rate of Xa generation with dramatic shortening of the lag phase, suggesting the formation of a "tenase" complex containing

all essential components. The substitution of pooled plasma with the cold activated preparation showed no significant changes in the rate. Under these conditions the optimal Ca^{++} concentration was 0.70 mM. Alterations in phospholipid to suboptimal levels also resulted in apparent changes in the VIII amidolytic levels.

B. Significance of Tenase Complex(es)

The term "tenase" for Xa generation implies a similar meaning as for prothrombinase in IIa generation, having identical characteristics:

1.   VIII in "tenase" plays the equivalent co-factor role as compared to V in prothrombinase.
2.   Calcium/phospholipid are the essential components in both systems where one Vitamin K dependent protein serves as the substrate and another as the enzyme (IXa/X as compared to Xa/II).
3.   VIII like V is activated and then inactivated by trace amounts of Xa and/or IIa and also inactivated by protein C_a. The rate of inactivation of protein C_a is reduced by the formation of tenase or prothrombinase complexes.[49]
4.   It is likely that the intracellularly released VIII like V is in the activated form,[50] accounting for the elevated levels of VIII:C in hypercoagulability.
5.   Like prothrombinase there must be practically endless variation for the control, modulation, and acceleration of tenase, and variable degrees of inhibition by circulating protease inhibitors.

It should be noted that a "ternary" tenase complex,[26] consisting of VII/VIIa, TF, and IXa (IXa-TF-VII/VIIa) has been reported with high catalytic activity for Xa generation. The effect of TF on Coatest VIII has not been investigated. Since Vitamin K dependent coagulation factors are preferentially adsorbed on $Al(OH)_3$, we have compared the effect of TF, at variable concentrations, on the rate of Xa generation using both $Al(OH)_3$ adsorbed and nonadsorbed samples. The disparity between results will provide some indication of the relative contribution of tenase complexes if present in the test samples.

C. Effect of $Al(OH)_3$ Adsorption

Pretreatment of plasma and concentrate standard with $Al(OH)_3$ prolonged the lag phase and decreased the reaction rate, as measured either by one-stage or two-stage amidolytic assay, as shown in Figure 2. This confirms that $Al(OH)_3$ not only removes Vitamin K dependent proteins, but also adsorbs some forms of VIII present in the concentrate.[43,44] Furthermore, $Al(OH)_3$ is also known to generate a strong anti-Xa effect.[51]

The time required to reach a set absorbancy (i.e., 0.5 or 0.75) in the linear part of the curve can be used as the "adsorption index" of various test preparations based on the APTT type assay. This is of particular relevance to manufacturers of factor VIII concentrates as $Al(OH)_3$ adsorption is one of the steps used to remove Vitamin K dependent proteins in the intermediate stage of VIII concentrate preparation. The presence of heparin in the test sample may alter the binding capacity of Vitamin K dependent proteins. Heparin also inhibits VIII amidolytic activity. In fact, ATIII with or without heparin inhibits Xa generation. The presence of 0.5 to 1.0 U of heparin in the test plasma leads to a 5 to 20% decrease in VIII amidolytic activity. This might contribute to some of the discrepancies observed in the assay and clinical VIII concentrates against a plasma standard containing ATIII or concentrates containing heparin.

D. Tissue Factor or Phospholipid as Variables

Porcine brain phospholipid and bovine IXa/X are used by the manufacturers of the Coatest VIII Kit. Species difference could account for the high rate of Xa generation seen using this reagent as compared to earlier reagents used by the present author.[7-9] It is important to investigate the effect of various types of phospholipid, including tissue factor and/or platelet components, on the reaction rate of Xa generation.

1. The Influence of Tissue Factor

Substitution of porcine phospholipid with various concentrations of TF renders the Coatest reagent suitable for TF/IXa/VIIa-induced activation of X as seen in Figures 3A and B. In both Al(OH)$_3$ adsorbed and nonadsorbed samples, increasing concentrations of TF led to a faster rate of Xa generation in both one-stage and two-stage amidolytic systems. This provided convincing evidence that the phospholipid moiety of TF is an excellent source of the active lipid. Furthermore, VII/VIIa may contribute to a great extent in the conversion of X to Xa, following the formation of a ternary complex as indicated earlier.[26] This observation is of particular importance when using chromogenic substrate assays to measure VIII:C levels in samples that may contain traces of TF. The dose-response relationship for TF-induced Xa generation can be investigated at fixed incubation times (Figure 3B).

2. The Influence of Phospholipid(s)

The nature of the added phospholipid(s) is also of prime importance. It is generally agreed that active phospholipids (i.e., phosphatidyl serine, phosphatidyl inositol) carry a negative charge and are active in the thromboplastin generation test. On the other hand, phosphatidylcholine and phosphotidyl ethanolamine and plasma lipid(s) are inactive in tenase/prothrombinase complexes. The fact that 95% of plasma lipids can be removed without a significant change in the recalcification time supports the view that active phospholipids are not present in the plasma.

Cell membranes, lipoproteins, and phospholipids are surface active agents. They can be replaced by certain bile salts, at concentrations required for micelle formation. However, in contrast to active phospholipids, bile salts conjugated with sodium dehydrocholate appear to be ineffective in thrombin generation tests.[52-54] This supports the notion that the property to form micelles does not imply effectiveness in the coagulation system and the number of hydroxyl groups in lipid is of significance.[52-54]

Platelets are the main source of phospholipid needed for blood coagulation. However, only stimulated platelets, with exposed platelet factor 3 are relevant. This is due to the phosphatidyl serine exposure to the outer layer of membrane bilayer following stimulation. In our experience, the addition of nonstimulated washed platelets to the Coatest VIII system appears to decrease the rate of Xa generation, possibly by providing an ineffective surface, supporting earlier observation by other investigators.[37]

The inner surface of red cell membranes exposed as a consequence to hemolysis as well as to the isolated peripheral blood monocytes and lymphocytes[55] and TF itself (thromboplastin) are also excellent sources of active phospholipids.

This raises the questions as to whether the changes apparent in VIII:C with varying amounts of added phospholipids are due to the complete tenase production in the assay system or to a specific phospholipid-VIII complex formation that enhances Xa generation with altered assay kinetics.

Two approaches may be adopted to answer this question:

1. Examination of Xa generation can be performed in a reaction mixture containing suboptimal concentrations of phospholipid, followed by the sequential sampling from this mixture and the addition of increasing concentrations of phospholipid. The rate of Xa generation measured in each case is compared with the optimal condition. Half maximum values of the reaction can be calculated to assess the relevance of the additional phospholipid. An increase in Xa generation is seen under these subsampling

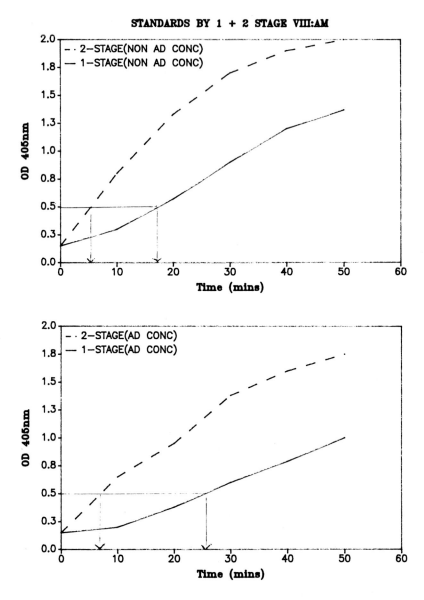

FIGURE 2.   The rate of Xa generation in VIII:Am$_1$ and VIII:Am$_2$, using adsorbed or
nonadsorbed concentrate and plasma standard(s). Substantial variations in the lag phase were
observed, in particular, subsequent to Al(OH)$_3$ adsorption. APPT-type assays (the time required for a fixed absorbancy, i.e., O.D. $\simeq 0.5$) are applicable. These times are prolonged
following adsorption of concentrate with Al(OH)$_3$, suggesting that some forms of VIII are
possibly adsorbed, or Al(OH)$_3$ adsorption has produced a strong anti-Xa in the test sample.
Divergence between one-stage and two-stage curves suggests that thrombin and Vitamin K
dependent proteins, to some degree, contribute to the enhanced VIII-mediated Xa generation
in the two-stage procedure.

circumstances, but values approximating the optimal condition can only be obtained
by the further addition of VIII, suggesting that VIII-phospholipid complex formation
is a prerequisite to complete tenase production. This procedure does not differentiate
VIII from VIIIa, which can be generated during the incubation period.
2.   A second approach involves a more direct evaluation of Xa generation whereby various
concentrations of phospholipid are incubated with the test samples in the presence of

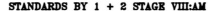

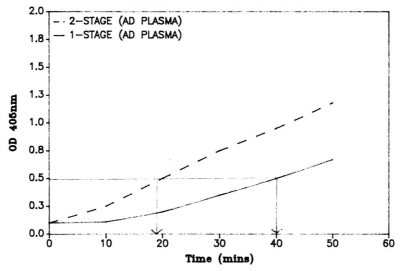

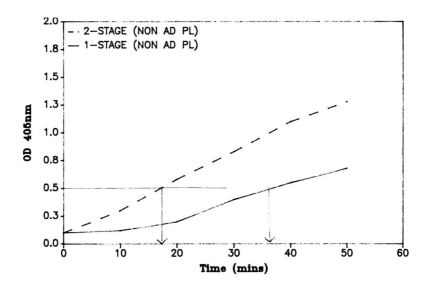

FIGURE 2 (continued)

the chromogenic substrate containing thrombin inhibitor (I-2581). The latter confers additional specificity to the test, by inhibiting the trace of thrombin which might be generated during the incubation period.

Using this system we have observed that at a fixed concentration of TF (Manchester Comparative Reagent [MCR] 1/25), the addition of porcine phospholipid as supplied by the Coatest Kit enhances the reaction rate whereas the addition of washed, non-stimulated platelets, under identical conditions, results in a reduction in the rate of Xa generation (Figure 4) and a modified lag phase.

These effects were apparent in both adsorbed and nonadsorbed plasma samples, indicating that both ternary and quarternary tenase complexes contribute to Xa generation under the two-stage experimental conditions. Therefore, caution should be exercised when intepreting with precision data from VIII amidolytic assays where undefined components are suspected to be present in the test samples.

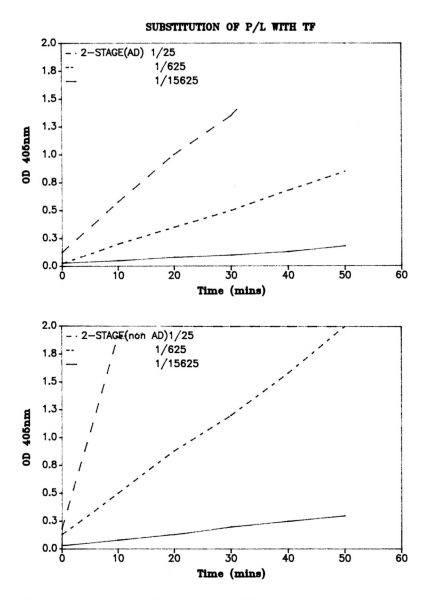

FIGURE 3A.   Tissue factor (TF), as variable in VIII amidolytic assays. Substitution of phospholipid in the Coatest VIII system, with various dilutions of the Manchester Comparative Reagent also leads to a dose-dependent increase in Xa generation. This suggests that (1) TF is a good source of phospholipid, (2) an alternative pathway is also involved in Xa generation, and (3) the optimal levels of TF or phospholipid of different origin can be standardized by this method. In both adsorbed and nonadsorbed samples, the lag phase is shortened and the reaction rate is increased with increasing concentrations of TF.

IV. ELEVATED VIII IN HYPERCOAGULABLE STATES

A. The Nature of VIII Amidolytic Activity in Pregnancy

It is well established that in certain pathophysiological states associated with hypercoagulability, i.e., in women taking the contraceptive pill, in pregnancy, and in the early stage of anticoagulant therapy, there is a systematic increase in VIII:C.

Several physiological events could be proposed to explain the elevated VIII:C levels in hypercoagulable states. These include:

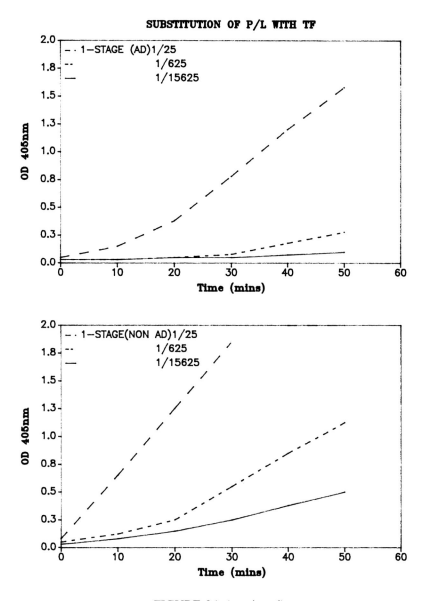

FIGURE 3A (continued)

1. Increased synthesis of the native form of VIII/von Willebrand factor (vWf)
2. Increased cellular release of native/activated VIII
3. Formation of phospholipid-VIII complexes
4. Generation of a circulating form of tenase complexes with high VIII:C-like activity
5. *In vivo* or *in vitro* activation of VIII:C due to imbalance between procoagulant and anticoagulant proteins

Earlier investigations to define the activation stage of VIII:C in hypercoagulable states were limited to coagulation assays and were based on:

1. Multiple dose response bioassay of test samples against a nonactivated standard to investigate parallelism

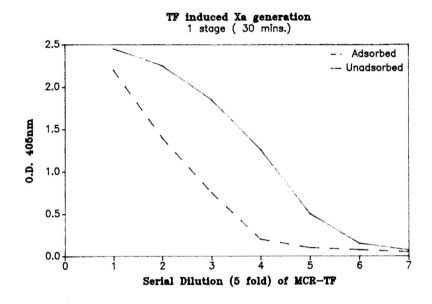

TF induced Xa generation
1 stage (30 mins.)

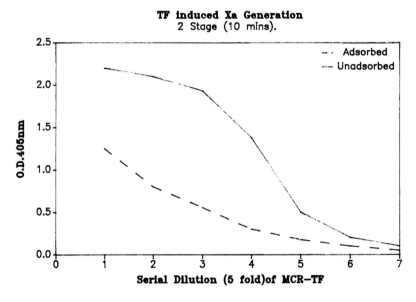

TF induced Xa Generation
2 Stage (10 mins).

FIGURE 3B.   The dose response curves for fivefold serial dilutions of MCR are shown. The greater disparity between adsorbed and nonadsorbed samples in the two-stage system as compared to the one-stage system emphasizes the potential role of Vitamin K dependent proteins in thrombin-induced activation of VIII. In the one-stage procedure, the presence of I2581 in the reaction mixture makes the assay highly specific to Xa-induced activation of VIII.

2.   Assessment of the VIII:C ratio of one-stage against two-stage assays, the former having a greater sensitivity to thrombin and thrombin-activated VIII
3.   Assessment of disparity between VIII:C levels following adsorption on $Al(OH)_3$ which, apart from removing Vitamin K dependent coagulation proteins, is thought to remove activated factor VIII[43,44]

Although considerable differences in the results from the above parameters provide some indication as to changes in the activation stage of VIII, there is, however, some uncertainty

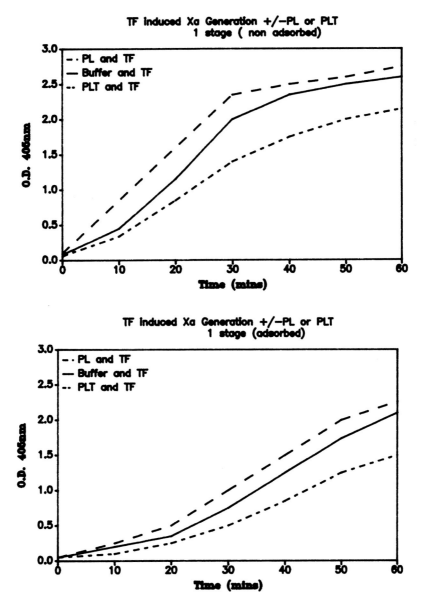

FIGURE 4. The synergistic effect of porcine phospholipid (at half recommended concentration) and the inhibitory effect of washed platelet concentrate (225×10^9 per liter) on a 1/25 dilution of TF-induced Xa generation, using both adsorbed and nonadsorbed samples. The lag phase is shortened and the Xa generation rate is increased with the addition of phospholipid, whereas in both adsorbed and nonadsorbed samples these are inhibited with the addition of platelets. The same trend was observed for serial 1/5 dilutions of phospholipid on platelets. These results suggest that both the nature of phospholipid and the additional binding of VIII to noncoagulant phospholipids of cell surfaces can alter the kinetic parameters of Xa generation.

inherent to the coagulant assays which renders such procedures for the assessment of the hypercoagulable state of limited use in general coagulation laboratories.

More recently the *in vitro* fibrinopeptide A (FPA) generation test and the direct assessment of the total circulating activated factors in plasma[57] by chromogenic assay (IIa-like activity) have been adopted. These methods attempt to provide an index for the presence of activated factors. The lack of specificity makes their use also limited. Nevertheless, these tests are of value to predict and/or provide an indication for the presence of low grade activated factors.

Another approach which is thought to be useful in differentiating the activated from of VIII from native forms is the use of the classical VIII:Am$_2$. As in the conventional two-stage amidolytic procedure, the presence of thrombin in the test sample may lead to changes in the activation of some components of the reaction. Both one-stage and two-stage procedures were used in our study to evaluate the nature of the rise in the VIII:C activity during pregnancy. For comparative analyses ("like with like" assays), the results were expressed in terms of direct absorbance, as the standards were not calibrated against an amidolytic VIII assay.

Finally, the trend in the elevation of the one-stage and two-stage amidolytic activities during pregnancy was compared with the trend in the increased values of VIII:C and vWf:antigen (Ag) (Figures 5 and 6).

In both nonadsorbed one-stage and two-stage amidolytic assays, the rate of Xa generation is increased substantially in late pregnancy as compared to samples taken at 7 weeks after delivery. Furthermore, although only slight differences between the adsorbed and nonadsorbed samples were evident in the two-stage procedure, the disparity between the results of the same samples measured by the one-stage amidolytic method is more pronounced. This would indicate the presence of activated VIII or variable levels of activated II, VII, IX, X, and/or proteolytic inhibitors contributing to different degrees to the observed variations. The absence of a lag phase in both adsorbed and nonadsorbed late pregnancy samples using the one-stage procedure, as shown in Figure 5, also suggests that VIII in these samples is probably circulating as tenase complex(es).

In a larger study of 78 pregnant women, we have shown[58] that there is a steady increase in VIII:C and VII:C levels during pregnancy. Interestingly, these elevated levels of VIII:C correlate well with the increased level of thrombin-like activity (TLA) in plasma,[57] measured under standardized conditions using the synthetic substrate for thrombin S2238. Up to fivefold increases over the basal TLA levels have been observed, using the 7-weeks postnatal sample from the same individuals as the presumed basal control. Other small peptide substrates specific for Kallikrein, IXa, protein C$_a$, and Xa were also cleaved more rapidly by these samples indicating the presence of potentially activated factors. These observations suggest that the observed increases in VIII:C may be related to activation and/or formation of circulating tenase complexes.

It remains, nevertheless, to establish whether the increase in synthesis and/or release of VIII are responsible for hypercoagulability or whether the formation of Xa and/or IIa is contributing to the activation of VIII, thus affecting the test procedure. Formation of a ternary complex of VII/VIIa with IIa-induced release TF *in vivo* and the low grade circulating intrinsic activator (IXa) could also contribute to hypercoagulability.

Both VIII:C and vWf:Ag are known to increase dramatically (three- to tenfold) during late pregnancy and then fall sharply post delivery.[58] In absolute terms, in late pregnancy the increase in VIII:C does not compare well with either the increase in vWf:Ag or the values of VIII amidolytic activities (Figure 6). The observed discrepancy between various VIII assays in late pregnancy could be due to the fact that large amounts of α_1 antitrypsin are present in late pregnancy[58] which might affect the rate of Xa generation.

Dalaker and Prydz[59] proposed the formation of a circulating "placenta phospholipid-factor VIII complex" during pregnancy. Their studies were based on the elevated levels of VII:C and a reduction of VII:C levels to normal subsequent to phospholipase C treatment. A similar interpretation could be pertinent to VIII:C or VIII amidolytic levels in pregnancy, as it is known that binding to phospholipid potentiates the co-factor activity of VIII, accounting for a higher rate of Xa generation. Nevertheless, the formation of such a complex does not

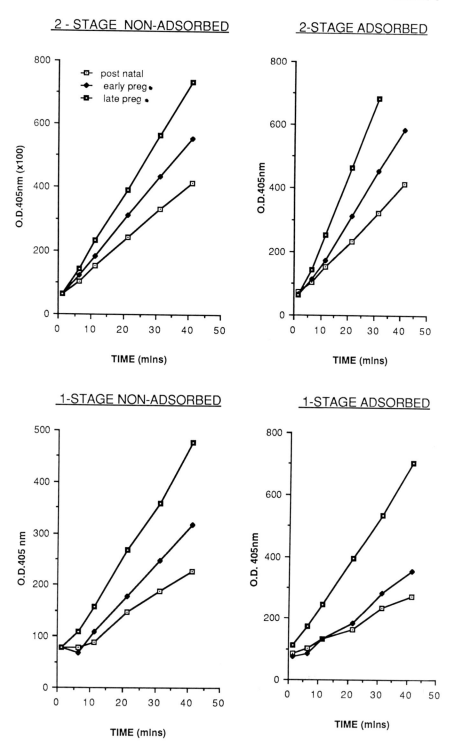

FIGURE 5. The rate of Xa generation of three plasma samples from the same individual at various stages of pregnancy, by one-stage and two-stage methods. In both adsorbed and nonadsorbed samples, the lag phase is abolished in late pregnancy samples, indicating the presence of a circulating "tenase", contributing to the increase in the reaction rate without the lag phase.

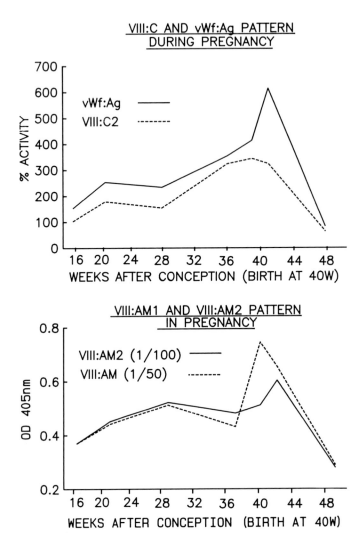

FIGURE 6.   Comparison between the distribution patterns of plasmatic levels of VIII and vWf during pregnancy. VIII is measured by a two-stage clotting and one-stage/two-stage amidolytic assay. vWf:Ag values are expressed in percent of a plasma standard. Similar increased patterns in VIII/vWf levels by all four methods support the view that elevated VIII/vWf during late pregnancy could be due to thrombin-induced activation/release of VIII/vWf components.

explain the high levels of nonspecific TLA, which are consistently observed[57] together with the high levels in VIII:C in VIII amidolytic assays. It is, therefore, postulated that the formation of ternary (IXa-TF-VII/VIIIa) or quaternary (IXa-phospholipid-X-VIII/VIIIa-Ca^{++}) complexes could account for both the elevated levels of TLA and VIII during late pregnancy. The formation of such complexes could protect the activated IXa in tenase and possibly Xa in the prothrombinase form from plasmatic inhibitors such as antithrombin III and activated protein C.[49]

Elevated levels of FPA are consistently observed in conjunction with the elevated VIII:C during pregnancy.[58] This supports the view that thrombin is formed and possibly protein C becomes activated locally compensating for a decrease in fibrinolytic activity due to release of plasminogen activator inhibitors.[58]

The increase in vWf:Ag is probably due to either thrombin-induced release of vWf from the endothelial cells or to further fragmentation of vWf by some cellular protease.[60] It is well established that vWf:Ag fragments migrate at a faster rate in agarose electrophoresis systems and also express altered antigenic determinants.[60] By implication the presence of these fragments may give falsely high values.

B. VIII Amidolytic Activity in Oral Anticoagulant Therapy

It is well established that abnormal Vitamin K proteins with impaired functional activities are produced during oral anticoagluant therapy. However, Vitamin K antagonists do not completely inactivate all the biological activities of these "des-Gla" proteins. This is due to the fact that the active sites responsible for the catalytic activities of Vitamin K dependent proteins are situated on the heavy chains.[61] The γ-carboxy residues, which are situated on the light chain, have no direct influence on the property of the catalytic sites. Changes in the primary structure of the light chains may, however, impair activation of the zymogen forms and could lead to the production of an enzyme with altered catalytic efficiency.[62] Furthermore, as exemplified by X, the binding of Vitamin K dependent proteins to phospholipid is essential in the facilitation of the exposure of a secondary cleavage bond (arginyl-glycine) in the carboxy-terminal end of the heavy chain. This leads to the removal of a degradation peptide containing the carbohydrate moiety. Nevertheless, the procoagulant activity of the carbohydrate-free form of factor Xa, the so-called β-Xa, is identical to α-Xa. However, if the proteolytic reaction continued, the loss of activity may occur concomitantly with the appearance of γ-Xa.[63] This inactive derivative is thought to compete with the native X for intrinsic and extrinsic activators, but is no longer capable of yielding a catalytically active enzyme. Therefore, autocatalysis may to some extent represent a restrictive path for uncontrolled generation of Xa in blood.

C. Possible Causes of Elevated VIII:C in Oral Anticoagulant Therapy

VIII activity as determined by two-stage clotting assay is relatively higher in oral anticoagulant patients as compared to the normal population. The comparison of the VIII:C results in samples obtained in the early phase of anticoagulant therapy with VIII:C levels of pretreatment samples from the same individuals also shows a considerable difference. Theoretically, it is possible that a modest but sharp fall in the level of protein C which occurs in the early phase of anticoagulant therapy might be responsible for the elevated VIII:C levels. Alternatively, the variation in the ratio of general procoagulant/anticoagulant protein during anticoagulation therapy could contribute to variability in the rate of IXa, Xa, Va, and IIa formation, hence affecting indirectly the rate of VIII activation. This, nevertheless, does not explain the rise in vWf:Ag in the early phase of oral anticoagulant therapy.

Experimentally, the ratio of V:C/V:Ag, VII:C/VII:T (based on the tritiated peptide assay) appeared to be increased in the early phase of oral anticoagulant therapy suggesting thrombin generation. The observed increase in vWf:Ag can also be explained on the basis of a similar mechanism as IIa is able to release vWf from endothelial cells. Anecdotal reports also suggest that both V and VIII, in early anticoagulant therapy, are in their activated forms. The reactions of des-Gla on either Xa generation and/or on small substrate (S2222) may not be the same as indicated in Table 1.

To investigate whether VIII in oral anticoagulant patients is in activated form, samples from 20 normal individuals and 20 patients on anticoagulant therapy, with INR values in the range of 1.29 to 7.46, were compared by various methods. The results, which are summarized in Table 2, indicate:

1.   Increased VIII:C and VIII amidolytic activity whether one-stage or two-stage assays were performed on either adsorbed or nonadsorbed samples

Table 1
MOLECULAR FORMS AND PROPERTIES OF FACTOR X AND ITS DERIVATIVES

Species (molecular weight)	Modifying enzyme	Properties
1. Human α-X (59,000-75,000)	Several physiological and nonphysiological activators	Native enzyme with unchanged primary structure
Bovine α-X (55,000)	Several physiological and nonphysiological activators	Native enzyme with unchanged primary structure
2. Bovine β-X (51,000)	Xa, trypsin, and all other activators,	Degradation peptide is removed; species differences will lead to variable products with different reaction rate
3. Human α-X (59,000)	Xa	Unactivatable (C-terminal peptide containing active serine is removed from H-chain
4. Bovine α-X (40,500)	RVV (acutin)	
5. Autoprothrombin (51,000)	Thrombin	Activate with RVV but not physiological activators
6. Bovine decarboxy-X (55,000)	Activate slowly with RVV but not by physiological activators	Lacks Gla residues due to abnormal synthesis
7. Bovine des-Gla X (49,000)	α-chromotrypsin and bacterial enzymes	(As above); residue 1-44 removed from L-chain
8. Human (54,000) and bovine α-Xa (45,300)	VIIa, IXa, and RVV; trypsin	Fully active enzyme without activation peptide
9. Human (50,000) and bovine (42,600) β-Xa	Xa and other Xa forming enzymes	Fully active enzyme without activation and degradation peptide
10. Bovine decarboxy-Xa (43,000—47,000)	RVV	Peptide(s) removed active on small substrates

Table 2
COMPARISON OF VIII PROCOAGULANT ACTIVITIES, DETERMINED BY TWO-STAGE CLOTTING AND ONE- AND TWO-STAGE AMIDOLYTIC ASSAYS

Method	VIII:C2	Adsorbed		Nonadsorbed	
		VIII:Am$_2$	VIII:Am$_1$	VIII:Am$_2$	VIII:Am$_1$
			Normal		
M	102	106	73	85	76
SD	19.3	23	8.3	19.2	27
Range	69—138	69—137	57—81	59—116	50—117
			Oral Anticoagulant		
M	260	125	91	158	107
SD	143	65	18.8	48	47
Range	121—524	41—234	63—120	105—252	50—184

Note: The lower amidolytic activity in the one-stage amidolytic procedure is possibly due to the fact that thrombin, which does not require surface binding, can act on VIII during the incubation period in the two-stage procedure whereas the presence of I-2581 in the incubation period during one-stage inhibits thrombin action on VIII, resulting in a lower value of pNA for the same duration of assay. Variable levels of thrombin like enzymes (TLA) were found in both normal and patients' samples as compared to standard. This might contribute to disparity between adsorbed and nonadsorbed samples.

2. Higher VIII amidolytic activity is consistently observed by two-stage assay as compared with one-stage assay
3. Disparity between VIII related activities was also apparent in both adsorbed and nonadsorbed samples from anticoagulant patients as compared to normal; this suggests that the presence of des-Gla protein in the test system can affect the final results

Further support for these observations is provided by evaluating the total pNA at a fixed time and/or at time intervals (the initial rate of Xa generation) using either two-stage or one-stage VIII amidolytic procedures. The same trend in activity changes was observed by two-stage clotting and amidolytic methods. However, a large discrepancy was observed when INR values were greater than 3.0. No direct comparison between two-stage and one-stage amidolytic assays was made as the lag phase was greatly prolonged in anticoagulant samples, thus requiring much longer activation times to obtain the same O.D. reading as demonstrated in Figure 7.

The reason for the large differences in the Xa generation rates is not clear, but might be related to the interaction and/or the intervention of partially des-Gla proteins in tenase complex formation. The co-factor activity of VIII might be abnormal when abnormal Vitamin K dependent proteins are present in the test systems. It has been reported[61,63] that the release of the peptide 1—44 from X inhibits the binding of Vitamin K dependent proteins to phospholipid which is essential for expression of their optimal catalytic activities. The binding of IIa which does not require phospholipid surfaces and acts in solution is not affected. This might account for the large discrepancy observed between one-stage and two-stage amidolytic Xa generation rates. In the former, thrombin-induced activation of VIII is expectedly blocked by the presence of I-2581 in the assay, giving a slower rate of Xa generation. In the two-stage assay, however, thrombin is present during the incubation period giving rise to VIIIa generation and thus increasing its catalytic activity. Although Xa, like thrombin, is able to activate VIII, Xa is a less potent enzyme for this purpose. At an equivalent concentration, Xa produces fivefold less VIIIa as identified by X generation.[64]

In the Coatest VIII assay system, bovine IXa/X plays the major role in the intrinsic Xa generation. Nevertheless, the importance of Vitamin K dependent proteins in the test sample, in particular VII/VIIa, should not be ignored. The latter indirectly enhances the rate of Xa generation. This view is substantiated experimentally by evaluating the Xa generation activity due to TF-VII/VIIa in a system consisting of purified bovine X, TF (1/25 MRC), and 1/100 dilution of native or cold activated plasma. The results as shown in Figure 8 indicated that in this system both the original VII:C level and cold/surface activation affect the lag phase and Xa generation rates. These observations further emphasize the importance of a "like with like" assay, particularly when using amidolytic substrates to measure VIII levels in samples that might contain TF.

V. SOME USEFUL APPLICATIONS OF COATEST FACTOR VIII

The procoagulant activity of VIII in clinical situations is most commonly determined by the one-stage clotting assay. This method requires VIII deficient plasma from patients with severe hemophilia A as substrate. In view of current concern over the potential infectivity of reagents from human origin, alternative principles must be considered.

Although immune depleted substrate plasmas are becoming increasingly available, they are not necessarily as good as human substrate plasma. In our experience some of these preparations contain VIII levels in excess of 1% of normal and sometimes appear to be depleted of other components, normally present in plasma, such as fibrinogen. Furthermore, they may contain low levels of activated factors, as determined by chromogenic methods using thrombin substrates.

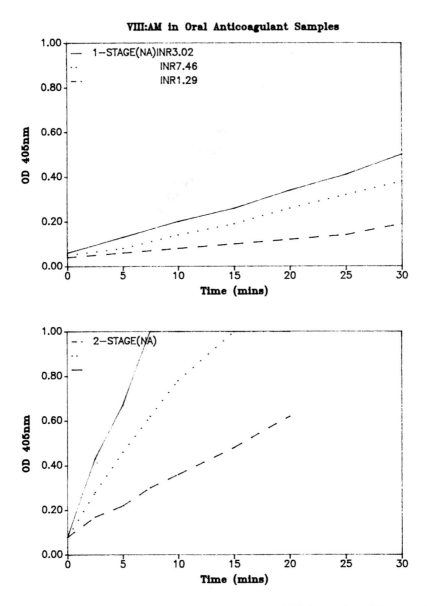

FIGURE 7.   The rate of Xa generation by one-stage and two-stage amidolytic procedures. Three samples with different levels of VIII:C and INR are compared:

VIII:C$_2$	VIII:Am$_2$	INR
524	233	3.02
292	193	7.46
103	83	1.29

The kinetics of Xa generation of ''Des-Gla'' proteins in the VIII amidolytic assay systems are clearly different from that observed with high levels of VIII:C in normals or during pregnancy. The greater degree of disparity between one-stage and two-stage results is possibly due to the lack of surface binding of ''Des-Gla'' forms and the thrombin-induced activation of VIII in the one-stage procedure.

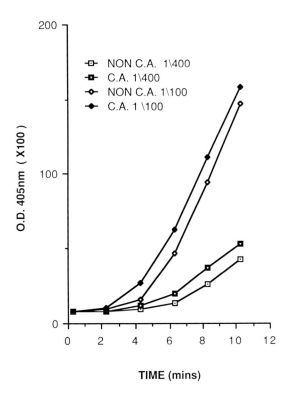

FIGURE 8. Formation of pNA in an extrinsic Xa generation system consisting of plasma dilutions, TF/calcium (at concentrations giving a PT of 17 s), and purified bovine X (1 U/ml). The progressive rate of Xa generation is measured with S2337, without thrombin inhibitor. The system represents one-stage VIII amidolytic acitvity which correlates well with VII:C levels in the test plasma. One-stage VIII amidolytic activity is reduced to a great extent in oral anticoagulated samples (not shown). The lag phase for VII-induced Xa generation is much shorter than for VIII-induced Xa generation, using reagents provided for the Coatest VIII assay. The cold activation of plasma shortens the lag phase in VII amidolytic assay without substantial change in the reaction rates. Species differences in reagents (the type of TF or X as shown in Table 1) contribute to increased reaction rates, hence making this system particularly suitable for standardization of various TFs and/or of reagents for amidolytic assay of VII or VIII.

Several two-stage clotting procedures have been developed and are frequently used in some laboratories. Although the two-stage clotting procedure has eliminated the use of hemophilic plasma as substrate, in common with other tests which are based on clotting principles these methods have poor reproducibility with coefficients of variation of 30% on occasion.

Furthermore, it is essential to preadsorb the test and standard plasma samples with $Al(OH)_3$, hence introducing a further factor of uncertainty. Other variables such as the source of phospholipid, the type and the concentration of the activator, as well as the nature of substrate plasma as the source of fibrinogen, may influence accuracy and precision of these clotting assays.

With the development of commercially available kits[12] (Coatest Factor VIII) offering greater sensitivity and reproducibility and a wider range of measurements, several laboratories have evaluated this system.[16]

The "Chromogenic Factor VIII Kit" which contains optimal levels of the various components of the tenase complex does not require any substrate plasma or catalytic enhancement of VIII. The high dilutions of plasma used in the procedure also reportedly reduce any interference attributable to Vitamin K dependent proteins in the coagulation cascade. Thus, the need for an $Al(OH)_3$ adsorption step is eliminated.

Table 3

CORRELATION OF VIII:C$_1$ AND VIII:Am$_2$ IN DIFFERENT GENETIC VARIANTS OF VIII DEFICIENCY STATES AND SUBSEQUENT TO INTRANASAL ADMINISTRATION OF DDAVP TO vWD[65,73]

Type of deficiency state	n	r
1. Moderate and mild hemophilia	52	0.97
a. Type I (no VIII:Ag)	15	0.89
b. Type IIA (VIII:Ag/VIII:C < 1)	16	0.95
c. Type IIB (VIII:Ag/VIII > 1.5)	21	0.98
d. Severe (below limit)	11	(All below limit)
2. Patients with different genetic variants of vWD		
a. All variants vWd	48	0.93
b. Type IA	17	0.96
c. Type IB	10	0.88
d. Severe recessive type 1	3	0.98
e. Type IIA	3	0.92
f. Type IIB	6	0.98
g. All types/type IIC, IID	11	0.96
h. vWD (type 4) after DDAVP	20	0.94

Note: There is a good correlation between the two tests in all cases, including the monitoring of DDAVP treatment.

A. Some Diagnostic Applications of Coatest Factor VIII

Earlier reports[12,18] by the manufacturer of Coatest Factor VIII have indicated a good correlation between this and clotting assays used in the evaluation of VIII in various deficient plasma samples. However, in some cases large discrepancies among results have been observed, as shown below.

	Deficiency state				
	XII	**XI**	**IX**	**VII**	**V**
VIII:C$_1$ (U/ml)	0.22	0.44	1.16	1.34	0.88
VIII:Am$_2$ (U/ml)	0.28	0.58	0.85	1.33	0.72

More recently, four leading laboratories[16] have evaluated the Coatest Kit, as compared with their own local one-stage assay procedure for clinical use.

The clinical material consisted of healthy individuals, patients with severe or mild hemophilia A or von Willebrand's disease (vWD), and hemophilia carriers. In all 385 cases, a significant correlation was observed between the two methods ($r = 0.96$ to 0.99). The chromogenic assay was found to be more precise. However, in some severe hemophilia samples, value discrepancies between the two methods were observed.

The results of a recent comparative[65] study using the Coatest and an in-house one-stage clotting assay are shown in Table 3. The data confirm the observation that VIII amidolytic assays can be successfully used in the diagnosis of all variants of hemophilia A and vWD irrespective of co-existing VIII:Ag or vWf:Ag levels. This study also indicates that the Coatest can be used to monitor VIII levels after 1-desamino-8-D-arginine-vasopressin (DDAVP) treatment.

Tripodi and Mannucci[66] in an independent study have also compared VIII:Am$_2$ and VIII one-stage clotting method (VIII:C$_1$) values in 12 hemophiliacs with severe to mild VIII deficiency (<1 to 34 U/dl) and 10 hemophilia A patients receiving therapeutic doses of commercial VIII concentrates (VIII:C 60 to 150 U/dl). The results obtained from the untreated hemophiliacs were significantly correlated (r = 0.97), but in 2/12 of these patients the amidolytic assay demonstrated lower values than the clotting assay (8 and 14 U/dl against 19 and 34 U/dl). In the treated patients no significant difference between the methods were observed (92 ± 30% in amidolytic against 95 ± 30 VIII:C [U/dl]). The C.V. at normal and low levels for the amidolytic and clotting assays were 7 to 5% and 11 to 12%, respectively. The linearity of VIII amidolytic assay calibration curves was found to be good, but the C.V.s of the optical densities, particularly at low VIII levels, were greater than 20% indicating poor reproducibility.

Discrepant results in some hemophilia A patients have also been reported by the present author in earlier investigations using different types of reagents[7,8] and independently by Rosen,[12] and Rosen et al.[16] using the Coatest Factor VIII Kit on three hemophilia samples. Higher VIII amidolytic assay values were, however, reported by both groups of investigators. Until the possible causes of their discrepant results are fully elucidated it is recommended that both assays should be run in parallel for clinical use.

On the basis of the reported insensitivity of VIII amidolytic assay to pretreatment of VIII by thrombin, Millar et al.[67] have studied the value of the Coatest VIII system for the prenatal diagnosis of hemophilic plasma from 21 fetuses at 18 to 20 weeks when assayed by one-stage clotting and the two-stage amidolytic methods. According to these investigators, the observed good correlation between the assays (r = 0.85) indicated the potential value of the amidolytic assay in prenatal diagnosis.

B. Assay Discrepancy in Potency Determination of Clinical Concentrates

An earlier study[18] on the potency estimation of VIII concentrates by five methods consisting of one-stage clotting, two-stage clotting, and amidolytic assays has indicated a good correlation among various methods. However, in a recent study performed by Hubbard et al.[19] on a large number of heat treated VIII concentrates, it has been shown that significant differences among the methods still exist. These observed differences are reportedly unrelated to the specific methods of processing and/or to the mode of heat treatment of the final material.

With the advances in the use of recombinant DNA (rDNA) technology for the production of VIII (DNA-VIII), Pancham et al.[17] have attempted to characterize the functional activity of various forms of VIII/vWf complex, VIII-derived from plasma free from vWf, and the rDNA-VIII from mammalian cell cultures. From the differing results obtained these investigators have suggested that the rate of tenase complex formation is altered when vWf is present in the test system.

Furthermore, the residual VIII activity of mixtures of monoclonal antibodies specific to 90- or 80-kDa subunits and plasma derived VIII or rDNA-VIII demonstrated discrepant values.[17] These differences were considered to be the consequence of varying degrees of inhibition of VIII as influenced by the presence or absence of vWf in the samples and the method of assay.

C. Assay Discrepancies in the Evaluation of Factor VIII Inhibitors

The accurate measurement of specific antibodies (inhibitors) to the procoagulant part of the VIII/vwF complex is of great importance for classification and therapeutic purposes. A recent study of interlaboratory determinations of VIII inhibitors has shown large variations in the observed measurement of inhibitor titers, irrespective of the clotting or amidolytic method, or the nature of the VIII added to the system.[68]

Variables contributing to the observed discrepancies include the use of different methodologies, variable stabilities of VIII:C in the source plasma or concentrates, and the nature or types of the inhibitors. Attempts at method standardization by using a reference inhibitor sample have improved, but not entirely eliminated the large differences among results. In

Table 4

VIII:C INHIBITOR STUDY — STOCKHOLM — MALMO

Sample	Chromogenic substrate assay		One-stage clotting assay	
	Lab. 1	Lab. 2	Lab. 1	Lab. 2
A	3	2	4	2
B	10	9	10	11
C	101	173	166	342
D	40	38	76	53
E	2	5	11	5
F	4	3	40	5
G	3	2	18	2
H	2375	1734	3300	2200
I	7	5	23	25
J	1	1	1	1
K	131	143	188	233
L	4	2	6	12
M	1	3	16	4
N	141	143	150	220

Note: Results in New Oxford Units.

	Chromogenic assay	One-stage clot
Lab 1 (Karolinska)	Cobas Bio	Phosphol. + kaolin
Lab 2 (Malmo Sjukhus)	Microplate	Platelet-rich plasma

earlier investigations using the combined reagent for the two-stage clotting in both VIII:C and VIII amidolytic assay methods and with the use of VIII-depleted cryosupernatant as diluent for the concentrate, Mackie and Seghatchian[69] have reported that residual VIII activity could be accurately measured by either the Bethesda or the New Oxford method over a wide range of inhibitor levels (1 to 10,000).

More recently, using Coatest kits, but different experimental conditions, Blomback et al.[70] have reported satisfactory results as shown in Table 4, but large discrepancies were reported by both groups of investigators.

The introduction of porcine VIII as an alternative treatment in inhibitor patients led to attempts to quantitate porcine VIII-antibody titers against human inhibitor standards. Considerable differences among inhibitors in their ability to inactivate human and porcine VIII are observed.

The nature of VIII inhibitors and their site of action can be further investigated using an analytical agarose electrophoretic method, with simultaneous analyses of various forms of VIII by clotting and amidolytic assays in gel slices.[71,72] Multiple peaks of VIII-like activity could be identified by both methods in certain conditions.[71]

Spontaneous inhibitor and hemophilic inhibitors may differ from each other on the basis of clotting, amidolytic, and immunoradiometric assay values. This was further substantiated on the basis of VIII amidolytic neutralization assay and electrophoretic migration of their complexes.[72]

Furthermore, using this procedure, plasma could be directly compared with concentrates and/or the residual VIII amidolytic activities. Such studies may demonstrate whether the presence of vWf could protect various forms of VIII either from inactivation or inhibitor neutralization. The high sensitivity and specificity of Coatest VIII would make it useful in such a system and may provide a better insight on the nature of observed discrepancies.

D. VIII Amidolytic Activity Levels in Various Pathophysiological States

The level of VIII:C is not only reduced in congenital diseases but also in some acquired disorders, e.g., in patients with fibrinolytic states and intravascular coagulation. However, it is more common to observe increased values of VIII:C in various pathophysiological states. In these conditions[60] the increase in VIII:C levels is accompanied by an increase in vWf. However, in certain conditions, such as widespread cancer, renal disease with uremia, nephrotic syndrome, severe burns, some cases of leukemia, myelomatosis, macroglobulinaemia (Waldenström), hemolytic uremic syndrome, and chronic liver disease, two- to threefold higher levels of vWf:Ag than VIII:C are documented. A less striking increase, nevertheless, may occur in myocardial infarction, patients with thrombotic thrombocytopenic purpura, and some other pathophysiological states.[60]

It is not clear whether the increased levels of vWf:Ag affect the procoagulant activity of VIII or the observed disproportionality is due to differential proteolytic fragmentation of VIII/vWf components. The latter is supported by the finding that in some of the above mentioned cases, altered forms of vWf:Ag, the so-called vWf fragment, could be observed.[60] There is also a good correlation between the elevated VIII:C, elevated vWf:Ag, and TLA.[58] Alternatively, the raised VIII:C levels could be due to higher sensitivity of clotting methods to thrombin, hence having a different origin than vWf:Ag.

VIII/vWf is also increased by at least two- to fourfold, after treatment of normal subjects with a single i.v. infusion (0.3 μg/kg) of DDAVP.[73] There is a good correlation between VIII:C and VIII amidolytic activity.

Tripodi and Mannucci[66] have compared the results of VIII amidolytic and one-stage clotting assays in ten patients with liver disease and in ten normal subjects treated with DDAVP. The results of this study are shown below.

Groups	VIII:Am$_2$ (U/dl)	VIII:C$_1$ (U/dl)	Ratio
DDAVP-treated	227 ± 87	292 ± 91	0.77
Liver disease	292 ± 101	278 ± 98	1.05

The low ratio of VIII:Am$_2$/VIII:C$_1$ as compared to either normal or liver disease groups having the same VIII:C-like activity strongly suggests that different forms of VIII are measured to a variable degree by these methods. Much remains to be resolved before the VIII amidolytic assay completely replaces clotting assays.

It should be noted that in all clinical applications of the VIII amidolytic assay that the potency is expressed against an international plasma standard or concentrate standard for VIII:C (NIBSC). Since these standards are not calibrated in terms of VIII amidolytic assays, one assumes that the pooled plasma used as standard arbitrarily contains equivalent VIII:C and VIII amidolytic activity potencies. The first step in the standardization of the VIII amidolytic assay would be to calibrate standard plasma and concentrate in terms of proteolytic enzymes, amidolytic VIII, and subsequently perform the assay according to biometric principles. Multiple point assays are of value in differentiating the presence or absence of partially ctivated and/nonactivated forms of VIII in either a standard or tests.

VI. FUTURE TRENDS/CONCLUDING REMARKS

New technology and sophisticated equipment make diagnostic tests more rapid, simpler,and more accurate. As a result, diagnostic testing in the near future could be expected to leave the laboratory environment and become more applicable to bedside use. The higher sensitivity, specificity, and accuracy of VIII amidolytic assays as compared to clotting procedures will not only improve the effective diagnosis of VIII deficiency states and the monitoring of therapy, but can also help in differentiating the activity state of VIII in various pathophysiological states. The ratio of VIII:Am_1/VIII:Am_2 could provide further insight in the role played by thrombin. Further studies into the mechanism of the lag phase of Xa generation by VIII:Am_1 may be of value in the assessment of the mode of action of various VIII inhibitors. Of immediate useful application is the APTT-type VIII:Am_1, which is applicable to automated technologies and could be adopted for large-scale screening programs. Moreover, the easy adaptation of this technique to centrifugal analyzers permits the direct conversion of absorbance to potency values. Such methodology, apart from higher sensitivity and precision, provides greater throughput of samples for analysis. In general, VIII amidolytic methods compare well with clotting methods. However, some discrepancies are observed. In principle there is no easy way of ensuring that the results of either amidolytic or clotting assays are the correct values. Each assay has its own intrinsic error which can only be determined by statistical assessment of repeated measurements. In this respect amidolytic assays can be considered as a method of choice, which in addition to improved sensitivity and specificity also reduce the unresolved problems associated with VIII:C standardization.

The use of control samples as a "check" on the correctness of test results in amidolytic assays may be misleading. However, the inclusion of control samples is a prerequisite for essential internal quality control. Assignment of an amidolytic potency on the international plasma and the use of heat treated standard concentrates are also essential to reduce interlaboratory variation in the assay of clinical VIII concentrates.

Finally, it is in the screening of blood donors and in the in-process validation of blood products that VIII amidolytic assays using microtiter procedures may have major contributions. It is not inconceivable that in the near future a donor panel for high VIII levels may be created for plasmapheresis to obtain a single unit cryoprecipitate from 600 ml of plasma, from appropriately screened donors, following intranasal DDAVP administration. With the aims of optimization of VIII potency both VIII:Am and IIa-like activity of such preparations should be evaluated. Only by doing so without complacency we can improve the safety and the quality of final products in a standardized manner.

ACKNOWLEDGMENTS

I am indebted to Miss J. A. Smith for typing this manuscript and to Mr. P. Harrison for his assistance with computer graphics.

REFERENCES

1. **Stormorken, H.,** A new-era in the laboratory evaluation of coagulation and fibrinolysis, *Thromb. Haemost.,* 36, 299, 1976.
2. **Seghatchian, M. J.,** The value of chromogenic substrates in the improvement of diagnostic tests for haemostatic function, *Ric. Clin. Lab.,* 2, 2, 1981.
3. **Austen, D. E. G., Rhynes, I. R., and Rizza, C. R.,** Factor VIII concentrate: what the label says, *Lancet,* I, 279, 1981.
4. **Seghatchian, M. J. and Sterling, Y.,** Factor VIII concentrates: what the label says and standardization, *Lancet,* I, 279, 1982.
5. **Heldebrant, C., Kleszysni, R., Short, M., Aronson, D., Brown, L., Barrowcliffe, T., Thomas, D., Jacoby, J., Leem, Howell, I., and Johnson, R. C.,** Assay of AHF concentrates and standards: failure to eliminate variability with a monographed assay, *Thromb. Res.,* 30, 337, 1983.
6. **Seghatchian, M. J. and Miller-Anderson, M.,** Assay of F.VIII using chromogenic substrate proceeding, in ICTH Symp. Synthetic Substrates and Inhibitors, International Committee on Thrombosis and Hemostasis, Kyoto, 1976, 51.
7. **Seghatchian, M. J. and Miller-Anderson, M.,** A colorimetric evaluation of F.VIII:C potency, *Med. Lab. Sci.,* 35, 347, 1978.

8. **Seghatchian, M. J.,** *The Usefulness of Chromogenic Substrates in the Diagnosis of Haemophilia and Control of Blood Products in Chromogenic Peptide Substrate,* Scully, M. F. and Kakkar, V. V., Eds., Churchill Livingstone, London, 1979, 102.

9. **Seghatchian, M. J.,** Recent advances in the use of chromogenic substrates in the control of blood products and the treatment of haemophilia, in *Chromogenic Substrate Assay,* Fareed, J., Ed., CRC Press, Boca Raton, Fla., to be published.

10. **Friberger, P. and Vinazzer, H.,** Assay of F.VIII:C with a chromosubstrate in *Trans. 1st Danube Symp. on Thromb. Haemost.,* Vinazzer, H., Ed., Medicus Verlag, Berlin, 1979, 117.

11. **Van Dieijien, G., Tans, G., Rosing, J., and Hemker, H. C.,** The role of phospholipid and F.VIIIa in the activation of bovine F.X, *J. Biol. Chem.,* 256, 3433, 1981.

12. **Rosen, S.,** Assay of F.VIII:C with a chromogenic substrate, *Scand. J. Haematol.,* 33 (Suppl. 41), 139, 1984.

13. **Beeser, H. and Baden, W.,** A new chromogenic F.VIII:C assay based on the two stage method, *Thromb. Haemost.,* 54, 250, 1985.

14. **Rosing, J. P., Amiral, J., and Martinoli, J. L.,** Amidolytic assay of F.VIII:C influence of phospholipids, *Thromb. Haemost.,* 54, 250, 1985.

15. **Ikesawa, J., Yamashite, T., Ohara, T., Taeemoto, K., Mimura, K., Matsuoka, A., and Okamoto, S.,** An improvement of F.VIII:C chromogenic method with combination use of the specific synthetic thrombin inhibitors. MD. 805 and I-2581, *Thromb. Haemost.,* 52, 250, 1985.

16. **Rosen, S., Anderson, M., Blomback, M., Hagglund, U., Larrieu, M. J., Woolf, M., Boyer, C., Rothschild, C., Nilsson, I. M., Sjorin, E., and Vinazzer, H.,** Clinical application of a chromogenic substrate method for determination of F.VIII activity, *Thromb. Haemost.,* 54, 818, 1985.

17. **Pancham, N., Dang, N., Madant, T., Cowgill, C., and Shroeder, C.,** Comparison of chromogenic and clotting activities in recombinant DNA and plasma derived F.VIII:C bound to or free of von Willebrand protein, *Thromb. Haemost.,* 54, 250, 1985.

18. **Mikaelsson, M. and Oswaldsson, V.,** Standardization of VIII:C assays: a manufacturer's view, *Scand. J. Haematol.,* 33 (Suppl. 41), 79, 1984.

19. **Hubbard, A. R., Curtis, A. D., Barrowcliffe, T. W., Edwards, S. J., Jennings, C. A., and Kembel-Cook, G.,** Assay of F.VIII concentrates: comparison of the chromogenic and two stage clotting assays, *Thromb. Res.,* 44, 887, 1986.

20. **Griffin, J. H. and Cochrane, C. G.,** Recent advances in the understanding of the contact activation reactions, *Semin. Thromb. Haemost.,* 5, 254, 1979.

21. **Rapaport, S.,** The activation of F.IX by the tissue factor pathway, in *Haemophilia and Haemostasis,* Menache, D., MacSurgenor, N., and Anderson, H., Eds., Alan R. Liss, New York, 1981, 57.

22. **Nemerson, Y.,** Regulation of the initiation of coagulation by factor VII, *haemostasis,* 13, 150, 1983.

23. **Nemerson, Y. and Zur, M.,** Is haemophilia a disease of the tissue factor pathway?, In *Haemophilia and Haemostasis,* Menache, D., MacSurgenor, N., and Anderson, H., Eds., Alan R. Liss, New York, 1981, 77.

24. **Østerud, B. and Rapaport, S. I.,** Activation of F.IX by the reaction product of tissue factor and F.VII: additional pathway for initiating blood coagulation, *Proc. Natl. Acad. Sci. U.S.A.,* 74, 5260, 1977.

25. **Seligsohn, U., Østerud, B., Griffin, J. H., and Rapaport, S. I.,** Evidence for the participation of both activated F.XII and activated F.IX in cold promoted activation of factor VII, *Thromb. Res.,* 13, 1049, 1978.

26. **Jesty, J., Spencer, A. I. C., and Nemerson, Y.,** The mechanism of activation of F.X kinetic control of alternative pathways leading to the formation of activated F.Xa, *J. Biol. Chem.,* 249, 5614, 1974.

27. **Radcliffe, R., Bagdasarian, A., and Colman, R. W.,** Activation of F.VII by Hageman factor fragments, Blood, 50, 611, 1977.

28. **Saito, H. and Ratnoff, O. D.,** Activation of F.VII activity by activated Fletcher factor (a plasma Kallikrein): a potential link between the intrinsic and extrinsic blood clotting systems, *J. Lab. Clin. Med.,* 85, 405, 1975.

29. **Walsh, P. N. and Griffin, J. H.,** Platelet dependent proteolytic activation of F.XI, *Thromb. Haemost.,* 42, 236, 1979.

30. **Nawroth, P. and Stern, D. M.,** A pathway of coagulation on endothelial cells, *J. Cell Biochem.,* 28, 253, 1985.

31. **Stern, D. M., Nawroth, P. P., Handley, D., and Kisiel, W.,** An endothelial cell-dependent pathway of coagulation, *Proc. Natl. Acad. Sci. U.S.A.,* 82, 2523, 1985.

32. **Rodgers, G. and Schuman, M.,** Prothrombin is activated on vascular endothelial cells by F.Xa and calcium, *Proc. Natl. Acad. Sci. U.S.A.,* 80, 7001, 1983.

33. **Golucci, M., Balconi, G., Lorenret, R., Pietra, A., Locati, D., Donati, M., and Sermeramo, P.,** Cultured endothelial cells express tissue factor, *J. Clin. Invest.,* 71, 1893, 1983.

34. **Bevilacqua, M., Pober, J. S., Majeau, G. R., Cotran, R. S., and Gimbourne, M. A.,** Interleukin I induces procoagulant activity in human vascular endothelial cells, *J. Exp. Med.,* 160, 618, 1984.

35. **Stern, D. M., Bank, I., Nawroth, P. P., Cassimeris, J., Kisiel, W., Fenton, J. W., Dinarello, C., Jaffe, E. A., and Chess, L.,** Self regulation of procoagulant events on the endothelial surface, *J. Exp. Med.*, 162, 1223, 1985.

36. **Stern, D. M., Nawroth, P. P., Misiel, W., Vehar, G., and Esmon, C. T.,** The binding of F.IXa to cultured bovine aortic endothelial cells: induction of a specific site in the presence of F.VIII and X, *J. Biol. Chem.*, 260, 6717, 1985.

37. **Elodi, S. and Varadi, K.,** Formation of the factor IXa/factor VIII complex on the surface of endothelial cells, *Thromb. Haemost.*, 54, 251, 1985.

38. **Nawroth, P., Kisiel, W., and Stern, D. M.,** Anti-coagulant and antithrombic pupentis of a α-carboxy glutamic acid-rich peptide derived from the light chain of blood coagulation factor X, *Thromb. Res.*, 44, 625, 1986.

39. **Prowse, C., Hornsey, V., MacKay, A., and Waterston, Y.,** Room temperature, micro chromogenic assay of F.VIII:C, *Vox Sang.*, 50, 21, 1986.

40. **Lollar, D., Knutson, G. J., and Fass, D. N.,** Stabilization of thrombin activated porcine F.VIII:C by F.IXa and phospholipid, *Blood*, 63, 1303, 1984.

41. **Bartl, K., Becker, U., and Lill, H.,** Application of several of chromogenic substrate assays to automated instrumentation for coagulation analysis, *Semin. Thromb. Haemost.*, 9, 301, 1983.

42. **Yamada, K. and Meguro, T.,** A new APTT assay employing substrate and a centrifugal autoanalyzer, *Thromb. Res.*, 15, 351, 1979.

43. **Seghatchian, M. J., Kemball-Cook, G., and Barrowcliffe, T. W.,** Adsorption of F.VIII by aluminium hydroxide, *Haemostasis*, 8, 106, 1979.

44. **Seghatchian, M. J. and Mackie, I. J.,** Aluminum hydroxide adsorption and factor VIII clotting assays, *Lancet*, II, 38, 1980.

45. **Suomela, H., Blomback, M., and Blomback, B.,** The activation of F.X evaluated by using synthetic substrates, *Thromb. Res.*, 10, 267, 1977.

46. **Seegers, W. H.,** Factor X (antithrombin III), *Semin. Thromb. Haemost.*, 7, 223, 1981.

47. **Seegers, W. H. and Ghosh, A.,** The activation of F.X and X B with F.VII or protein M, *Thromb. Res.*, 17, 501, 1980.

48. **Hultin, M. B. and Nemerson, Y.,** Activation of F.X by F.Xa by F.IXa and VIII: a specific assay for F.IXa in the presence of thrombin-activated F.VIII, *Blood*, 52, 928, 1978.

49. **Bertina, R. M., Gupers, R., and Van Wunaarden, A.,** F.IXa protects activated F.VIII against inactivation by activation protein C, *Biochem. Biophys. Res. Comp.*, 125, 177, 1984.

50. **Østerud, B., Rapaport, S. I., and Lavine, K. K.,** The F.V activity of platelets: evidence for an activated F.V molecular for a platelet activator, *Blood*, 49, 819, 1977.

51. **Marciniak, E. and Tsukamura, S.,** Two progressive inhibitors of factor Xa in human blood, *Br. J. Haematol.*, 22, 341, 1972.

52. **Bajaj, S. and Hanahan, D. J.,** Interaction of short chain and long chain fatty acid, phosphoglycerides and bile salts with prothrombin, *Biochem. Biophys. Acta*, 444, 118, 1976.

53. **Barthels, M. and Seegers, W. H.,** Substitution of lipid with bile salts in the formation of thrombin, *Thromb. Diath. Haemorrh.*, 22, 13, 1969.

54. **Mann, K. G. and Fass, D. H.,** The molecular biology of blood coagulation, in *Haematology*, Vol. 2, Fairbanks, V. F., Ed., John Wiley & Sons, New York, 1983, 347.

55. **Tracy, P. B., Rohrback, M. S., and Mann, K. G.,** Functional prothrombinase complex assembly on isolated monocytes and lymphocytes, *J. Biol. Chem.*, 258, 7264, 1983.

56. **Kockum, C. and Frebelius, S.,** Rapid radioimmunoassay of human fibrinopeptide A, removal of cross-reacting fibrinogen with bentonite, *Thromb. Res.*, 19, 589, 1980.

57. **Seghatchian, M. J.,** Enzymology of thrombin: purification procedure characterization, surface binding, stability unitage and standardization, in, *Thrombin*, Vol. 1, Machovich, R., Ed., CRC Press, Boca Raton, Fla., 1984, 102.

58. **Stirling, Y., Woolf, L., North, W. R. S., Seghatchian, M. J., and Meade, T. W.,** Haemostasis in normal pregnancy, *Thromb. Haemost.*, 52, 176, 1984.

59. **Dalaker, K. and Prydz, H.,** The coagulation factor VII in pregnancy, *Br. J. Haematol.*, 56, 233, 1984.

60. **Lombardi, R., Mannucci, P. M., Seghatchian, M. J., Vincente Garcia, V., and Coppola, R.,** Alterations of factor VIII von Willebrand factor in clinical conditions associated with an increase in its plasma concentration, *Br. J. Haematol.*, 49, 61, 1981.

61. **Morita, T. and Jackson, C.,** Structural and functional characterization of a proteolytically modified "Gla-domainless" bovine factor X and Xa (Des-light chain residue 1-44), in *Vitamin K Metabolism and Vitamin K-Dependent Protein*, Suttie, J. W., Ed., University Park Press, Baltimore, 1980, 124.

62. **Fujikawa, K., Coan, M. H., Legaz, M. E., and Davie, E. W.,** The mechanism of activation of bovine factor X by intrinsic and extrinsic pathways, *Biochemistry*, 13, 5290, 1974.

63. **Mertens, K., Wortelboer, M., Van Dieijen, G., and Bertina, R. M.,** Proteolysis of blood coagulation factor X by activated factor X. Difference between the bovine and human proteins, *FEBS Lett.,* 139, 174, 1982.

64. **Fass, D. N. and Lollar, P.,** Physiological modulator of factor VIII activity, in *Factor VIII von Willebrand Factor,* Ciavarella, N. L., Ruggeri, Z. M., and Zimmerman, T. S., Eds., Wichtig Editore, Milan, 1986, 224.

65. **Lethagen, S., Østergaard, H., and Nilsson, I. M.,** Clinical application of the chromogenic assay of factor VIII in haemophilia A and different variants of von Willebrand's disease, *Scand. J. Haematol.,* to be published.

66. **Tripodi, A. and Mannucci, P. M.,** Factor VIII activity as measured by an amidolytic assay compared with a one-stage clotting assay, *Ricerca,* 16, 132, 1986.

67. **Millar, D. S., Mibashan, R. S., Rodek, C. H., and Nicolaides, K. H.,** Chromogenic factor VIII:C assay for prenatal diagnosis of haemophilia A, *Ricerca,* 16, 93, 1986.

68. **Austen, D. E. G.,** The Oxford antibody assay and a comparison of methods, in *Activated Prothrombin Complex,* Mariani, G., Russo, M. A., and Mondelli, F., Eds., Prager, New York, 1982, 22.

69. **Mackie, I. J. and Seghatchian, M. J.,** Amidolytic end-point methods for factor VIII:C inhibitors, *Med. Lab. Sci.,* 39, 345, 1982.

70. **Blomback, M., Carlebjork, G., Dahlback, B., Nilsson, I. M., and Rosen, S.,** Photometric determination of factor VIII:C inhibitors in haemophilia A patients with Coatest factor VIII, *Ricerca,* 16, 93, 1986.

71. **Seghatchian, M. J.,** An agarose gel method for evaluating F.VIII procoagulant electrophoretic distribution, *Ann. N.Y. Acad. Sci.,* 370, 236, 1981.

72. **Seghatchian, M. J. and Mackie, I. J.,** The association of VIII:C with the various molecular forms of VIII/vWf present in clinical concentrates, *Thrombin. Res.,* 29, 447, 1983.

73. **Nilsson, I. M., Felding, P., Timberg, L., Jonsson, S., and Harris, A.,** Clinical experience with DDAVP, in *Factor VIII/von Willebrand Factor,* Ciavarella, N. L., Ruggeri, Z. M., and Zimmerman, T. S., Eds., Wichtig Editore, Milan, 1986, 63.

Chapter 6

PROGRESS IN vWf METHODOLOGY AND ITS RELEVANCE IN vWD

R. G. Dalton and G. F. Savidge

TABLE OF CONTENTS

I.   Introduction 130

II.   *In Vivo* Assessment — The Bleeding Time 130

III.   *In Vitro* Assessment 131
        A.   Sample Preparation 131
        B.   Functional Assays 132
                1.   Platelet Adhesion/*In Vitro* Bleeding Time 132
                2.   Ristocetin Dependent Tests 132
                        a.   Ristocetin Induced Platelet Aggregation in PRP 132
                        b.   Ristocetin Co-Factor Activity 133
                        c.   Ristocetin Induced Platelet Binding of vWf 133
                        d.   Alternatives to Ristocetin 133
                3.   Collagen Binding Assays 134
        C.   Immunologic Assays for vWf:Ag 134
                1.   Quantitative Assays 134
                        a.   Electroimmunoassay (EIA) 134
                        b.   Immunologic Assays Using Radioisotopes 135
                        c.   Enzyme Linked Immunosorbent Assays (ELISA) 136
                        d.   Monoclonal Antibody Assays 136
                2.   Crossed (or Two Dimensional) Immunoelectrophoresis 136
                3.   Multimer Sizing Techniques 137

IV.   Summary 141

References 141

I. INTRODUCTION

Von Willebrand originally described an autosomally inherited bleeding diathesis with a prolonged bleeding time. Advances made since then have established that a reduction in the activity of a large polymeric glycoprotein in plasma — von Willebrand factor (vWf) — is a critical diagnostic feature of the disease in many patients, including the original kindred. This reduction of activity may be expressed as a quantitative deficiency or as a qualitative alteration in vWf.

Recent advances reviewed elsewhere in this volume suggest that the disease will be understood at a genetic and molecular level in the foreseeable future, and diagnosis may be possible using genetic techniques. At present, however, the diagnosis rests upon the recognition of the abnormal phenotype, and the initial diagnostic screening of patients is likely to remain so.

vWf is synthesized and stored in endothelial cells and megakaryocytes/platelets whence it is released into the plasma. Its principle functions appear to be that of a carrier for the procoagulant protein VIII:C and as an adhesive protein in primary hemostasis. In the latter case the exact role of vWf has yet to be fully elucidated. It is clear, however, that vWf is able to bind to collagen and possibly other subendothelial structures and mediate the adhesion of platelets through binding to the surface receptor glycoprotein Ib. This is of particular importance in the adhesion of platelets at high shear rates. vWf may also play a role in platelet-platelet interaction through binding to the glycoprotein IIb/IIIa.

The diagnostic tests for vWD consist of an *in vivo* assessment of primary hemostasis, the bleeding time, and *in vitro* tests designed to assess the vWf on both a quantitative and qualitative basis. Due to the low concentrations of vWf in plasma and platelets, these tests rely on detection of either functional and/or antigenic properties of the factor.

In this chapter we attempt to briefly but critically review the methods currently available for the diagnosis and evaluation of vWD. The application of these techniques is discussed elsewhere.

II. *IN VIVO* ASSESSMENT — THE BLEEDING TIME

The bleeding time has been defined as the time taken for the cessation of bleeding from a small standard incision.[1] The bleeding time is widely held to correlate most closely with the hemorrhagic risk in vWD but, this belief is difficult to substantiate.

Since its inception early this century when the bleeding time was measured following an incision made in the ear lobe,[2] a number of modifications have been proposed to the original method. Most notably such modifications have included the use of the forearm with a tourniquet to elevate venous pressure and increase sensitivity[3] and the use of a blade[4] with a template to ensure a uniform cut.

A recent working party[6] observed that the bleeding time was found to vary with site, direction, and length of incision as well as the level of venous pressure. It recommended that the lateral aspect of the volar surface of the forearm should be used with venous pressure elevated to 40 mm Hg, as described by Ivy et al.[3]

A survey in 1984 of practice in British hospitals showed a wide variation of techniques in clinical use.[7] The single most popular technique makes use of the commercially available Simplate II (Organon Teknika, Cambridge, U.K.).[8,9] This convenient disposable device incorporates two spring loaded blades and template. It makes two incisions 6 mm long and 1 mm deep and is most frequently used in the manner described by Kumar et al.[9] in the use of the forearm with a tourniquet pressure of 40 mm Hg, longitudinal direction of the incisions, and blotting of extruded blood every 30 sec without contact with the wound. The use of the "longitudinal" incision (parallel to the long axis of the arm) is reported to produce shorter bleeding times than the "horizontal" incision,[10] but it is debatable whether this significantly affects the sensitivity of the test.

The bleeding time remains the most important and convenient screening test for vWD. However, the template method leaves a scar in the majority of patients[9] and is difficult to use in children if they are noncompliant. Alternative techniques have been described[11,12] which attempt to overcome these disadvantages by reversion to the use of lancets. These, however, have yet to be evaluated in vWD. Furthermore, despite efforts to standardize the test, a large normal range is still observed with a considerable overlap between the recorded bleeding times in normal volunteers and in vWD patients.[13] The observation that the bleeding time is principally dependent upon the concentration of platelet vWf[14] rather than plasma levels of vWf, which hitherto have been primarily used to establish the diagnosis, may explain this overlap, particularly since platelet vWf concentrations in mild type I vWD are frequently normal. The measurement of bleeding time following an oral dose of aspirin[15] may increase the sensitivity of the test for the detection of vWD,[16] but this modification has not been widely used.[7] The usual template methods retain an element of operator dependency. This can be avoided by an automated technique for recording the bleeding time,[17] but this requires elaborate apparatus. In practice, it is important that an adequate number of normal controls should be recruited. Since it is a test of all aspects of primary hemostasis, the bleeding time obviously lacks specificity, and in the absence of the appropriate clinical and family history, an observed prolongation is unlikely to be due to vWD.[18]

III. *IN VITRO* ASSESSMENT

A. Sample Preparation

vWf circulates in plasma but is also present in platelets, endothelial cells, and the sub-endothelium. As plasma is most readily available, most diagnostic tests have primarily been performed on this material. It is, however, becoming increasingly apparent that subendothelial[19] and platelet vWf[14] are of significance in hemostatic mechanisms and that platelet studies are also important in the classification of vWD.

Plasma studies are usually performed on citrated samples. A recent report, however, has suggested that the small multimer size detected in type IIA vWD is due to *in vitro* cleavage of large multimers by a calcium ion dependent protease and may be corrected by the collection of blood into EDTA.[20] In contrast, others have found this correction to be only partial and not present in all patients.[21]

Platelets are usually investigated either in autologous citrated plasma (PRP), or platelet vWf may be studied independently of plasma. The latter method involves washing the platelets, followed by lysis and collection of the supernatant. In this case, it is important to avoid activation of the platelets by the washing step which would result in release of stored vWf or the binding of plasma vWf to surface platelet glycoproteins. For this reason a membrane stabilizing agent, commonly EDTA, is often used.[22-24] The washing procedure may be performed using a gradient of albumin,[25] or arabinogalactan,[24] to prevent mechanical trauma to the platelets. Platelet lysis has been achieved by a variety of techniques including repeated freeze-thawing,[22,23] hypotonic glycerol lysis,[26] or by treatment with detergents such as Triton-X100.[24] Higher values of platelet vWf have been reported using lytic techniques with detergent rather than freeze-thawing,[27,28] possibly due to binding of the high molecular weight (HMW) multimers by the platelet membrane after freeze-thawing. The supernatant of the platelet lysate can be assayed for vWf in a similar manner to plasma, although platelet vWf demonstrates qualitative differences from plasma vWf.[29] Quantitation may be performed using a plasma standard and expressed as units per 10^9 platelets or units per milligram platelet protein.

B. Functional Assays

1. Platelet Adhesion/In Vitro Bleeding Time

Several *in vitro* methods have been described to facilitate the study of the primary phase of hemostasis. Methods to quantify the adhesion of platelets to everted rabbit[30] or human arterial subendothelium, or to isolated components of vessel walls in perfusion chambers,[31] have proven to be of greater value in the elucidation of fundamental physiological processes of hemostasis than in patient evaluation.

Alternative techniques relying on platelet adhesion/aggregation induced by foreign surfaces such as platelet adhesiveness,[32,33] or the methods for *in vitro* "bleeding times",[34-36] are more readily applicable on a routine basis, although they require special apparatus. The experimental data using these methods tend to correlate with the bleeding time as determined by established methods and, furthermore, avoid the risk of scarring the patient and the problems associated with poor patient compliance. Although the surfaces initiating platelet adhesion are nonphysiological, these tests do incorporate the additional function of shear stress between platelets and the adherent surface which appears increasingly to be of importance in normal hemostasis.[37] Nevertheless, such tests remain nonspecific and are not generally used for diagnostic purposes as there is little evidence that they yield additional information to the *in vivo* bleeding time.

2. Ristocetin Dependent Tests

By far the most widely applied functional tests of vWf depend on the ability of vWf to bind and aggregate platelets in the presence of the cationic antibiotic ristocetin. Historically, this antibiotic was withdrawn from therapeutic use following the high incidence of thrombocytopenia in those treated. Howard and Firkin[38] reported that ristocetin induced platelet aggregation in PRP in normal individuals but not vWD patients. Weiss and colleagues[39] demonstrated that this effect was due to a plasma factor. The precise mechanism of action of ristocetin remains uncertain but is known to depend on the binding of the largest multimeric forms of vWf to the platelet glycoprotein Ib.[40] Interestingly similar vWf enhanced platelet aggregation is caused by a number (albeit not all) of disparate polycations.[41,42]

Possibly two separable characteristics of ristocetin are necessary for its action, i.e., the ability to enhance the binding of high molecular weight vWf to platelets and second the ability to reduce the net negative charge of platelets[43] thus permitting platelet-platelet interaction. This is supported by the observation that vancomycin (a closely related, but less positively charged molecule) promotes vWf binding to platelets,[44] but inhibits ristocetin induced aggregation.[45] Conversely, reduction in the negative charge alone by the action of neuraminidase on platelets does not produce platelet aggregation.[46]

a. Ristocetin Induced Platelet Aggregation in PRP(RIPA)

Ristocetin induced platelet aggregation in autologous platelet rich plasma may be used as an initial screen for vWD by demonstration of failure or reduced aggregation compared to a normal control preparation, using final concentrations of 1.5 to 2.0 mg/ml of ristocetin. However, it is not quantitative. It lacks specificity, since it is abnormal in many normal blacks due to the presence of an inhibitor in the plasma[47] and in Bernard Soulier syndrome. It also lacks sensitivity compared to the ristocetin co-factor assay discussed below.

Apart from the demonstration of other defects, the principal reason for performing RIPA in von Willebrand's disease (vWD) is for the detection of certain variants of the disease. Patients with these variants have platelets demonstrating an increased sensitivity to ristocetin with aggregation occurring at ristocetin concentrations as low as 0.5 mg/ml. This is due to an increased affinity of variant vWf to platelets. When this is observed it is necessary to determine whether the abnormality producing the increased affinity is inherent to the vWf (e.g., type IIB)[48] or to the platelet receptor ("pseudo-vWD" or "platelet-type vWD").[49]

b. Ristocetin Co-Factor Activity

The use of ristocetin in a quantitative assay of vWf with test plasma and donor platelets was described in 1973 by Weiss et al.[50] This method is comprised of a measurement of the total aggregation of washed donor platelets in an aggregometer produced by ristocetin in dilutions of standard pooled normal plasma or test plasma. Standard results were plotted graphically as a log-linear function and the test results were interpolated. Since then many variations in this method have been proposed and many different modifications remain in current use in the U.K.[51] The main variations involve the method of the end point determination and the type of platelet preparation used.

End point determinations include measurement of the initial kinetics of aggregation in an aggregometer,[52] the counting of platelets using a particle counter,[53] or, to preclude the use of expensive equipment, determination of the time take for the production of visible aggregates in entirely manual systems.[54,55] Washed viable platelets are laborious to produce and require fresh preparations each time the method is used. Furthermore, they progressively release their own vWf over a period of 2 to 3 h during the performance of the test. This problem has been circumvented by the use of formalin-fixed[56,57] or paraformaldehyde-fixed[58] platelets which can be stored satisfactorily for several months and can be prepared in relatively large quantities at any one time.

Whichever method is used, there is usually good agreement between laboratories in the recognition of severe vWD, and at normal levels of vWf the coefficient of variation (CV) is small.[59] However, at the most critical intermediate levels there is a large interlaboratory variation (CV 60%) posing considerable problems in the diagnosis of mild vWD. A consistent finding is that of higher levels of ristocetin co-factor (vWf:RCo) activity when fresh rather than fixed or lyophilized platelets are used.[60]

As the demonstration of vWf:RCo requires the presence of HMW multimers, which are functionally most important, the method is useful as an indicator of plasma vWf activity. It is, however, not synonymous with the total vWf activity mediating hemostatic processes *in vivo*, although it has been used as such in the past. It would seem unlikely that a single finite figure could be used to define the activity of this heterogeneous and multifunctional protein.

c. Ristocetin Induced Platelet Binding of vWf

Rather then relying upon platelet aggregation as an end point for the vWf assay, the platelets may be used as a ligand in a competitive radioreceptor assay. The analytical principle is based upon competitive binding of ^{125}I vWf and an unlabeled sample of vWf to formalin-fixed platelets in the presence of ristocetin. Although this method was described previously for quantitation of vWf in column eluates,[61] it has subsequently been shown to be of value in plasma samples.[62] The value of the method for diagnostic purposes is limited by technical difficulties in producing ^{125}I vWf with retained biological activity and also the narrow range of dilutions of plasma showing competition in the standard dose response curve.

d. Alternatives to Ristocetin

While many polycations induce vWf enhanced platelet aggregation, the only reagent proposed as an alternative to ristocetin is the extract of snake venom — "botrocetin" or "coagglutinin".[63,64] This reagent also causes platelet aggregation dependent on the presence of vWf, and at least partly on the presence of the platelet receptor glycoprotein IB. Unlike ristocetin, however, it does cause aggregation of platelets in assorted animals models, is not inhibited by vancomycin, and induces the binding of all molecular size forms of the vWf glycoprotein. As a consequence of the latter property, the botrocetin co-factor activity correlates well with vWf levels measured antigenically, and the method may thus fail to detect some variants deficient in the higher molecular weight forms.[65]

Thus, while botrocetin is a useful reagent in animal models, it appears to be less sensitive than ristocetin in screening tests in man while offering no substantial advantages.

3. Collagen Binding Assays

Assessment of the physiologically relevant ability of vWf to bind to collagen has proven difficult. The principal reasons are the diversity of forms of collagen (and other possibly relevant subendothelial structures) and the problems of separation and purification of these notoriously insoluble substances while maintaining the important aspects of their tertiary and quaternary structure. The molecular structure of the collagen used in collagen binding studies is of great relevance and must be considered in the interpretation of binding data. The nature of the collagen will vary with species and organ of origin as well as with the purification procedure. Preparation procedures may often include proteolysis and can result in insoluble, amorphous, or assorted fibrillary forms of collagen. An extreme example of the problems encountered in the interpretation of results is illustrated by a recent report of the assessment of commercially available collagen preparations for platelet aggregation studies. Amino acid analysis of one preparation revealed an absence of proline residues.[66]

Notwithstanding these difficulties there is evidence that a variety of fibrillary collagens can bind vWf[67] and that reconstituted native fibrils of acid soluble collagen from rat skin preferentially bind high molecular weight multimers.[68]

A simple assay technique for the binding of vWf to collagen has recently been described.[69] This method reports the use of a soluble preparation of type I collagen from bovine tendon bound to microtiter plates for vWf capture in a solid phase assay. Interestingly, when used for the investigation of type II vWD plasma and for evaluation of factor VIII concentrates, the experimental data correlated more closely with vWf:RCo activity than with vWf antigen (vWf:Ag) as assessed by enzyme linked immunoabsorbent assay (ELISA) or by electroimmunoassay (EIA). The authors have, therefore, indicated that this assay could be used as a substitute for the ristocetin co-factor method in the laboratory evaluation of vWD.

C. Immunologic Assays for vWf:Ag

For the purpose of diagnosis, immunologic methodology tends to be simpler and more specific than functional assays. However, the quantitation of vWf is difficult since the glycoprotein is heterogeneous as it consists of a population of multimers of varying molecular size.[70-72] Furthermore, it appears likely that antigenic determinants may also vary with the individual size of the molecular form.[28]

Immunologic assays may be used to give an overall quantitation of both plasma and platelet vWf. Alternatively, the variously sized multimers of vWf may be separated by electrophoresis and independently assessed, albeit only semiquantitatively, using crossed immunoelectrophoresis or "multimeric sizing" techniques.

Until recently, the antibodies used in immunologic assays were usually derived from polyclonal heterologous antisera raised against purified higher molecular weight forms of vWf. The antibodies were further purified by absorption against plasma obtained from severe vWD patients or against cryosupernatant which is known to lack higher molecular weight forms of vWf. In recent years monoclonal antibodies have become increasingly available for assay purposes.

1. Quantitative Assays
a. Electroimmunoassay (EIA)

The most convenient and frequently used method to quantitate vWf:Ag is by EIA.[73] In EIA, dilutions of plasma undergo electrophoresis into agarose containing a heterologous precipitating antibody. The vWf is electrophoresed into the gel with a progressive fall in concentration as antigen is precipitated at the sides of the migration path. When the vWf concentration in the center of the rocket is equivalent to that of the antibody, precipitation prevents further migration. The height of the rocket is approximately proportional to the concentration of the antigen, and quantitation is made by comparing the height of unknown samples with those obtained with dilutions of a standard, usually pooled normal plasma.

This method, although convenient and technically simple, lacks precision and sensitivity. The lower limit of sensitivity is approximately 12%, with a coefficient of variation of 20% at that level.[74] The sensitivity can be increased, however, by concentrating plasma vWf prior to electrophoresis.[75]

The precipitation in EIA depends on the concentration of molecules which will form a stable lattice with the precipitating antibody. The assay method is known to tend to underestimate the concentration of vWf:Ag when polymerization of antigenic subunits occurs with reduction in the total number of molecules. This is particularly important with higher molecular weight molecules.[76] It will, therefore, overestimate vWf levels of the low molecular weight forms if high molecular weight forms are used as a standard. Although the increased mobility of low molecular weight forms is used as an explanation for this effect, differences in electrophoretic mobilities should only affect the time taken to reach a steady state, not the final distance of migration.

b. Immunologic Assays Using Radioisotopes

The use of radioligands permits much greater sensitivity of immunoassays. Radioimmunoassays (RIAs) for vWf have been described by several investigators.[77-80] However, one of the major technical difficulties in adapting competitive RIAs in general use is the problem encountered in producing reproducible amounts of purified vWf with a specific radioactivity high enough for efficient counting and with preserved antigenic and functional properties after radiolabeling. As heterologous antibody to vWf can be prepared with relative ease and the radiolabeling of IgG is far simpler,[81] it is more likely to be successful than the radioiodination of vWf, and immunoradiometric assays (IRMAs) which have been preferred for general diagnostic use.

The most popular IRMA methods in current use are either the single site fluid phase assay[82,83] or the two-site solid phase assay.[84,85] The one-site method depends on the reaction of dilutions of vWf in test samples or standards with an excess of ^{125}I labeled antibody, and the separation of antigen bound from free antibody by selective precipitation of the bound moiety with ammonium sulfate or polyethylene glycol. The principle of the two-site IRMA involves the adsorption of unlabeled antibody onto a solid phase matrix, addition of dilutions of the test plasma samples or standard, and the detection of the bound vWf by application of a second ^{125}I radiolabeled antibody to vWf. Solid phase IRMAs are generally more time consuming than fluid phase assays since longer incubation periods are necessary. Two-site solid phase systems are considered to be more sensitive and will detect levels as low as 2.10^{-5} U/ml vWf:Ag,[83] compared with 5.10^{-4} U/ml vWf:Ag by the fluid phase assay, where there is often difficulty in achieving complete separation of bound from free ^{125}I antibody moieties.

As with EIA, quantitation is achieved through construction of radioactivity binding curves as a function of dilutions of a standard plasma. Radioactivity binding of dilutions of the test sample is then read from the standard curve in terms of the equivalent concentration of standard vWf:Ag. The use of standard curves for vWf:Ag quantitation for diagnostic purposes may, on occasion, be difficult, since in samples where the vWf is in predominantly a low molecular weight form (such as some variants of vWD or cryosupernatant), the dose response curve of the test sample is not parallel to that of the standard curve[86-88] and such differences cannot be altered by using plot transforms. This observation of nonparallel dose response may be explained on the basis that the vWf present in the test samples demonstrates lower affinity for the antibody than the native form of vWf in the standard sample. This is not surprising if one accepts that the different molecular weight forms of vWf can conceivably exhibit slightly different antigenic epitopes (despite being formed from the same subunits) and given the high molecular forms of vWf are specifically used as the immunogen for the preparation of antibody. Furthermore, as plasma cryosupernatant or severe vWD plasma is used to absorb other heterologous antibodies in the preparation of monospecific vWf antisera, assay anomalies to samples containing low molecular weight vWf:Ag may be seen since these materials for antibody absorbtion may not be completely devoid of vWf containing some low molecular weight material. High molecular weight vWf is often used for affinity purifications.

c. Enzyme Linked Immunosorbent Assay (ELISA)

In recent years the use of enzyme conjugated antibodies in immunoassays has rapidly increased. These techniques have been applied to the assay of vWf with some success.[89-92] In the method described by Short et al.,[90] polyclonal rabbit antibody is adsorbed onto the wells of a plastic microtiter plate and dilutions of vWf:Ag are incubated in the wells for 1 h. Unbound protein is removed by washing and peroxidase conjugated antibody is added. After further washing the second antibody is detected by spectrophotometry following addition of a chromogenic substrate for the peroxidase. This method consumes more antibody and is less sensitive than IRMA. Values as low as 10^{-2} U/ml can be assayed, which is adequate for all routine diagnostic purposes. Alternatively, by the use of $F(ab')_2$ fractions[91] of the antibody which has less nonspecific binding, the sensitivity can be increased to 3×10^{-4} U/ml. ELISA has the considerable advantage of avoiding the use of radioisotopes and can be performed within 1 working day. One might expect type II vWD plasma to give nonparallel assay results, but this has not to our knowledge been reported.

d. Monoclonal Antibody Assays

Monoclonal antibodies to vWf have been described by a number of laboratories.[93] These monoclonal preparations offer an infinite source of antibody of consistent specificity that can replace polyclonal antibodies in IRMAs and ELISAs without the need for protracted purification procedures.

The highly specific nature of the idiotype of these antibodies may usefully be exploited. The monoclonal antibody RFF-VIII:R1 (and RFF-VIII:R2 directed at the same epitope)[94,28] when used in IRMAs or ELISAs gives values which correlate closely with vWf:RCo activity. The explanation for this is uncertain, but may be due to the specificity of the monoclonal antibodies for an epitope only present on the larger multimeric forms which expresses the vWf:RCo activity. Immunoassays making use of the specificity of such antibodies could perhaps replace vWf:RCo assays as screening tests. Another monoclonal antibody has been described with specificity to the reduced and alkylated subunit of vWf. By the reduction cleavage of all multimers to their constituent subunits prior to assay, problems with immunoassays arising from nonparallel dose response curves of dissimilar molecules may be avoided. Comparative studies using this antibody and monoclonal antibodies raised against the higher molecular weight forms of vWf may be of value in the assessment of the degree of multimerization of vWf. A critical degree of reduction will need to be consistently achieved to produce reproducible subunit forms without loss of antigenicity.

2. Crossed (or Two Dimensional) Immunoelectrophoresis

In crossed immunoelectrophoresis (IEP), simple electropheresis is initially carried out in agarose in the absence of antibody to separate the different sized multimers of vWf. A second electrophoreresis is then performed at right angles to the initial run so that the proteins enter a further gel containing precipitating antibody to vWf.[95,96] Using this technique, it is possible to demonstrate under nondenaturing conditions the molecular size heterogeneity of the vWf in normal plasma, and that variants (type II) of vWD demonstrate a predominance of smaller and hence more rapidly anodally migrating forms of the molecule.[87,88,97] The technique may be made more sensitive by incubation of radiolabeled purified antibody to vWf in the second dimension and subsequently performing autoradiography to visualize the precipitation arcs.[27] A more recent report has described a modification of crossed IEP in which autoradiography has been combined with performance of the initial electrophoresis in high concentration agarose (2 to 3%) permitting separation and identification of the smaller individual multimers of vWf:Ag.[98] The method of crossed IEP has now largely been superceded for diagnostic purposes by higher resolution "multimeric sizing" techniques.

3. Multimeric Sizing Techniques

In recent years identification of the multimers of vWf in plasma has become the established method for the classification of the various types of vWD following reports by Hoyer and Shainoff[72] and by Ruggeri and Zimmerman.[99] Since the original publications a large number of variations in the method have been described, but the principle of the technique is the same. Samples of test plasma are incubated for a short period of time in sodium dodecyl sulfate at approximately 60°C to disaggregate the vWf molecules and impart a uniform negative charge to the multimers. Electrophoresis is then performed in a large pore gel, usually on a flat-bed electrophoretic system for convenience. The multimers are identified by the use of ^{125}I labeled antibodies raised against high molecular weight vWf. The use of sensitive immunologic methods permits the detection of the very low concentrations of vWf in normal plasma and patient samples. This eliminates the need for sample concentration which had previously been necessary,[70,100] when nonspecific protein stains had been used. An alternative nonimmunologic method has recently been described[101] in which the multimers in polyacrylamide gels are detected nonspecifically by the use of the very sensitive silver stain technique. Unfortunately this method is unsuitable when applied to agarose gels.

The single most common modification is that of Ruggeri and Zimmerman[102] who used a discontinuous buffer system with a stacking gel of dilute (0.8%) agarose.

A number of different running gels have been used. In general, agarose at lower concentrations (<2%) allows separation of the highest molecular weight multimers. Reduction of the pore size by the use of higher concentrations (2 to 3%)[103,104] of agarose or by the addition of polyacrylamide improves the resolution of lower molecular weight bands permitting the discrimination of at least three (a triplet) and up to five or six subbands within each multimer. The type of agarose is important; many laboratories follow the example of Zimmerman and use highly purified Seakem HGT(P) (FMC) agarose, but satisfactory results may be obtained with a variety of products.[103-106] In particular it should be noted that the use of a low gelling temperature agarose (Sigma) at 1.4% concentration produces a high resolution gel.[107] We have obtained similar results using 1.6% Seaplaque LGT agarose. These gels are easier to pour than the alternative higher concentration high gelling temperature agarose gels. However, they have less tensile strength and require careful handling.

The vWf subcommittee of the International Committee on Thrombosis and Haemostasis (ICTH) has suggested[105] that for the purpose of diagnosis a low resolution gel should be used to screen plasma samples. If a type II picture is found (i.e., the absence of high molecular weight multimers), then a high resolution gel should be used to subclassify this variant of vWD. However, the techniques are not easy, and even superficially similar methods apparently can produce different degrees of resolution in different "expert" centers.

Visualization of the multimers may be achieved either directly on the running gel or after electrophoretic transfer to a nitrocellulose membrane.[108] When identification is directly on the gel it is customary to fix the proteins to the gel. This is usually performed by immersion of the gel in a solution of acetic acid and isopropanol. Alternatively, fixation can be achieved by the inclusion of glyoxyl modified agarose in the running gel and subsequent elevation of the pH (with a solution of sodium carbonate containing sodium carbohydride and Triton-

X100) which produces a linkage through the aldehyde groups on the gel with the electrophoresed proteins.[72] A recent report, however, suggests that fixation may not be necessary,[109] presumably because of the high molecular weights of the multimers, of vWf particularly, after their complex formation with antibody. The most frequently used method of visualization of multimers, at least up to this time of writing, is the use of autoradiography (Figure 1A). The gel is incubated with ^{125}I radioiodinated antibody to vWf while nonspecific binding is inhibited by "blocking" with nonspecific immunoglobulin or other protein. After extensive washing in saline and distilled water, the gel is placed in contact with a suitable photographic film. The speed of the autoradiography can be enhanced by use of intensifying screens and incubation at −70°C. The latter stabilizes the latent image centers found in exposed silver halide grains produced by the low level of light emitted from the intensifying screen.

Autoradiography is an extremely sensitive method and has the advantage that varying degrees of sensitivity can be obtained from the same gel. This is achieved by the simple expedient of reexposure of the gel for different periods to the X-ray film.

The major disadvantages of this method are the need to handle radioisotopes and the time necessitated by the extensive washing and exposure of the autoradiograph. The use of enzymatically labeled antibodies with a suitable chromogenic substrate can circumvent the use of radioligands. However, due to the lower sensitivity of these enzyme labels it is necessary to amplify the chromogenic signal used as the assay end point for visualization. This has been achieved by the use of a primary unlabeled antibody and its subsequent amplification with a bridging antibody with the peroxidase-antiperoxidase[110] or avidin-biotin-peroxidase methods.[109] These methods are also time consuming since each layer of antibody or peroxidase complex requires prolonged incubation (often overnight) and intensive washing.

The use of immunoenzymatic methods has been more effectively[106,111-113] exploited following electroblotting onto nitrocellulose membranes. The multimers of vWf:Ag adsorbed to the nitrocellulose are more concentrated and accessible to applied solutions. This allows reduction of antibody concentration and greatly shortened incubaton and washing times (see Figure 1B). The antibody systems used to demonstrate the multimers include direct application of peroxidase conjugated antibody to vWf,[111] addition of peroxidase or galactosidase conjugated second antibody following an unlabeled first antibody,[106,112] and use of a biotinylated second antibody followed by an avidin-biotin-peroxidase complex. Substrates used for the detection of peroxidase include *o*-dansidine, diaminobenzidine, barbazole, and chloronaphthol.

One problem with electroblotting is that the efficiency of transfer of proteins falls as the molecular weight increases.[114] This, in view of the large size of vWf multimers, necessitates the use of significantly longer blotting times or higher current density than is usual for the blotting of most proteins or protein digests. It may also cause relatively inefficient transfer of high molecular weight multimers compared to low molecular weight multimers. This implies that, by comparison with autoradiographic identification of the multimers directly on the gel, quantitation of the multimers will be inaccurate. However, in view of difficulties of immunological quantitation of dissimilar molecules (discussed above), any form of multimeric sizing is at best semiquantitative. The only aspect of classification which depends on quantitation is the recognition of types IA and IB.[115] As a multicenter study[105] showed, a minority of "expert" laboratories were able to distinguish these types; the value of this classification is debatable.

The real value of multimeric sizing for diagnostic purposes is essentially qualitative in the detection of the presence or the absence of the high and intermediate molecular weight multimers and resolution of the internal structure of the smallest multimers. In both of these aspects, blotting/immunoenzymatic methods give similar information to autoradiography. In our experience the enzymatic method tends to give better results with clearer resolution of triplets even using a "low resolution" gel for electrophoresis (Figure 1).

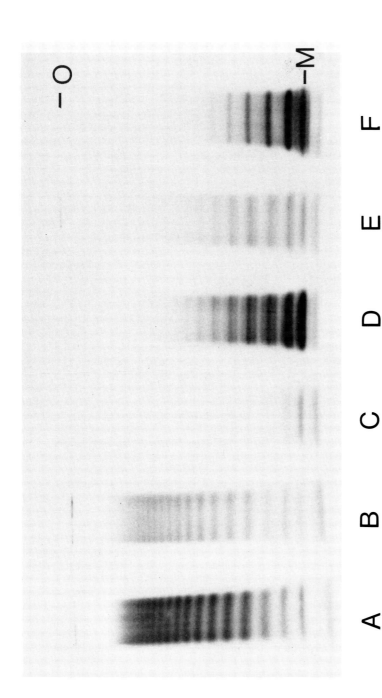

FIGURE 1A.   Multimeric sizing using 1.6% HGT(P) agarose and visualization by autoradiograph using the method of Ruggeri and Zimmerman.[102] Samples: lane A, normal plasma; lane B, type 1 vWD; lane C, type IIA vWD; lane D, type IIA vWD after DDAVP; lane E, type IIB; lane F, type IID. −0, origin of running gel. −M, position of IgM.

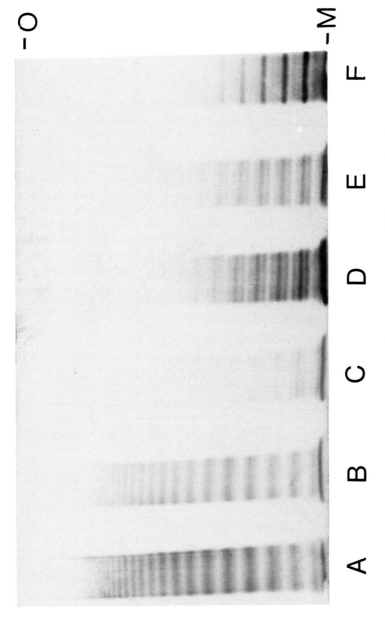

FIGURE 1B.   Multimeric sizing using the same samples and electrophoretic conditions as in Figure 1A. Multimeric detection was by electroblotting onto nitrocellulose and sequential addition of rabbit anti-vWf antibody, biotinylated goat anti-rabbit antibody, and streptavidin-biotinylated-peroxidase complex. The nitrocellulose was incubated with each reagent for 1 h followed by washing for 5 min. Color development was with diaminobenzidine and hydrogen peroxidase for 20 min.

For use outside well-staffed "expert" centers blotting/immunoenzymatic methods can be performed using commercially available purified and labeled antibodies. The rapid nature of the procedure is of great benefit both in evaluating a multimeric sizing technique and in subsequent clinical use. The long shelf life of the reagents without the problems of storage and disposal of radioisotopes makes these techniques more appropriate than autoradiography for intermittent routine use.

In conclusion, while autoradiograph has advantages as a research tool, immunoenzymatic methods are more convenient and will greatly facilitate the use of multimeric sizing as a diagnostic test.

IV. SUMMARY

No single all-embracing diagnostic test currently exists for vWD. However, the vWf:RCo assay can be considered the closest approximation to such, although it is clearly nonphysiological and its mechanism is poorly understood.

In the diagnosis of vWD it is convenient to perform the evaluation in three stages.

Stage I — Patients referred for investigation are screened by means of a detailed clinical and family history, including a careful evaluation of all current medication. First line tests including the platelet count, bleeding time, prothrombin time, and partial thromboplastin time are performed.

Stage II — In the event of a clinical history suggestive of a congenital bleeding disorder or a prolongation of the bleeding time inexplicable on the basis of thrombocytopenia or medication, further tests are performed. Quantitative assays of VIII:C, vWf:RCo, and vWf:Ag are undertaken as are platelet function studies including RIPA. For reasons previously discussed, the ELISA for vWf:Ag is most convenient. Equivocal test results necessitate resampling and repeated assay measurements including the bleeding time since characteristic parameters in vWD are known to demonstrate variability in any one individual.

Stage III — Following the tentative diagnosis of vWD from Stage II tests, further evaluation is performed by means of miltimer sizing of plasma vWf and quantitation and multimer sizing of platelet vWf. In our hands, blotting/enzymatic methods for multimer sizing are more rapid and convenient for routine diagnostic purposes than autoradiography. Finally, and of most importance with respect to the future management of the patient with vWD, is the evaluation of the clinical response to 1-desamino-8-D-arginine-vasopressin (DDAVP) infusion and an objective assessment of its hemostatic efficacy as monitored by the bleeding time and vWf:RCo activity.

REFERENCES

1. **O'Brien, J. R.**, The bleeding time in normal and abnormal subjects, *J. Clin. Pathol.*, 4, 272, 1951.
2. **Duke, W. W.**, The relation of blood platelets to hemorrhagic disease, *JAMA*, 55, 1185, 1910.
3. **Ivy, A. C., Nelson, D., and Bucher, G.**, The standardization of certain factors in the cutaneous "venostasis" bleeding time technique, *J. Lab. Clin. Med.*, 26, 1812, 1940—41.
4. **Borchgrevink, C. F. and Waaler, B. A.**, The secondary bleeding time. A new method for the differentiation of hemorrhagic diseases, *Acta Med. Scand.*, 162, 361, 1958.
5. **Mielke, C. H., Kaneshiro, M. M., Maher, I. A., and Weiner, J. M.**, The standardised normal bleeding time and its prolongation by asprin, *Blood*, 34, 204, 1969.
6. **Mielke, C. H.**, Measurement of the bleeding time, *Thromb. Haemost.*, 52, 210, 1984.
7. **Poller, L., Thomson, J. M., and Tomenson, J. A.**, The bleeding time: current practice in the UK, *Clin. Lab. Haematol.*, 6, 369, 1984.

8. **Babson, S. R. and Babson, A. L.,** Development and evaluation of a disposable device for performing simultaneous duplicate bleeding time determinations, *Am. J. Clin. Pathol.*, 70, 406, 1978.

9. **Kumar, R., Ansell, J. E., Canoso, R. T., and Deykin, D.,** Clinical trial of a new bleeding-time device, *Am. J. Clin. Pathol.*, 70, 642, 1978.

10. **Mielke, C. H.,** Asprin prolongation of the template bleeding time: influence of venostasis and direction of incision, *Blood*, 60, 1139, 1982.

11. **Rennie, J. M., Gibson, T., and Cooke, R. W. I.,** Micromethod for bleeding time in the newborn, *Arch. Dis. Child.*, 60, 51, 1985.

12. **Toomey, K. C., Kim, H. C., Kosmin, M., and Saidi, P.,** Clinical trial of a new disposable bleeding-time device, *Am. J. Clin. Pathol.*, 85, 610, 1986.

13. Italian Working Group, Spectrum of von Willebrand's disease: a study of 100 cases, *Br. J. Haematol.*, 35, 101, 1977.

14. **Gralnick, H. R., Rick, M. E., McKeown, L. P., Williams, S. B., Parker, R. I., Maisonneuve, P., Jenneau, C., and Sultan, Y.,** Platelet von Willebrand factor: an important determinant of bleeding time in type I von Willebrand's disease, *Blood*, 68, 58, 1986.

15. **Quick, A. J.,** Acetylsalicylic acid as a diagnostic aid in haemostasis, *Am. J. Med. Sci.*, 254, 392, 1967.

16. **Stuart, M. J., Miller, M. L., Davey, F. R., and Wolk, J. A.,** The post aspirin bleeding time: a screening test for evaluating haemostatic disorders, *Br. J. Haematol.*, 43, 649, 1979.

17. **Sutor, A. H., Bowie, E. J. W., Thompson, J. H., Didisheim, P., Mertens, B., and Owen, C. A.,** Bleeding from standardised skin punctures: automated technic for recording time, intensity and pattern of bleeding, *Am. J. Clin. Pathol.*, 55, 541, 1971.

18. **Barber, A., Green, D., Galluzzo, T., and Ts'ao, C.,** The bleeding time as a preoperative screening test, *Am. J. Med.*, 78, 761, 1985.

19. **Stel, H. V., Sakariassen, K. S., de Groot, P. G., van Mourik, J. A., and Sixma, J. J.,** Von Willebrand factor in the vessel wall mediates platelet adherence, *Blood*, 65, 85, 1985.

20. **Gralnick, H. R., Williams, S. B., McKeown, L. P., Maisonneuve, P., Jenneau, C., Sultan, Y., and Rick, M. E.,** In vitro correction of the abnormal multimeric structure of von Willebrand factor in type IIa von Willebrand's disease, *Proc. Natl. Acad. Sci. U.S.A.*, 82, 5968, 1985.

21. **Batlle, J., Lopez-Fernandez, M. F., Campos, M., Justica, B., Berges, C., Navarro, J. L., Diaz Cremades, J. M., Kasper, C. K., Dent, J. A., Ruggeri, Z. M., and Zimmerman, T. S.,** The heterogeneity of type IIA von Willebrand's disease: studies with protease inhibitors, *Blood*, 68, 1207, 1986.

22. **Howard, M. A., Montgomery, D. C., and Hardisty, R. M.,** Factor VIII-related antigen in platelets, *Thromb. Res.*, 4, 617, 1974.

23. **Bouman, B. M., Hordijk-Hos, J. M., de Graaf, S., and Sixma, J. J.,** Presence of factor VIII-related antigen in blood platelets of patients with von Willebrand's disease, *Nature*, 257, 510, 1975.

24. **Gralnick, H. R., Williams, S. B., McKeown, L. P., Krizek, D. M., Shafer, B. C., and Rick, M. E.,** Platelet von Willebrand factor: comparison with plasma von Willebrand factor, *Thromb. Res.*, 38, 623, 1985.

25. **Walsh, P. N.,** Albumin density gradient separation and washing of platelets and the study of platelet coagulant activities, *Br. J. Haematol.*, 22, 205, 1972.

26. **Ruggeri, Z. M., Mannucci, P. M., Bader, R., and Barbui, T.,** Factor VIII-related properties in platelets from patients with von Willebrand's disease, *J. Lab. Clin. Med.*, 91, 132, 1978.

27. **Koutts, J., Walsh, P. N., Plow, E. F., Fenton, J. W., Bouma, B. N., and Zimmerman, T. S.,** Active release of human platelet factor VIII-related antigen by adenosine diphosphate, collagen, and thrombin, *J. Clin. Invest.*, 62, 1255, 1978.

28. **Chand, S., McCraw, A., Hutton, R., Tuddenham, E. G. D., and Goodall, A. H.,** A two-site, monoclonal antibody-based immunoassay for von Willebrand factor — demonstration that vWF function resides in a conformational epitope, *Thromb. Haemost.*, 55, 318, 1986.

29. **Lopez-Fernandez, M. F., Lopez-Berges, C., Nieto, J., Martin, R., and Batlle, J.,** Platelet and plasma von Willebrand factor: structural differences, *Thromb. Res.*, 44, 125, 1986.

30. **Baumgartner, H. R.,** The role of blood flow in platelet adhesion, fibrin deposition, and formation of mural thrombi, *Microvasc. Res.*, 5, 167, 1973.

31. **Sakariassen, K. S., Aarts, P. A. M. M., de Groot, P. G., Houdijk, W. P. M., and Sixma, J. J.,** A perfusion chamber developed to investigate platelet interaction in flowing blood with human vessel wall cells, their extracellular matrix, and purified components, *J. Lab. Clin. Med.*, 102, 522, 1983.

32. **Salzman, E. W.,** Measurement of platelet adhesiveness: a simple in vitro technique demonstrating an abnormality in von Willebrand's disease, *J. Lab. Clin. Med.*, 62, 124, 1963.

33. **Bowie, E. J. W., Owen, C. A., Thompson, J. H., and Didisheim, P.,** Platelet adhesiveness in von Willebrand's disease, *Am. J. Clin. Pathol.*, 52, 69, 1969.

34. **Blakely, J., Prchal, J. T., and Glynn, M. F.,** An in vitro measurement of bleeding time, *J. Lab. Clin. Med.*, 89, 1306, 1977.

35. **Uchiyama, S., Bach, M. L., Didisheim, P., and Bowie, E. J. W.,** Clinical evaluation of a new test of hemostasis: the filter bleeding time, *Thromb. Res., 34,* 397, 1984.
36. **Gorog, P. and Ahmed, A.,** Haemostatometer: a new in vitro technique for assessing haemostatic activity of blood, *Thromb. Res., 34,* 341, 1984.
37. **Meyer, D. and Baumgartner, H. R.,** Role of von Willebrand factor in platelet adhesion to the subendothelium, *Br. J. Haematol., 54,* 1, 1983.
38. **Howard, M. A. and Firkin, B. G.,** Ristocetin — a new tool in the investigation of platelet aggregation, *Thromb. Diath. Haemorrh., 262,* 362, 1971.
39. **Weiss, H. J., Rogers, J., and Brand, H.,** Defective ristocetin-induced platelet aggregation in von Willebrand's disease and its correction by factor VIII, *J. Clin. Invest., 52,* 2697, 1973.
40. **Doucet-de Bruine, M. H. M., Sixma, J. J., Over, J., and Beeser-Visser, N. H.,** Heterogeneity of human factor VIII binding to platelets in the presence of ristocetin, *J. Lab. Clin. Med., 92,* 96, 1978.
41. **Rosborough, T. K.,** Von Willebrand factor, polycations, and platelet agglutination, *Thromb. Res., 17,* 481, 1980.
42. **Coller, B. S.,** Polybrene-induced platelet agglutination and reduction in electrophoretic mobility: enhancement by von Willebrand factor and inhibition by vancomycin, *Blood, 55,* 276, 1980.
43. **Coller, B. S.,** The effects of ristocetin and von Willebrand factor on platelet electrophoretic mobility, *J. Clin. Invest., 61,* 1168, 1978.
44. **Suzuki, K., Nishioka, J., and Hashimoto, S.,** Vancomycin as well as ristocetin facilitates von Willebrand factor binding to platelets, *Thromb. Res., 19,* 287, 1980.
45. **Moake, J. L., Cimo, P. L., Peterson, D. M., Roper, P., and Natelson, E. A.,** Inhibition of ristocetin-induced platelet agglutination by vancomycin, *Blood, 50,* 397, 1977.
46. **Tanoue, K., Jung, S. M., Yamamoto, N., and Yamazaki, H.,** Neutralization of the local negative charge carried by glycoprotein (GP)-Ib in ristocetin-induced platelet agglutinatination, *Thromb. Haemost., 51,* 79, 1984.
47. **Buchanan, G. R., Holtkamp, C. A., and Levy, E. N.,** Racial differences in ristocetin-induced platelet aggregation, *Br. J. Haematol., 49,* 455, 1981.
48. **Ruggeri, Z. M., Pareti, F. I., Mannucci, P. M., Ciavarella, N., and Zimmerman, T. S.,** Heightened interaction between platelets and factor VIII/von Willebrand factor in a new subtype of von Willebrand's disease, *New Engl. J. Med., 302,* 1047, 1980.
49. **Miller, J. L. and Castella, A.,** Platelet-type von Willebrand's disease: characterization of a new bleeding disorder, *Blood, 60,* 790, 1982.
50. **Weiss, H. J., Hoyer, L. W., Rickles, F. R., Varma, A., and Rogers, J.,** Quantitative assay of a plasma factor deficient in von Willebrand's disease that is necessary for platelet aggregation, *J. Clin. Invest., 52,* 2708, 1973.
51. U.K. National External Quality Assurance Scheme in Blood Coagulation, Annual Review, 1986.
52. **Macfarlane, D. E., Stibbe, J., Kirby, E. P., Zucker, M. B., Grant, R. A., and McPherson, J. A.,** A method for assaying von Willebrand factor (ristocetin cofactor), *Thromb. Diath. Haemorrh., 34,* 306, 1975.
53. **Evans, R. J. and Austen, D. E. G.,** Assay of ristocetin co-factor using fixed platelets and a platlet counting technique, *Br. J. Haematol., 37,* 289, 1977.
54. **Brinkhous, K. M., Graham, J. E., Cooper, H. A., Allain, J. P., and Wagner, R. H.,** Assay of von Willebrand factor in von Willebrand's disease and haemophilia: use of a macroscopic platelet aggregation test, *Thromb. Res., 6,* 267, 1975.
55. **Reisner, H. M., Katz, H. J., Goldin, L. R., Barrow, E. S., and Graham, J. B.,** Use of a simple visual assay of von Willebrand factor for diagnosis and carrier identification, *Br. J. Haematol., 40,* 339, 1978.
56. **Zuzel, M., Nilsson, I. M., and Aberg, M.,** A method for measuring plasma ristocetin cofactor activity, *Thromb. Res., 12,* 745, 1978.
57. **Brinkhous, K. M. and Read, M. S.,** Preservation of platelet receptors for platelet aggregating factor/von Willebrand factor by air drying, freezing, or lyophilization: new stable platelet preparations for von Willebrand factor assays, *Thromb. Res., 13,* 591, 1978.
58. **Allain, J. P., Cooper, H. A., Wagner, R. H., and Brinkhous, K. M.,** Platelets fixed with paraformaldrhyde: a new reagent for assay of von Willebrand factor and platelet aggregating factor, *J. Lab. Clin. Med., 85,* 318, 1975.
59. **Nilsson, I. M., Peake, I. R., Bloom, A. L., Veltkamp, J., and Green, D.,** Report of the working party on factor VIII-related antigens. Addendum: the relationship between ristocetin co-factor activity (VIIIR:Cof) and factor VIII related antigen (VIIIR:Ag), *Thromb. Haemost., 43,* 167, 1980.
60. **Kelton, J. G., Bishop, J., Carter, C. J., and Hirsh, J.,** A comparison of the quantitative ristocetin von Willebrand factor assay by using fresh and fixed platelets, *Thromb. Res., 18,* 477, 1980.
61. **Kao, K.-J., Pizzo, S. V., and McKee, P. A.,** A radioreceptor assay for quantitating FVIII/von Willebrand protein, *Blood, 57,* 579, 1981.

62. **Savidge, G. F., Mahmood, N. M., and Saundry, R. H.,** Variable ristocetin-induced platelet binding affinity of FVIII/von Willebrand protein in von Willebrand's disease, *Thromb. Haemost.,* 50, 192, 1983.

63. **Brinkhous, K. M. and Read, M. S.,** Use of venom coagglutinin and lyophilized platelets in testing for platelet-aggregating von Willebrand factor, *Blood,* 55, 517, 1980.

64. **Brinkhous, K. M., Fricke, W. A., and Read, M. S.,** Determinants of von Willebrand factor activity elicited by ristocetin and botrocetin: studies on a human von Willebrand factor-binding antibody, *Semin. Thromb. Haemost.,* 11, 337, 1985.

65. **Howard, M. A., Perkin, J., Salem, H. H., and Firkin, B. G.,** The agglutination of human platelets by botrocetin: evidence that botrocetin and ristocetin act at different sites on the factor VIII molecule and platelet membrane, *Br. J. Haematol.,* 57, 25, 1984.

66. **Fauvel, F., Karniguian, A., Leger, D., Pignaud, G., and Legrand, Y. J.,** Collagen induced platelet aggregation: a comparison between several commercially available collagens, *Thromb. Res.,* 38, 707, 1985.

67. **Morton, L. F., Griffin, B., Pepper, D. S., and Barnes, M. J.,** The interaction between collagens and factor VIII/von Willebrand factor: investigation of the structural requirements for interaction, *Thromb. Res.,* 32, 545, 1983.

68. **Santoro, S. A.,** Preferential binding of high molecular weight forms of von Willebrand factor to fibrillar collagen, *Biochim. Biophys. Acta,* 756, 123, 1983.

69. **Brown, J. E. and Bosak, J. O.,** An ELISA test for the binding of von Willebrand antigen to collagen, *Thromb Res.,* 43, 303, 1986.

70. **van Mourik, J. A., Bouma, B. N., LaBruyere, W. T., de Graaf, S., and Mochtar, I. A.,** Factor VIII, a series of homologous oligomers and a complex of two proteins, *Thromb. Res.,* 4, 155, 1974.

71. **Counts, R. B., Paskell, S. L., and Elgee, S. K.,** Disulfide bonds and the quaternary structure of factor VIII/von Willebrand factor, *J. Clin. Invest.,* 62, 702, 1978.

72. **Hoyer, L. W. and Shainoff, J. R.,** Factor VIII-related protein circulates in normal human plasma as high molecular weight multimers, *Blood,* 55, 1056, 1980.

73. **Laurel, C. B.,** Quantitative estimation of proteins by electrophoresis is agarose gel containing antibodies, *Anal. Biochem.,* 15, 45, 1966.

74. **Zimmerman, T. S., Hoyer, L. W., Dickson, L., and Eddington, T. S.,** Determination of the von Willebrand's disease antigen (factor VIII-related antigen) in plasma by quantitative electrophoresis, *J. Lab. Clin. Invest.,* 86, 152, 1974.

75. **Holmberg, L. and Nilsson, I. M.,** Genetic variants of von Willebrand's disease, *Br. Med. J.,* 3, 317, 1972.

76. **Laurel, C. B.,** Electroimmuno assay, *Scand. J. Clin. Lab. Invest.,* 29 (Suppl. 24), 21, 1972.

77. **Kasten, B. L., Vaitutaitis, J. L., and Gralnick, H. R.,** A new factor VIII radioimmunoassay, *Clin. Res.,* 21, 558, 1973.

78. **Paulssen, M. M. P., van de Graaf-Wildschut, M., Kolhorn, A., and Planje, M. C.,** Radioimmunoassay of antihaemophilic factor (factor VIII) antigen, *Clin. Chim. Acta.,* 63, 349, 1975.

79. **Green, D. and Reynolds, N.,** Double-antibody radioimmunoassay for factor VIII-related antigen, *Clin. Chem.,* 23, 1648, 1977.

80. **Savidge, G. F. and Carleborg, G.,** An optimised radioimmunoassay of FVIII related antigen (FVIII R:Ag) in plasma and eluates, *Thromb. Res.,* 14, 363, 1979.

81. **Greenwood, F. C., Hunter, W. M., and Glover, J. S.,** The preparation of ^{131}I-labelled human growth hormone of high specific radioactivity, *Biochem. J.,* 89, 114, 1963.

82. **Hoyer, L. W.,** Immunologic studies of antihemophilic factor (AHF, factor VIII). IV. Radioimmunoassay of AHF antigen, *J. Lab. Clin. Med.,* 80, 822, 1972.

83. **Girma, J. P., Ardaillou, N., Meyer, D., Lavergne, J. M., and Larrieu, M. J.,** Fluid-phase immunoradiometric assay for the detection of qualitative abnormalities of factor VIII/von Willebrand factor in variants von Willebrand's disease, *J. Lab. Clin. Med.,* 93, 926, 1979.

84. **Counts, R. B.,** Solid-phase immunoradiometric assay of factor VIII protein, *Br. J. Haematol.,* 31, 429, 1975.

85. **Ruggeri, Z. M., Mannucci, P. M., Jeffcoate, S. L., and Ingram, G. I. C.,** Immunoradiometric assay of factor VIII related antigen, with observations in 32 patients with von Willebrand's disease, *Br. J. Haematol.,* 33, 321, 1976.

86. **Peake, I. R., Bloom, A. L., and Giddings, J. C.,** Inherited variants of factor VIII-related protein in von Willebrand's disease, *New Engl. J. Med.,* 291, 113, 1974.

87. **Kernoff, P. B. A., Gruson, R., and Rizza, C. R.,** A variant of factor VIII related antigen, *Br. J. Haematol.,* 26, 435, 1974.

88. **Ardaillou, N., Girma, J. P., Meyer, D., Lavergne, J. M., Shoa'i, I., and Larrieu, M. J.,** "Variants" of von Willebrand's disease Demonstration of a decreased antigenic reactivity by immunoradiometric assay, *Thromb. Res.,* 12, 817, 1978.

89. **Bartlett, A., Dormandy, K. M., Hawkey, C. M., Stableforth, P., and Voller, A.,** Factor VIII-related antigen: measurement by enzyme immunoassay, *Br. Med. J.,* 1, 994, 1976.

90. **Short, P. E., Williams, C. E., Picken, A. M., and Hill, F. G. H.,** Factor VIII related antigen: an improved immunoassay, *Med. Lab. Sci.,* 39, 351, 1982.

91. **Silveira, A. M. V., Yamamoto, T., Adamson, L., Hessel, B., and Blomback, B.,** Application of an enzyme-linked immunosorbent assay (ELISA) to von Willebrand factor (vWF) and its derivatives, *Thromb. Res.,* 43, 91, 1986.

92. **Yorde, L. D., Hussey, C. V., Yorde, D. E., and Sasse, E. A.,** Competitive enzyme-linked immunoassay for factor VIII antigen, *Clin. Chem.,* 25, 1924, 1979.

93. **Goodall, A. H. and Meyer, D.,** Registry of monoclonal antibodies to factor VIII and von Willebrand factor, *Thromb. Haemost.,* 54, 878, 1985.

94. **Goodall, A. H., Jarvis, J., Chand, S., Rawlings, E., O'Brien, D. P., McGraw, A., Hutton, R., and Tuddenham, E. G. D.,** An immunoradiometric assay for human factor VIII/von Willebrand factor (VIII:vWF) using a monoclonal antibody that defines a functional epitope, *Br. J. Haematol.,* 59, 565, 1985.

95. **Laurel, C. B.,** Antigen-antibody crossed electrophoresis, *Anal. Biochem.,* 10, 358, 1965.

96. **Ganrot, P. O.,** Crossed immunoelectropheresis, *Scand. J. Clin. Lab. Invest.,* 29 (Suppl. 124), 39, 1972.

97. **Gralnick, H. R., Coller, B. S., and Sultan, Y.,** Studies of the human factor VIII/von Willebrand factor protein III. Qualitative defects in von Willebrand's disease, *J. Clin. Invest.,* 56, 814, 1975.

98. **Lamb, M. A., Reisner, H. M., Cooper, H. A., and Wagner, R. H.,** The multimeric distribution of factor VIII-related antigen studies by an improved crossed-immunoelectropheresis technique, *J. Lab. Clin. Invest.,* 98, 751, 1981.

99. **Ruggeri, Z. M. and Zimmerman, T. S.,** Variant von Willebrand's disease. Characterisation of two subtypes by analysis of multimeric composition of factor VIII/von Willebrand factor in plasma and platelets, *J. Clin. Invest.,* 65, 1318, 1980.

100. **Meyer, D., Obert, B., Pietu, G., Lavergne, J. M., and Zimmerman, T. S.,** Multimeric structure of factor VIII/von Willebrand factor in von Willebrand's disease, *J. Lab. Clin. Med.,* 95, 590, 1980.

101. **Perret, B. A., Felix, R., Furlan, M., and Beck, E. A.,** Silver staining of high molecular weight proteins on large pore polyacrylamide gels, *Anal. Biochem.,* 131, 46, 1983.

102. **Ruggeri, Z. M. and Zimmerman, T. S.,** The complex multimeric composition of factor VIII/von Willebrand factor, *Blood,* 57, 1140, 1981.

103. **Mazurier, C., Samor, B., and Goudemand, M.,** Improved characterisation of plasma von Willebrand factor heterogeneity when using 2.5% agarose gel electropheresis, *Thromb. Haemost.,* 55, 61, 1986.

104. **Kinoshita, S., Harrison, J., Lazerson, J., and Abildgaard, C. F.,** A new variant of dominant type II von Willebrand's disease with aberrant multimeric pattern of factor VIII-related antigen (type IID), *Blood,* 63, 1369, 1984.

105. **Mannucci, P. M., Abildgard, C. F., Gralnick, H. R., Hill, F. G. H., Hoyer, L. W., Lombardi, R., Nilsson, I. M., Tuddenham, E., and Meyer, D.,** Multicentric comparison of von Willebrand factor multimeric sizing techniques, *Thromb. Haemost.,* 54, 873, 1985.

106. **Brosstad, F., Kjonniksen, I., Ronning, B., and Stormorken, H.,** Visualisation of von Willebrand factor multimers by enzyme-conjugated secondary antibodies, *Thromb. Haemost.,* 55, 276, 1986.

107. **Ciavarella, G., Ciavarella, N., Antoncecchi, S., De Mattia, d., Ranieri, P., Dent, J., Zimmerman, T. S., and Ruggeri, Z. M.,** High resolution analysis of von Willebrand factor multimeric composition deines a new variant of type I von Willebrand disease with aberrant structure but presence of all size multimers (type IC), *Blood,* 66, 1423, 1985.

108. **Furlong, B. L. and Peake, I. R.,** An electoblotting technique for the detection of factor VIII/von Willebrand factor multimers in plasma, *Br. J. Haematol.,* 53, 641, 1983.

109. **Aihara, M., Sawada, Y., Ueno, K., Morimoto, S., Yoshida, Y., de Serres, M., Cooper, H. A., and Wagner, R. H.,** Visualization of von Willebrand factor multimers by immunoenzymatic stain using avidin-biotin-peroxidase complex, *Thromb. Haemost.,* 55, 263, 1986.

110. **Chow, R. and Savidge, G. F.,** Enzyme linked antibody system for the visualisation of FVIII multimers, *Thromb. Haemost.,* 54, 75, 1985.

111. **Bukh, A., Ingerslev, J., Stenbjerg, S., and Hundahl, Moller, N. P.,** The miltimeric structure of plasma F VII:RAg studied by electroelution and immunoperoxidase detection, *Thromb. Res.,* 43, 579, 1986.

112. **Zaleski, A. and Henriksen, R. A.,** Visualisation of the multimeric structure of von Willebrand factor using a peroxidase-conjugated second antibody, *J. Lab. Clin. Med.,* 107, 172, 1986.

113. **Lombardi, R., Gelfi, C., Righetti, P. G., Lattuada, A., and Mannucci, P. M.,** Electroblot and immunoperoxidase staining for rapid screening of the abnormalities of the multimeric structure of von Willebrand factor in von Willebrand's disease, *Thromb. Haemost.,* 55, 246, 1986.

114. **Gershoni, J. M. and Palade, G. E.,** Protein blotting: principles and applications, *Anal. Biochem.,* 131, 1, 1983.

115. **Hoyer, L. W., Rizza, C. R., Tuddenham, E. G. D., Carta, C. A., and Armitage, F.,** Von Willebrand factor multimer patterns in von Willebrand disease, *Br. J. Haematol.,* 55, 493, 1983.

Chapter 7

ADVANCES IN IMMUNOCHEMICAL ASPECTS OF vWD

Alison H. Goodall

TABLE OF CONTENTS

I.   Introduction 148

II.   The vWf Molecule 148

III.   The Role of vWf in Primary Hemostasis 149

IV.   Monoclonal Antibodies (MAbs) and the Functions of vWf 151
        A.   MAbs that Inhibit Aggregation and Adhesion:
                The GP Ib Binding Site 151
        B.   MAbs that Inhibit Aggregation but Not Adhesion:
                The GP IIb/IIIa Binding Site 154
        C.   MAbs that Inhibit Adhesion but Not Aggregation:
                The Collagen Binding Site 154
        D.   MAbs that Have No Effect on vWF Function 154
        E.   MAbs with Other Functional Effects 154
        F.   Epitope Recognition by Anti-vWf MAbs 155

V.   Proteolytic Studies of vWf:
        Mapping of Functional Epitopes with MAbs 155

VI.   The Structure and Function of vWf: A Model 157

VII.   vWD 158
        A.   The Multimeric Structure of vWf 158
        B.   Diagnosis and Classification of vWD 159
        C.   MAbs in vWD Diagnosis 161
                1.   MAbs and Multimer Sizing 161
                2.   MAb Based Immunoassays 162

VIII.   Summary 163

Acknowledgments 163

References 166

I. INTRODUCTION

Von Willebrand's disease (vWD) is a severe hemorrhagic disorder characterized by a prolonged bleeding time and a decrease in factor VIII procoagulant activity (VIII:C) and von Willebrand factor (vWf). This deficiency in vWf leads to a failure in platelet thrombus formation in damaged blood vessels. Studies carried out more than 10 years ago by a variety of workers demonstrated that plasma from vWD patients gave a decreased adhesion of platelets to glass bead columns[1] or to the subendothelium,[2] and a decrease in platelet aggregation induced by the antibiotic ristocetin.[3,4] These defects can be corrected by normal plasma or by vWf.

The vWf molecule is a large, multimeric polymer which bears at least four distinct sites that are important in the functional role of this protein. In this chapter, the various functions of vWf will be outlined, and it will be demonstrated how recent advances in immunochemical methods, in particular, the development of monoclonal antibodies (MAbs), have helped to improve our understanding of the structure and and function of this molecule and have led to improved diagnostic methods for vWD.

II. THE vWF MOLECULE

This protein was, for many years, the object of some confusion, not the least in its nomenclature[5] for the vWf molecule coexists in plasma with the factor VIII procoagulant protein (VIII:C). When, in 1971, Zimmerman et al.[6] raised a precipitating rabbit antiserum to vWf (then termed factor VIII-related antigen), it was demonstrated that vWf could be differentiated from VIII:C, (which could be detected with human alloantibodies from inhibitor patients) and that vWf was reduced or absent in vWD. Subsequent biochemical and immunological studies confirmed that vWf and VIII:C were two separate entities, linked by electrostatic, ionic, and hydrophobic interactions.[7-11] Within the last 5 years we have seen the purification of human VIII:C,[12] the sequencing and cloning of the factor VIII gene,[13-16] and the demonstration that it is synthesized in the liver.[17] vWf, however, is unrelated to VIII:C in structure, site of synthesis, and function and has been known, for many years, to be synthesized by vascular endothelial cells[18,19] and by megakaryocytes[20] (hence its localization in the α granules of platelets). The basic subunit of vWf is a 220-kDa glycoprotein which is found in the plasma as a series of disulfide-bonded polymers ranging in size from the 850-kDa tetramer to large molecules of $>2 \times 10^7$ kDa[21,22] which can be visualized in sodium-dodecyl sulfate (SDS)-agarose gels as illustrated in Figure 1. Studies in isolated endothelial cells have demonstrated that vWf is synthesized as a larger 260-kDa precursor, or pro-vWf,[23,24] which assembles intracellularly into pro-vWf dimers. Before secretion these dimers undergo glycosylation and subsequent assembly and proteolytic cleavage of the pro-sequence into the array of multimers seen in normal plasma.[25,27] The pro-sequence also appears to be released from endothelial cells and can be detected in plasma[28] where it was originally described as vW-antigen II.[29]

Titani et al.[30] have reported the amino acid sequence of plasma vWf and vWf DNA has now been cloned from human endothelial cell gene libraries.[31-34] The vWf gene has been mapped to chromosome 12, and recently the entire vWf gene has been cloned and expressed in mammalian cells.[35] These studies show the vWf molecule to contain approximately 2800 amino acids, of which the 750 amino acid N-terminal sequence represents the pro-sequence. It has little or no homology to other proteins. There is a high concentration of cysteine residues at both the N-terminal (amino acids 34—1242) and C-terminal (amino acids 1948—2813). The N-terminal of the cDNA sequence of pro-vWf contains two repeating sequences with extensive homology, two of which form the 100-kDa pro-sequence, or vW-antigen II. The C-terminal, cysteine rich domain also contains a region with approximately

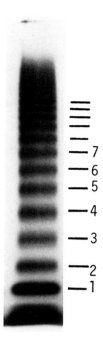

FIGURE 1.   The multimeric composition of vWf. Normal plasma electrophoresed in 1.8% agarose and visualized with ^{125}I-rabbit anti-vWf (Dako).

25% homology with the N-terminal repeat blocks. The central region consists of an approximately 600 amino acid sequence, arranged in three repeating sections, which are in contrast, poor in cysteine residues.

While there are some discrepancies in the vWf sequence described by different laboratories, these molecular studies correlate with the appearance of vWf seen by electron microscopy. Ohimori et al.[36] originally demonstrated that purified vWF consisted of a collection of strands of varying molecular weight with repeated, globular domains arranged along their lengths. A more detailed study from the same laboratory has shown structures, assumed to be the dimeric vWf protomer, which consist of globular domains at each end of a filamentous section with a smaller, central, globular domain.[37] Figure 2 illustrates a possible scheme for the assembly and organization of the vWf multimers.[38] This shows two monomers, joined symmetrically via the smaller, C-terminal, globular domains, and these dimers then linked symmetrically, via the N-terminal cysteine residues, to form multimers.

The function of vWf has been studied extensively for many years. Our understanding of the role(s) of the vWf molecule has been complemented by studies with MAbs that can block its various physiological functions, proteolytic digestion of vWf combined with MAb data, functional studies, and electron microscopy.

III. THE ROLE OF vWf IN PRIMARY HEMOSTASIS

Platelets in severe vWD plasma do not adhere to the subendothelium[2,39-41] and vWF appears to be the only plasma protein required for this attachment.[40] Platelet binding, via vWF, is maximal at high shear rates,[41,42] and it is the high molecular weight multimers of vWF ($>2 \times 10^6$ kDa) that are required for platelet attachment and spreading.[40,43,44] The binding to the subendothelium involves binding of vWF to collagen (types I and III),[45,46] although other ligands in the subendothelium may be involved.[47,48] Binding of vWf to the subendothelium has been shown to precede platelet adhesion and spreading,[40,49] and vWf appears to be present, attached to the subendothelium, prior to injury to the vessel wall,[50,51] presumably deposited by the vascular endothelial cells.

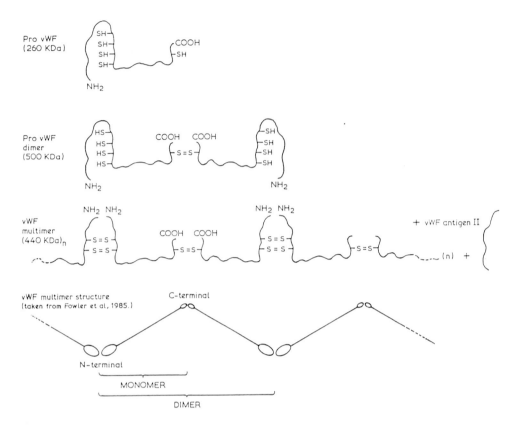

FIGURE 2.   Assembly and organization of the vWf molecule (redrawn from Fowler et al., 1985,[37] and Lynch et al., 1986[38]). Pro-vWf is synthesized by endothelial cells and linked within the cell, into dimers via their C-terminal regions. The pro-sequence (vWf:antigen II) is cleaved, and the dimers are assembled into multimers via N-terminal, before secretion. The large and small globular domains seen in the electron miscroscope may thus represent, respectively, the cysteine rich N-terminal and C-terminal regions of the molecule.

vWf, bound to the subendothelium, attaches to platelets via the platelet membrane glycoprotein Ib (GP Ib) receptor since platelets from patients with Bernard Soulier syndrome (BSS), which lack the GP Ib antigen, fail to adhere.[2,41,52,53] Platelets from patients with Glanzmann's thrombasthaenia, on the other hand, which lack the platelet glycoprotein IIb/IIIa (GP IIb/IIIa) complex do bind to the subendothelium.[54]

Normal, unstimulated platelets do not aggregate spontaneously or bind vWf.[55] The observation that the antibiotic ristocetin had a thrombocytopenic effect led to the discovery that ristocetin causes platelet aggregation in normal plasma. This aggregation is not seen with severe vWD plasma.[3,4] Ristocetin induces the binding of vWf to the GP Ib receptor as evidenced by the observation that platelets from BSS patients fail to respond in this assay[56-58] and monoclonal antibodies to GP Ib can block ristocetin-induced platelet aggregation.[59,60] As with platelet-subendothelium adhesion, the larger molecular weight multimers of vWf are required for this aggregation.[61-63] vWf can also bind to the GP IIb/IIIa antigen on platelets. This receptor complex (which is the primary binding site for fibrinogen) binds vWf on activation of platelets with adenosine diphosphate (ADP), thrombin, or collagen.[55,64,65] Platelets from BSS patients, although lacking the GP Ib molecule, can bind vWf when thus activated.[65] In addition, plasma from patients with congenital afibrinogenemia can produce the first phase of platelet aggregation despite the absence of fibrinogen in the plasma, and this aggregation is associated with the binding of vWf to platelets.[66]

One of the earliest laboratory observations of vWD was that the VIII:C level was reduced in patient's plasma.[67,68] This could be corrected by infusion of plasma,[69] but it was seen that the plasma half-life of VIII:C was shorter in vWD patients than in hemophilia A patients.[70] vWf, which is present in the plasma in vast excess over VIII:C, is seen to protect the VIII:C molecule from degradation.[71] Hamer et al.[72] have shown that VIII:C bound to vWf is less susceptible to activation by factor Xa than is isolated VIII:C.

Thus, vWf has at least four roles in primary hemostatis. It binds to types I and III collagen (and possibly to additional as yet unidentified ligands) in the subendothelium. It can bind to the GP Ib receptor on platelets, and this would appear to be the major contribution of vWf to platelet subendothelium adhesion, but may also play a role in platelet-platelet aggregation, and it is this binding site that is detected in the vWf: ristocetin co-factor (vWf:RCo) laboratory test for vWf activity. vWf also binds to the GP IIb/IIIa complex on platelets activated by thrombin or ADP and thus, together with fibronogen, causes the platelet-platelet aggregation required for thrombus formation. vWf also associates noncovalently with VIII:C, protecting it and acting as a carrier molecule.

IV. MONOCLONAL ANTIBODIES (MAbs) AND THE FUNCTIONS OF vWF

Many groups of workers have reported MAbs to vWf.[73] It is a highly immunogenic molecule, and many antibodies have been raised in the search for MAbs to VIII:C as well as in deliberate immunizations with vWf. Table 1 lists some selected antibodies that have enhanced our understanding of vWf function and have clarified the physiological observations described in the preceding section. MAbs to vWf fall broadly into five categories, which will be discussed in detail.

A. MAbs that Inhibit Aggregation and Adhesion: The GP Ib Binding Site

Several MAbs have been described that cause total inhibition of platelet aggregation induced by ristocetin.[73-77,80,82] Two laboratories have studied the effects of such antibodies on platelet adhesion,[74,75] and in both investigations, the antibodies gave marked inhibition (>80%) of platelet adhesion to the subendothelium which was particularly apparent at high shear rates. Both the CLB-RAg 35 antibody produced in Amsterdam[74] and the RFF-VIII:R/1 and R/2 antibodies produced in our laboratory[75] also inhibit ristocetin induced binding of vWf to platelets.[74,75,78,79] These antibodies do not inhibit platelet aggregation or vWf-platelet binding induced by other agonists[75,78,79] nor do they inhibit vWf-collagen binding.[78] Competition binding studies show that these three antibodies are directed against closely related epitopes of the vWf molecule, as shown in Figure 3. Conversely a MAb that affects platelet adhesion but not aggregation (CLB-RAg-201) showed no cross-reaction with these antibodies. The reactivity of these three MAbs is consistent with an epitope on vWf that binds to the GP Ib receptor on platelets.

MAb H9, produced by Meyer et al.,[80] also interacts with the GP Ib binding site of vWf, but gives only 10 to 20% inhibition of ristocetin induced platelet aggregation or vWf-platelet binding. This antibody, however, causes marked inhibition of platelet adhesion to the subendothelium at high shear rates.[80]

Other laboratories have described MAbs that appear to recognize the GP Ib receptor binding epitope of vWf, but have reported them in less detail. For example, Ogata et al.[76] described a MAb with a reactivity that resembled that seen with CLB-RAg-35 or RFF-VIII:R/1. Thomas et al.[77] have described a MAb that inhibits ristocetin induced platelet aggregation by 100%, but this antibody differs from other similar MAbs in its recognition of variant vWD plasma, as discussed later in this chapter. Sultan and her co-workers have described two antibodies that give partial inhibition of ristocetin induced platelet aggregation after prolonged incubation[81,82] which again seem to bind at, or around, the GP Ib binding site on vWf.

Thus, binding of vWf to GP Ib may involve a relatively large domain on the vWf molecule that is recognized by these various MAbs which are directed against overlapping or non-

Table 1
A SELECTION OF ANTI-vWf MAbs THAT INHIBIT FUNCTION

MAb	Inhib. of platelet aggregation by		Inhib. of platelet vWf binding by		Inhibition of platelet subendothelial adhesion	Inhibition of vWf collagen binding	Ref.
	Ristocetin	ADP/thrombin	Ristocetin	ADP/thrombin			
CLB-RAg 35	100%	None	100%	None	95%	None	74,78
RFF-VIII:R/1	100%	None	100%	None	80%	None	75,79,123
H9	20%	None	—	None	95%	None	79,80,84
202 D3	70%[a]	—	—	—	—	—	81,82
9	None	90%	None	90%	—	—	79,84
CLB-RAg 201	None	None	None	None	33%	Yes	74,78
B203	None	None	None	None	60%	50%	84
ESvWF 5	600% Enhancement	None	Enhancement	None	—	—	87

[a] Slow-acting.

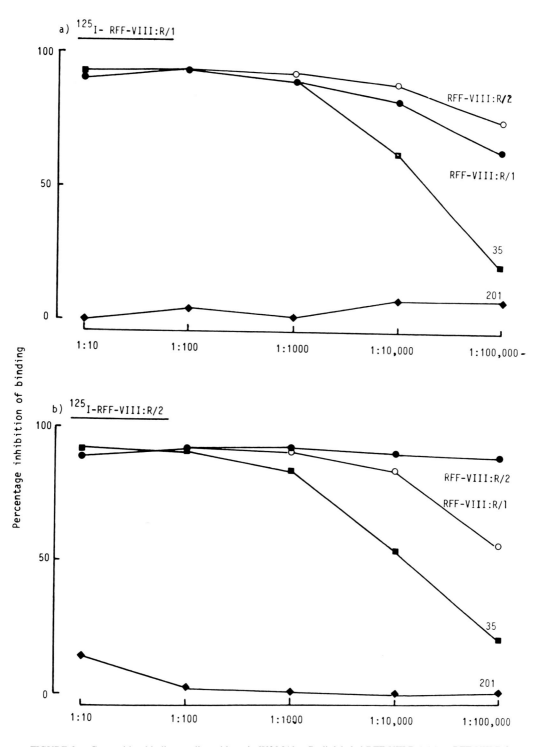

FIGURE 3. Competition binding studies with anti-vWf MAbs. Radiolabeled RFF-VIII:R/1 (a) or RFF-VIII:R/2 (b) was coincubated with normal plasma and with various dilutions of ascites containing unlabeled anti-vWf MAbs. Bound antibody was precipitated with ammonium sulfate (see Reference 75). RFF-VIII:R/1 and 2 competed with each other, and the binding of both antibodies was inhibited, to a lesser extent, by CLB-RAg-35. No inhibition of either antibody was produced by MAb CLB-RAg-201, which inhibits platelet adhesion but has no effect on platelet aggregation.

competing epitopes. It is generally agreed that a single antibody recognizes a relatively small site on an antigen consisting of no more than six amino acids thus suggesting that the GP Ib binding site on vWf may be greater than 10 to 12 amino acid residues. MAbs to the GP Ib receptor on platelets also inhibit ristocetin induced platelet aggregation and confirm the interaction of vWf with this antigen.[59,60] Recent studies suggest vWf binds to the glycocalicin fragment of the GP Ib receptor.[83]

B. MAbs that Inhibit Aggregation but Not Adhesion: The GP IIb/IIIa Binding Site

Meyer et al.[80] have described a MAb that inhibits platelet aggregation induced by thrombin but has no effect on ristocetin induced platelet aggregation or on platelet adhesion. This antibody (MAb 9) which has been extensively studied, also inhibits thrombin induced binding of vWf to platelets. No other well-characterized MAbs to this GP IIb/IIIa binding site have been reported.

C. MAbs that Inhibit Adhesion but Not Aggregation: The Collagen Binding Site

Stel et al.,[74] Meyer et al.,[80] and Girma et al.[84] have reported several MAbs that inhibit platelet adhesion, but have no effect on platelet aggregation induced by either ristocetin or thrombin. These MAbs, best represented by CLB-RAg-201[74,78] and by MAb B203,[84] have been shown to inhibit the binding of vWf to both subendothelium and to types I and III collagen.

D. MAbs that Have No Effect on vWf Function

Many MAbs have been produced that apparently have no interaction with functional sites on the vWf molecule.[73] Good examples of such antibodies have been described by Lamme et al.[85] and by Bradley et al.[86] These MAbs have been used in immunoassays for vWf antigen (vWf:Ag), substituting for polyclonal antisera, and as such, represent extremely useful reagents.

E. MAbs with Other Functional Effects

Two MAbs have been reported that enhance ristocetin induced platelet aggregation.[87] This effect was dose dependent and was most pronounced when small molecular weight multimers of vWf were used. It did not appear to involve cross-linking of the vWf molecules by the MAbs as Fab′ preparations were equally as active as intact MAb IgG. The mechanism of this increase in aggregation remains unclear. Enhancement of aggregation by MAbs to porcine vWf has also been seen (personal observation). A group of MAbs raised against porcine vWf, by Katzmann et al.,[88] has enabled studies on their effects on the bleeding times in pigs.[89,90] No clear correlation between the effects of these antibodies *in vivo* and their performance in laboratory tests for vWf activity was seen. Indeed, the one MAb that inhibited ristocetin induced aggregation of washed human platelets (MAb W1-2) while prolonging bleeding time in an *in vitro* test system produced relatively little prolongation of bleeding time *in vivo*, although ''rebleeding'' (i.e., bleeding from the incision following an initial cessation) occurred. In constrast, MAb W1-8, which did not cross-react with human vWf had a marked effect in prolonging bleeding time *in vivo* and *in vitro*. Microscopical examination of damaged tissue from normal pigs infused with W1-8 antibody indicated the formation of platelet aggregates with little or no adhesion to the damaged vessel wall, a pattern analogous to that seen in vWD pigs.[90] While a precise correlation between the results of these studies and those with MAbs to human vWf cannot be made due to the lack of species cross-reactivity, the W1-8 antibody may recognize an epitope analogous to the collagen binding site on human vWf. No MAbs to vWf have been shown to interfere with the interactions of vWf and VIII:C; however, it is worth noting that MAbs to the light (80-kDa) chain of VIII:C have been raised which inhibit the binding to vWf.[72]

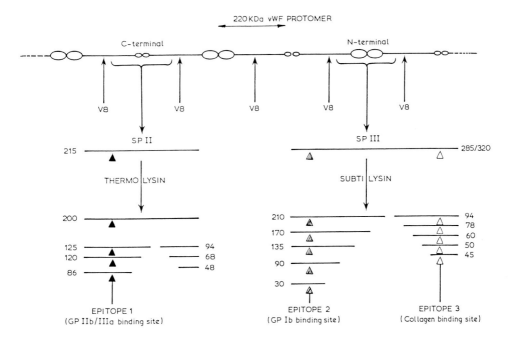

FIGURE 4. Digestion of vWf with *Staphylococcus* V8 protease. The location of the GPIb, GPIIb/IIIa, and collagen binding sites.[84,92,94]

F. Epitope Recognition By Anti-vWf MAbs

Large-scale epitope mapping studies with MAbs produced in different laboratories have not been undertaken. However, cross-reactivity studies with selected MAbs have demonstrated that the sites on vWf that bind to the platelet GP Ib and GP IIb/IIIa receptors and to subendothelium/collagen are separate epitopes as shown in Figure 3.

V. PROTEOLYTIC STUDIES OF vWF: MAPPING OF FUNCTIONAL EPITOPES WITH MAbs

Proteolytic enzymes have been used to cleave the vWf molecule in a controlled way, and the proteolytic fragments so formed have been examined for their ability to bind to platelets and/or collagen, or to bind to well-characterized MAbs.[78,84,91-94]

These studies have been carried out in several laboratories, using different proteolytic enzymes and different approaches to the identification of the functional epitopes on vWf. There are, of necessity, discrepancies in the data arising from this work, but, in general, the different groups arrive at similar conclusions, and differences can be ascribed to either variations in the methods of proteolysis or in the molecular weight determinations, or to different sensitivities of the test systems used to assay the vWf fragments. An attempt to summarize the findings has been made in Figures 4 and 5.

Two laboratories have used *Staphylococcus* V8 protease (which cleaves the C-terminal end of glutamyl and aspartyl residues) to digest vWf. Girma et al.[84] report two fragments of vWf of molecular weights 215 and 320 kDa which have been termed SP II and SP III, respectively. The SP III fragment is reported as a dimer of 320 and 285 kDa, the 285-kDa fragment being thought to be a product of further *S. aureus* V8 protease digestion. This fragment, which on reduction formed a doublet or triplet of around 170 kDa, contains the GP Ib and collagen binding sites, as identified with MAbs H9 and 203, respectively. Further proteolysis of SP III, with increasing amounts of subtilisin yielded a series of molecular weight fragments (see Figure 4), and blotting studies with the GP Ib binding site MAb, H9

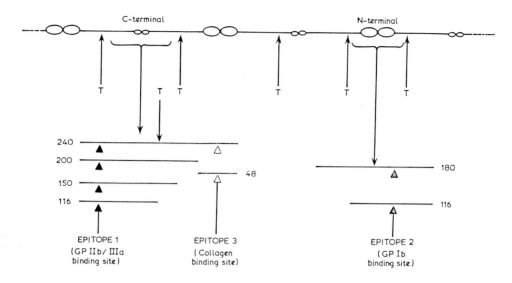

FIGURE 5.   Digestion of vWf with trypsin. The location of the GPIb, GPIIb/IIIa, and collagen binding sites.[78,91,93]

demonstrated this epitope to be on fragments of 210, 170, 135, and 90 kDa. A 30-kDa fragment, present after extensive proteolysis, also reacted with H9. Immunoabsorbtion of *S. aureus* V8 protease-digested SP III on an H9 affinity column also yielded fragments of around 30 kDa. A collagen binding epitope, localized with MAb 203, was found on additional subtilisin fragments of molecular weights 94,78,60,50, and 45 kDa.

The SP II fragment can be reduced by SDS to two 110-kDa fragments which have identical C-terminal sequences to native vWf. Western blotting studies, with MAb9 which recognizes the GP IIb/IIIa binding site on vWf, locate this epitope on the SP II fragment. Proteolytic digestion of the 215-kDa SP II dimer, with thermolysin, produced first a 200-kDa poly-peptide, then a series of peptides of molecular weights 125, 120, 98, and 86 kDa, which further reduced to two 64- and 48-kDa fragments. MAb9, bound to the 215-, 200-, 125-, 120-, and 86-kDa polypeptides.

The reactivity of the SP II and SP III proteolytic fragments with platelets was established in direct and competition binding studies,[84] as was the reactivity of SP III with collagen.[94]

Similar studies by Bockenstedt et al.,[92] in which vWf was reduced in SDS and alkylated before subjection to proteolysis with *S. aureus* V8 protease, produced a 285-kDa fragment that bound to heparin and thus could be separated from the remaining 225 and 210-kDa fragments. The 285-kDa fragment would seem to be analogous to the SP III fragment reported by Girma et al. as it could compete with ^{125}I-vWf in binding studies with ristocetin stimulated platelets. Neither the 225- or 210-kDa fragment(s) nor the 220-kDa monomer obtained from the reduced vWf competed for collagen binding with ^{125}I-vWf, but this may be due to a lower sensitivity in the binding assay used in this study. In general, in all of these studies the proteolytic fragments of vWf bound less avidly to their various receptors than did the native protein.

Sixma et al.[78] have used the MAbs described by Stel et al.[74] to identify the GP Ib and collagen binding sites on tryptic fragments of vWf, as shown in Figure 5. Unreduced vWf was incubated with trypsin (which cleaves the C-terminal bonds of lysine or arginine residues) for varying lengths of time, then immunoprecipitated with CLB-RAg-35 (which recognizes the GP Ib binding site) or CLB-RAg-201 (which recognizes a collagen binding site).

A 10-min incubation with trypsin produced a 240-kDa fragment which was precipitated with CLB-RAg-201 and a 180-kDa fragment which reacted with CLB-RAg-35. The CLB-RAg-201 binding site was located, on further proteolysis, on a 48-kDa fragment. The GP Ib binding site was found, following more than 6-h incubation with trypsin, to be on a 116-

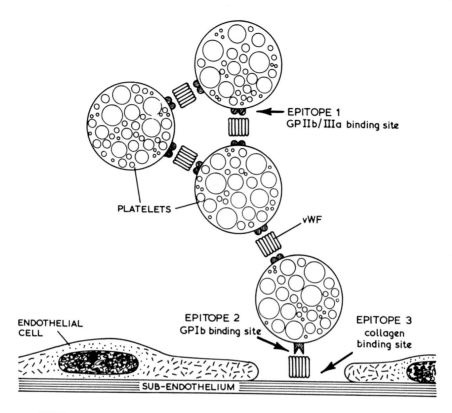

FIGURE 6. A model for the role of vWf in platelet adhesion and platelet aggregation.

kDa fragment of vWf. On reduction this fragment was seen to consist of two polypeptides of molecular weight 50 to 55 kDa (which reacted with CLB-RAg-35) and one of 14 kDa (which did not). The reactivities of these tryptic fragments have been confirmed in direct binding studies.[91]

Reduction, alkylation, and tryptic digestion of vWf have been reported by Fujimura et al.[93] They observed a 52- to 48-and 46-kDa doublet, with identical N-terminal sequences, which could inhibit ristocetin induced platelet aggregation and vWf binding and which reacted with three MAbs with anti-GP Ib characteristics. The peptide possibly represents a fragment of the N-terminal portion of vWf beginning at amino acid 449. Allowing for minor inter-laboratory variations, this fragment is undoubtedly analogous to the reduced 52- to 56-kDa fragment reported by Sixma et al.[78] as bearing the GP Ib binding epitope.

Further evidence for the location of the GP Ib binding site on vWf comes from the studies of Katzmann et al.[88] Mice were immunized with 48- to 52-kDa tryptic fragments of vWf and MAbs were subsequently produced. Of the 24 MAbs raised from these mice, 5 inhibited ristocetin induced platelet aggregation.

VI. THE STRUCTURE AND FUNCTION OF vWF:A MODEL

It is possible to construct a model for the location of three functional sites on the vWf molecule. The epitopes, which are designated as epitope 1 (the GP IIb/IIIa receptor binding site), epitope 2 (the GP Ib receptor binding site), and epitope 3 (one candidate for a collagen binding site), are shown schematically in Figure 6. This illustrates the three distinct and separate roles of these three epitopes in the formation of the hemostatic plug. Damage to the vessel wall causes retraction of the vascular endothelial cells and exposure of the sub-endothelium. vWf, either released from platelets and/or endothelial cells in response to injury or already present in the subendothelium, is attached to the subendothelium via epitope 3. This forms a bridge between the subendothelium and platelets, binding predominantly to the GP Ib receptor via epitope 2. Thrombin and/or ADP stimulation of platelets induces the binding of vWf to the GP IIb/IIIa receptor to cause platelet-platelet aggregation. Molecules other than vWf are undoubtedly involved in platelet aggregation (e.g., fibrinogen), and platelet aggregates can occur in severe vWD. Platelet adhesion to the vessel wall is, however, not observed in severe vWD.[2,90] From the studies described in the preceding section, these three epitopes appear to be present on the individual monomers of vWf as well as on the multimers. It is established that the maximum activity of vWf lies in the large molecular weight multimers.[43-45,61-63] Low molecular weight forms of the molecule and peptide fragments can, however, bind to stimulated platelets and to the subendothelium.[91,93,94] The larger, polymeric forms of the molecule may be necessary to effect the strong, multivalent associations required to cause platelet adhesion and platelet aggregation in fast flowing blood. From the various studies on partially proteolysed vWf,[78,84,91-94] it would appear that epitope 1, the GP IIb/IIIa binding site, is found nearest to the carboxy-terminal of the vWf monomer with epitope 2, the GP Ib binding site being found near to the amino-terminal, and the collagen binding site (epitope 3) being located relatively centrally in the molecule. Further sequencing of the various proteolytic fragments of vWf will undoubtedly clarify the locations of these epitopes and allow a more complete map of vWf to be constructed.

The sequence of vWf shows it to be an unusual protein in that it lacks homology with other molecules.[30-35,38] In particular, vWf has little homology with other molecules that are involved in cell attachment and adhesion, for example, fibrinogen, fibronectin, and the fibroblast binding protein vitronectin (all of which show sequence homology), although vWf does have a similar, trinodular structure to fibrinogen when viewed by electron microscopy.[96] vWf does, however, contain the sequence of amino acids consisting of arginine-glycine-asparagine (RGD) found in both fibrinogen and fibronectin as well as in vitronectin, which is associated with adhesion.[97] Synthetic peptides containing this sequence can block the attachment of fibroblasts to fibronectin or vitronectin[97,98] and can block the binding of vWf to the platelet GP IIb/IIIa receptor.[99]

The evolutionary conservation in many of these adhesion proteins is mirrored by similarities in the structure and amino acid sequences of their cell membrane receptors. The GP IIb/IIIa complex consists of a two-subunit, integral membrane protein.[100] Similar di- or tri-polypeptide structures are seen in the fibronectin receptor (integrin) and vitronectin receptor isolated from human osteosarcoma cells or from fibroblasts[97] and in the LFA-1 antigen complex that mediates lymphocyte contact in man and mouse.[101,102]

VII. vWD

A. The Multimeric Structure of vWf

As illustrated earlier, in Figure 1, the appearance of vWf in normal plasma is of a series of high molecular weight multimers, ranging from the 850-kDa tetramer and increasing logarithmically to complexes of more than 2×10^6 kDa. Biochemical and amino acid sequence data all indicate that the higher molecular weight forms of vWf consist of polymers of the vWf protomer.[38,63] Well-resolved SDS-agarose gels show, in addition to the presence of the basic multimer structure, a characteristic "triplet"[103] (as illustrated in Figures 1 and 7) in which each strongly stained band in the gel is flanked by two fainter bands. The reason for this pattern is not clear. Fowler et al.[37] have proposed that vWf can be cleaved *in vivo* by an unidentified protease at sites adjacent to the globular C-terminal and N-terminal domains, thus leading to polymerized vWf fragments of slightly differing lengths. This picture would correspond to the variant ends of vWf filaments seen in their electron microscopy studies. No specific protease has been identified although at least two platelet

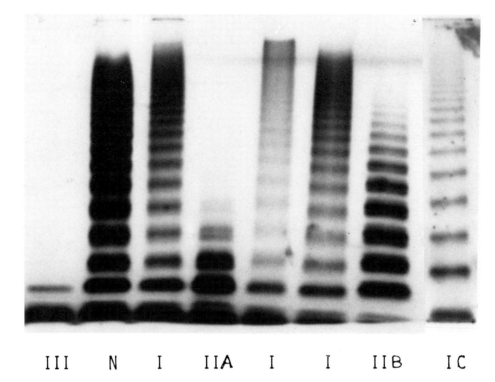

III   N   I   IIA   I   I   IIB   IC

FIGURE 7.   Multimer patterns in vWD.

derived proteases are thought to be capable of degrading vWf *in vivo*.[104,105] Plasmin has been investigated,[37] but like the platelet drived enzymes, this only causes a reduction in the size of the multimers and does not lead to an increase in the appearance of the triplet structure.

B. Diagnosis and Classification of vWD

vWD is, normally, a mild disorder in which patients have a lowered production of normal vWf. This form of the disease, which has been classified as type I vWD, has an autosomal dominant inheritance. Rare homozygous patients have a total lack of vWf and have a severe form of the disease.[11,103,106-108] In the laboratory vWD is normally diagnosed in three ways. vWf activity is determined in the ristocetin induced platelet aggregation assay.[3,4] vWf:Ag is measured immunologically, using polyclonal antisera (usually rabbit in origin) in either Laurell immunoelectrophoresis (IEP) systems[6] or in immunoradiometric assays.[109,110] In addition, the multimeric composition of vWf analyzed in agarose gels is also increasingly employed as a diagnostic test for the disease.

In type I vWD the levels of vWf and vWf:Ag are comparably low, and the multimer pattern is normal, albeit with a reduced amount of vWf present.[22,103,106-108]

A percentage of patients, however, have anomalous values for vWf and vWf:Ag,[111] and their vWf has an increased mobility in crossed, two dimensional immunoelectrophoresis.[112,113] These variant vWD patients also show abnormal multimer patterns[22,103,106-108,114] with lack of the higher molecular weight multimers and/or abnormalities in their triplet structure, as illustrated in Figure 7. Following the description by Ruggeri and Zimmerman of the type IIA and IIB forms of variant vWD, at least nine forms of vWD have been described which vary in the levels of vWf activity and vWf:Ag and in their multimeric pattern,[22,103,106-108,114-118] plus a variant with an apparent defect in the VIII:C binding site.[119] Table 2 attempts to summarize the current classification of vWD. Type IIA patients have

Table 2
THE CLASSIFICATION OF vWD

Variant	Inheritance	VIII:C	vWf:Ag	vWf:RCo	Multimers
Type IA	Autosomal, dominant	↓	↓	↓	Normal but all forms reduced in proportion
Type IB	Autosomal, dominant	↓	↓	↓	All multimers present but high molecular weight reduced relative to the rest
Type IC	Autosomal, dominant	N or ↓	N or ↓	↓	All multimers present but abnormal — no triplet structure
Type INY and Type I Malmo	Autosomal, dominant	N or ↓	N or ↓	↓	Normal multimeric structure
Type IIA	Autosomal, dominant	N or ↓	N or ↓	↓↓	Large and intermediate multimers absent
Type IIB	Autosomal, dominant	N or ↓	N or ↓	N or ↓	Large molecular weight multimers absent; platelet vWf normal
Type IIC	Autosomal, recessive	N	N	↓↓	Large multimers absent and abnormal triplets (prominent lower band)
Type IID	Autosomal, dominant	N	N	↓	Large multimers absent and abnormal triplet structure (some intermediate bands)
Type III	Autosomal, recessive	↓	↓	↓	No vWf present

Note: N, normal.

Table 3
EXAMPLES OF MAbs USED IN vWf MULTIMER STUDIES

Epitope specificity/activity	Mab	Multimer binding	Ref.
GPIb binding site	CLB-RAg-7	No	74
	RFF-VIII:R/1	No	75
	RFF-VIII:R/2	No	75
	CLB-RAg-35	Yes	74
	H9	Yes	80
GPIb binding site-related	F4	Yes	77
	4Fg	Yes	81
	202 D3	Yes	81
	CLB-RAg-21	No	74
GPIIb/IIIa binding site	9	Yes	80
Collagen binding site	CLB-RAg-1	Yes	74
	CLB-RAg-20	Yes	74
	CLB-RAg-201	Yes	74
	B203	Yes	80
No detected effect on vWf function	CLB-RAg-36	Yes	74
	D7	Yes	86
	B7	No	80
	B2A	No	73
Enhancement of ristocetin induced platelet aggregation and vWf binding	EsvWF-5	Yes	87
50% inhibition of vWf:RCo but no effect on vWf binding	EsvWF-1	Partial	87
50% enhancement of botrocetin-induced platelet aggregation	21-42	Yes	73

normal or reduced levels of vWf:Ag with little or no detectable vWf activity. They lack the large and intermediate vWf multimers. Type IIB patients have variable levels of vWf and vWf:Ag, show an increased ability to aggregate platelets at low concentrations of ristocetin, and lack the large vWf multimers. Additional variants have been described, for example, type IC vWD in which all multimers are present but no triplet structure is seen. Abnormal triplet structure has also been reported in variants of vWD classified as type IIC and IID (see Table 2), and this can be examined in more detail in high resolution SDS-agarose gels. Additional variants will undoubtedly be described. The reduction in higher molecular multimers of vWF in variant vWD has been proposed to be due to an increased sensitivity to platelet derived proteases in these patients.[122]

In summary, it is clear that vWD comprises a variable defect in which the vWf molecule can be both deficient and defective. So far genetic studies have proved uninformative as to the nature of the defect,[38] although this situation will undoubtedly alter.

C. MAbs in vWD Diagnosis

MAbs are obvious candidates for use in diagnostic assays as they represent a source of highly specific, standard antibody. In addition, the specificity of MAbs for particular epitopes on vWf that are of functional relevance has been exploited for the diagnosis of vWD.

1. MAbs and Multimer Sizing

The analysis of vWf multimers normally employs a polyclonal (rabbit) anti-vWf antiserum to visualize the multimers. Several laboratories have investigated the use of MAbs to replace the rabbit antiserum, with variable results. Much of this work is unpublished and comes from data reported to the International Committee on Thrombosis and Haemostasis (ICTH) subcommittee on factor VIII and vWf.[73] In general, many MAbs have been reported to bind to vWf multimers in SDS-agarose gels and some of these are listed in Table 3. Where data are available it would appear that these MAbs bind to all multimers. In general, MAbs that recognize the GP IIb/IIIa receptor and the collagen binding sites on vWf can react with vWf in SDS-agarose gels whereas many MAbs directed towards the GP Ib binding site do not. For example, RFF-VIII:R/1 and RFF-VIII:R/2 do not bind to any multimers in SDS gels, and this has been shown to be due to the effects of SDS and urea on the vWf molecule.[123] Treatment of plasma vWf with these agents, which cause conformational changes and unfolding of the vWf molecule, totally inhibited the binding of vWf by the MAbs. Thus, the GP Ib receptor binding site on vWf, recognized by these two MAbs would appear to be a conformationally dependent epitope.

In summary, the use of MAbs to vWf in multimer analysis would not seem to have added to a greater understanding of vWf structure, other than to reinforce the fact that the vWf multimers are comprised of repeated subunits of identical composition.

2. MAb Based Immunoassays

MAbs used in immunoassays have advantages of availability and reproducibility over polyclonal antisera. In addition, MAbs facilitate the development of immunobinding assays which are, in general, more reproducible and more sensitive than immunoprecipitation methods. Added to this, the fact that MAbs which recognize antigenic epitopes of functional significance can be used means that MAbs can prove extremely powerful diagnostic tools.

Several groups have reported the use of MAbs in immunoradiometric assays (IRMAs) for vWf:Ag. Ogata et al.[76] and Thomas et al.[77] have reported IRMAs that use MAbs which appear to be directed at or around the GP Ib binding site on vWf. The two-site assay described by Ogata et al.[76] used one MAb. This assay gave a good correlation with vWf activity in 16 samples of vWD plasma (r = 0.687). It was not clear from this report, however, whether any variant vWD samples were included in this survey. The study by Thomas et al.[77] indicated a poor correlation with vWf activity for variant vWD plasma. In this paper, two different MAbs were used in a two-site, solid phase IRMA. Both inhibited ristocetin induced platelet aggregation, but the two antibodies were directed against different epitopes. This assay showed classical nonparallel curves with variant vWD plasma of the type seen when polyclonal antisera are used. Very similar data were obtained if only one of the MAbs was used as a tracer in a two-site IRMA in which a polyclonal antiserum formed the solid phase. It is not known whether either MAb had any effect on platelet subendothelium interactions, and thus it is not clear whether these MAbs were specific for the GP Ib receptor binding site.

Two MAbs have been described by Sola et al.[81] which, on prolonged incubation, gave either 95 or 30% inhibition of ristocetin induced vWf activity. Using these two MAbs in a two-site IRMA,[82] a good correlation was seen between vWf:Ag measured in the MAb assay and in a polyclonal IRMA for normals and type I vWD, whereas the assay gave considerably lower values of vWf:Ag for type IIA vWD plasma.

Two groups have reported MAb based assays that employ MAbs with no functional activity. In both cases, these assays gave a good correlation with the vWf:Ag levels detected with polyclonal antisera.[85,86] Such MAbs would offer convenient and standardized replacements for polyclonal antisera for the detection of vWf:Ag.

Our group has described the use of the RFF-VIII:R/1 and/or RFF-VIII:R/2 antibodies in IRMAs (or ELISA) enzyme linked immunoabsorbent assays.[75,123,124] These two competing antibodies are directed against the same GP Ib receptor binding site on vWf. They both give total inhibition of ristocetin induced platelet aggregation and vWf-binding to platelets and inhibit vWf-subendothelial adhesion at high shear rates, but have no effect on thrombin, ADP, or collagen induced platelet aggregation.[75,79] As shown in Figure 8, the MAb assay has been used to study a large group of vWD patients,[124] of whom 71 were classified as type I vWD, 4 had homozygous severe type I vWD, and 37 had a variant form of vWD (31 — IIA, 5 — IIB, and 1 — IID vWD).

In all samples, whether from normal individuals, from type I, or from variant vWD patients, the levels of vWf detected in the MAb assay were comparable to the levels of vWf activity detected by ristocetin induced platelet aggregation. The MAb assay was highly reproducible and sensitive, detecting vWf at <0.05 U/ml plasma. Such an assay can substitute for the tedious ristocetin induced platelet aggregation assay for measuring vWf activity. Both MAbs have a comparable sensitivity for vWf and give identical results with variant vWD plasma when used in either a one-site[75,124] or two-site IRMA, or in ELISA.[123] Both the one-site IRMA and two-site ELISA can be performed in 5 to 6 h, and many samples can be analyzed simultaneously.

The remarkable degree of correlation (r = 0.950) between vWf activity and the level of vWF detected in this MAb assay in all types of vWD was consistent with the recognition by these antibodies of an epitope on the GP Ib binding site on vWf.

VIII. SUMMARY

MAbs to vWf have improved our understanding of the structure and function of this molecule. MAbs directed against separate sites, located on different regions of the vWf protomer, have shown that this molecule bears at least three epitopes which have distinct and separate roles in platelet aggregation and platelet adhesion (Figure 6). Two of these epitopes form the binding sites for collagen and for the platelet GP Ib receptor, respectively, and, via these interactions, bind platelets to the subendothelium. The third epitope on vWf is the binding site for the platelet GP IIb/IIIa receptor, important in causing platelet-platelet aggregation.

MAbs have also proved extremely useful in the development of laboratory assays for vWf. MAbs with no effect on vWF activity can be used as substitutes for polyclonal antisera in IRMA or ELISA assays or in multimer analysis while MAbs to epitopes of functional importance, and in particular to the GP Ib binding site, can be used in IRMA or ELISA systems to replace the ristocetin co-factor (RCo) platelet aggregation assay for vWf activity.

ACKNOWLEDGMENTS

I would like to thank Kathy Matthews for running the vWf multimer gels.

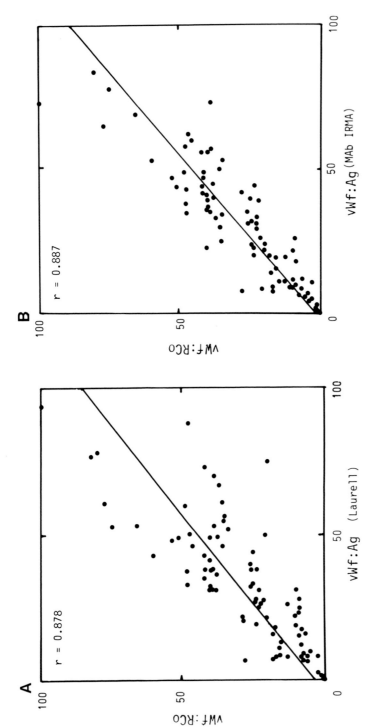

FIGURE 8. Immunoassay for vWf activity using MAbs. Plasma samples were assayed for vWf activity by ristocetin induced platelet aggregation (vWf:RCo) and for vWf:Ag by Laurell IEP. The plasma samples were also assayed for vWf in the MAb based IRMA (see References 75 and 124) using RFF-VIII:R/2 (MAb-IRMA). (A/B) Type I vWD. (C/D) Type II (variant) vWD.

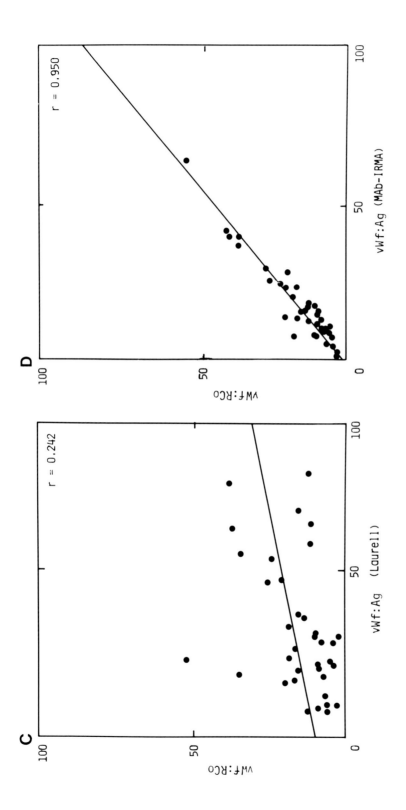

REFERENCES

1. **Salzman, E. W.,** Measurement of platelet adhesiveness. A simple in vitro technique demonstrating an abnormality in von Willebrand's disease, *J. Lab. Clin. Med.,* 62, 724, 1963.
2. **Tschopp, T. B., Weiss, H. J., and Baumgartner, H. R.,** Decreased adhesion of platelets to subendothelium in von Willebrand's disease, *J. Lab. Clin. Med.,* 83, 296, 1974.
3. **Howard, M. A. and Firkin, B. G.,** Ristocetin — a new tool in the investigation of platelet aggregation, *Thromb. Diath. Haemorrh.,* 26, 362, 1971.
4. **Weiss, H. J., Rogers, J., and Brand, H.,** Defective ristocetin-induced platelet aggregation in von Willebrand's disease and its correction by factor VIII, *J. Clin. Invest.,* 52, 2697, 1973.
5. **Marder, V. J., Mannucci, P. M., Firkin, B. G., Hoyer, L. W., and Meyer, D.,** Standard nomenclature for factor VIII and von Willebrand factor: a recommendation by the International Committee on Thrombosis and Haemostasis, *Thromb. Haemost.,* 54, 871, 1985.
6. **Zimmerman, T. S., Ratnoff, O. D., and Powell, A. E.,** Immunologic differentiation of classic haemophilia (factor VIII deficiency) and von Willebrand's disease, *J. Clin. Invest.,* 50, 244, 1971.
7. **Cooper, H. A., Griggs, T. R., and Wagner, R. H.,** Factor VIII recombination after dissociation by CaCl$_2$, *Proc. Natl. Acad. Sci. U.S.A.,* 70, 2326, 1973.
8. **Zimmerman, T. S. and Edgington, T. S.,** Factor VIII coagulant activity and factor VIII-like antigen: independent molecular entities, *J. Exp. Med.,* 138, 1015, 1973.
9. **Hougie, C., Sargeant, R. B., Brown, J. E., and Baugh, R. F.,** Evidence that factor VIII and ristocetin aggregating factor are separate molecular entities, *Proc. Soc. Exp. Biol. Med.,* 147, 58, 1974.
10. **Koutts, J., Lavergne, J.-M., and Meyer, D.,** Immunological evidence that human factor VIII is composed of two linked moieties, *Br. J. Haematol.,* 37, 415, 1977.
11. **Tuddenham, E. G. D., Trabold, N. C., Collins, J. A., and Hoyer, L. W.,** The properties of factor VIII coagulant activity prepared by immunoabsorbant chromatography, *J. Lab. Clin. Med.,* 93, 40, 1979.
12. **Rotblat, F., O'Brien, D. P., O'Brien, F. J., Goodall, A. H., and Tuddenham, E. G. D.,** Purification of human FVIII:C and its characterisation by Western blotting using monoclonal antibodies, *Biochemistry,* 241, 4924, 1985.
13. **Gitschier, J., Wood, W. I., Goralka, T.-M., Wian, K.-L., Chen, E. Y., Eaton, D. H., Vehar, G. A., Capan, D. J., and Lawn, R. M.,** Characterization of the human factor VIII gene, *Nature,* 312, 326, 1984.
14. **Wood, W. I., Capon, D. J., Simonsen, C. C., Eaton, D. L., Gitschier, J., Keyt, B., Seeburg, P. H., Smith, D. H., Hollingshead, P., Wian, K. -L., Delwart, E., Tuddenham, E. G. D., Vehar, G. A., and Lawn, R. M.,** Expression of active human factor VIII from recombinant DNA clones, *Nature,* 312, 330, 1984.
15. **Vehar, G. A., Keyt, B., Eaton, D., Rodriguez, H., O'Brien, D. P., Rotblat, F., Opperman, H., Keck, R., Wood, W. I., Harkins, R. N., Tuddenham, E. G. D., Lawn, R. M., and Capon, D. J.,** Structure of human factor VIII, *Nature,* 312, 337, 1984.
16. **Toole, J. J., Khopf, V. L., Wozney, J. M., Sultzman, L. A., Buecker, J. L., Pittman, D. D., Kaufman, R. J., Brown, E., Shoemaker, C., Orr, E. C., Amphlett, G. W., Foster, W. B., Coe, M. L., Kuntson, G. J., Fass, D. N., and Hewick, R. M.,** Molecular cloning of a cDNA encoding human antihaemophililic factor, *Nature,* 312, 342, 1984.
17. **Wion, K. L., Kelly, D., Summerfield, J. A., Tuddenham, E. G. D., and Lawn, R. M.,** Distribution of factor VIII mRNA and antigen in human liver and other tissues, *Nature,* 317, 726, 1985.
18. **Jaffe, E. A., Hoyer, L. W., and Nachman, R. L.,** Synthesis of von Willebrand factor by cultured human endothelial cells, *Proc. Natl. Acad. Sci. U.S.A.,* 71, 1906, 1974.
19. **Shearn, S. A. M., Peake, I. R., Giddings, J. C., Humphreys, J., and Bloom, A. L.,** The characterisation and synthesis of antigens related to factor VIII in vascular endothelium, *Thromb. Res.,* 11, 43, 1977.
20. **Nachman, R., Levine, R., and Jaffe, E. A.,** Synthesis of factor VIII by cultured guinea pig megakaryocytes, *J. Clin. Invest.,* 60, 914, 1979.
21. **Hoyer, L. W. and Shainoff, J. R.,** Factor VIII related protein circulates in normal human plasma as high molecular weight multimers, *Blood,* 55, 1056, 1980.
22. **Ruggeri, Z. M. and Zimmerman, T. S.,** Variant von Willebrand's disease. Characterization of two subtypes by analysis of multimeric composition of factor VIII/von Willebrand factor in plasma and platelets, *J. Clin. Invest.,* 65, 1318, 1980.
23. **Wagner, D. D. and Marder, V. J.,** Biosynthesis of von Willebrand protein by human endothelial cells: identification of a larger precursor polypeptide chain, *J. Biol. Chem.,* 258, 2065, 1983.
24. **Lynch, D. C., Williams, R., Zimmerman, T. S., Kirby, E. P., and Livingston, D. M.,** Biosynthesis of the subunit of factor VIIIR by bovine aorta endothelial cells, *Proc. Natl. Acad. Sci. U.S.A.,* 80, 2738, 1983.
25. **Lynch, D. C., Zimmerman, T. S., Kirby, E. P., and Livingston, D. M.,** Subunit composition of oligomeric human von Willebrand factor, *J. Biol. Chem.,* 258, 12757, 1983.

26. **Wagner, D. D. and Marder, V. J.,** Biosynthesis of human von Willebrand protein by human endothelial cells: processing steps and their intracellular localization, *J. Cell Biol.,* 99, 2123, 1984.

27. **Wagner, D. D., Mayadas, T., Urban-Pickering, M., Lewis, B. H., and Marder, V. J.,** Inhibition of disulphide bonding of von Willebrand protein by monesin results in small, functionally defective multimers, *J. Cell Biol.,* 101, 112, 1985.

28. **Fay, R. J., Kawal, Y., Wagner, D. D., Ginsburg, D., Bonthron, D., Ohlnsson-Wilhelm, B. M., Chavin, S. I., Abraham, G. N., Handin, R. I., Orkin, S. H., Montgomery, R. R., and Marder, V. J.,** The molecular identity of a 100 Kd plasma glycoprotein and the von Willebrand's antigen II (vW AGII) with the protein encoded by the 5′ end of the cDNA for pro-vWF, *Blood,* 66, (Suppl.), 333a, 1985.

29. **Montgomery, R. R. and Zimmerman, T. S.,** von Willebrand's disease antigen II: a new plasma and platelet antigen deficient in severe von Willebrand's disease, *J. Clin. Invest.,* 61, 1498, 1978.

30. **Titani, K., Ericsson, L. H., Takio, K., Kumar, S., Chopek, M. W., and Fujikawa, K.,** Chemical characterization of human von Willebrand factor, *Thromb. Haemost.,* 54, 123, 1985.

31. **Verweij, C. L., de Vries, C. J. M., Distel, B., van Zonnefeld, A.-J., van Kessel, A. G., van Mourik, J. A., and Pannokoek, H.,** Construction of cDNA coding for human von Willebrand factor using antibody probes for colony-screening and mapping of the chromosomal gene, *Nucleic Acids Res.,* 13, 4699, 1985.

32. **Ginsburg, D., Handin, R. I., Bonthron, D. T., Donlon, T. A., Bruns, G. A. P., Latt, S. A., and Orkin, S. H.,** Human von Willebrand factor (vWF): isolation of complementary DNA (cDNA) clones and chromosomal localization, *Science,* 228, 1401, 1985.

33. **Lynch, D. C., Zimmerman, T. S., Collins, C. J., Brown, M., Morin, M. J., Ling, E. H., and Livingston, D. M.,** Molecular cloning of cDNA for human von Willebrand factor: authentication by a new method, *Cell,* 41, 49, 1985.

34. **Sadler, J. E., Shelton-Inholes, B. B., Sorace, J. M., Hardan, J. M., Titani, K., and Davie, E. W.,** Cloning and characterization of two cDNAs coding for human von Willebrand factor, *Proc. Natl. Acad. Sci. U.S.A.,* 82, 6394, 1985.

35. **Bonthron, D. T., Handin, R. I., Kaufman, R. J., Wasley, L. C., Orr, E. C., Mitsock, L. M., Ewenstein, B., Loscalzo, J., Ginsburg, D., and Orkin, S. H.,** Structure of pre-pro-von Willebrand factor and its expression in heterologous cells, *Nature,* 324, 270, 1986.

36. **Ohimoro, K., Fretto, L. J., Harrison, R. L., Switzer, M. E. P., Erickson, H. P., and McKee, P. A.,** The electron microscopy of human factor VIII/von Willebrand factor glycoprotein: effect of reducing agents on structure and function, *J. Cell Biol.,.* 95, 632, 1982.

37. **Fowler, W. E., Fretto, L. J., Hamilton, K. K., Erickson, H., P., and Mckee, P. A.,** Substructure of human von Willebrand factor, *J. Clin. Invest.,* 76, 1491, 1985.

38. **Lynch, D. C., Zimmerman, T. S., and Ruggeri, Z. M.,** von Willebrand factor, now cloned, *Br. J. Haematol.,* 64, 15, 1986.

39. **Weiss, H. J., Baumgartner, H. R., Tschopp, T. B., Turitto, V. T., and Cohen, D.,** Correction by factor VIII of the impared platelet adhesion to subendothelium in von Willebrand's disease, *Blood,* 51, 267, 1978.

40. **Sakariassen, K. S., Bolhuis, P. A., and Sixma, J. J.,** Adhesion of human blood platelets to human artery subendothelium is mediated by factor VIII—von Willebrand factor bound to subendothelium, *Nature,* 279, 636, 1979.

41. **Weiss, H. J., Turitto, V. T., and Baumgartner, H. R.,** Effect of shear rate on platelet interaction with subdenothelium in citrated and native blood. I. Shear rate dependent decrease of adhesion in von Willebrand's disease and the Bernard-Soulier syndrome, *J. Lab. Clin. Med.,* 92, 750, 1979.

42. **Baumgartner, H. R., Tschopp, T. B., and Meyer, D.,** Shear rate dependent inhibition of platelet adhesion and aggregation on collagenous surfaces by antibodies to human factor VIII/von Willebrand factor, *Br. J. Haematol.,* 44, 127, 1980.

43. **Santoro, S. A.,** Preferential binding of high molecular weight forms of von Willebrand factor to fibrillar collagen, *Biochem. Biophys. Acta,* 756, 123, 1983.

44. **Sixma, J. J., Sakariassen, K. S., Beeser-Visser, N. H., Ottenhof-Rovers, M., and Bolhuis, P. A.,** Adhesion of platelets to human artery subendothelium: effect of factor VIII-von Willebrand factor of various multimeric composition, *Blood,* 63, 128, 1984.

45. **Kessler, C. M., Floyd, C. M., Rick, M. E., Krizek, D. M., Lee, S. L., and Gralnick, H. R.,** Collagen-factor VIII/von Willebrand factor protein interaction, *Blood,* 63, 1291, 1984.

46. **Houdikj, W. P. M., Sakariassen, K. S., Nievelstein, P. F. E. M., and Sixma, J. J.,** Role of factor VIII-von Willebrand factor and fibronectin in the intraction of platelets in flowing blood with monomeric and fibrillar human collagen types I and III, *J. Clin. Invest.,* 75, 531, 1985.

47. **Fauvel, F., Grant, M. E., Legrand, Y. J., Sanchon, S., Tobelem, G., Jackson, D. S., and Caen, J. P.,** Interaction of blood platelets with a microfibrillar extract from adult bovine aorta: requirement for von Willebrand factor, *Proc. Natl. Acad. Sci. U.S.A.,* 80, 551, 1983.

48. **Wagner, D. D., Urban-Pickering, M., and Marder, V. J.,** von Willebrand protein binds to extracellular matrices independently of collagen, *Proc. Natl. Acad. Sci. U.S.A.,* 81, 471, 1984.

49. **Bolhuis, P. A., Sakariassen, K. S., Sander, H. J., Bouma, B. N., and Sixma, J. J.,** Binding of factor VIII-von Willebrand factor to human artery subendothelium precedes increased platelet adhesion and enhances platelet spreading, *J. Lab. Clin. Med.,* 97, 568, 1981.

50. **Rand, J. H., Sussman, I. I., Gordon, R. E., Chu, S. V., and Solomon, V.,** Localization of factor VIII related antigen in human vascular subendothelium, *Blood,* 55, 752, 1980.

51. **Stel, H. V., Sakariassen, K. S., de Groot, P. G., van Mourik, J. A., and Sixma, J. J.,** von Willebrand factor in the vessel wall mediates platelet adherance, *Blood,* 65, 85, 1985.

52. **Weiss, H. J., Tschopp, T. B., Baumgartner, H. R., Sussman, I. I., Johnson, M. M., and Egan, J. J.,** Decreased adhesion of giant (Bernard-Soulier) platelets to subendothelium: further implication of the role of the von Willebrand factor in haemostatis, *Am. J. Med.,* 57, 920, 1974.

53. **Caen, J. P., Nurden, A. T., Jeanneau, C., Michael, H., Tobelem, G., Levy-Toledano, S., Sultan, Y., Valensi, F., and Bernard, J.,** Bernard-Soulier syndrome: a new platelet glycoprotein abnormality. Its relationship with platelet adhesion to subendothelium and with the factor VIII/von Willebrand protein, *J. Lab. Clin. Med.,* 87, 586, 1976.

54. **Tschopp, T. B., Weiss, H. J., and Baumgartner, H. R.,** Interaction of platelets with subendothelium in thrombasthenia: normal adhesion, impared aggregation, *Experentia,* 31, 113, 1975.

55. **Fujimoto, T., Ohara, S., and Hawinger, J.,** Thrombin-induced exposure and prostacyclin inhibition of the receptor for factor VIII/von Willebrand factor on human platelets, *J. Clin. Invest.,* 69, 1212, 1982.

56. **Kao, K.-J., Pizzo, S. V., and McKee, P. A.,** Demonstration and characterization of specific binding sites for factor VIII/von Willebrand factor on human platelets, *J. Clin. Invest.,* 62, 656, 1979.

57. **Zucker, M. B., Kian, S. J. A., McPherson, J., and Grant, R. A.,** Binding of factor VIII to platelets in the presence of ristocetin, *Br. J. Haematol.,* 35, 535, 1977.

58. **Moake, J. L., Olson, J. D., Troll, J. H., Tang, S. S., Funicella, T., and Peterson, D. M.,** Binding of radiodinated human von Willebrand factor to Bernard-Soulier, thrombasthenic and von Willebrand platelets, *Thromb. Res.,* 19, 21, 1980.

59. **Ruan, C., Tobelem, G., McMichael, A. J., Drouet, L., Lewgrand, Y., Degos, L., Kieffer, N., Lee, H., and Caen, J. P.,** Monoclonal antibody to human platelet glycorprotein 1. II. Effects on human platelet function, *Br. J. Haematol.,* 49, 511, 1981.

60. **Coller, B. S., Peerschke, E. I., Scudder, L. E., and Sullivan, C. A.,** Studies with a murine monoclonal antibody that abolishes ristocetin-induced binding of von Willebrand factor to platelets: additional evidence in support of GPIb as a platelet receptor for von Willebrand factor, *Blood,* 61, 99, 1983.

61. **Zimmerman, T. S., Robert, J., and Edgington, T. S.,** Factor VIII related antigen: multiple molecular forms in plasma, *Proc. Natl. Acad. Sci. U.S.A.,* 72, 5121, 1975.

62. **Doucet-de Bruine, M. H. M., Sixma, J. J., Over, J., and Beeser-Visser, N. H.,** Heterogeneity of human factor VIII: characterization of forms of factor VIII binding to platelets in the presence of ristocetin, *J. Lab. Clin. Med.,* 92, 96, 1978.

63. **Counts, R. B., Paskel, S. L., and Elgee, S. K.,** Disulphide bonds and the quatenary structure of factor VIII-von Willebrand factor, *J. Clin. Invest.,* 62, 702, 1978.

64. **Fujimoto, J. and Hawinger, J.,** Adenosine diphosphate induces binding of von Willerband factor to human platelets, *Nature,* 297, 154, 1982.

65. **Ruggeri, Z. M., de Marco, L., Gatti, L., Bader, R., and Montgomery, R. R.,** Platelets have more than one binding site for von Willebrand factor, *J. Clin. Invest.,* 72, 1, 1983.

66. **de Marco, L., Girolami, A., Zimmerman, T. S., and Ruggeri, Z. M.,** von Willebrand factor interaction with the glycoprotein IIb/IIIa complex. Its role in platelet function as demonstrated in patients with congenital afibrinogenaemia, *J. Clin. Invest.,* 77, 1272, 1986.

67. **Larrieu, M. J. and Soulier, J. P.,** Deficit en facteur antihemophilique a chez une fille associe a un trouble de sangnement, *Rev. Hematol.,* 8, 361, 1953.

68. **Jurgens, R., Lehmann, W., Wegelius, O., Eriksson, A. W., and Hiepler, E.,** Mitteilung uber der Mangel an Antihaemophilen Globulin (factor VIII) bei der Aalandischefn Thrombopathie, *Thromb. Diath. Haemorrh.,* 1, 257, 1957.

69. **Nilsson, I. M., Blomback, M., Jorpes, E., Blomback, B., and Johansson, S. A.,** von Willebrand's disease and its correction with human fraction I-0, *Acta Med. Scand.,* 159, 179, 1957.

70. **Cornu, P., Larrieu, M. J., Caen, J., and Bernard, J.,** Transfusion studies in von Willebrand's disease: effect on bleeding time and factor VIII, *Br. J. Haematol.,* 9, 189, 1963.

71. **Weiss, H. J., Sussman, I. I., and Hoyer, L. W.,** Stabilisation of factor VIII in plasma by the von Willebrand factor. Studies on post transfusion and dissociated factor VIII in patients with von Willebrand's disease, *J. Clin. Invest.,* 60, 390, 1977.

72. **Hamer, R. J., Houkijk, W. P., and Sixma, J. J.,** The physiology and pathophysiology of the factor VIII complex, *CRC Crit. Rev. Oncol. Hematol.,* 6, 19, 1986.

73. **Goodall, A. H. and Meyer, D.,** Registry of monoclonal antibodies to factor VIII and von Willebrand factor, *Thromb. Haemost.,* 54, 878, 1985.

74. **Stel, H. V., Sakariassen, K. S., Scholte, B. J., Veerman, E. C. I., van der Kwast, T. H., de Groot, P. G., Sixma, J. J., and van Mourik, J. A.,** Characterisation of 25 monoclonal antibodies to factor VIII-von Willebrand factor: relationship between ristocetin induced platelet aggregation and platelet adherence to subendothelium, *Blood,* 63, 1408, 1984.

75. **Goodall, A. H., Jarvis, J., Chand, S., Rawlings, E., O'Brien, D. P., McCraw, A., Hutton, R., and Tuddenham. E. G. D.,** An immunoradiometric assay for human factor VIII/von Willebrand factor (VIII:vWF) using a monoclonal antibody that defines a functional epitope, *Br. J. Haematol.,* 59, 565, 1985.

76. **Ogata, K., Saito, H., and Ratnoff, O. D.,** The relationship of the properties of antihaemophilic factor (factor VIII), that support ristocetin-induced platelet agglutination (factor VIIIR:RC) and platelet retention by glass beads as demonstrated by a monoclonal antibody, *Blood,* 61, 27, 1983.

77. **Thomas, J. E., Peake, I. R., Giddings, J. C., Welch, A. N., and Bloom, A. L.,** The application of a monoclonal antibody to factor VIII related antigen (VIII:Rag) in immunoradiometric assays for factor VIII, *Thomb. Haemost.,* 53, 143, 1985.

78. **Sixma, J. J., Sakariassen, K. S., Stel, H. V., Houdikj, W. P. M., In der Maur, D. W., Hamer, R. J., de Groot, P. G., and van Mourik, J. A.,** Functional domains on von Willebrand factor. Recognition of discrete tryptic fragments by monoclonal antibodies that inhibit direct interaction of von Willebrand factor with platelets and with collagen, *J. Clin. Invest.,* 74, 736, 1984.

79. **Nokes, T. J. C., Mahmoud, N. A., Savidge, G. F., Goodall, A. H., Meyer, D., Edgington, T. S., and Hardisty, R. M.,** von Willebrand factor has more than one binding site for platelets, *Thromb. Res.,* 34, 361, 1984.

80. **Meyer, D., Baumgartner, H. R., and Edgington, T. S.,** Hybridoma antibodies to human von Willebrand factor. II. Relative role of intramolecular loci in mediation of platelet adhesion to the subendothelium, *Br. J. Haematol.,* 57, 609, 1984.

81. **Sola B., Avner, P., Sultan, Y., Jeanneau, C., and Maisonneuve, P.,** Monoclonal antibodies against human factor VIII molecule neutralize antihemophilia factor and ristocetin cofactor activities, *Proc. Natl. Acad. Sci. U.S.A.,* 79, 183, 1982.

82. **Sultan, Y., Avner, P., Maisonneuve, P., Arnaud, D., and Jeanneau, C.,** An immunoradiometric assay for factor VIII related antigen (VIII:RAg) using two monoclonal antibodies — comparison with polyclonal rabbit antibodies for use in von Willebrand's disease diagnosis, *Thromb. Haemost.,* 52, 250, 1984.

83. **Michelson, A. D., Loscalzo, J., Melnick, B., Coller, B. S., and Handin, R. I.,** Partial characterization of a binding site for von Willebrand factor on glycocalicin, *Blood,* 67, 19, 1986.

84. **Girma, J.-P., Kalafatis, M., Pietu, G., Lavergne, J.-M., Chopek, M. W., Edgington, T. S., and Meyer, D.,** Mapping of distinct von Willerband factor domains interacting with platelet GPIb and GPIIb/IIIa and with collagen using monoclonal antibodies, *Blood,* 67, 1356, 1986.

85. **Lamme, S., Wallmark, A., Holmberg, L., Nilsson, I. M., and Sjogren, H.-O.,** The use of monoclonal antibodies in measuring factor VIII/von Willebrand factor, *Scand. J. Clin. Lab. Invest.,* 45, 17, 1985.

86. **Bradley, L. A., Franco, E. L., and Reisner, H. M.,** Use of monoclonal antibodies in an enzyme immunoassay for factor VIII-related antigen, *Clin. Chem.,* 30, 87, 1984.

87. **Hornsey, V., Micklem, R. R., McCann, M. C., James, K., Dawes, J., McClelland, D. B. L., and Prowse, C. V.,** Enhancement of factor VIII-von Willebrand factor ristocetin cofactor activity by monoclonal antibodies, *Thromb. Haemost.,* 54, 510, 1985.

88. **Katzmann, J. A., Mujwid, D. K., Miller, R. S., and Fass, D. N.,** Monoclonal antibodies to von Willebrand's factor: reactivity with porcine and human antigens, *Blood,* 58, 530, 1981.

89. **Bowie, E. J. W., Fass, D. N., and Katzmann, J. A.,** Functional studies of Willebrand factor using monoclonal antibodies, *Blood,* 62, 146, 1983.

90. **Sawada, Y., Fass, D. N., Katzmann, J. A., Bahm, R. C., and Bowie, E. J. W.,** Hemostatic plug formation in normal and von Willebrand pigs: the effect of administration of cryoprecipitate and a monoclonal antibody to Willebrand factor, *Blood,* 62, 1229, 1986.

91. **Houdijk, W. P. M., Schiphorst, M. E., and Sixma, J. J.,** Identification of functional domains on von Willebrand factor by binding of tryptic fragments to collagen and to platelets in the presence of ristocetin, *Blood,* 67, 1498, 1986.

92. **Bockenstedt, P., Greenberg, J. M., and Handin, R. I.,** Structural basis of von Willebrand factor binding to platelet glycoprotein Ib and collagen. Effects of disulphide reduction and limited proteolysis of polymeric von Willebrand factor, *J. Clin. Invest.,* 77, 743, 1986.

93. **Fujimura, Y., Titani, K., Holland, L. Z., Russell, S. R., Roberts, J. R., Elder, J. H., Ruggeri, Z. M., and Zimmerman, T. S.,** Von Willebrand factor. A reduced and alkylated 52/48 kDa fragment beginning at amino acid 449 contains the domain interacting with platelet glycoprotein Ib, *J. Biol. Chem.,* 261, 381, 1986.

94. **Sakariassen, K. S., Fressinaud, E., Girma, J.-P., Baumgartner, H. R., and Meyer, D.,** Mediation of platelet adhesion to fibrillar collagen in flowing blood by a proteolytic fragment of human von Willebrand factor, *Blood,* 67, 1515, 1986.

95. **Fulcher, C. A. and Zimmerman, T. S.,** Characterisation of the human factor VIII procoagulant protein with a heterologous precipitating antibody, *Proc. Natl. Acad. Sci. U.S.A.,* 79, 1648, 1982.

96. **Fowler, W. E. and Erickson, H. P.,** The trinodular structure of fibronogen: confirmation by both shadowing and negative stain electron microscopy, *J. Mol. Biol.,* 134, 241, 1979.

97. **Ruoslahti, E. and Pierschbacher, M. D.,** Arg-gly-asp: a versatile cell recognition signal, *Cell,* 44, 517, 1986.

98. **Pierschbacher, M. D. and Ruoslahti, E.,** Cell attachment activity of fibronectin can be duplicated by small synthetic fragments of the molecule, *Nature,* 309, 30, 1984.

99. **Pytela, R., Pierschbacher, M. D., Ginsberg, M. H., Plow, E. F., and Ruoslahti, E.,** Platelet membrane glycoprotein IIb/IIIa: member of a family of arg-gly-asp-specific adhesion receptors, *Science,* 231, 1559, 1986.

100. **Barn, M. C. and Phillips, D. R.,** Platelet membrane proteins: composition and receptor function, in *Platelets in Biology and Pathology,* Gordon, J. L., Ed., Elsevier, New York, 1981, 43.

101. **Hildreth, J. E., Gotch, F. M., Hildreth, P. D., and McMichael, A. J.,** A human lymphocyte-associated antigen involved in cell-mediated lympholysis, *Eur. J. Immunol.,* 13, 202, 1983.

102. **Sanchez-Madrid, F., Krensky, A. M., Ware, C. F., Robbins, E., Strominger, J. W., Burakoff, S. J., and Springer, T. A.,** Three distinct antigens associated with human T-lymphocyte-mediated cytolysis; LFA-1, LFA-2, and LFA-3, *Proc. Natl. Acad. Sci., U.S.A.,* 79, 7489, 1982.

103. **Ruggeri, Z. M. and Zimmerman, T. S.,** The complex multimeric composition of factor VIII/von Willebrand factor, *Blood,* 57, 1140, 1981.

104. **Kunicki, T. J., Montgomery, R. R., and Schullek, J. R.,** Cleavage of human von Willebrand factor by platelet calcium-activated protease, *Blood,* 65, 352, 1984.

105. **Thompson, E. A. and Howard, M. A.,** Proteolytic cleavage of human von Willebrand factor induced by enzyme(s) released from polymorphonuclear cells, *Blood,* 67, 1281, 1986.

106. **Ruggeri, Z. M. and Zimmerman, T. S.,** Variant von Willebrand's disease. Characterization of two subtypes by analysis of multimeric composition of factor VIII/von Willebrand factor in plasma and platelets, *J. Clin. Invest.,* 65, 1318, 1980.

107. **Hoyer, L. W., Rizza, C. R., Tuddenham, E. G. D., Carta, C. A., Armitage, H., and Rotblat, F.,** von Willebrand factor multimer patterns in von Willebrand's disease, *Br. J. Haematol.,* 55, 493, 1983.

108. **Tuddenham, E. G. D.,** The varieties of von Willebrand's disease, *Clin. Lab. Haematol.,* 6, 307, 1984.

109. **Hoyer, L. W.,** Immunologic studies of antihemophilic factor (AHF, factor VIII). IV radioimmunoassay of AHF antigen, *J. Lab. Clin. Med.,* 80, 822, 1972.

110. **Counts, R. B.,** Solid-phase immunoradiometric assay for factor VIII-protein, *Br. J. Haematol.,* 31, 429, 1975.

111. **Holmberg, L. and Nilsson, I. M.,** Genetic variants of von Willebrand's disease, *Br. Med. J.,* 3, 317, 1972.

112. **Kernoff, P. B., Gruson, A. R., and Rizza, C. R.,** A variant of factor VIII related antigen, *Br. J. Haemtol.,* 26, 435, 1974.

113. **Peake, I. R., Bloom, A. L., and Giddings, J. C.,** Inherited variants of factor VIII-related protein in von Willebrand's disease, *N. Engl. J. Med.,* 291, 113, 1974.

114. **Ruggeri, Z. M., Nilsson, I. M., Lombardi, R., Holmberg, L., and Zimmerman, T. S.,** Aberrant multimer structure of von Willebrand factor in a new variant of von Willebrand disease (Type IIc), *J. Clin. Invest.,* 70, 1124, 1982.

115. **Mannucci, P. M., Lombardi, R., Pareti, F. I., Solinas, S., Mazzucconi, M. G., and Mariani, G.,** A variant of von Willebrand's disease characterized by recessive inheritance and missing triplet structure of von Willebrand factor multimers, *Blood,* 62, 1000, 1983.

116. **Ciavarella, G., Giavarella, N., Antonecchi, S., de Mattia, D., Ranieri, P., Dent, J., Zimmerman, T. S., and Ruggeri, Z. M.,** High resolution analysis of von Willebrand factor multimeric composition defines a new variant of type I von Willebrand disease with aberrant structure but presence of all size multimers (type Ic), *Blood,* 66, 1423, 1985.

117. **Weiss, H. J. and Sussman, I. I.,** A new von Willebrand variant (type I, New York): increased ristocetin-induced platelet aggregation and plasma von Willebrand factor containing the full range of multimers, *Blood,* 68, 149, 1986.

118. **Mannucci, P. M., Abildgaard, C. F., Gralnick, H. R., Hill, F. G. H., Hoyer, L. W., Lombardi, R., Nilsson, I. M., Tuddenham, E. G. D., and Meyer, D.,** Multicenter comparison of von Willebrand factor multimer sizing technique, *Thromb. Haemost.,* 54, 873, 1985.

119. **Montgomery, R. R., Hathaway, W. E., Johnson, J., Jacobson, L., and Munstean, W.,** A variant of von Willebrand's disease with abnormal expression of factor VIII, procoagulant activity, *Blood,* 60, 201, 1982.

120. **Zimmerman, T. S., Dent, J. A., Federici, A. B., Ruggeri, Z. M., Nilsson, I. M., Holmberg, L., Abilgaard, C. A., and Nannini, L. H.,** High resolution NaDod SO$_4$ agarose electrophoresis identifies new molecular abnormalities in von Willebrand's disease, *Clin. Res.,* 32, A501, 1984.

121. **Mazurier, C., Samor, B., and Goudemand, M.,** Improved characterization of plasma von Willebrand factor heterogeneity when using 2.5% agarose gel electrophoresis, *Thromb. Haemost.,* 55, 61, 1986.

122. **Gralnick, H. R., Williams, S. B., McKeown, L. P., Maisonneuve, P., Jeanneau, C., Sultan, Y., and Rick, M. E.,** *In vitro* correction of the abnormal multimeric structure of von Willebrand factor in type IIa von Willebrand's disease, *Proc. Natl. Acad. Sci. U.S.A.,* 82, 5968, 1985.

123. **Chand, S., McCraw, A., Hutton, R., Tuddenham, E. G. D., and Goodall, A. H.,** A two-site, monoclonal antibody-based immunoassay for von Willebrand factor: demonstration that vWF function resides in a conformational epitope, *Thromb. Haemost.,* 55, 318, 1986.

124. **McCraw, A., Chand, S., Tuddenham, E. G. D., O'Callaghan, U., and Goodall, A. H.,** A monoclonal antibody based immunoassay for von Willebrand factor: survey of a large patient group, *Thromb. Res.,* 45, 101, 1987.

Chapter 8

VON WILLEBRAND FACTOR AND THE VESSEL WALL

Jan A. van Mourik and Jan Hendrik Reinders

TABLE OF CONTENTS

I.   Introduction 174

II.   Biosynthesis, Secretion, and Storage of von Willebrand factor 175

III.   Concluding Remarks 183

IV.   Acknowledgments 183

References 184

I. INTRODUCTION

In the early 1970s, when antibodies to the factor VIII-von Willebrand factor (VIII/vWf) complex became available, immunofluorescence studies revealed that the vascular endothelium of a variety of human tissues contain immunoreactive material.[1,2] Soon it became clear that most normal endothelial cells synthesize and secrete (vWf) or vWf-like material, including endothelial cells isolated from large and smaller veins, capillaries, aorta, and arteries.[3-8] Endothelial cells do not synthesize the VIII moiety of the VIII/vWf complex. Until recently, investigations on the site of synthesis of VIII were unsuccessful. Northern blotting analysis of factor VIII-mRNA demonstrated that VIII is synthesized by a variety of organs and cells and not by the endothelium.[9]

Thus, the assembly of the VIII/vWf complex from its constituent units most likely does not occur in the vascular endothelium, but should take place elsewhere in the body. This is a most challenging and intriguing problem, not only from a scientific but also from a clinical point of view. Although the synthesis of vWf and VIII is encoded by different genes located on different chromosomes, the plasma concentration of VIII seems to be governed by the rate of synthesis and secretion of vWf by endothelial cells. Except in hemophilia A, there is a close correlation between the plasma concentration of VIII and the concentration of vWf. Insight into the biosynthesis of vWf and processes that regulate its secretion from endothelial cells is, therefore, of importance for a better understanding of the role of vWf in maintaining an adequate hemostatic balance.

Pertinent to this point is the finding that vWf may act as a hemostatic compound itself. One of the initial responses to vascular injury is the adhesion of platelets to the damaged vessel wall. In the early 1970s, Tschopp et al.[10] observed that platelets in the blood of patients with von Willebrand's disease (vWD) were less adhesive to subendothelium than were platelets in blood of healthy volunteers. This key observation, together with other observations using purified blood constituents,[11] led to the generally accepted view that vWf is an essential co-factor for platelet adhesion to natural surfaces, such as subendothelium and collagen. These observations are even more interesting if one considers that endothelial cells not only secrete vWf in a constitutive way by the default pathway, but also may act as regulated secretory cells and rapidly release their vWf content upon exposure to certain stimuli, such as thrombin.[12,13] Thus, appropriate stimulation of endothelial cells in the vicinity of vascular injury could aid in attaining effective hemostatis.

Apparently, endothelial cells serve as a storage pool for vWf. If one considers that the entire vasculature contains about 90% of vWf in the human body,* the contribution of the endothelium in maintaining an effective hemostatis could, therefore, be of more importance than previously appreciated.

Another aspect of vWf as a biosynthetic product of endothelial cells deserves special attention.

vWf is not a single chain polypeptide but possesses a rather complex quarternary structure. The vWf activity seems only fully expressed if single chain polypeptides encoded by the vWf gene polymerize. The assembly of the vWf molecule takes place intracellularly. This process and several posttranslocational modifications associated with it are, as yet, poorly understood. In this chapter, we will review in more detail our present understanding of the biosynthetic pathways of the vWf polypeptide and its assembly to a mature set of polymers. We will describe the property of the endothelial cell to serve as a storage pool and secretory

---

*   The total surface area of the vascular bed is approximately 1000 m^2. This surface area is covered with about
     $5 \cdot 10^{11}$ endothelial cells, assuming $5 \cdot 10^4$ cells per square centimer. Upon stimulation, 10^6 endothelial cells
     may release 0.5 to 1 μg of vWf. Thus, $5 \cdot 10^{11}$ cells may secrete 250 to 500 mg vWf. The circulating blood
     contains about 35 mg vWf, assuming a plasma volume of 3 l containing 10 mg vWf/ml and $3 \cdot 10^{11}$ circulating
     platelets containing about 5 mg vWf (0.4 mg per 10^{11} platelets).[15]

cell for vWf. All the studies described here were performed with cultured endothelial cells from umbilical veins. It seems reasonable to assume that the present findings may be extrapolated to more physiological conditions.

II. BIOSYNTHESIS, SECRETION, AND STORAGE OF vWf

As many kinds of cells, endothelial cells behave as secretory cells. Many endothelial proteins, including fibronectin, thrombospondin, and collagens, travel from their site of synthesis, the rough endoplasmic reticulum, through the Golgi apparatus and are subsequently delivered to the outside of the cell. During this journey, the newly synthesized proteins undergo several processing steps, including signal peptide cleavage, glycosylation, and intersubunit interactions. The molecular events associated with the biosythesis and secretion of vWf are, to a large extent, similar to the processing steps and routing of proteins destined to be externalized. First, a precursor polypeptide chain is synthesized which then forms dimers, undergoes carbohydrate processing, limited proteolysis, and further polymerization before vWf is delivered to the outside of the cell.

Recently, it became apparent that, with respect to vWf secretion, endothelial cells should be classified as both constitutive and regulated secretory cells. The constitutive secretory nature of the endothelium is reflected by the observation that soon after synthesis vWf (and many other proteins) accumulates extracellularly in the absence of a stimulus.[3] No external stimulus or trigger is required for this type of secretion. On the other hand, if endothelial cells are exposed to stimuli, such as thrombin, ionophore A23187, or phorbol esters, vWf rapidly (within minutes) accumulates outside the cells.[12,13] The rate of this so-called regulated secretion[16] is much higher (tenfold or more) than the synthetic rate of vWf as shown in Figure 1. The regulated vWf secretion is not or only mildly affected by pretreatment of endothelial cells with a protein sythesis inhibitor. In contrast, constitutive vWf secretion is, as expected, virtually abolished by cycloheximide.

These observations indicate that vWf, released when the endothelial cell receives an appropriate signal, originates from a storage pool. This view is supported by the observation that simulus induced secretion of vWf is correlated with the disappearance of the typical granular staining pattern, as observed by immunofluorescence microscopy using antibodies against vWf as demonstrated in Figure 2. The latter observation suggests that vWf is packed in secretory vesicles which are transported to the cell surface when endothelial cells are exposed to stimuli.

Another line of evidence confirms that endothelial cells indeed condense vWf in secretory vesicles. Fractionation of endothelial cell homogenates by density centrifugation yields two fractions that are relatively rich in vWf, a buoyant protein rich fraction containing a variety of cell organelles, such as mitochondria, Golgi apparatus, rough endoplasmic reticulum, and a dense fraction virtually devoid of known cell constituents as shown in Figure 3. In both the buoyant and dense fraction, vWf is present in vesicle-like structures: when these fractions are subjected to freeze-thawing, and subsequently this material is refractionated by density centrifugation, vWf remains on the top of the gradient.[17] The dense vesicles, then, are apparently involved in regulated secretion. Stimulation of endothelial cells depletes the dense fractions of vWf whereas the vWf content of the buoyant fraction is largely unaffected by stimulation.[17] The latter fraction may represent a vWf pool associated with the plasma membrane, rough endoplasmic reticulum, or Golgi apparatus.

Previously, it has been shown that vWf is located intracellularly in the endothelial cell-specific Weibel-Palade bodies.[18] These rod-shaped vesicles, which most likely originate from the Golgi apparatus,[19] contain vWf in a highly condensed form and, as observed by immunofluorescence staining, disappear from endothelial cells upon stimulation.[17] In addition, the secretory vesicles containing vWf that sediment at high density (cf. Figure 3)

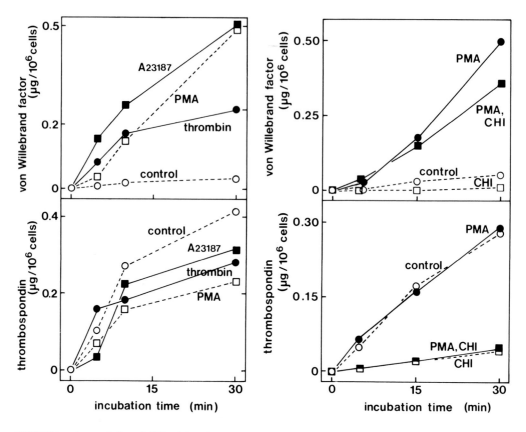

FIGURE 1.   Accumulation of vWf and thrombospondin in conditioned medium of cultured endothelial cells; influence of thrombin, ionophore A23187, and the phorbol ester PMA. Endothelial cells were incubated with serum-free medium in the presence of thrombin, 2 U/ml; ionophore A23187, 10 μM; PMA, 10 ng/ml, or no additions (control). In addition, the influence of preincubation of cultured endothelial cells with cycloheximide on the PMA-induced secretion of vWf and thrombospondin is shown. Cells were incubated with serum-free medium containing 10 μg/ml cycloheximide for 6 h, followed by incubation with 10 ng/ml PMA. The values are the mean of three incubations. (From Reinders, J. H., de Groot, Ph.G., Dawes, J., Hunter, N. R., van Heugten, H. A. A., Zandbergch, J., Gonsalves, M. D., and van Mourik, J. A., *Biochim. Biophys. Acta,* 844, 306, 1985. With permission.)

are morphologically similar to Weibel-Palade bodies examined *in situ* by electron microscopy.[20]

Taking these findings together, it seems justifiable to conclude that the Weibel-Palade body serves as the secretory vesicle involved in regulated secretion of vWf, whereas other vesicles, which most likely also originate from the Golgi apparatus, are involved in a passive flow of vWf to the cell surface. As has been shown with other cell types, it is to be expected that both the transport vesicles of the constitutive and the regulated pathway fuse with the plasma membrane to release their contents by exocytosis.[21] Unlike the vesicles of the constitutive pathway, the secretion of Weibel-Palade bodies is prevented from fusing until the level of cytoplasmic calcium is raised.[22]

The knowledge that there are two pathways of vWf secretion leads to a number of questions. For instance, is vWf externalized by the constitutive route structurally different from vWf secreted by the regulated pathway? What is the mechanism that leads to the apparent sorting of vWf molecules into separate secretion pathways? What is the physiological significance of the diversity of vWf secretion? Although at present these questions are difficult to answer, it seems clear now that constitutively secreted vWf molecules are indeed structurally, and most likely also functionally, different from vWf released from

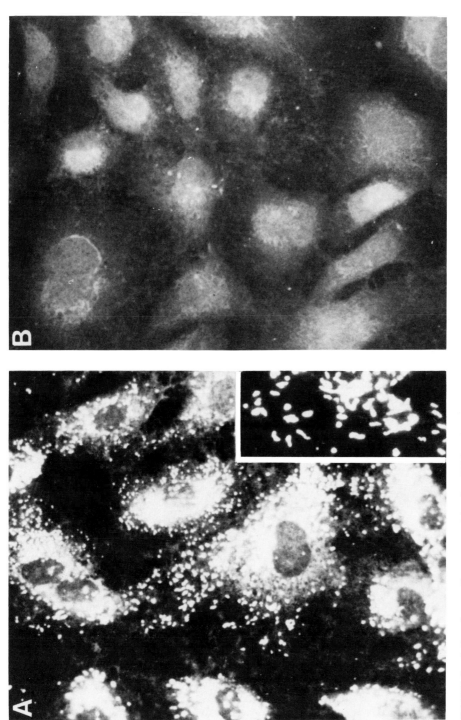

FIGURE 2. Indirect immunoflourescent staining for vWf in cultured human endothelial cells with a monoclonal antibody to vWf and FITC-labeled goat anti-murine IgG. (A) endothelial cells and (B) endothelial cells treated with the phorbol ester PMA, 100 ng/ml for 1 h. For experimental details, see Reference 17. Insert represents an enlarged detail.

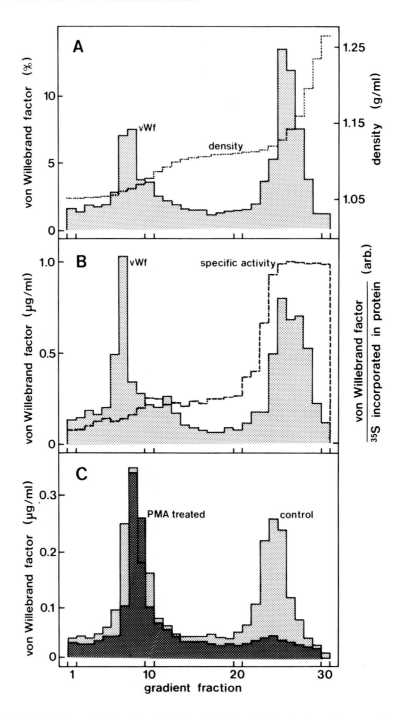

FIGURE 3 (A,B,C).   Isolation of endothelial cell vWf vesicles by density gradient centrifugation. Cultured endothelial cells were harvested with trypsin and homogenized by pottering; the homogenate was layered on colloidal silica and centrifuged for 75 min at 100 000 × g. (A) The distribution of vWf as measured in an immunoradiometric assay (% total gradient contents) and the density profile after centrifugation. (B) Distribution in the density gradient of vWf and the quotient of vWf and ^{35}S-methionine labeled endothelial cell proteins: the ''specific activity'' of vWf (arbitrary units). (C) The distribution of vWf after density centrifugation of endothelial cells before and after treatment with the phorbol ester PMA, 100 ng/ml for 1 h.

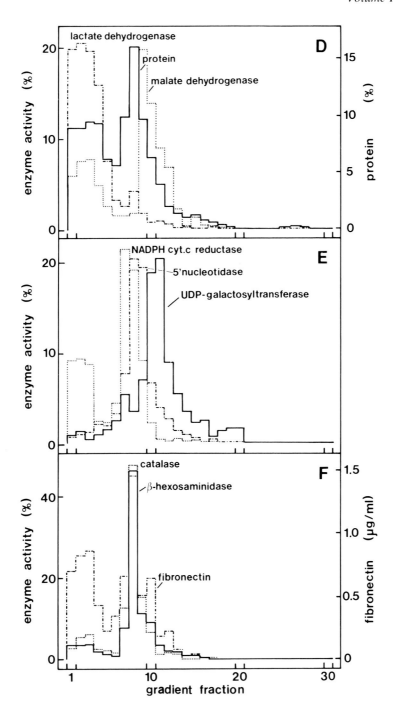

FIGURE 3 (D,E,F).   Distribution of marker enzymes of cytosol (lactate dehydrogenase), cytosol and mitochondria (malate dehydrogenase), microsomes and endoplasmic reticulum fragments (NADPH cyt c. reductase), plasma membrane fragments (5′ nucleotidase), Golgi apparatus (UDP-galactosyltransferase), peroxisomes (catalase), lysosomes (β-hexosaminidase), protein, and fibronectin after density centrifugation of endothelial cells. (Adapted from Reinders, J. H. et al., *Biochim. Biophys. Acta,* 804, 361, 1984. With permission.)

Molecular species		Molecular size	Cellular localization

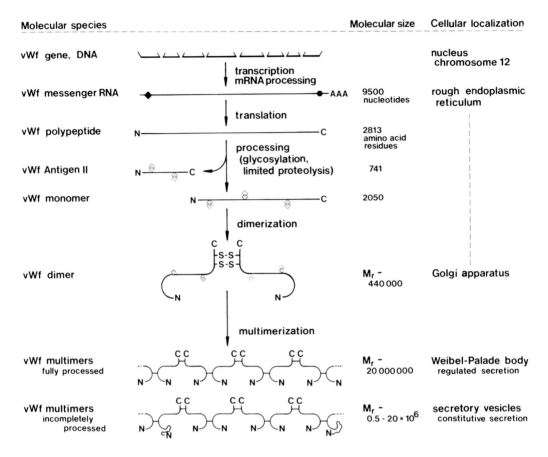

FIGURE 4.   Schematic representation of vWf synthesis in endothelial cells. For explanation, see text.

Weibel-Palade bodies after stimulation. These differences can most readily be explained if one considers our present knowledge of the synthesis, processing, and assembly of vWf as shown in Figure 4.

First, the primary translation product, a precursor subunit (pro-vWf, Mr = 309,000*),[23,24] undergoes N-linked glycosylation and dimer formation in the rough endoplasmic reticulum.[25] These dimers, then, are transferred to the Golgi apparatus. During the travel through the Golgi compartments, several more processing steps may occur. These include processing of the mannose-type carbohydrate to the complex type, proteolytic cleavage of a Mr = 83,000 precursor polypeptide,* which is identical to von Willebrand antigen (vWf:Ag) II,[26] and interdimer disulfide bond formation to form multimers.[25] Mature dimers, dimers consisting of pro-vWf, and (hetero-)dimers may undergo multimerization.[25-28] Two lines of evidence indicate that only mature vWf is packed as biologically active multimers in the Weibel-Palade bodies and is secreted upon demand. First, vWf released by endothelial agonists, such as thrombin or the calcium ionophore A23187, only consists of large multimers composed of mature subunits[29] and second, isolated Weibel-Palade bodies contain biologically active vWf[20] which is composed of mature subunits as shown in Figure 5. Thus, vWf secreted by the regulated pathway seems mature, both in terms of its subunit composition and its degree of polymerization. In contrast, constitutively secreted vWf is composed of

---

*   This value is calculated from the complete amino acid sequence of pro-vWf.[26,27] Apparently, previously reported molecular weights estimated by sodium-dodecyl sulfate (SDS)-polyacrylamide gel electrophoresis are not correct.

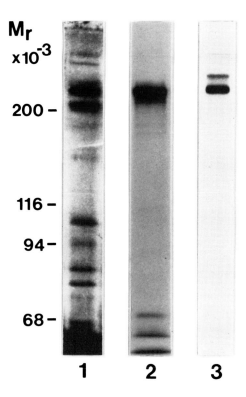

Mr
x10⁻³

200 –

116 –

94 –

68 –

1   2   3

FIGURE 5.   SDS-polyacrylamide gel electrophoresis of metabolically labeled proteins associated with Weibel-Palade bodies. Human endothelial cells were metabolically labeled by incubating cells with ^{35}S-methionine for 3 d. Cells were then fractionated by density centrifugation (see Figure 3), and the dense fraction containing Weibel-Palade bodies was subjected to electrophoresis (lane 1). Lane 2 represents vWf immunoisolated with a monoclonal antibody to vWf; lane 3 shows vWf immunoisolated from the conditioned medium.

both mature and immature (pro-) vWf subunits[29] (cf. Figure 5). In addition, the degree of polymerization of these homo- and heterodimers seems lower than the extent of polymerization of vWf secreted by the regulated pathway.[28,29]

In summary, the accumulated data so far indicate that stored vWf consists of mature, fully processed vWf subunits assembled as biologically active multimers, whereas constitutively secreted vWf consists of a significant proportion of precursor subunits which are polymerized to a lesser extent.

As to the mechanism of vWf sorting and subsequent storage of the protein on the one hand and constitutive release on the other, we can only speculate. As limited proteolysis is apparently one of the steps that precedes regulated secretion, one might expect that this process is a factor that contributes to sorting. Most likely this is not the case. Together with mature vWf, the 83-kDa propiece is present in the Weibel-Palade bodies,[30] indicating that proteolysis may occur after sorting has taken place. It seems more likely that (pro-)vWf, when present in its aggregated condensed form in the Golgi cisternae or trans-Golgi network, preferentially associates with a Golgi membrane "sorting" protein or receptor which then buds out of the Golgi. In other words, this hypothesis proposes that self-association of vWf protomers is a driving force for the formation of Weibel-Palade bodies; non- or partially aggregated protomers are released by the constitutive bulk flow of secreting proteins. This view is supported by the finding that inhibition of polymer formation leads to defective storage of vWf.[31] Studies on the fine localization of vWf should indicate whether this budding model is correct. Morphological evidence in favor of such a mechanism has recently appeared for insulin-secreting cells.[32] This model implies that only a limited number of other secretory proteins, together with a subpopulation of Golgi membrane proteins, are expected to be in the Weibel-Palade bodies. Indeed, this appears to be the case. In addition to (pro-)vWf, only a few proteins are associated with Weibel-Palade bodies as shown in Figure 5.

Although the molecular events associated with intracellar sorting of vWf are as yet poorly understood, it seems clear that besides carbohydrate processing, limited proteolysis and polymerization are steps along the pathways of vWf secretion. As vWf processing, sorting, and secretion seem to require a complex machinery to accomplish these events, one might expect that only endothelial cells possess the capacity to handle newly synthesized vWf in a proper way. This is apparently not the case. Megakaryocyte-derived vWf is in terms of cellular and secreted subunit composition and degree of multimerization very similar to that produced by endothelial cells.[33] In addition, megakaryocytes store vWf in granules that are most likely identical to platelet α-granules.[34-36] As platelet α granules contain proteins, including fibronectin and thrombospondin.[37,38] which are constitutively secreted by endothelial cells, it seems that the vWf sorting in the Golgi apparatus of the megakaryocytes is different from the sorting mechanism in endothelial cells. However, recently it has been shown that within the platelet α granules vWf is present in condensed form in tubular structure, which closely resemble Weibel-Palade bodies.[39] Thus, also in megakaryocytes vWf seems to be sorted in a selective way.

Another line of evidence suggests that the machinery required for processing, assembly, and secretion of vWf is not unique for endothelial cells. When cDNA encoding the complete pre-pro-vWf sequence is expressed in heterologous cells, such as monkey kidney and Chinese hamster ovary cells, these cell types correctly process, assemble, and secrete disulfide bonded vWf multimers.[40] Although it is not known whether these cells also possess the capacity to store recombinant vWf, it seems likely now that the information required for processing, assembly, and secretion resides largely within the primary structure of vWf itself and is not primarily restricted to the specialized cells that normally secrete vWf. It may be clear, then, that site-directed mutagenesis and expression of the cDNA in cultured cells will provide a powerful means to delineate structural features of the (pro-)vWf molecules that are essential for its processing, assembly, storage, and secretion.

The knowledge that endothelial cells have the ability to store a pool of biologically active vWf multimers which are readily available for release after endothelial cell stimulation and, in addition, may constitutively release vWf which, in terms of degree of multimerization and subunit composition, is different from stored vWf, also leads to a number of questions as to the physiological significance of these phenomena. To answer these questions, one should first consider the functional properties of vWf as described elsewhere in this volume.

vWf serves at least two major functions: first, it serves as a carrier molecule for VIII[41-44] and, second, it supports platelet adhesion to the damaged vessel wall.[10,11] As VIII is not produced by endothelial cells but in other tissues,[9] it seems likely that VIII and vWf form (reversible) complexes after secretion of these proteins into the circulating blood. This view is supported by the finding that purified VIII may form complexes with vWf, both *in vitro*[43] and *in vivo*.[45]

In addition, it might be possible that VIII travels directly from VIII-producing cells to endothelial cells that are in close contact. For instance, VIII produced by hepatocytes[9] might be delivered by exocytosis to the cell surface, subsequently be taken up by endocytosis by the sinusoidal endothelial cells, and form complexes with vWf inside the sinusoidal cells. The newly formed complexes may be stored or directly secreted into the bloodstream. Indeed, immunoelectron microscopy studies have shown that VIII is not only located in hepatocytes but also in sinusoidal endothelial cells, in the latter case together with vWf.[46]

It is also possible that VIII forms complexes with vWf that is bound to the endothelial cell surface. Recenlty, it has been reported that endothelial cells synthesize a glycoprotein complex that is structurally related to the platelet glycoprotein IIb/IIIa complex.[47,48] This heterodimer is exposed at the outer surface of the endothelial plasma membrane and may, as its platelet counterpart, function as a receptor for adhesive proteins that contain the RGD sequence, including fibronectin, fibrinogen, and also vWf.[49] Indeed, it has been shown that vWf may be associated with the endothelial cell membrane[29], possibly via the putative RGD-receptor. It is tempting to assume, therefore, that VIII may bind to membrane associated vWf. The membrane bound complexes thus formed could be of significant importance in contributing to local hemostasis. So far, this is speculation only and it remains to be established whether these hypotheses are correct. There is little doubt, however, that indeed VIII and vWf may form noncovalently linked complexes, either *in vitro* or *in vivo*. Which part or domain of the vWf molecule interacts with VIII is not known at present. It has been suggested that pro-vWf is responsible for VIII binding.[26] Although pro-vWf is most likely present in the circulation,[28,30] there is no experimental evidence to support this view. It is also unknown whether or not VIII preferentially binds to polymerized vWF.

As vWf secreted either by the constitutive pathway or the regulated route may equal well contribute to hemostasis in terms of functioning as a carrier protein for VIII, this is probably not the case if one considers the function of vWf as a protein (whether or not associated with VIII) that mediates platelet adhesion to the damaged vessel wall. It is likely that the storage pool of vWf serves an important function in supporting platelet adhesion. This pool is biologically active,[20] whereas constitutively secreted vWf, because of its limited degree of polymerization, is probably less effective in supporting platelet adhesion. Upon activation of endothelial cells (for instance, by thrombin formed locally as a result of vascular damage), local accumulation of stored vWf could, therefore, be of importance in attaining effective hemostatis. Pertinent to this point could be our recent finding that vWf secreted by the regulated pathway is predominantly released to the luminal site of the endothelium,[50] thus providing a subset of biologically active polymers that is readily available in the vicinity of the injured vessel.

III. CONCLUDING REMARKS

More than 10 years after the discovery that endothelial cells produce vWf, it has become clear that these cells do not simply release this hemostatic component in a constitutive way, but, in addition, may release mature and biologically active vWf immediately upon exposure to stimuli that are generated in response to vascular injury, as shown in Figure 6. These observations, then, have led us to reconsider the physiological function of vWf. vWf is not only an omnipresent plasma protein that functions as a carrier protein for VIII on the one hand and serves as an adhesive protein to support platelet adhesion on the other. It may also be recruited under conditions where its presence is badly needed. Endothelial cells, then, serve as a storage pool for vWf which becomes readily available upon demand. Since these cells are now readily accessible for detailed cell-biological studies and, in addition, techniques are now available to study the biology of vWf at the molecular level in detail, we are convinced that many of the questions and points that have been raised will be solved in the near future.

IV. ACKNOWLEDGMENTS

This study was supported in part by grants from the Foundation for Medical Research (MEDIGON), which is subsidized by the Netherlands Organization for the Advance of Pure Research (ZWO) (Grant no. 13-30-31) and the Netherlands Heart Foundation (Grant no. 28.004).

The authors gratefully acknowledge the secretarial assistance of Mrs. J. Gerritsen.

Endothelial cell von Willebrand factor

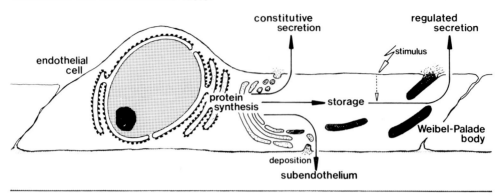

FIGURE 6. Schematic view of the routing of vWf in endothelial cells. This view proposes that vWf is externalized by two pathways: (1) transport vesicles (Weibel-Palade bodies) containing mature, biologically active vWf bud from the Golgi apparatus and are, after appropriate stimulation, delivered to the luminal site of the endothelial cell (regulated secretion); (2) transport vesicles containing immature vWf are delivered to the luminal site of the endothelium (constitutive secretion). In addition, vWf (mature and/or immature) is delivered to the subendothelial compartment.[51] Transport vesicles fuse with the plasma membrane to release their contents. Secretion of vWf by Weibel-Palade bodies is preceded by Ca-influx.[22]

REFERENCES

1. **Bloom, A. L., Giddings, J. C., and Wilks, C. J.,** Factor VIII on the vascular intima: possible importance in hemostatis and thrombosis, *(London) Nature New Biol.,* 241, 217, 1973.
2. **Hoyer, L.W., de los Santos, R. P., and Hoyer, J. R.,** Antihemophilic factor antigen. Localization in endothelial cells by immunofluorescent microscopy, *J. Clin. Invest.,* 52, 2737, 1973.
3. **Jaffe, E. A., Hoyer, L. W., and Nachman, R. L.,** Synthesis of antihemophilic factor antigen by cultured human endothelial cells, *J. Clin. Invest.,* 52, 2757, 1973.
4. **Jaffe, E. A., Hoyer, L. W., and Nachman, R. L.,** Synthesis of von Willebrand factor by cultured human endothelial cells, *Proc. Natl. Acad. Sci. U.S.A.,* 71, 1906, 1974.
5. **Maciag, T., Weinstein, R., Stemmerman, M. B., and Gilchrest, B. A.,** Selective growth of human endothelial cells from both papillary and reticular dermis, *J. Invest. Dermatol.,* 74, 256, 1980.
6. **Folkman, J., Haudenschild, C. C., and Zetter, B. R.,** Long-term culture of capillary endothelial cells, *Proc. Natl. Acad. Sci. U.S.A.,* 76, 5217, 1979.
7. **Johnson, A. R.,** Human pulmonary endothelial cells in culture. Activity of cells from arteries and cells from veins, *J. Clin. Invest.,* 65, 841, 1980.
8. **Booyse, F. M., Sedlak, B. J., and Rafelson, M. E.,** Culture of arterial endothelial cells. Characterization and growth of bovine aortic endothelial cells, *Thromb. Diathes. Haemorrh.,* 34, 825, 1975.
9. **Wion, K. L., Kelly, D., Summerfield, J. A., Tuddenham, E. G. D., and Lawn, R. M.,** Distribution of factor VIII mRNA and antigen in human liver and other tissues, *Nature,* 317, 726, 1985.
10. **Tschopp, T. B., Weiss, H. J., and Baumgartner, H. R.,** Decreased adhesion of platelets to subendothelium in von Willebrand's disease, *J. Lab. Clin. Med.,* 83, 296, 1974.
11. **Sakariassen, K. S., Bolhuis, P. A., and Sixma, J. J.,** Human blood platelet adhesion to artery subendothelium is mediated by factor VIII-von Willebrand factor bound to the subendothelium, *Nature,* 279, 636, 1979.
12. **Levine, J. D., Harlan, J. M., Harker, L. A., Joseph, M. L., and Counts, R. B.,** Thrombin-mediated release of factor VIII antigen from human umbilical vein endothelial cells in culture, *Blood,* 60, 531, 1982.
13. **Loesberg, C., Gonsalves, M. D., Zandbergen, J., Willems, Ch., van Aken, W. G., Stel, H. V., van Mourik, J. A., and de Groot, Ph.G.,** The effect of calcium on the secretion of factor VIII-related antigen by cultured human endothelial cells, *Biochim. Biophys. Acta,* 763, 160, 1983.
14. **Reinders, J. H., de Groot, Ph.G., Dawes, J., Hunter, N. R., van Heugten, H. A. A., Zandbergen, J., Gonsalves, M. D., and van Mourik, J. A.,** Comparison of secretion and subcellular localization of von Willebrand protein with that of thrombospondin and fibronectin in cultured human vascular endothelial cells, *Biochim. Biophys. Acta,* 844, 306, 1985.

15. **Bouma, B. N., Hordijk-Hos, J. M., de Graaf, S., Sixma, J. J., and van Mourik, J. A.,** Presence of factor VIII-related antigen in blood platelets of patients with von Willebrand's disease, *Nature,* 257, 5526, 1975.

16. **Kelly, R. B.,** Pathways of protein secretion in eukaryotes, *Science,* 230, 25, 1985.

17. **Reinders, J. H., de Groot, Ph.G., Gonsalves, M. D., Zandbergen, J., Loesberg, C., and van Mourik, J. A.,** Isolation of a storage and secretory organelle containing von Willebrand protein from cultured human endothelial cells, *Biochim. Biophys. Acta,* 804, 361, 1984.

18. **Wagner, D. D., Oluisted, J. B., and Marder, V. J.,** Immunolocalization of von Willebrand protein in Weibel-Palade bodies of human endothelial cells, *J. Cell Biol.,* 95, 355, 1982.

19. **Sengel, A. and Stoebner, P.,** Golgi origin of tubular inclusions in endothelial cells, *J. Cell Biol.,* 44, 223, 1970.

20. **Reinders, J. H., de Groot, Ph.G., van den Berg, A., Vervoorn, R. C., Sixma, J. J., and van Mourik, J. A.,** The Weibel-Palade body is the storage vesicle for von Willebrand factor in endothelial cells, in press.

21. **McNiff, J. M. and Gil, J.,** Secretion of Weibel-Palade bodies observed in extra-alveolar vessels of rabbit lung, *J. Appl. Physiol. Respir. Environ. Exercise Physiol.,* 54, 1284, 1983.

22. **De Groot, Ph.G., Gonsalves, M. D., Loesberg, C., van Buul-Wortelboer, M. F., van Aken, W. G., and van Mourik, J. A.,** Thrombin-induced release of von Willebrand factor from endothelial cells is mediated by phospholipid methylation. Prostacyclin synthesis is independent of phospholipid methylation, *J. Biol. Chem.,* 259, 13329, 1984.

23. **Wagner, D. D. and Marder, V. J.,** Biosynthesis of von Willebrand protein by human endothelial cells: identification of a large precursor protein, *J. Biol. Chem.,* 258, 2065 1983.

24. **Lynch, D. C., Williams, R., Zimmerman, T. S., Kirby, E. P., and Livingston, D. M.,** Biosynthesis of the subunits of factor VIIIR by bovine aortic endothelial cells, *Proc. Natl. Acad. Sci. U.S.A.,* 80, 2738, 1983.

25. **Wagner, D. D. and Marder, V. J.,** Biosynthesis of von Willebrand protein by human endothelial cells: processing steps and their intracellular localization, *J. Cell Biol.,* 99, 2123, 1984.

26. **Fay, P. J., Kawai, Y., Wagner, D. D., Ginsburg, D., Bonthron, D., Ohlsson-Wilhelm, B. M., Chavin, S. I., Abraham, G. N., Handin, R. I., Orkin, S. H., Montgomery, R. R., and Marder, V. J.,** Propolypeptide of von Willebrand factor circulates in blood and is identical to von Willebrand antigen II, *Science,* 232, 995, 1986.

27. **Verweij, C. L., Diergaarde, P. J., Hart, M., and Pannekoek, H.,** Full-length von Willebrand factor (vWf) cDNA encodes a highly repetitive protein considerably larger than the mature vWf subunit, *EMBO J.,* 5, 1839, 1986.

28. **Lynch, D. C., Zimmerman, T. S., Ling, E. H., and Browning P. J.,** An explanation for minor multimer species in endothelial cell-synthesized von Willebrand factor, *J. Clin. Invest.,* 77, 2048, 1986.

29. **Sporn, L. A., Marder, V. J., and Wagner, D. D.,** Inducible secretion of large, biologically potent von Willebrand factor multimers, *Cell,* 46, 185, 1986.

30. **McCaroll, D. R., Levin, E. G., and Montgomery, R. R.,** Endothelial cell synthesis of von Willebrand antigen II, von Willebrand factor, and von Willebrand factor/von Willebrand antigen-II complex, *J. Clin. Invest.,* 75, 1089, 1985.

31. **Wagner, D. D., Mayades, T., Urban-Pickering, M., Lewis, B. H., and Marder, V. J.,** Inhibition of disulfide bonding of von Willebrand protein by monensin results in small, functionally defective multimers, *J. Cell Biol.,* 101, 112, 1985.

32. **Orci, L., Halban, P., Armherdt, M., Ravazzola, M., Vassalli, J.-D., and Perrelet, A.,** A clathrin-coated, Golgi-related compartment of the insulin secreting cell accumulates proinsulin in the presence of monesin, *Cell,* 39, 39, 1984.

33. **Sporn, L. A., Chavin, S. I., Marder, V. J., and Wagner, D. D.,** Biosynthesis of von Willebrand protein by human megakaryocytes, *J. Clin. Invest.,* 76, 1102, 1985.

34. **Slot, J. W., Bouma, B. N., Montgomery, R. M., and Zimmerman, T. S.,** Platelet factor VIII-related antigen: immunofluorescent localization, *Thromb. Res.,* 13, 871, 1978.

35. **Koutts, J., Walsh, P. N., Plow, E. F., and Fenton, J. W., II, Bouma, B. N., and Zimmerman, T. S.,** Active release of human platelet factor VIII-related antigen by adenosine diphosphate, collagen, and thrombin, *J. Clin. Invest.,* 62, 1255, 1978.

36. **Zucker, M. B., Broekman, M. J., and Kaplan, K. L.,** Factor VIII-related antigen in human blood platelets. Localization and release by thrombin or collagen, *J. Lab. Clin. Med.,* 94, 675, 1979.

37. **Zucker, M. B., Moseson, M. W., Broekman, M. J., and Kaplan, K. L.,** Release of platelet fibronectin (cold-insoluble globulin) from alpha granules induced by thrombin or collagen: lack of requirement for plasma fibronectin in ADP-induced platelet aggregation, *Blood,* 54, 8, 1979.

38. **Wencel-Drake, J. D., Plow, E. F., Zimmerman, T. S., Painter, R. G., and Ginsberg, M. H.,** Immunofluorescent localization of adhesive glycoproteins in resting and thrombin-stimulated platelets, *Am. J. Pathol.,* 115, 156, 1984.

39. **Cramer, E. M., Meyer, D., Le Menn, R., and Breton-Gorius, J.,** Eccentric localization of von Willebrand factor in an internal structure of platelet α-granule resembling that of Weibel-Palade bodies, *Blood,* 66, 710, 1985.

40. **Bonthron, D. T., Handin, R. I., Kaufman, R. J., Wasley, L. C., Orr, E. C., Mitsock, L. M., Ewenstein, B., Loscalzo, J., Ginsburg, D., and Orkin, S. H.,** Structure of pre-pro-von Willebrand factor and its expression in heterologous cells, *Nature,* 324, 270, 1986.

41. **Bouma, B. N., Wiegerinck, Y., Sixma, J. J., van Mourik, J. A., and Mochtar, I. A.,** Immunological characterization of purified anti-hemophilic factor A (factor VIII) which corrects abnormal platelet retention in von Willebrand's disease, *Nature (London) New Biol.,* 236, 104, 1972.

42. **Owen, W. G. and Wagner, R. H.,** Antihemophilic factor: separation of an active fragment following dissociation by salts or detergents, *Thromb. Diath Haemorrh.,* 27, 502, 1972.

43. **Cooper, H. A., Griggs, T. R., and Wagner, R. H.,** Factor VIII recombination after dissociation by CaCl$_2$, *Proc. Natl. Acad. Sci. U.S.A.,* 70, 2326, 1973.

44. **Zimmerman, T. S. and Edgington, T. S.,** Factor VIII-coagulant activity and factor VIII-like antigen: independent molecular entities, *J. Exp. Med.,* 138, 1015, 1973.

45. **Brinkhous, K. M., Sandberg, H., Garris, J. B., Mattson, C., Palm, M., Griggs, T., and Read, M. S.,** Purified human factor VIII-procoagulant protein: comparative hemostatic response after infusions into hemophilic and von Willebrand disease dogs, *Proc. Natl. Acad. Sci. U.S.A.,* 82, 8752, 1985.

46. **Zelechowska, M. G., van Mourik, J. A., and Brodniewicz-Proba, T.,** Ultrastructural localization of factor VIII-procoagulant antigen in human liver hepatocytes, *Nature,* 317, 729, 1985.

47. **Fitzgerald, L. A., Charo, I. F., and Phillips, D. R.,** Human endothelial cells synthesize membrane glycoproteins similar to platelet membrane GP IIb and GP IIIa, *J. Biol. Chem.,* 260, 10893, 1985.

48. **Leeksma, O. C., Zandbergen-Spaargaren, J., Giltay, J. C., and van Mourik, J. A.,** Cultured human endothelial cells synthesize a plasma membrane protein complex immunologically related to the platelet glycoprotein IIb/IIIa complex, *Blood,* 67, 1176, 1986.

49. **Pytela, R., Pierschbacher, M. D., Ginsberg, M. H., Plow, E. F., and Ruoslahti, E.,** Platelet membrane glycoprotein IIb/IIIa: member of a family of Arg-Gly-Asp-specific adhesion receptors, *Science,* 231, 1559, 1986.

50. **Van Buul-Wortelboer, M. F., Brinkman, H.-J., Reinders, J. H., van Aken, W. G., and van Mourik, J. A.,** Polar secretion of von Willebrand factor by perturbed endothelial cells, submitted 1987.

51. **De Groot, Ph.G., Reinders, J. H., and Sixma, J. J.,** Perturbation of human endothelial cells by thrombin or PMA changes the reactivity of their extracellular matrix towards platelets, *J. Cell Biol.,* in press 1987.

Chapter 9

vWf, PLATELETS, AND MEGAKARYOCYTES

R. M. Hardisty

TABLE OF CONTENTS

I.   Introduction 188

II.   Synthesis of vWf by Megakaryocytes 188

III.   Platelet vWf 188
       A.   Intracellular Location of Platelet vWf 188
       B.   Secretion of vWf by Platelets 189

IV.   Interaction of vWf with the Platelet Membrane 189
       A.   Effect of Ristocetin 189
       B.   Effect of Thrombin and Other Agonists 190
       C.   Asialo-vWF 190

V.   Characterization of Binding Sites on Platelets and vWf 191
       A.   Ristocetin-Induced Binding 191
             1.   Platelet Receptor 191
             2.   vWf Receptor 191
       B.   Thrombin and ADP-Induced Binding 192
             1.   Platelet Receptor 192
             2.   vWf Receptor 192

VI.   Physiological Significance of Platelet-vWf interactions 192
       A.   Adhesion to Subendothelium 192
       B.   Platelet Aggregation 193

VII.   Summary 193

References 194

I. INTRODUCTION

The von Willebrand factor (vWf) and the platelets are intimately related in many respects: not only is vWf essential for platelet-vessel wall interaction through its binding to at least two different sites on the platelet membrane as well as to vascular subendothelium, but it is synthesized in megakaryocytes, stored and transported in circulating platelets, and secreted from them in response to various physiological stimuli. In this chapter, the intracellular synthesis and distribution of vWf in megakaryocytes and platelets are considered first, followed by their interactions in the course of the hemostatic process.

II. SYNTHESIS OF vWf BY MEGAKARYOCYTES

Following the demonstration of vWf within platelets and the observation that the deficiency of vWf in the platelets of patients with severe von Willebrand's disease (vWD) was not corrected by transfusion, Nachman et al.[1] showed that cultured guinea pig megakaryocytes synthesized vWf antigen (vWf:Ag) with the same polypeptide subunit structure as that present in guinea pig plasma. Kupinski and Miller[2] have subsequently shown that the multimeric structure of guinea pig megakaryocyte vWf is essentially identical with that isolated from platelets, both sources containing a subset of very high molecular weight forms not seen in plasma. It may, therefore, be inferred that the vWf within circulating platelets is synthesized in the megakaryocyte, while that bound to the platelet plasma membrane is derived partly from this source (after secretion from within the platelets) and partly from the plasma pool secreted from vascular endothelial cells. Both morphologically recognizable megakaryocytes and their mononuclear precursors (promegakaryoblasts), whether obtained directly from human bone marrow or grown in culture, can be shown by immunofluorescent or immuno histochemical techniques to contain vWf:Ag.[3-5] This has a granular distribution in the morphologically recognizable cells,[4,5] while megakaryoblasts show a diffuse pattern of labeling, most prominent in the region of the Golgi apparatus.[4] It would seem, therefore, that platelet vWf is synthesized by promegakaryoblasts and subsequently packaged into α granules when these mature into morphologically recognizable megakaryocytes.

III. PLATELET vWf

Normal human platelets contain no factor VIII procoagulant activity[6-9] but do contain large amounts of vWf:Ag, estimates ranging from about 0.1 to 0.6 U per 10^9 platelets.[6-8,10,11] This represents between 5 and 25% of the vWf:Ag in whole blood, of which the platelets constitute only about 0.2% by volume. Platelet vWf is functionally active, as assessed by the ristocetin co-factor assay — indeed, more so than plasma vWf in terms of its activity:antigen ratio.[12] This higher specific activity is presumably attributable to the presence of larger multimers in platelet than in plasma vWf,[12-14] which are known to be hemostatically more effective. Platelet and plasma vWf appear to have the same polypeptide subunit structure,[7] but peptide mapping has revealed some minor differences:[15] 2 peptides were more intensely labeled in platelet than in plasma vWf, 32 ethers were shared, and 7 were seen in the plasma but not the platelet protein. It cannot yet be concluded, however, that plasma and platelet vWf are two distinct gene products: the observed differences may have been due to a posttranslational change, or even to proteolytic modification.

A. Intracellular Location of Platelet vWf

While normal platelets bind vWf avidly to their plasma membranes in response to a variety of stimuli, it is difficult to be certain, for technical reasons, whether unstimulated platelets carry any membrane-associated vWf. Perhaps the best evidence that they do is that of Parker et al.[16] There is no doubt, however, that the chief, if not the only, intracellular location of vWf is the platelet α granules,[10,17-19] from which it is secreted, together with other α granule proteins, in response to thrombin, collagen, and other stimuli. Cramer et al.,[20] using a sensitive immunogold method, found that vWf was distributed eccentrically within the α granules, opposite to the nucleoids. This distribution corresponded to that of tubular structures of 200—250-Å diameter, similar to those seen in the Weibel-Palade bodies of endothelial cells, where vWf is also located:[21] Cramer and colleagues have suggested that these structures may represent the vWf molecule itself.

B. Secretion of vWf by Platelets

Platelet vWf is secreted, together with other α granule proteins, in response to stimulation of the platelets by thrombin, collagen, and other agonists.[10,22,23] Since the same agonists also expose receptor sites for vWf on the platelet membrane, a proportion of the secreted protein is rapidly bound to the membrane,[13,24] not more than about 30% of the activity being recovered in the supernatant fluid. The binding is divalent cation dependent,[24] occurs more rapidly than that of exogenous vWf,[25] and requires the presence of the glycoprotein (GP) IIb/IIIa complex:[25,26] thrombasthenic platelets thus secrete vWf normally in response to thrombin, but fail to bind it to the membrane. In response to thrombin, though much less so in response to collagen, the larger multimers are preferentially bound, this effect being more pronounced with increasing thrombin concentrations.[13] This reassociation with the platelet membrane suggests an important hemostatic role for platelet vWf: Lopez Fernandez et al.[13] have calculated that the vWf concentration in the interstices of a thrombin induced platelet aggregate might reach about 50 times that in normal plasma. There is also some evidence that thrombin may enhance the surface exposure of vWf by a separate, calcium independent mechanism, possibly related to plasma membrane rearrangement.[16]

IV. INTERACTION OF vWf WITH THE PLATELET MEMBRANE

A. Effect of Ristocetin

In 1971, Howard and Firkin[27] first showed that the antibiotic ristocetin agglutinated normal platelets in their own plasma, but failed to agglutinate those of patients with vWD. It was soon firmly established that platelet agglutination by ristocetin depended on the presence of vWf,[28-30] and determination of the "ristocetin co-factor" of plasma, using either fresh[31] or fixed[32-33] normal platelets, became a standard method for the diagnosis of vWD. Subsequently, Howard et al.[34] showed that ristocetin-induced platelet agglutination was also defective in the Bernard Soulier syndrome, but that this was due to a platelet rather than a plasma defect. With the demonstration of a deficiency of GP Ib in the plasma membrane of Bernard Soulier platelets,[35] it became apparent that ristocetin-induced agglutination involved an interaction between plasma vWf and GP Ib. There is now abundant evidence that ristocetin promotes the binding of vWf to normal platelets in a dose-dependent manner,[36] and that the vWf receptor sites involved are situated on GP Ib.[37-39] Binding assays on normal platelets for both vWf and monoclonal antibodies to GP Ib reveal about 25,000 to 35,000 binding sites per platelet.[36,39,40]

The binding of vWf and agglutination of platelets in response to ristocetin requires neither metabolically active platelets nor the presence of divalent cations,[36] though if these are present, platelet adenylate cyclase is inhibited,[40a] and secretion and secondary aggregation result. The action of ristocetin appears to depend on its positive electrical charge, which promotes its binding to the platelets, with a resultant lowering of their net negative charge and consequent binding of vWf.[41,42] Other polycations, including protamine sulfate, polylysine, and polybrene, also induce platelet-vWf interaction,[43,44,44a] but the positively charged platelet factor 4, though it binds to the platelet surface on secretion, evidently has no such effect.[45] Vancomycin, an antibiotic resembling ristocetin in structure and peptide-binding properties, but with a lower positive charge, inhibits platelet agglutination in response to both ristocetin[46] and polybrene,[44] presumably by competing for binding sites on the platelet membrane.[46a]

There is abundant evidence, from experiments with various purified preparations of vWf and from the study of patients with variant forms of vWD, that the larger multimeric forms of vWF bind more readily to the platelets in response to ristocetin and support ristocetin induced agglutination more effectively than the smaller mutimers.[47-50] The carbohydrate side chains of the vWf molecule, particularly the penultimate galactose residues, have been held necessary for both optimal polymerization[51,52] and ristocetin co-factor activity,[52-54] but the work of Federici et al.[55] suggests that they confer these properties indirectly by protecting the molecule against proteolytic degradation. Removal of the terminal sialic acid residues alone results in spontaneous binding to the platelet membrane without the mediation of ristocetin.

Botrocetin (venom coagglutinin), an active principle derived from snake venom of the *bothrops* species, also induces platelet agglutination in the presence of vWf,[56] but differs from ristocetin in that its activity is independent of the vWf multimer size, so that preparations containing only small multimers support botrocetin induced agglutination as well as the high molecular weight forms.[57] Botrocetin induced agglutination is not completely defective in the Bernard-Soulier syndrome and is not inhibited by vancomycin.[58]

B. Effect of Thrombin and Other Agonists

In the attempt to find a physiological counterpart to ristocetin, Fujimoto and Hawiger[59] and Fujimoto et al.[60] showed that adenosine diphosphate (ADP) and thrombin were both able to stimulate the binding of vWf to normal platelets. In contrast to ristocetin induced binding, however, binding in response to ADP and thrombin required metabolically active platelets and the presence of divalent cations.[60] Other platelet activating agents, including arachidonic acid, collagen, and the endoperoxide analogue U46619, also induce vWf binding by a similar mechanism.[61] Experiments on platelets of patients with Glanzmann's thrombasthenia and the Bernard-Soulier syndrome, and on normal platelets exposed to monoclonal antibodies against specific membrane glycoproteins, have clearly shown that thrombin and ADP induce receptors for vWF not on GP Ib, like ristocetin, but on the GP IIb/IIIa complex.[62,63] The binding of vWf in response to these agonists is inhibited competitively by fibrinogen,[64-66] which also binds to the same or a closely adjacent site on GP IIb/IIIa in response to the same agonists. Since fibrinogen is present in the plasma in great molar excess over vWf, this competition for binding sites has thrown doubt on the physiological significance of thrombin induced vWf binding. It may be, however, that vWf is present in relative excess in the immediate environment of a platelet plug, owing to its secretion from the platelets themselves and from adjacent vascular endothelial cells.

The use of monoclonal antibodies has also shown that two different sites on the vWf molecule are involved in binding to GP Ib and GP IIb/IIIa.[67] The properties of the binding sites on both vWf and the platelets involved in their interaction are considered in more detail below.

C. Asialo-vWf

Vermylen and colleagues[68-70] were the first to observe that neuraminidase-treated human vWf, like native bovine vWf, aggregated human platelets directly in the presence of plasma, but without the addition of ristocetin or other agonists. De Marco and Shapiro[71] then showed that purified asialo-vWf bound directly to the platelet membrane in a saturable manner and caused aggregation of normal, but not Bernard-Soulier platelets, in the absence of ristocetin. They therefore suggested that asialo-vWf, like native vWf in the presence of ristocetin, bound to platelet GP Ib, though in contrast to ristocetin-induced agglutination, aggregation by asialo-vWf requires the presence of divalent cations and fibrinogen.[70,71] Subsequent work using monoclonal antibodies to platelet glycoproteins has shown that asialo-vWf does indeed bind initially to GP Ib, but that this reaction exposes receptors on the GP IIb/IIIa complex for both fibrinogen and asialo-vWf itself.[72,73] The resulting aggregation depends chiefly on the binding of fibrinogen rather than asialo-vWf to GP IIb/IIIa.[73]

Native bovine vWf behaves very similarly to human asialo-vWf in that it binds to formalin-fixed normal human platelets and agglutinates them, but fails to agglutinate Bernard-Soulier platelets;[34,74,75] it appears to share a common binding site on GP Ib with human vWf.[76,77]

V. CHARACTERIZATION OF BINDING SITES ON PLATELETS AND vWf

Since the recognition that vWf and platelets both possess two distinct classes of binding sites involved in their interaction, much effort has been devoted to the detailed identification of these sites and their relationship to those involved in the reactions between platelets and other proteins.

A. Ristocetin-Induced Binding
1. Platelet Receptor
Platelet GP Ib is a sialic acid rich transmembrane glycoprotein composed of two glyco-peptides connected by a disulfide bridge.[78] Most of the extracellular part of the larger α chain can be cleaved from the remainder by an endogenous platelet Ca^{2+}-activated protease[79] to yield the hydrophilic glycoprotein known as glycocalicin.[80] Besides the ristocetin induced vWf receptor, GP Ib carries receptors for quinine/quinidine-dependent antibodies,[81,82] for the Fc fragment of IgG,[83] and for thrombin.[84,85] Proteolytic cleavage of the molecule with various enzymes removes the vWf receptor and leaves little doubt that it is situated on the glycocalicin part of the α chain;[86-88] furthermore, purified glycocalicin has been shown to inhibit the binding to platelets of whole vWf in response to ristocetin, and of a monoclonal antibody to GP Ib which itself blocks ristocetin induced vWf binding.[89] These properties of glycocalicin were not affected by removal of sialic acid and galactose residues, but removal of N-acetyl glucosamine residues greatly reduced its inhibitor effect on vWf binding to platelets, suggesting that this part of the oligosaccharide chains of glycocalicin contributes to vWf binding.[89] Wicki and Clemetson[90] have shown that both vWf and thrombin receptors lie on a 45-kDa fragment cleaved from the exterior end of the α chain of GP Ib by leukocyte elastase; activation of the platelets by thrombin, however, involves at least one other receptor, probably situated on GP V.

2. vWf Receptor
Although large multimers of vWf are the most effective in promoting ristocetin induced agglutination, this property is retained not only by the basic vWf subunit but also by some of its proteolytic digestion fragments.[91,92] Martin et al.[93] observed residual ristocetin co-factor activity on a 116-kDa peptide derived by tryptic digestion, and Sixma et al.[94] found that a similar fragment was immunoprecipitated by a monoclonal antibody to vWf which inhibited ristocetin induced binding to platelets. Reduction of this peptide showed that the antibody bound to chains of 58/53 kDa. Girma et al.[95,96] have shown that cleavage of vWf by *Staphylococcus aureus* V-8 protease produces a 215-kDa C-terminal fragment and an approximately 310-kDa N-terminal fragment, the latter chiefly composed of 170-kDa peptide chains: a monoclonal antibody which blocked ristocetin-induced binding of vWf also inhibited binding of the N-terminal fragment to platelets and bound to the fragment and to 33- and 23-kDa peptides derived from it by digestion with subtilisin. An antibody to the collagen binding site of vWf also recognized the main N-terminal fragment, but bound to different domains after cleavage with subtilisin, while a monoclonal antibody to the GP IIb/IIIa binding

site of vWf bound to the C-terminal fragment.[96] Fujimura et al.[97] purified a reduced and alkylated tryptic fragment of 52/48 kDa from vWf which not only bound monoclonal antibodies recognizing the ristocetin induced binding sites, but itself inhibited ristocetin induced binding of intact vWf to platelets. Amino-terminal sequencing of this fragment showed that it began at residue 449 of the approximately 2050-residue vWf subunit. All these observations combine to show that the vWf receptor for platelet GP Ib can be located to a limited peptide sequence towards the N-terminal end of the vWf subunit.

B. Thrombin and ADP-Induced Binding

The vWf is only one of several adhesive proteins which are known to bind to the platelet GP IIb/IIIa complex in the presence of divalent cations when its receptors are exposed in response to thrombin, ADP, and other agonists. Evidence is accumulating that the binding sites for GP IIb/IIIa on these proteins are closely similar, if not identical, and that they attach to closely adjacent or identical sites on the platelet glycoprotein.

1. Platelet Receptor

In response to thrombin, receptors are exposed on platelet GP IIb/IIIa for fibrinogen,[98-100] fibronectin,[101] and thrombospondin,[102] as well as for vWf; though these receptors have not been characterized in biochemical terms, their close spatial relationship can be inferred from the closely similar effects of monoclonal antibodies recognizing different epitopes on the GP IIb/IIIa complex, or its components, on the binding of the various proteins.[65,103-105] The possibility that the vWf receptor is not identical with that for fibrinogen, but merely adjacent to it, is suggested by the work of Lombardo et al.[106] who raised a monoclonal antibody of which the monovalent Fab fragments inhibited vWf but not fibrinogen binding. Since both this and another antibody, which inhibited the binding of both proteins, bound to unstimulated platelets, however, on which the receptors are not exposed, their epitopes cannot be identified directly with the receptors: the selective inhibition of vWf binding might be a steric effect related to the much larger size of the vWf multimers than the fibrinogen molecule.

2. vWf Receptor

Fibrinogen binds to the platelet membrane through the carboxy-terminal portion of its γ chain, and synthetic peptides of 10 to 12 amino acids corresponding to this region (γ 400—411, γ 402—411) inhibit thrombin and ADP induced binding not only of fibrinogen but also of vWf and fibronectin.[107,108] Similarly, the amino acid sequence Arg-Gly-Asp in fibronectin is involved in its cell attachment function, and synthetic peptides containing this sequence inhibit not only the binding of fibronectin to fibroblasts[109] and to thrombin stimulated platelets,[110] but also the binding of both fibrinogen and vWf to platelets stimulated by thrombin or ADP.[111-113] vWf has indeed been shown to contain an Arg-Gly-Asp sequence,[114] and fibrinogen has two such sequences on its α chain, which also appears to react with the platelet membrane.[115] There is thus evidence for the involvement of two distinct small peptides in the binding of vWf and other adhesive proteins to GP IIb/IIIa, though the functional and spatial relationships between these sequences remains to be elucidated. A monoclonal antibody to vWf which inhibits thrombin induced binding to platelets was found to bind to a C-terminal proteolytic fragment of 215 kDa, which itself inhibited the thrombin induced binding to whole vWf and to an 86-kDa piece derived from it by further proteolysis with thermolysin.[96]

VI. PHYSIOLOGICAL SIGNIFICANCE OF PLATELET-vWf INTERACTIONS

A. Adhesion to Subendothelium

It has been abundantly demonstrated, by the study in perfusion systems of blood from patients with vWD[116-118] and the Bernard Soulier syndrome,[117,119,120] that the adhesion of platelets to subendothelium, particularly at high shear rates, requires the presence of both vWf and GP Ib. The adhesion of platelets in flowing blood to subendothelium is also blocked by antibodies against these two components.[121-125] The question of the trigger mechanism by which the receptors on vWf and/or GP Ib are activated *in vivo* remains unresolved: ristocetin has no obvious physiological analog, but perhaps the prior binding of vWf to the exposed subendothelium[126] induces a similar functional change to disialylation, enabling the molecule to bind to otherwise unstimulated platelets.

The observation that vWf binds to platelets at the GP IIb/IIIa complex as well as GP Ib raises the question whether this interaction also has a role in the adhesion of platelets to subendothelium. The original observations of Tschopp et al.[127] that thrombasthenic platelets adhere normally, though they fail to form thrombi, would seem to argue against this idea. Their experiments, however, were performed by perfusion for 10 min at the low shear rate of 800 s^{-1}. Weiss et al.[128] have recently carried out similar experiments over shorter perfusion times at shear rates up to 2600 s^{-1} and have found a significant defect of adhesion of thrombasthenic platelets and of normal platelets in the presence of a monoclonal antibody to GP IIb/IIIa, most marked at the higher shear rates. This defect appeared to involve the spreading of platelets on the exposed vascular surface rather than their initial attachment to it: this contrasts with the situations in vWD, in which the attachment phase is defective.[118] It seems possible, therefore, that the binding of vWf to GP Ib is chiefly involved in the initial attachment of platelets to the subendothelium, while their subsequent spreading on the subendothelial surface depends mainly on vWf binding to GP IIb/IIIa. This interpretation is consistent with the observation that only the latter stage of adhesion is Ca^{2+} dependent.[129]

Another theoretical objection to this physiological role of vWf binding to GP IIb/IIIa comes from the fact that it is competitively inhibited by fibrinogen,[64-66] of which the molar concentration in plasma is two or three orders of magnitude greater than that of vWf: very little binding occurs in response to thrombin at normal plasma fibrinogen concentrations.[66] When platelets are activated on contact with a damaged vessel wall, however, they secrete their intrinsic vWf; not only does this contain larger multimeric forms than plasma vWf, which may bind more avidly to GP IIb/IIIa as well as to GP Ib, but it has been calculated that the concentration in the immediate environment of the platelets might reach about 50 times that in plasma.[13] The platelets will also secrete their fibrinogen, but the molar ratio of fibrinogen to vWf in platelets is much less than that in plasma.[127] The local concentration of vWf will be further enhanced by that secreted from adjacent endothelial cells and bound to the subendothelium.

B. Platelet Aggregation

The binding of vWf to the platelet membrane is not required for aggregation by ADP, thrombin, or collagen *in vitro,* as evidenced by the fact that the platelets of patients with severe vWD respond normally to these agonists. In the particular case of afibrinogenemia, however, vWf appears to substitute for fibrinogen in supporting aggregation by binding to GP IIb/IIIa.[130] It remains an open question whether vWf may contribute in this way to aggregation in the special circumstances of hemostatic plug formation *in vivo.*

VIII. SUMMARY

About 5 to 25% of the vWf in whole blood is synthesized by the megakaryocytes and transported in the platelets. Synthesis begins in the megakaryocyte precursors, and the vWF is packaged into α granules at the morphologically recognizable megakaryocyte stage. Platelet vWf differs from plasma vWf in comprising a proportion of higher multimers of the basic subunit, which are hemostatically more active. It is secreted from the platelet α granules

Table 1
TWO TYPES OF PLATELET-vWf BINDING

Agonists	Ristocetin (bovine vWf, human asialo-vWf)	Thrombin, ADP, collagen, arachidonic acid, etc.
Requirement for:		
Platelet metabolic activity	—	+
Ca^{2+}	—	+
Inhibited by	Vancomycin	Fibrinogen, fibronectin
Platelet receptor	GB Ib α (glycocalicin)	GP IIb-IIIa
vWf receptor	N-terminal	C-terminal
	Valine 449 →	Arg-Gly-Asp γ 400—411
Probable physiological function	Initial attachment to subendothelium	Spreading on subendothelium

in response to thrombin, collagen, and other agonists, and the larger multimers are preferentially bound to GP IIb/IIIa on the platelet membrane. Plasma vWf binds to GP Ib and agglutinates normal platelets when these are stimulated by ristocetin, and similar binding and agglutination result from the exposure of normal human platelets to bovine vWf or human asialo-vWf in the absence of ristocetin. In response to thrombin or ADP, vWf binds to GP IIb/IIIa, and this is competitively inhibited by fibrinogen, which binds to the same or a closely adjacent receptor. The properties of these two distinct types of platelet-vWf interaction are set out in Table 1.

REFERENCES

1. **Nachman, R., Levine, R., and Jaffe, E. A.,** Synthesis of factor VIII antigen by cultured guinea pig megakaryocytes, *J. Clin. Invest.,* 60, 914, 1977.
2. **Kupinski, J. M. and Miller, J. L.,** Multimeric analysis of von Willebrand factor in megakaryocytes, *Thromb. Res.,* 38, 603, 1985.
3. **Rabellino, E. M., Levene, R. B., Leung, L. L. K., and Nachman, R. L.,** Human megakaryocytes. II. Expression of platelet proteins in early marrow megakaryocytes, *J. Exp. Med.,* 154, 88, 1981.
4. **Vinci, G., Tabilio, A., Deschamps, J. F., Van Haeke, D., Henri, A., Guichard, J., Tetteroo, P., Lansdorp, P. M., Hercend, T., Vainchenker, W., and Breton-Gorius, J.,** Immunological study of in vitro maturation of human megakaryocytes, *Br. J. Haematol.,* 56, 589, 1984.
5. **Beckstead, J. H., Stenberg, P. E., McEver, R. P., Shuman, M. A., and Bainton, D. F.,** Immunohistochemical localization of membrane and α-granule proteins in human megakaryocytes: application to plastic-embedded bone marrow biopsy specimens, *Blood,* 67, 285, 1986.
6. **Howard, M. A., Montgomery, D. C., and Hardisty, R. M.,** Factor VIII-related antigen in platelets, *Thromb. Res.,* 4, 617, 1974.
7. **Nachman, R. L. and Jaffe, E. A.,** Subcellular platelet factor VIII antigen and von Willebrand factor, *J. Exp. Med.,* 141, 1101, 1975.
8. **Bouma, B. N., Hordijk-Hos, J. M., De Graaf, S., and Sixma, J. J.,** Presence of factor VIII-related antigen in blood platelets of patients with von Willebrand's disease, *Nature,* 257, 510, 1975.
9. **Meucci, P., Peake, I. R., and Bloom, A. L.,** Factor VIII-related activities in normal, haemophilic and von Willebrand's disease platelet fractions, *Thromb. Haemost.,* 40, 288, 1978.
10. **Zucker, M. B., Broekman, M. J., and Kaplan, K. L.,** Factor VIII-related antigen in human blood platelets. Localization and release by thrombin and collagen, *J. Lab. Clin. Med.,* 94, 675, 1979.
11. **Shearn, S. A. M., Giddings, J. C., Peake, I. R., and Bloom, A. L.,** A comparison of five different rabbit antisera to factor VIII-related antigen in normal and von Willebrand's disease platelets, *Thromb. Res.,* 5, 585, 1974.
12. **Gralnick, H. R., Williams, S. B., McKeown, L. P., Krizek, D. M., Shafer, B. C., and Rick, M. E.,** Platelet von Willebrand factor: comparison with plasma von Willebrand factor, *Thromb. Res.,* 38, 623, 1985.
13. **Lopez Fernandez, M. F., Ginsberg, M. H., Ruggeri, Z. M., Batlle, F. J., and Zimmerman, T. S.,** Multimeric structure of platelet factor VIII/von Willebrand factor: the presence of larger multimers and their reassociation with thrombin stimulated platelets, *Blood,* 60, 1132, 1982.

14. **Ruggeri, Z. M., Mannucci, P. M., Lombardi, R., Federici, A. B., and Zimmerman, T. S.,** Multimeric composition of factor VIII/von Willebrand factor following administration of DDAVP: implications for pathophysiology and therapy of von Willebrand's disease subtypes, *Blood,* 59, 1272, 1982.

15. **Nachman, R. L., Jaffe, E. A., and Ferris, B.,** Peptide map analysis of normal plasma and platelet factor VIII antigen, *Biochem. Biophy. Res. Commun.,* 92, 1208, 1980.

16. **Parker, R. I., Rick, M. E., and Gralnick, H. R.,** Effect of calcium on the availability of platelet von Willebrand factor, *J. Lab. Clin. Med.,* 106, 336, 1985.

17. **Slot, J. W., Bouma, B. N., Montgomery, R., and Zimmerman, T. S.,** Platelet factor VIII-related antigen: immunofluorescent localization, *Thromb. Res.,* 13, 871, 1978.

18. **Giddings, J. C., Brookes, L. R., Piovella, F., and Bloom, A. L.,** Immunohistological comparison of platelet factor 4 (PF4), fibronectin (Fn) and factor VIII related antigen (VIIIR:Ag) in human platelet granules, *Br. J. Haematol.,* 52, 79, 1982.

19. **Wencel-Drake, J. D., Painter, R. G., Zimmerman, T. S., and Ginsberg, M. H.,** Ultrastructural localization of human platelet thrombospondin, fibrinogen, fibronectin and von Willebrand factor in frozen thin section, *Blood,* 65, 929, 1985.

20. **Cramer, E. M., Meyer, D., Le Menn, R., and Breton-Gorius, J.,** Eccentric localization of von Willebrand factor in an internal structure of platelet α-granule resembling that of Weibel-Palade bodies, *Blood,* 66, 710, 1985.

21. **Wagner, D. D., Olmsted, J. B., and Marder, V. J.,** Immunolocalization of von Willebrand protein in Weibel-Palade bodies of human endothelial cells, *J. Cell Biol.,* 95, 355, 1982.

22. **Koutts, J., Walsh, P. N., Plow, E. F., Fenton, J. W., II, Bouma, B. N., and Zimmerman, T. S.,** Active release of human platelet factor VIII-related antigen by adenosine diphosphate, collagen and thrombin, *J. Clin. Invest.,* 62, 1255, 1978.

23. **Sultan, Y., Maisonneuve, P., and Angeles-Cano, E.,** Release of VIIIR:Ag and VIIIR:WF during thrombin and collagen induced aggregation, *Thromb. Res.,* 15, 415, 1979.

24. **George, J. N. and Onofre, A. R.,** Human platelet surface binding of endogenous secreted factor VIII-von Willebrand factor and platelet factor 4, *Blood,* 59, 194, 1982.

25. **Ruggeri, Z. M., Bader, R., Pareti, F. I., Mannucci, L., and Zimmerman, T. S.,** High affinity interaction of platelet von Willebrand factor with distinct platelet membrane sites, *Thromb. Haemost.,* 50, 35, 1983.

26. **Furby, F. H., Berndt, M. C., Castaldi, P. A., and Koutts, J.,** Characterization of calcium-dependent binding of endogenous factor VIII/von Willebrand factor to surface activated platelets, *Thromb. Res.,* 35, 501, 1984.

27. **Howard, M. A. and Firkin, B. G.,** Ristocetin — a new tool in the investigation of platelet aggregation, *Thromb. Diath. Haemorrh.,* 26, 362, 1971.

28. **Howard, M. A., Sawers, R. J., and Firkin, B. G.,** Ristocetin: a means of differentiating von Willebrand's disease into two groups, *Blood,* 41, 687, 1973.

29. **Meyer, D., Jenkins, C. S. P., Dreyfus, M., and Larrieu, M. J.,** Experimental model for von Willebrand's disease, *Nature,* 243, 293, 1973.

30. **Weiss, H. J., Rogers, J., and Brand, H.,** Defective ristocetin-induced platelet aggregation in von Willebrand's disease and its correction by factor VIII, *J. Clin. Invest.,* 52, 2697, 1973.

31. **Weiss, H. J., Hoyer, L. W., Rickles, F. R., Varma, A., and Rogers, J.,** Quantitative assay of a plasma factor deficient in von Willebrand's disease that is necessary for platelet aggregation. Relationship to factor VIII procoagulant activity and antigen content, *J. Clin. Invest.,* 52, 2708, 1973.

32. **Allain, J. P., Cooper, H. A., Wagner, R. H., and Brinkhous, K. M.,** Platelets fixed with paraformaldehyde: a new reagent for assay of von Willebrand factor and platelet aggregating factor, *J. Lab. Clin. Med.,* 85, 318, 1975.

33. **Macfarlane, D. E., Stibbe, J., Kirby, E. P., Zucker, M. B., Grant, R. A., and McPherson, J.,** A method for assaying von Willebrand factor (ristocetin cofactor), *Thromb. Diath. Haemorrh.,* 34, 306, 1975.

34. **Howard, M. A., Hutton, R. A., and Hardisty, R. M.,** Hereditary giant platelet syndrome: a disorder of a new aspect of platelet function, *Br. Med. J.,* 2, 586, 1973.

35. **Nurden, A. T. and Caen, J. P.,** Specific roles for surface glycoproteins in platelet function, *Nature,* 255, 720, 1975.

36. **Kao, K.-J., Pizzo, S. V., and McKee, P. A.,** Demonstration and characterization of specific binding sites for factor VIII/von Willebrand factor on human platelets, *J. Clin. Invest.,* 63, 656, 1979.

37. **Zucker, M. B., Kim, S.-J. A., McPherson, J., and Grant, R. A.,** Binding of factor VIII to platelets in the presence of ristocetin, *Br. J. Haematol.,* 35, 535, 1977.

38. **Moake, J. L., Olson, J. D., Troll, J. H., Tang, S. S., Funicella, T., and Peterson, D. M.,** Binding of radio-iodinated human von Willebrand factor to Bernard-Soulier, thrombasthenic and von Willebrand's disease platelets, *Thromb. Res.,* 19, 21, 1980.

39. **Coller, B. S., Peerschke, E. I., Scudder, L. E., and Sullivan, C. A.,** Studies with a murine monoclonal antibody that abolishes ristocetin-induced binding of von Willebrand factor to platelets: additional evidence in support of GPIb as a platelet receptor for von Willebrand factor, *Blood,* 61, 99, 1983.

40. **Montgomery, R. P., Kunicki, T. J., Taves, C., Pidard, D., and Corcoran, M.,** Diagnosis of Bernard-Soulier syndrome and Glanzmann's thrombasthenia with a monoclonal assay on whole blood, *J. Clin. Invest.,* 71, 385, 1983.

40a. **Kao, K.-J., Tsai, B.-S., McKee, P. A., Lefkowitz, R. J., and Pizzo, S. V.,** Inhibitory effect of ristocetin and factor VIII/von Willebrand factor protein on human platelet adenylate cyclase activity, *Thromb. Res.,* 30, 301, 1983.

41. **Coller, B. S. and Gralnick, H. R.,** Studies on the mechanism of ristocetin-induced platelet agglutination. Effects of structural modification of ristocetin and vancomycin, *J. Clin. Invest.,* 60, 302, 1977.

42. **Coller, B. S.,** The effects of ristocetin and von Willebrand factor on platelet electrophoretic mobility, *J. Clin. Invest.,* 61, 1168, 1978.

43. **Rosborough, T. K. and Swaim, W. R.,** Abnormal polybrene-induced platelet agglutination in von Willebrand's disease, *Thromb. Res.,* 12, 937, 1978.

44. **Coller, B. S.,** Polybrene-induced platelet agglutination and reduction in electrophoretic mobility: enhancement by von Willebrand factor and inhibition by vancomycin, *Blood,* 55, 276, 1980.

44a. **Rosborough, T. K.,** von Willebrand factor, polycations and platelet agglutination, *Thromb. Res.,* 17, 481, 1980.

45. **Levine, S. P. and Moake, J. L.,** Platelet factor 4 does not promote von Willebrand factor binding to human platelets, *Thromb. Res.,* 36, 233, 1984.

46. **Moake, J. L., Cimon, P. L., Peterson, D. M., Roper, P., and Natelson, E. A.,** Inhibition of ristocetin-induced platelet agglutination by vancomycin, *Blood,* 50, 397, 1977.

46a. **Baugh, R. F., Jacoby, C., Brown, J. E., and Hougie, C.,** Effect of vancomycin on ristocetin and bovine PAF-induced agglutination of human platelets, *Thromb. Res.,* 12, 511, 1978.

47. **Doucet-De Bruine, M. H. M., Sixma, J. J., Over, J., and Beeser-Visser, N. H.,** Heterogeneity of human factor VIII. II. Characterization of forms of factor VIII binding to platelets in the presence of ristocetin, *J. Lab. Clin. Med.,* 92, 96, 1978.

48. **Ruggeri, Z. M. and Zimmerman, T. S.,** Variant von Willebrand's disease: characterization of two subtypes by analysis of multimeric composition of factor VIII/von Willebrand factor in plasma and platelets, *J. Clin. Invest.,* 65, 1318, 1980.

49. **Meyer, D., Obert, B., and Pietu, G.,** Multimeric structure of factor VIII/von Willebrand factor in von Willebrand's disease, *J. Lab. Clin. Med.,* 95, 590, 1980.

50. **Gralnick, H. R., Williams, S. B., and Morisato, D. K.,** Effect of the multimeric structure of the factor VIII/von Willebrand factor protein on binding to platelets, *Blood,* 58, 387, 1981.

51. **Gralnick, H. R., Williams, S. B., and Rick, M. E.,** Role of carbohydrate in multimeric structure of factor VIII/von Willebrand factor protein, *Proc. Natl. Acad. Sci. U.S.A.,* 80, 2771, 1983.

52. **Goudemand, J., Mazurier, C., Samor, B., Bouquelet, S., Montreuil, J., and Goudemand, M.,** Effect of carbohydrate modifications of factor VIII/von Willebrand factor on binding to platelets, *Thromb. Haemost.,* 53, 390, 1985.

53. **Gralnick, H. R.,** Factor VIII/von Willebrand factor protein. Galactose, a cryptic determinant of von Willebrand factor activity, *J. Clin. Invest.,* 62, 496, 1978.

54. **Sodetz, J. M., Paulson, J. C., Pizzo, S. V., and McKee, P. A.,** Carbohydrate on human factor VIII/von Willebrand factor. Impairment of function by removal of specific galactose residues, *J. Biol. Chem.,* 253, 7202, 1978.

55. **Federici, A. B., Elder, J. H., De Marco, L., Ruggeri, Z. M., and Zimmerman, T. S.,** Carbohydrate moiety of von Willebrand factor is not necessary for maintaining multimeric structure and ristocetin cofactor activity but protects from proteolytic degradation, *J. Clin. Invest.,* 74, 2049, 1984.

56. **Read, M. S., Shermer, R. W., and Brinkhous, K. M.,** Venom coagglutinin: an activator of platelet aggregation dependent on von Willebrand factor, *Proc. Natl. Acad. Sci. U.S.A.,* 75, 4514, 1978.

57. **Brinkhous, K. M., Read, M. S., Fricke, W. A., and Wagner, R. H.,** Botrocetin (venom coagglutinin): reaction with a broad spectrum of multimeric forms of factor VIII macromolecular complex, *Proc. Natl. Acad. Sci. U.S.A.,* 80, 1436, 1983.

58. **Howard, M. A., Perkin, J., Salem, H. H., and Firkin, B. G.,** The agglutination of human platelets by botrocetin: evidence that botrocetin and ristocetin act at different sites on the factor VIII molecule and platelet membrane, *Br. J. Haematol.,* 57, 25, 1984.

59. **Fujimoto, T. and Hawiger, J.,** Adenosine diphosphate induces binding of von Willebrand factor to human platelets, *Nature,* 297, 154, 1982.

60. **Fujimoto, T., Ohara, S., and Hawiger, J.,** Thrombin-induced exposure and prostacyclin inhibition of the receptor for factor VIII/von Willebrand factor on human platelets, *J. Clin. Invest.,* 69, 1212, 1982.

61. **Di Minno, G., Shapiro, S. S., Catalano, P. M., De Marco, L., and Murphy, S.,** The role of ADP secretion and thromboxane synthesis in factor VIII binding to platelets, *Blood,* 62, 186, 1983.

62. **Ruggeri, Z. M., Bader, R., and De Marco, L.,** Glanzmann thrombasthenia: deficient binding of von Willebrand factor to thrombin-stimulated platelets, *Proc. Natl. Acad. Sci. U.S.A.,* 79, 6038, 1982.

63. **Ruggeri, Z. M., De Marco, L., Gatti, L., Bader, R., and Montgomery, R. R.,** Platelets have more than one binding site for von Willebrand factor, *J. Clin. Invest.,* 72, 1, 1983.

64. **Piétu, G., Cherel, G., Marguerie, G., and Meyer, D.,** Inhibition of von Willebrand factor-platelet interaction by fibrinogen, *Nature,* 308, 648, 1984.

65. **Gralnick, H. R., Williams, S. B., and Coller, B. S.,** Fibrinogen competes with von Willebrand factor for binding to the glycoprotein IIb/IIIa complex when platelets are stimulated with thrombin, *Blood,* 64, 797, 1984.

66. **Schullek, J., Jordan, J., and Montgomery, R. R.,** Interaction of von Willebrand factor with human platelets in the plasma milieu, *J. Clin. Invest.,* 73, 421, 1984.

67. **Nokes, T. J. C., Mahmoud, N. A., Savidge, G. F., Goodall, A. H., Meyer, D., Edgington, T. S., and Hardisty, R. M.,** von Willebrand factor has more than one binding site for platelets, *Thromb. Res.,* 34, 361, 1984.

68. **Vermylen, J., Donati, M. B., De Gaetano, G., and Verstraete, M.,** Aggregation of human platelets by bovine or human factor VIII: role of carbohydrate side chains, *Nature,* 244, 167, 1973.

69. **Vermylen, J., De Gaetano, G., Donati, M. B., and Verstraete, M.,** Platelet-aggregating activity in neuraminidase-treated human cryoprecipitates: its correlation with factor VIII-related antigen, *Br. J. Haematol.,* 26, 645, 1974.

70. **Vermylen, J., Bottecchia, D., and Szpilman, H.,** Factor VIII and human platelet aggregation. III. Further studies on aggregation of human platelets by neuraminidase-treated human factor VIII, *Br. J. Haematol.,* 34, 321, 1976.

71. **De Marco, L. and Shapiro, S. S.,** Properties of human asialo-factor VIII, a ristocetin-independent platelet aggregating agent, *J. Clin. Invest.,* 68, 321, 1981.

72. **De Marco, L., Girolami, A., Russell, S., and Ruggeri, Z. M.,** Interaction of asialo-von Willebrand factor with glycoprotein Ib induces fibrinogen binding to the glycoprotein IIb-IIIa complex and mediates platelet aggregation, *J. Clin. Invest.,* 75, 1198, 1985.

73. **Gralnick, H. R., Williams, S. B., and Coller, B. S.,** Asialo von Willebrand factor interactions with platelets. Interdependence of glycoproteins Ib and IIb/IIIa for binding and aggregation, *J. Clin. Invest.,* 75, 19, 1985.

74. **Kirby, E. P. and Mills, D. C. B.,** The interaction of bovine factor VIII with human platelets, *J. Clin. Invest.,* 56, 491, 1975.

75. **Kirby, E. P.,** The agglutination of human platelets by bovine factor VIII:R, *J. Lab. Clin. Med.,* 100, 963, 1982.

76. **Cooper, H. A., Clemetson, K. J., and Lüscher, E. F.,** Human platelet membrane receptor for bovine von Willebrand factor (platelet aggregating factor): an integral membrane glycoprotein, *Proc. Natl. Acad. Sci. U.S.A.,* 76, 1069, 1980.

77. **Suzuki, K., Nishioka, J., and Hashimoto, S.,** Identical binding site on human platelets for von Willebrand factor and bovine platelet aggregating factor, *Thromb. Res.,* 17, 215, 1980.

78. **Clemetson, K. J.,** Platelet membrane glycoprotein I: structure and function. The domain of glycoprotein I involved in the von Willebrand receptor, *Blood Cells,* 9, 319, 1983.

79. **Phillips, D. R. and Jakabova, M.,** Ca^{2+}-dependent protease in human platelets, *J. Biol. Chem.,* 252, 2121, 1977.

80. **Okumura, T. and Jamieson, G. A.,** Platelet glycocalicin. I. Orientation of glycoproteins of the human platelet surface, *J. Biol. Chem.,* 251, 5944, 1976.

81. **Kunicki, T. J., Johnson, M. M., and Aster, R. H.,** Absence of the platelet receptor for drug dependent antibodies in the Bernard-Soulier syndrome, *J. Clin. Invest.,* 62, 716, 1978.

82. **Kunicki, T. J., Russell, N., Nurden, A. T., Aster, R. H., and Caen, J. P.,** Further studies on the human platelet receptor for quinine- and quinidine-dependent antibodies, *J. Immunol.,* 126, 398, 1981.

83. **Moore, A., Ross, G. D., and Nachman, R. L.,** Interaction of platelet membrane receptors with von Willebrand factor, ristocetin and the Fc region of immunoglobulin G, *J. Clin. Invest.,* 62, 1053, 1978.

84. **Okumura, T., Hasitz, M., and Jamieson, G. A.,** Platelet glycocalicin III. Interaction with thrombin and role as thrombin receptor of the platelet surface, *J. Biol. Chem.,* 253, 3435, 1978.

85. **Ganguly, P. and Gould, N. L.,** Thrombin receptors of human platelets: thrombin binding and antithrombin properties of glycoprotein I, *Br. J. Haematol.,* 42, 137, 1979.

86. **Jenkins, C. S. P., Phillips, D. R., Clemetson, K. J., Meyer, D., Larrieu, M.-J., and Lüscher, E. F.,** Platelet membrane glycoproteins implicated in ristocetin-induced aggregation, *J. Clin. Invest.,* 57, 112, 1976.

87. **Cooper, H. A., Bennett, W. P., White, G. C., II, and Wagner, R. H.,** Hydrolysis of human membrane glycoproteins with a *Serratia marcescens* metalloprotease: effect on response to thrombin and von Willebrand factor, *Proc. Natl. Acad. Sci. U.S.A.,* 79, 1433, 1982.

88. **Adelman, B., Michelson, A. D., Loscalzo, J., Greenberg, J., and Handin, R. I.,** Plasmin effect on platelet glycoprotein Ib-von Willebrand factor interactions, *Blood,* 65, 32, 1985.

89. **Michelson, A. D., Loscalzo, J., Melnick, B., Coller, B. S., and Handin, R. I.,** Partial characterization of a binding site for von Willebrand factor on glycocalicin, *Blood,* 67, 19, 1986.

90. **Wicki, A. N. and Clemetson, K. J.,** Structure and function of platelet membrane glycoproteins Ib and V. Effects of leukocyte elastase and other proteases on platelet response to von Willebrand factor and thrombin, *Eur. J. Biochem.*, 153, 1, 1985.

91. **Pasquini, R. and Hershgold, E. J.,** Effects of plasmin on human factor VIII (AHF), *Blood*, 41, 105, 1973.

92. **Guisasola, J. A., Cockburn, C. G., and Hardisty, R. M.,** Plasmin digestion of factor VIII: characterization of the breakdown products with respect to antigenicity and von Willebrand activity, *Thromb. Haemost.*, 40, 302, 1978.

93. **Martin, S. E., Marder, V. J., Francis, C. W., Loftus, L. S., and Barlow, E. H.,** Enzymatic degradation of the factor VIII-von Willebrand protein: a unique tryptic fragment with ristocetin cofactor activity, *Blood*, 55, 848, 1980.

94. **Sixma, J. J., Sakariassen, K. S., Stel, H. V., Houdijk, W. P. M., In der Maur, D. W., Hamer, R. J., de Groot, P. G., and van Mourik, J. A.,** Functional domains on von Willebrand factor: recognition of discrete tryptic fragments by monoclonal antibodies inhibiting interaction of von Willebrand factor with platelets and with collagen, *J. Clin. Invest.*, 74, 736, 1984.

95. **Girma, J.-P., Chopek, M. W., Titani, K., and Davie, E. W.,** Limited proteolysis of human von Willebrand factor by S. aureus V-8 protease: isolation and partial characterization of a platelet-binding domain, *Biochemistry*, 25, 3156, 1986.

96. **Girma, J.-P., Kalafatis, M., Pietu, G., Lavergne, J.-M., Chopek, M. W., Edgington, T. S., and Meyer, D.,** Mapping of distinct von Willebrand factor domains interacting with platelet GP Ib and GP IIb/IIIa and with collagen using monoclonal antibodies, *Blood*, 67, 1356, 1986.

97. **Fujimura, Y., Titani, K., Holland, L. Z., Russell, S. R., Roberts, J. R., Elder, J. H., Ruggeri, Z. M., and Zimmerman, T. S.,** von Willebrand factor. A reduced and alkylated 52/48-kDa fragment beginning at amino acid residue 449 contains the domain interacting with platelet glycoprotein Ib, *J. Biol. Chem.*, 261, 381, 1986.

98. **Bennet, J. S. and Vilaire, G.,** Exposure of platelet fibrinogen receptors by ADP and epinephrine, *J. Clin. Invest.*, 64, 1393, 1979.

99. **Marguerie, G. A., Plow, E. F., and Edgington, T. S.,** Human platelets possess an inducible and saturable receptor specific for fibrinogen, *J. Biol. Chem.*, 254, 5357, 1979.

100. **Peerschke, E. I., Zucker, M. B., Grant, R. A., Egan, J. J., and Johnson, M. M.,** Correlation between fibrinogen binding to human platelets and platelet aggregability, *Blood*, 55, 841, 1980.

101. **Plow, E. F. and Ginsberg, M.,** Specific and saturable binding of plasma fibronectin to thrombin-stimulated human platelets, *J. Biol. Chem.*, 256, 9477, 1981.

102. **Wolff, R., Plow, E. F., and Ginsberg, M. H.,** Interaction of thrombospondin with resting and stimulated human platelets, *J. Biol. Chem.*, 261, 6840, 1986.

103. **Pidard, D., Montgomery, R. R., Bennett, J. S., and Kunicki, T. J.,** Interaction of AP-2, a monoclonal antibody specific for the human platelet glycoprotein IIb-IIIa complex, with intact platelets, *J. Biol. Chem.*, 258, 12582, 1983.

104. **Jones, D., Fritschy, J., Garson, J., Nokes, T. J. C., Kemshead, J. T., and Hardisty, R. M.,** A monoclonal antibody binding to human medulloblastoma cells and to the platelet glycoprotein IIb-IIIa complex, *Br. J. Haematol.*, 57, 621, 1984.

105. **Plow, E. F., McEver, R. P., Coller, B. S., Woods, V. L., Marguerie, G. A., and Ginsberg, M. H.,** Related binding mechanisms for fibrinogen, fibronectin, von Willebrand factor, and thrombospondin on thrombin-stimulated human platelets, *Blood*, 66, 724, 1985.

106. **Lombardo, V. T., Hodson, E., Roberts, J. R., Kunicki, T. J., Zimmerman, T. S., and Ruggeri, Z. M.,** Independent modulation of von Willebrand factor and fibrinogen binding to the platelet membrane glycoprotein IIb/IIIa complex as demonstrated by monoclonal antibody, *J. Clin. Invest.*, 76, 1950, 1985.

107. **Plow, E. F., Srouji, A. H., Meyer, D., Marguerie, G., and Ginsberg, M. H.,** Evidence that three adhesive proteins interact with a common recognition site on activated platelets, *J. Biol. Chem.*, 259, 5388, 1984.

108. **Timmons, S., Kloczewiak, M., and Hawiger, J.,** ADP-dependent common receptor mechanism for binding of von Willebrand factor and fibrinogen to human platelets, *Proc. Natl. Acad. Sci. U.S.A.*, 81, 4935, 1984.

109. **Pierschbacher, M. D. and Ruoslahti, E.,** Cell attachment activity of fibronectin can be duplicated by small synthetic fragments of the molecule, *Nature*, 309, 30, 1984.

110. **Ginsberg, M., Pierschbacher, M. D., Ruoslahti, E., Marguerie, G., and Plow, E.,** Inhibition of fibronectin binding to platelets by proteolytic fragments and synthetic peptides which support fibroblast adhesion, *J. Biol. Chem.*, 260, 3931, 1985.

111. **Gartner, T. K. and Bennett, J. S.,** The tetrapeptide analogue of the cell attachment site of fibronectin inhibits platelet aggregation and fibrinogen binding to activated platelets, *J. Biol. Chem.*, 260, 11891, 1985.

112. **Haverstick, D. M., Cowan, J. F., Yamada, K. M., and Santoro, S. A.,** Inhibition of platelet adhesion to fibronectin, fibrinogen and von Willebrand factor substrates by a synthetic tetrapeptide derived from the cell-binding domain of fibronectin, *Blood*, 66, 946, 1985.

113. **Plow, E. F., Pierschbacher, M. D., Ruoslahti, E., Marguerie, G. A., and Ginsberg, M. H.,** The effect of Arg-Gly-Asp-containing peptides on fibrinogen and von Willebrand factor binding to platelets, *Proc. Natl. Acad. Sci. U.S.A.,* 82, 8057, 1985.

114. **Sadler, J. E., Shelton-Inloes, B. B., Sorace, J. M., Harlan, J. M., Titani, K., and Davie, E. W.,** Cloning and characterization of two cDNAs coding for human von Willebrand factor, *Proc. Natl. Acad. Sci. U.S.A.,* 82, 6394, 1985.

115. **Hawiger, J., Timmons, S., Kloczewiak, M., Strong, D. D., and Doolittle, R. F.,** γ and α chains of human fibrinogen possess sites reactive with human platelet receptors, *Proc. Natl. Acad. Sci. U.S.A.,* 79, 2068, 1982.

116. **Tschopp, T., Weiss, H. J., and Baumgartner, H. R.,** Decreased adhesion of platelets to subendothelium in von Willebrand's disease, *J. Lab. Clin. Med.,* 83, 296, 1974.

117. **Weiss, H. J., Turitto, V. T., and Baumgartner, H. R.,** Effect of shear rate on platelet interaction with subendothelium in citrated and native blood. Shear-dependent decrease of adhesion in von Willebrand's disease and the Bernard-Soulier syndrome, *J. Lab. Clin. Med.,* 92, 750, 1978.

118. **Turitto, V. T., Weiss, H. J., and Baumgartner, H. R.,** Decreased platelet adhesion on vessel segments in von Willebrand's disease: a defect in initial platelet attachment, *J. Lab. Clin. Med.,* 102, 551, 1983.

119. **Weiss, H. J., Tschopp, T. B., Baumgartner, H. R., Sussman, I. I., Johnson, M. M., and Egan, J. J.,** Decreased adhesion of giant (Bernard-Soulier) platelets to subendothelium — further implication on the role of the von Willebrand factor in haemostasis, *Am. J. Med.,* 57, 920, 1974.

120. **Caen, J. P., Nurden, A. T., Jeanneau, C., Michel, H., Tobelem, G., Levy-Toledano, S., Sultan, Y., Valensi, F., and Bernard, J.,** Bernard-Soulier syndrome: a new platelet glycoprotein abnormality. Its relationship with platelet adhesion to subendothelium and with the factor VIII von Willebrand protein, *J. Lab. Clin. Med.,* 4, 586, 1976.

121. **Baumgartner, H. R., Tschopp, T. B., and Meyer, D.,** Shear rate dependent inhibition of platelet adhesion and aggregation on collagenous surfaces by antibodies to human factor VIII/von Willebrand factor, *Br. J. Haematol.,* 44, 127, 1980.

122. **Meyer, D., Baumgartner, H. R., and Edgington, T. S.,** Hybridoma antibodies to human von Willebrand factor. II. Relative role of intramolecular loci in mediation of platelet adhesion to the subendothelium, *Br. J. Haematol.,* 57, 609, 1984.

123. **Stel, H. V., Sakariassen, K. S., Scholte, B. J., Veerman, E. C. I., van der Kwast, Th., H. de Groot, Ph. G., Sixma, J. J., and von Mourik, J. A.,** Characterization of 25 monoclonal antibodies to factor VIII-von Willebrand factor: relationship between ristocetin-induced platelet aggregation and platelet adherence to subendothelium, *Blood,* 63, 1408, 1984.

124. **Tobelem, G., Levy-Toledano, S., Bredoux, R., Michel, H., Nurden, A., and Caen, J. P.,** New approach to determination of specific functions of platelet membrane sites, *Nature,* 263, 427, 1976.

125. **Ruan, C., Tobelem, G., McMichael, A. J., Drouet, L., Legrand, Y., Degos, L., Kieffer, N., Lee, H., and Caen, J. P.,** Monoclonal antibody to human platelet glycoprotein I. II. Effects on human platelet function, *Br. J. Haematol.,* 49, 511, 1981.

126. **Sakariassen, K. S., Bolhuis, P. A., and Sixma, J. J.,** Human blood platelet adhesion to artery subendothelium is mediated by factor VIII-von Willebrand factor bound to the subendothelium. *Nature,* 279, 636, 1979.

127. **Tschopp, T. B., Weiss, H. J., and Baumgartner, H. R.,** Interaction of platelets with subendothelium in thrombasthenia: normal adhesion, impaired cohesion, *Experientia,* 31, 113, 1975.

128. **Weiss, H. J., Turitto, V. T., and Baumgartner, H. R.,** Platelet adhesion and thrombus formation on subendothelium in platelets deficient in glycoproteins IIb-IIIa, Ib, and storage granules, *Blood,* 67, 322, 1986.

129. **Sakariassen, K. S., Ottenhof-Rovers, M., and Sixma, J. J.,** Factor VIII-von Willebrand factor requires calcium for facilitation of platelet adherence, *Blood,* 63, 996, 1984.

130. **De Marco, L., Girolami, Z., Zimmerman, T. S., and Ruggeri, Z. M.,** von Willebrand factor interaction with the glycoprotein IIb/IIIa complex. Its role in platelet function as demonstrated in patients with congenital afibrinogenemia, *J. Clin. Invest.,* 77, 1272, 1986.

Chapter 10

ELECTRON MICROSCOPIC STUDIES OF vWf IN PLATELETS AND MEGAKARYOCYTES

Elisabeth M. Cramer

TABLE OF CONTENTS

I.   Introduction 202

II.   Electron Microscopic Studies of vWf Distribution in Normal Cells 202
       A.   Substructure of vWf 202
       B.   Endothelial Cells 202
       C.   Normal Human Platelets 203
       D.   Porcine Platelets 204
       E.   Normal Megakaryocytes 206
            1.   Cultured Megakaryocytes 206
            2.   Bone Marrow Megakaryocytes 207

III.   Electron Microscopic Studies of vWf in Disease States 208
       A.   Gray Platelet Syndrome 208
       B.   von Willebrand's Disease 209

IV.   Conclusions 210

Acknowledgments 211

References 211

I. INTRODUCTION

In normal platelets, four different types of granules have been recognized which differ in their content and their ultrastructural appearances.

1. Alpha-granules are the principal storage site of hemostatic proteins which are present in both the platelets and the plasma. These include von Willebrand factor (vWf), fibrinogen, and thrombospondin, or platelet-specific proteins such as β-thromboglobulin and platelet factor 4. α-Granules also store some proteins with other functions as exemplified by platelet derived growth factor and immunoglobulins.[14,18,19]
2. Dense bodies store serotonin, calcium, and the nonmetabolic pool of adenine nucleotides.[46]
3. Peroxisomes contain catalase.[5]
4. Lysosomes contain hydrolases such as acid phosphatase and aryl-sulfatase.[3]

α-Granules, the contents of which are released during platelet activation, represent the largest population and play a prominent role in the hemostatic process. The analysis of their content has been performed by several techniques, mainly by biochemical methods using subcellular fractionation[3,18,19] or by immunological techniques relying on light microscopy.[27,34,43]

Recently, electron microscopy (EM) has become a very useful tool following the development of immunocytochemistry and in particular immunogold staining methods. These techniques allow the demonstration of antigenic sites on thin sections of fixed and embedded intact cells.[7,12] The content of α-granules has thus been able to be specifically stained, each protein being the subject of an individual reaction and localization.[8-11,25,31,37,44] The ultrastructural study of vWf localization has lead to original and specific findings concerning this protein.[8] This technique has also been applied to the study of the appearance of vWf in the bone marrow precursors of platelets, the megakaryocytes.[10] Finally its study in bleeding disorders such as von Willebrand's disease (vWD)[11] or the gray platelet syndrome[9] has given new and interesting information and has thus contributed to further knowledge and understanding of these diseases.

II. ELECTRON MICROSCOPIC STUDIES OF vWf DISTRIBUTION IN NORMAL CELLS

vWf is a large glycoprotein of high molecular weight and complex multimeric structure[13] which plays a key role in the interaction between platelets and the vessel wall in primary hemostasis, arterial thrombosis, and possibly atherosclerosis. Its two main functions are (1) to transform the platelets from free circulating cells to adhesive cells which can stick to each other and adhere to the subendothelium of the vessel wall and (2) to act as the carrier protein for the coagulation protein factor VIII. vWf is a protein found in normal plasma and in platelets. It demonstrates duplicity of origin in that it is synthesized by endothelial cells,[39] presumably the source of plasma and subendothelium vWf, and by megakaryocytes[22] before circulating in platelets. *In vitro*, vWf can be detected by its antigenic determinants which bind to specific polyclonal or monoclonal antibodies.

A. Substructure of vWf

EM examination of vWf purified from fresh plasma and from factor VIII/vWf concentrates has shown strands of various lengths (100 to 1200 nm) consistent with the size heterogeneity of the vWf multimers.[24,33] The dimeric units also called promoters are formed of two 240-kDa subunits, and are polymerized linearly in an end-to-end pattern through disulfide bonds.

Each protomer is formed by two large globular ends (22 × 6.5 nm) connected to a small central node (6.4 × 3.4 nm) by two flexible rod domains each 34 nm long and 2 nm in diameter. However, the normal globular end is not always observed and may be either absent or elongated and twice the size of normal. This was interpreted by Fowler et al.[13] as being the consequence of a proteolytic action which could either be plasma derived or integral to platelets and endothelial cells. The protomer has a length of 120 nm when fully extended, and each of its two arms corresponds to one 240-kDa subunit. The two subunits are linked by disulfide bonds near their carboxyl end to form a protomer, and the protomers are linked by disulfide bonds through their amino-terminal extremity. The substructure of the protomer is reminiscent of the trinodular fibrinogen molecule, although it is twice as long as fibrinogen and its central node is smaller. The appearance of the protomer has also some similarities with fibronectin.[24]

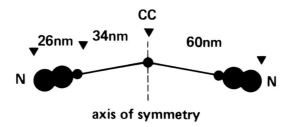

Diagram of Factor VIII/vWf substructure. N, amino-terminal extremity; C, carboxyl-terminal extremity. (Adapted from Fowler, W. E. et al., *J. Clin. Invest.*, 76, 1491, 1985.)

B. Endothelial Cells

In the endothelial cells, vWf is synthesized as a large precursor (260 kDa) which forms dimers, the predominant intracellular form of the protein, and which subsequently undergoes several changes before further multimerization.[39] vWf is stored in the endothelial cells within specific organelles called the Weibel-Palade bodies.[8,41] These are elongated rod-shaped single membrane-bound bodies containing several (up to 26) parallel tubular structures set in an electron dense matrix. They were first described by Weibel and Palade[42] and since then have been recognized in the endothelial cells of arteries, veins, capillaries, and endocardium of many vertebrates. They are found randomly scattered in the cytoplasm of the endothelial cells. Their length is difficult to determine since in EM thin sections, this organelle is rarely cut along its entire length. The longest one observed by Weibel and Palade measured 3.2 μ. The diamter of these bodies ranges from 0.1 to 0.5 μ (human about 0.15 μ) and that of the tubules in its substance from 150 to 270 Å (human about 200 Å). The tubules are parallel to each other and are generally disposed parallel to the long axis of the organelle. Sometimes they show a twisted spiral or whorled configuration. A central filament within the individual tubule has occasionally been observed.

These tubular figures seem first to appear in the Golgi saccules of the endothelial cells and are subsequently released by pinching off from the Golgi stacks.[32] Little is known of the fate of these bodies after secretion of vWf by the endothelial cells under appropriate stimuli (such as phorbol myristate acetate, Ca^{++} inophore A 23187, or cell irradiation). Furthermore, it is uncertain whether there is a parallel disappearance of the tubular structures of the entire Weibel-Palade bodies with their content or only of their content.[30,35] However, it seems that 2 d after the release of vWf from cultured endothelial cells the rod-shaped structures containing vWf are restored in the cells.[30]

C. Normal Human Platelets

In human platelets, the intracellular storage compartment of vWf is the α-granules. This has been shown by immunofluorescence,[27,34,43] subcellular fractionation studies,[3,18,19] and more recently by immuno-EM[8,44] The presence of vWf on the plasma membrane and on the membrane of the surface-connected canalicular system (SCCS) has been described,[20] but its origin is questionable. It is unknown whether the vWf is adsorbed from the plasma or released by slight platelet activation during isolation. Finally it seems that, in resting platelets, vWf is either absent or in very low concentrations on the membrane.

However, using a sensitive immunogold technique, we have shown a specific pattern of distribution of vWf within α-granules.[8] The technique involves fixation of platelets in 1% glutaraldehyde, freezing or embedding in plastic, and cutting ultra-thin sections of the cells. These sections are then incubated with a monospecific antibody to vWf, followed by an antiglobulin coupled to colloidal gold as the electron dense marker. They are counterstained and observed under EM.[12]

Fibrinogen and thrombospondin were found by ourselves,[9] as by others,[25,31,37] to be randomly and similarly distributed in the matrix of all the platelet α-granules as demonstrated in Figure 1b.

However vWf was detected in the α-granules in a focal and asymmetric distribution pattern and sparing the nucleoids as seen in Figure 1a and 2a. With this immunogold technique, plasma and SCCS membranes were not stained either in washed anticoagulated platelets or in platelets from whole fixed blood.

After careful EM examination of the platelets, labeling for vWF was sometimes observed over small tubular structures, either isolated or in groups of up to five, and located opposite the nucleoids as shown in Figure 2b. On standard EM examination, these tubules appeared to be located at the periphery of the α-granule in an electron luscent zone and away from the nucleoids, as demonstrated in Figure 2c and 2d. Their diameters ranged from 200 to 250 Å. These tubular structures were first observed by White[45] in human platelet α-granules and Behnke[1] in megakaryocyte α-granules. These structures look very similar in size and association pattern to those found within Weibel-Palade bodies. The fact that the tubules are only seldom found within the platelet α-granules can be explained by their apparent high sensitivity to fixation, and the relative difficulty of their visualization due to the electron density of the environmental matrix. White[45] found an increase in the occurrence of these tubules after digitonin treatment of platelets. We observed only 4 to 6 tubule profiles per 100 platelet sections. The relationship between these tubules and vWf remains to be defined. Their colocalization has been clearly demonstrated, and this could imply either that the tubular structure represents the vWf molecule itself, or that it corresponds to a structural carrier protein such as proteoglycans or, less likely, tubulin. However, these tubules display several morphological features allowing their distinction from microtubules. On the other hand, the factor VIII/vWf protomer, as observed in EM[13,24,33] has a large size compared to these structures.

D. Porcine Platelets

It is known that the pig can suffer from severe vWD,[4] and, therefore, normal porcine platelet vWf was studied by EM as a control.[11] Porcine platelets differ from human platelets by their smaller size and the uneven size of their α-granules which are generally larger. The most striking difference was observed by immuno-EM. The amount of vWf antigen detectable per α-granule was far greater than in human as seen in Figure 3a. The distribution of labeling was similar to that described in humans in that it showed polar localization or distribution at the periphery or along the long axis of the α-granule. However, the labeling was always intense. The standard EM aspect of the α-granule showed that, in accordance with the observations by immuno-EM, this extensive immunolabeling coincided with the presence of numerous tubules regularly spaced with an average diameter of 200 Å as seen in Figure 3b, c, and d. They were in groups of up to 30 per α-granule, disposed in parallel array, usually exhibiting a straight course, or, rarely, twisted along the periphery of the granule.

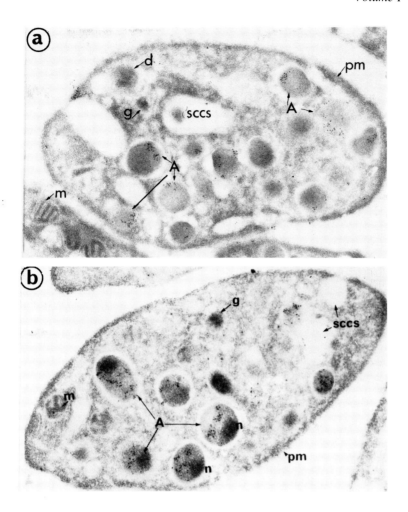

FIGURE 1. (a) Section of a platelet stained with an antibody raised against vWf and immunogold: the gold particles are eccentrically located in the α granules, generally labeling one of their poles (A). Plasma membrane (pm), SCCS, dense granules (d), and mitochondria (m), are not labeled. (Magnification × 33,000.) (b) Section of a platelet labeled with an anti-fibrinogen followed by immunogold: gold particles are randomly distributed over the entire light matrix of the α granules, in a different distribution pattern from vWf (A). The dark nucleoids (n) are devoid of labeling, as are the SCCS mitochondria (m), small granules (g), and plasma membrane (pm). (Magnification × 33,000.) (From Cramer, E. M., Vainchenker, W., Vinci, G., Guichard, J., and Breton-Gorius, J., *Blood*, 66, 1310, 1985. With permission.)

Thus, due to the prominence of these structures, the appearance of the pig platelet α-granule was very similar to that of Weibel-Palade bodies in endothelial cells. Sometimes slight morphological differences allow their distinction from microtubules as found in Figure 3c, in that their diameter was slightly less, 200 vs. 250 Å for microtubules. Furthermore, their wall was thinner and they were not surrounded by a clear halo although they sometimes displayed a central filament.

The significance of this distribution of vWf in the α-granules compared with that of other coagulation proteins of the α-granules is still unclear. However, it may explain some differences observed in the redistribution of these different components during platelet activation. Some authors found that fibrinogen was released from platelets, after thrombin stimulation while vWf was still associated with the platelets.[47] This association may also be

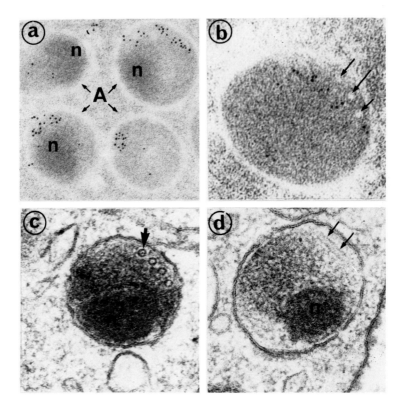

FIGURE 2.   High magnification of normal platelet α-granules. (a) Immunogold labeling
for vWf: the vWf is revealed by the gold particles gathered at one pole of the α-granules
(A), alongside the dark nucleoid (n). (Magnification × 66,300.) (b) Same preparation
as in (a): gold particles revealing vWf are eccentrically located over the α-granules. This
localization coincides with the presence of three tubular structures transversely sectioned
(arrows). (Magnification × 70,600.) (c) The tubular structures colocalized with vWf are
better seen by standard EM: they are located apart from the nucleoid (n) in an electron
luscent part of the α-granules, here a group of four with an average diameter of 200Å
and sometimes with a central filament (arrow). (Magnification × 113,100.) (d) The
longitudinal section of these tubules (arrow) can sometimes be seen in the α granule
beside the nucleoid (n). (Magnification × 83,500.) ([a] and [b] from Cramer, E. M.,
Meyer, D., Lemenn, R., and Breton-Gorius, J., *Blood*, 66, 710, 1985. With permission.
[c] and [d] courtesy of Breton-Gorius, J., Hopital H. Mondor, Créteil, France.)

involved in the reassociation and competition of vWf and fibrinogen for their common
plasma membrane receptor, glycoprotein IIb/IIIa,[26] or their respective receptors, glycoprotein
Ib and glycoprotein IIb/IIIa.

E. Normal Megakaryocytes
1. Cultured Megakaryocytes
The study of normal cultured megakaryocytes, as shown in Figure 4, demonstrated that
vWf is detected in small vesicles and granules in the Golgi area of the cell. In the immature
α-granules, the distribution of vWf is focal and asymmetrical similar to that which is found
in the mature α-granules of either platelet or megakaryocytes. In the latter cell type, vWf
antigen (vWf:Ag) is observed to be associated with the occurrence of tubules. This raises
the possibility that the function of these structures is related to the storage of vWf after
synthesis. The finding of labeled vWf in the Golgi region of megakaryocytes also supports
previous biochemical studies suggesting that vWf is synthesized by these cells.[22,36]

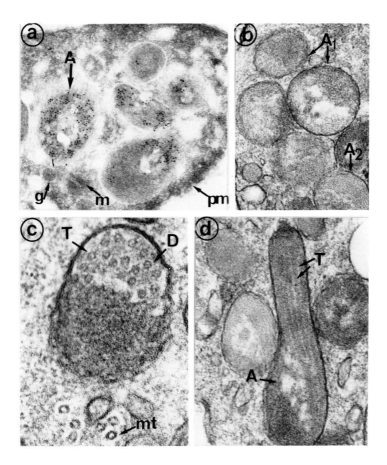

FIGURE 3.   Some characteristics of pig platelet α-granules (a) Immunolabeling for vWf is prominent in the α granules (A), distributed focally or along their periphery. The plasma membrane (pm) mitochondria (m), and small granules (g) are not labeled. (Magnification × 39,000.) (b) This corresponds to numerous tubular structures which can be seen in tranverse (A1) or longitudinal (A2) sections and generally grouped at one side of the granules. (Magnification × 31,600.) (c) This high magnification of an α granule section shows the large number of the tubules (T) in porcine species (displaying sometimes a central dense dot [D]). It also illustrates the slight morphological differences between the granule associated tubules and the cytoplasmic microtubules (mt) which have a slightly larger diameter and thicker wall, no central filament, and a clear surrounding halo. (Magnification × 110,600.) (d) Longitudinal section of an α granule (A) displaying numerous tubules (T) oriented parallel to the long axis of the granule and sectioned longitudinally. (Magnification × 50,000.) (From Cramer, E. M., Caen, J. P., Drouet, L., and Breton-Gorius, J., *Blood,* 68, 774, 1986. With permission.)

2. Bone Marrow Megakaryocytes

Some preliminary results obtained from cultured megakaryocytes can also be demonstrated *in vivo*. First, the appearance of immunolabeled vWf may be observed in the vesicles and small granules located in the Golgi zone, subsequently leading to the localization in the megakaryocyte α-granules with a distribution identical to that in platelet α-granules.[10] In parallel experiments, we have studied the appearance of thrombospondin which follows essentially the same sequential appearance, but which is, however, randomly distributed in the matrix of these organelles. It is interesting to note that vWf and thrombospondin, two α-granule components, are thought to be synthesized by megakaryocytes and that the EM studies support this hypothesis. Indeed, it has recently been demonstrated that circulating

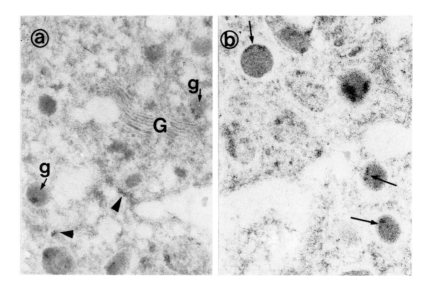

FIGURE 4.   Immunolocalization of vWf in normal cultured megakaryocytes. (a) Near the
Golgi complex (G) some dense vesicles (arrowheads) and small granules (g) are focally labeled
for vWf. (Magnification × 36,300.) (b) The megakaryocyte mature α-granules (arrows) also
display vWf according to the characteristic eccentric distribution observed in platelets. (Magnification × 36,300.) (From Cramer, E. M., Vainchenker, W., Vinci, G., Guichard, J., and
Breton-Gorius, J., *Blood,* 66, 1310, 1985. With permission.)

proteins can be removed from the plasma and then incorporated, via receptor coated vesicles,
into the α-granules of megakaryocytes.[16]

III. ELECTRON MICROSCOPIC STUDIES OF vWf IN DISEASE STATES

A. Gray Platelet Syndrome
The gray platelet syndrome is a rare congenital disease in which the bleeding symptoms
and the morphologic abnormalities of the platelet are associated.[29] The platelets lack α-
granules specifically and thus appear gray after Romanowsky stain. EM studies have shown
that these platelets do not contain α granules, but that they have a normal number of granules
of other types.[6,21] Biochemical studies have shown that the concentrations of proteins normally present in the α-granules are concomitantly very low.[15,23]
Immunostaining of fibrinogen and vWf in the platelets of three patients with this syndrome
revealed that these two proteins could be detected within small granules, the appearance,
size, and number of which could lead to confusion with lysosomes and peroxisomes as
demonstrated in Figure 5a. These structures were thus identified as abnormal α-granules. It
is another interesting observation that vWf was observed to be scattered within the whole
matrix of these granules instead of being localized eccentrically as in normal α-granules.
Further studies will be necessary to ascertain whether or not tubules are present within these
small granules, and to determine whether this pattern of vWf distribution corresponds to
some abnormality in its structure and multimerization.
The study of cultured megakaryocytes from these patients also allowed interesting observations as shown in Figure 6. Numerous vesicles carrying vWf and some small granules
identical with those found in blood platelets were observed within the Golgi zone. However,
despite an apparently normal synthesis of the α-granule content, the granules were not
normally formed and their contents were lost prior to storage. Indeed, some dense material
was found within the dilated cisternae of the demarcation membrane of the megakaryocytes
and also within the SCCS of platelets as demonstrated in Figure 5b. This dense material
was identified as lost α-granule content by its fibrinogen immunoreactivity.

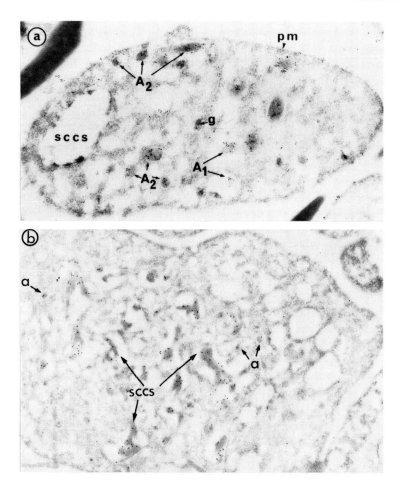

FIGURE 5.   Platelets from a patient with the gray platelet syndrome. (a) Immunolabeling for vWf reveals the presence of very small granules which can thus be identified
as abnormal α-granules (A2). Note the random distribution of vWf within these granules.
Some clear vacuoles are slightly labeled for vWf and thus seem to correspond to partially
empty α-granules (A1). No labeling is present in SCCS, plasma membrane (pm), and
small granules of other type (g). (Magnification × 26,800.) (b) Immunolabeling for
fibrinogen shows that some dense material present in the SCCS is probably the normal
content of α-granules which has been prematurely lost. Small abnormal α-granules (a)
can also be seen. (Modification × 16,200.) (From Cramer, E. M., Vainchenker, W.,
Vinci, G., Guichard, J., and Breton-Gorius, J., *Blood*, 66, 1310, 1985. With permission.)

This study led to two main conclusions: first, that the α-granule content is synthesized
but lost early in the megakaryocyte maturation and second, that gray platelets have some
abnormally small α-granules where vWf is distributed in a manner unlike that observed in
normal platelets.

B. von Willebrand's Disease

von Willebrand's disease (vWD) is characterized by quantitative and qualitative abnormalities of vWf.[17] The study of the platelet vWf by EM in the porcine homozygous disease
has provided some interesting observations. Indeed, the study of porcine platelets has shown
that the antigenic reactivity of vWf and the occurrence of tubular structures are both extensive.[11] On the basis of these findings, it was considered of interest to study porcine

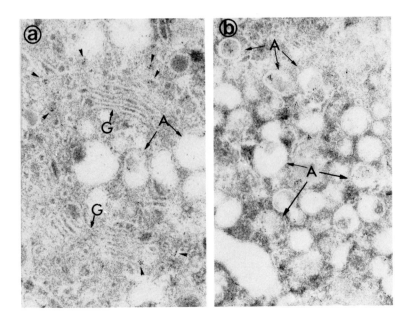

FIGURE 6.   (a) and (b) Cultured megakaryocytes from a patient with the gray platelet syndrome immunolabeled for vWf: some vesicles (arrowheads) located near the Golgi saccules (G) contain vWf, but this protein is not packed into the empty α-granules (A). (Magnification × 31,600 and 31,600.) (From Cramer, E. M., Vainchenker, W., Vinci, G., Guichard, J., and Breton-Gorius, J., *Blood*, 66, 1310, 1985. With permission.)

homozygous vWD since it is known that vWf is virtually absent both from platelets and plasma of these animals.[4]

Immunolabeling for vWf was negative and no antigenic reactivity was found in the α granules as shown in Figure 7a. In parallel, no tubular structures whatsoever could be detected as demonstrated in Figure 7b and c. In spite of this absence of vWf immunoreactivity, the elongated appearance of the granules was the same as observed in normal porcine platelets. Although the distribution was observed in the long axis of the granules, the tubules did not seem to be responsible for this elonaged shape. However, the circumferential band of cytoplasmic microtubules was still present in these platelets as shown in Figure 7c.

The absence of granule associated tubules in vWD, together with the lack of vWf, favors the hypothesis that vWf itself is the structural protein of these tubules. Further studies are being performed to compare the morphological EM aspects of the platelets with the quantitation of platelet vWf and its degree of multimerization in the different types of human vWD.

IV. CONCLUSIONS

Immuno-EM is a simple and reliable technique for studying the localization and distribution of vWf within different cell types. Some new findings have arisen from studies performed on platelets and megakaryocytes:

1. In platelets vWf is restricted to a compartment of the α granule distinct from the other coagulation proteins. This finding has led to the discovery of vWf associated tubules which are also present in megakaryocytes and endothelial cells, the nature and function of which remain to be elucidated.
2. Some specific abnormalities in the ultrastructural distribution of vWf have been found in diseases such as the gray platelet syndrome and vWD. These findings may lead to

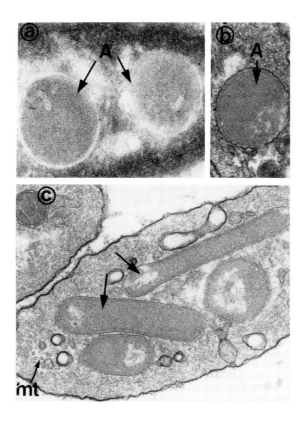

FIGURE 7. Platelets from a pig with homozygous vWD. (a) Immunolabeling for vWf detects no immunoreactivity within the α-granules (A). (Magnification × 20,000.) (b) and (c) In parallel, no granule associated tubules can be found (A). Note that some α-granules, however, have an elongated shape (arrows). The cytoplasmic microtubules (mt) are present. (Magnification × 37,350.) (From Cramer, E. M., Caen, J. P., Drouet, L., and Breton-Gorius, J., *Blood*, 68, 774, 1986. With permission.)

a new understanding of the function of vWf and its role in the pathophysiology of these diseases.

ACKNOWLEDGMENTS

The author gratefully acknowledges Patricia Dopping-Hepenstal (Wellcome Research Laboratories, Beckenham, England) for careful review of the manuscript and Josette Guichard (INSERM, Hopital H. Mondor, Creteil, France) for photographic assistance.

REFERENCES

1. **Behnke, O.,** An electron microscopic study of the megakaryocyte of the rat bone marrow. I. The development of the demarcation membrane system and the platelet surface coat, *J. Ultrastruct. Res.,* 24, 412, 1968.
2. **Bentfeld-Baker, M. F. and Bainton, D. F.,** Identification of primary lysosomes in human megakaryocytes and platelets, *Blood,* 59, 472, 1982.
3. **Bouma, B. N., Hardijk-Hos, J. M., de Graff, S., and Sixma, J. J.,** Presence of factor VIII related antigen in blood platelets of patients with von Willebrand's disease, *Nature,* 25, 510, 1975.
4. **Bowie, E. J. W., Owen, C. A., Jr., Zollman, P. E., Thompson, J. H., Jr., and Fass, D. N.,** Tests of hemostasis in swine: normal values and values in pig affected with von Willebrand's disease, *Am. J. Vet. Res.,* 34, 1405, 1973.

5. **Breton-Gorius, J. and Guichard, J.,** Two different types of granules in megakaryocytes and platelets as revealed by the diaminobenzidine reaction, *J. Micros C. Biol. Cell,* 23, 197, 1975.
6. **Breton-Gorius, J., Vainchenker, W., Nurden, A., Levy Toledano, S., and Caen, J.,** Defective α-granule production in megakaryocytes from gray platelet syndrome. Ultrastructural studies of bone marrow cells and megakaryocytes growing in culture from blood precursors, *Am. J. Pathol.,* 102, 10, 1981.
7. **Cramer, E., Pryzwansky, K. B., Villeval, J. L., Testa, U., and Breton-Gorius, J.,** Ultrastructural localization of lactoferrin and myeloperoxidase in human neutrophils by immunogold methods, *Blood,* 65, 423, 1985.
8. **Cramer, E. M., Meyer, D., Lemenn, R., and Breton-Gorius, J.,** Eccentric localization of von Willebrand factor within a tubular structure of platelet α-granule resembling that of Weibel-Palade bodies, *Blood,* 66, 710, 1985.
9. **Cramer, E. M., Vainchenker, W., Vinci, G., Guichard, J., and Breton-Gorius, J.,** Gray platelet syndrome: immunoelectron-microscopic localization of fibrinogen and von Willebrand factor in platelets and megakaryocytes, *Blood,* 66, 1310, 1985.
10. **Cramer, E. M., Breton-Gorius, J., Beesley, J. E., and Martin, J. F.,** Ultrastructural demonstration of tubular inclusions coinciding with von Willebrand factor in pig megakaryocytes, *Blood* 71(533), 1988.
11. **Cramer, E. M., Caen, J. P., Drouet, L., and Breton-Gorius, J.,** Absence of tubular structures and immunolabeling for von Willebrand factor in the platelet α-granules from porcine von Willebrand disease, *Blood,* 68, 774, 1986.
12. **De Mey, J.,** A critical review of light and electron microscopy immunocytochemical techniques used in neurobiology, *J. Neurosci. Methods,* 7, 1, 1983.
13. **Fowler, W. E., Fretto, L. J., Hamilton, K. K., Erickson, H. P., and McKee, P. A.,** Substructure of human von Willebrand factor, *J. Clin. Invest.,* 76, 1491, 1985.
14. **George, J. N., Saucerman, S., Levine, S. P., Knieriem, L. K., and Bainton, D. F.,** Immunoglobulin G is a platelet α-granule secreted protein, *J. Clin. Invest.,* 79, 1012, 1986.
15. **Gerrard, J. M., Philips, D. R., Radg, H. R., Plow, E. F., Walz, D., Ross, R., and Harker, L. A.,** Biochemical studies of two patients with the gray platelet syndrome, a selective deficiency of platelet α-granules, *J. Clin. Invest.,* 66, 102, 1982.
16. **Handagama, P. G., Georges, J. M., Shutian, M. A., McEver, R. P., and Bainton, D. F.,** Incorporation of a circulating protein into megakaryocytes and platelet granules, *Blood,* 68, 158a, 1986.
17. **Holmberg, L. and Nilsson, I. M.,** von Willebrand's disease, *Clin. Haematol.,* 14, 46, 1985.
18. **Howard, M. A., Montgomery, D. C., and Hardisty, R. M.,** Factor VIII related antigens in platelets, *Thromb. Res.,* 4, 617, 1974.
19. **Kaplan, D. R., Broekman, M. J., Chernoff, A., Lesznik, G. R., and Drillings, M.,** Platelet α-granules: studies on release and subcellular localization, *Blood,* 53, 1043, 1979.
20. **Jeanneau, C., Avner, P., and Sultan, Y.,** Use of monoclonal antibody and colloidal gold in E. M.: localization of von Willebrand factor in megakaryocytes and platelets, *Cell Biol. Int. Rep.,* 8, 841, 1984.
21. **Levy-Toledano, S., Caen, J. P., Breton-Gorius, J., Rendu, F., Cuwin, E. R., Golenzer, C., Dupuy, E., Legrand, Y., and Maclouf, J.,** Gray platelet syndrome: α-granule dificiency. Its influence on platelet function, *J. Lab. Clin. Med.,* 98, 831, 1981.
22. **Nachman, R., Levine, R., and Jaffe, E.,** Synthesis of factor VIII antigen by cultured guinea pig megakaryocytes, *J. Clin. Invest.,* 60, 914, 1977.
23. **Nurden, A. T., Kunicki, T. J., Dupuis, D., Soria, C., and Caen, J. P.,** Specific protein and glycoprotein deficiencies in platelets isolated from two patients with the gray platelet syndrome, *Blood,* 59, 709, 1982.
24. **Ohmori, K., Fretto, L. J., Harrison, R. L., Switzer, H. E. P., Erickson, H. P., and McKee, P.,** Electron microscopy of human factor VIII/von Willebrand glycoprotein: effect of reducing reagents on structure and function, *J. Cell Biol.,* 95, 632, 1982.
25. **Pham, T. D., Kaplan, K. L., and Butler, V. P., Jr.,** Immunoelectron microscopic localization of platelet factor 4 and fibrinogen in the granules of human platelets, *J. Histochem. Cytochem.,* 31, 905, 1983.
26. **Pietu, G., Cherel, G., Marguerie, G., and Meyer, D.,** Inhibition of von Willebrand factor - platelet interaction by fibrinogen, *Nature,* 308, 648, 1984.
27. **Piovella, F., Ascari, E., Sitar, G. M., Malamani, G. D., Catteno, G., Mactiulo, E., and Sorti, E.,** Immunofluorescent detection of factor VIII related antigen in human platelets and megakaryocytes, *Haemostasis,* 3, 288, 1974.
28. **Rabellino, E. M., Awidi, A., Sitar, G.,** et al., Human megakaryocytes synthesize platelet glycoproteins IIb, IIIa and thrombospondin, *Blood,* 64 (Suppl. 1), 250a, 1984.
29. **Racuglia, G.,** Gray platelet syndrome: a variety of qualitative platelet disorders, *Am. J. Med.,* 51, 818, 1971.
30. **Reinders, J. H., De Groot, P. G., Gonsalves, H. D., Zandbergen, J., Loesberg, C., and Van Mourik, J. A.,** Isolation of a storage and secretory organelle containing von Willebrand protein from cultured human endothelial cells, *Biochim. Biophys. Acta,* 804, 361, 1984.

31. **Sander, H. J., Slot, J. W., Bouma, B. N., Bolhuis, P. A., Pepper, D. S., and Sixma, J. J.,** Immunocytochemical localization of fibrinogen, platelet factor 4 and beta-thromboglobulin in thin frozen sections of human blood platelets, *J. Clin. Invest.,* 72, 1277, 1983.

32. **Siegel, A. and Stoebner, P.,** The origin of tubular inclusions in endothelial cells, *J. Cell Biol.,* 44, 223, 1970.

33. **Slauter, H., Loscalzo, J., Bockenstedt, P., and Handin, R. I.,** Native conformation of human von Willebrand protein. Analysis by electron microscopy and quasi-elastic light scattering, *J. Biol. Chem.,* 260, 8559, 1985.

34. **Slot, J. W., Bouma, B. N., Montgomery, R., and Zimmerman, T. S.,** Platelet factor VIII related antigen: immunofluorescent localization, *Thromb. Res.,* 13, 871, 1978.

35. **Sporn, L. A., Rubin, P., Harder, V. J., and Wagner, D. D.,** Irradiation induces release of von Willebrand protein from endothelial cells in culture, *Blood,* 64, 567, 1984.

36. **Spron, L. A., Chavin, S. I., Marder, V. J., and Wagner, D. D.,** Biosynthesis of von Willebrand protein by human megakaryocytes, *J. Clin. Invest.,* 60, 914, 1985.

37. **Stenberg, P. E., Shuman, M. A., Levine, S. P., and Bainton, D. F.,** Redistribution of alpha-granules and their contents in thrombin-stimulated platelets, *J. Cell Biol.,* 98, 748, 1984.

38. **Wagner, D. D., Olmsted, J. B., and Marder, V. J.,** Immunolocalization of von Willebrand protein in Weibel-Palade bodies of human endothelial cells, *J. Cell Biol.,* 95, 355, 1982.

39. **Wagner, D. D. and Marder, V. J.,** Biosynthesis of von Willebrand protein by human endothelial cells: processing steps and their intracellular localization, *J. Cell Biol.,* 19, 2123, 1984.

40. **Wagner, D. D., Hayada, S. T., Urban-Pickering, M., Lewis, B. H., and Marder, V. J.,** Inhibition of disulfide bonding of von Willebrand protein by monensin results in small, functionally defective multimers, *J. Cell Biol.,* 101, 112, 1985.

41. **Warhol, H. J. and Sweet, J.,** The ultrastructural localization of von Willebrand factor in endothelial cells, *Am. J. Pathol.,* 117, 310, 1984.

42. **Weibel, E. A. and Palade, G. E.,** New cytoplasmic components in arterial endothelia, *J. Cell Biol.,* 23, 101, 1964.

43. **Wencel-Drake, J. D., Plow, E. F., Zimmerman, T. S., Painter, R. G., and Ginsberg, M. H.,** Immunofluorescent localization of adhesive glycoproteins in resting and thrombin-stimulated platelets, *Am. J. Pathol.,* 115, 156, 1984.

44. **Wencel-Drake, J. D., Painter, R. G., Zimmerman, T. S., and Ginsberg, M. H.,** Ultrastructural localization of human platelet thrombospondin, fibrinogen, fibrinectin and von Willebrand factor in frozen thin section, *Blood,* 65, 929, 1985.

45. **White, J. G.,** Tubular elements in platelet granules, *Blood,* 32, 148, 1968.

46. **White, J. G.,** The dense bodies of human platelets: origin of serotonin storage particles from platelet granules, *Am. J. Pathol.,* 53, 791, 1968.

47. **Zucker, H., Broekman, M., and Kaplan, K.,** Factor VIII related antigen in human blood platelets: localization and release by thrombin and collagen, *J. Lab. Clin. Med.,* 94, 675, 1979.

Chapter 11

INTERACTION OF SURFACE-BOUND FACTOR VIII WITH OTHER COAGULATION FACTORS

S. Elödi

TABLE OF CONTENTS

I.   Introduction...216

II.   Assembly of the Factor IXa-VIII Complex 216
      A.   Activated Factor VIII..216
      B.   Effect of the Binding Surface 218
            1.   Phospholipid...218
            2.   Platelet Membrane 218
            3.   Endothelial Cells..219

III. Advantages of the Surface Binding of Factor VIII.............................220

IV.   Summary 222

References..223

I. INTRODUCTION

Blood coagulation is a localized process taking place at the site of vascular injury. The local character of blood clotting is ensured by surface-bound enzyme reactions occurring on the membrane of platelets aggregated on the damaged endothelium. In the intrinsic pathway of blood coagulation, factor X is activated by a molecular complex composed of factor IXa, VIII, phospholipid, and calcium.[1-5] Out of the components of the factor X activator complex, factor IXa is a serine protease containing γ-carboxy-glutamic acid residues at the amino-terminus of the molecule.[6-9] The γ-carboxy residues enable factor IXa to bind to the negatively charged groups of phospholipid through calcium ions. Factor VIII serves as a co-factor regulating the enzymatic activity of factor IXa.[4,5,10]

The formation of the IXa-VIII-phospholipid-calcium complex is a prerequisite for the efficient activation of factor X. Several observations indicate that the rate of formation of the IXa-VIII complex is determined by the binding rate of VIII. This latter process is apparently influenced by the protein structure of VIII, but is also dependent on the composition and quality of the phospholipid surface.

II. ASSEMBLY OF THE IXa-VIII COMPLEX

Studies on the intrinsic activation of factor X indicate that the formation of factor Xa is not an instantaneous reaction. The activation of factor X can be measured, depending on the experimental conditions, only after a lag phase of various length.[3,4,11-13] The lag phase is shortened, however, if VIII is preincubated with trace amounts of thrombin prior to the mixing of the components.[4,5,14] It is a matter of controversy as to whether pretreatment of VIII with thrombin is essential for the optimal formation of the IXa-VIII complex. Several authors claim that the "activation" of VIII with thrombin is vital for complex formation.[5,10,14] Others hold the view that the IXa-VIII complex also is built up in the presence of "native" VIII.[12,13,15,16]

A. Activated Factor VIII

Factor VIII is extremely sensitive even to minute concentrations of thrombin, with a consequential pronounced increase of activity. Thrombin-activated VIII (VIII_t) is labile and its activity rapidly diminishes, as seen in Figure 1.[17-19] Since VIII is not an enzyme, the meaning of the term "activation" is ill defined. After the cloning of the human factor VIII gene and with the knowledge of the predicted protein structure, the phenomenon of VIII "activation" could be interpreted. As deduced from the DNA sequence, intact VIII is a single polypeptide chain protein of Mr 265 kDa, comprising 2332 amino acid residues.[20,21] When the carbohydrate content is taken into account, the assumed molecular weight would be 330 kDa. Following the effect of thrombin, the molecular weight markedly decreases, and a protein composed of a heavy (Mr 90 kDa) and a light (Mr 80 kDa) chain is formed. Thrombin further cleaves the Mr 90-kDa chain into smaller fragments of Mr 54 and 43 kDa. The appearance of these small fragments coincides with the decrease of VIII_t activity.[22,23]

It is presumed that the smaller VIII_t fragment, because of its size, is incorporated more easily into the molecular complex formed on the phospholipid surface, and the faster binding shortens the lag phase preceding the activation of factor X.[65]

It is unclear during the course of physiological blood coagulation whether thrombin plays a role in the activation of VIII, as the formation of the IXa-VIII complex precedes the appearance of thrombin. Activation of VIII may, however, be brought about by other clotting proteases as well. Vehar and Davie[24] have shown that VIII is also activated by bovine factor Xa. A similar phenomenon has been observed also in purified and plasma systems with human factor Xa.[25,26] It appears, however, that VIII_t is a more efficient cofactor than the

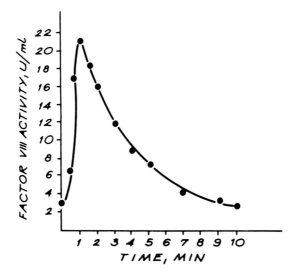

FIGURE 1.   Transient increase of VIII:C activity induced by the effect of 0.025 NIH U/ml thrombin.

Table 1
ENZYME CONCENTRATION
NEEDED TO ACTIVATE VIII

Protease	Concentration nM	Ref.
Thrombin	1.3	29
	0.27	27
Factor Xa	2.0	27
	0.5	25
Factor IXa	250	28

form activated by factor Xa. The initial rate of formation of factor Xa with VIII$_t$ was 18 nM min^{-1}, whereas with factor VIII$_{Xa}$ the same parameter reached only 6.7 nM min^{-1}.[27] Besides factor Xa and thrombin, factor IXa can also activate VIII.[28] The increase of factor VIII procoagulant activity (VIII:C) and the inactivation characteristics after reaching the peak value demonstrated the same profile as in the case of thrombin activation, but the extent of activation was somewhat less. Considerably larger amounts of factor IXa were needed to achieve the activation as compared with thrombin or even factor Xa.

Although the data obtained under different experimental conditions are difficult to compare, the values as shown in Table 1 indicate that thrombin and factor Xa are more effective activators of VIII than is factor IXa. It should be taken into account, however, that in the intrinsic pathway the formation of IXa precedes that of factor Xa and thrombin, i.e., factor IXa has an earlier availability to activate VIII than the other two enzymes. Furthermore, on the phospholipid surface, in the heterogeneous phase, the local concentration of proteins may be higher than in solution, and the spatial orientation of the two proteins on the phospholipid surface may favor the activation of VIII by factor IXa. As demonstrated in our experiments performed in the presence of phospholipid, about 5 min were needed for the development of maximum activity of the IXa-VIII complex.[4] According to Rick's[28] data a similar, about 4- to 5-min period, is required for the maximal activation of VIII under the influence of factor IXa. As the activity of the IXa-VIII complex develops, albeit slower, also in the presence of "native" VIII,[4,12,13,15,16] it can be assumed that during the lag phase, factor IXa slowly activates VIII. This, in turn, becomes incorporated into the complex

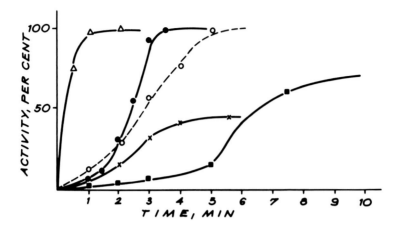

FIGURE 2.   Effect of the binding surface on the assembly rate of the IXa-VIII complex.
Time course of complex formation in the presence of factors IXa, VIII, calcium, and
thrombin aggregated platelets; 3×10^8 per milliliter ●-●, 3×10^7 per milliliter ×-×,
5×10^8 per milliliter ■-■, 3×10^8 per milliliter plus VIII, △-△, and phospholipid (20
μg/ml) ○-○. 100% activity equals the formation of 54 mol factor Xa per min per mol
factor IXa.[13,40]

proportional to the rate of activation. The positive feedback effects of factor Xa and thrombin,
produced either by the intrinsic or the extrinsic pathway, further accelerate the formation of
the IXa-VIII complex.

B. Effect of the Binding Surface
1. Phospholipid
The "procoagulant" activity of various phospholipids actually represents the optimal
composition for the binding of coagulation factors. The presence of phosphatidylserine is
essential, but the concentration and ratio of the other phospholipids also markedly influence
the formation of enzyme complexes.[30,31] Although the calcium-mediated binding of Vitamin
K dependent coagulation factors to the negatively charged phospholipids has been studied
in detail, much less is known of the forces and interactions influencing the binding of VIII
to the phospholipid surface. For the development of maximum activity, it is necessary that
factors VIII and IXa are bound in juxtaposition to the same phospholipid micelle.[32,33] Factor
VIII and von Willebrand factor (vWf) in the plasma are held together presumably by electrostatic interactions.[34] It appears from experiments performed with phospholipid mixtures
that the affinity to phospholipid is greater for VIII than for vWf. On incubation with
phospholipid, VIII and vWf dissociate, and VIII binds to the phospholipid.[35-37] The binding
is concentration dependent and also influenced by the composition of the phospholipid.[35-38]
Under identical conditions, VIII binds best to phosphatidylserine, then in decreasing order
to phosphatidylethanolamine and phosphatidylcholine.[38]

Native VIII bound to phospholipid can be activated by thrombin, although the extent of
activation is less than that of VIII in solution.[37-39]

2. Platelet Membrane
The various phospholipid preparations can only serve as models of the interactions occurring *in vivo,* since in the circulation the intrinsic factor X activator complex is formed
probably on the surface of the platelets.

In studies of the development of the IXa-VIII complex on the platelet surface, we have
established that the IXa-VIII complex is built up faster on the surface of thrombin stimulated
platelets than in the presence of phospholipid alone.[13] As shown in Figure 2, the shortest

lag phase was observed in the presence of platelets and VIII$_t$. Factor VIII$_t$ accelerated the development of maximal activity, but did not affect its extent. However, activity of the complex and also the rate of formation were influenced by the number of platelets present in the system. If the platelet number was below the optimum, only one half of maximum factor Xa formation could be measured, suggesting that the number of binding sites available to factors IXa and VIII is insufficient. At higher platelet counts the lag phase became strongly prolonged, about 80% of maximal activity developed only after 15 min. The excess of binding sites apparently may interfere with the proper steric fit of protein components. We assumed that a similar phenomenon may contribute to the paradoxical bleeding tendency of thrombocythaemic patients.[40]

It remains an open question which component of the membrane binds VIII. Zwaal[30] assumed that hydrophobic interactions play a predominant role in the binding of VIII. It appears that the activation of platelets is a prerequisite for the binding of VIII. In our experience, with nonactivated platelets, there was practically no activation of factor X.[13] Sewerin and Andersson[41] studied the binding of VIII by discontinuous albumin gradient centrifugation and found that nonactivated platelets bound only 3% of native VIII, whereas platelets activated by collagen or adenosine diphosphate (ADP) bound 10%. In the case of VIII$_t$, binding was 50%. These data are in good agreement with the rapid complex formation observed by us in the presence of thrombin-activated platelets and VIII$_t$ (Figure 2). Rosing et al.[42] have recently shown that on the surface of platelets, stimulated by the combined effect of thrombin plus collagen, there are about 20,000 binding sites per platelet for the factor IXa-VIII complex, in contrast to the 920 binding sites calculated for the nonstimulated platelets. The activation of factor X, i.e., the development of binding sites for the IXa-VIII complex was marginal if the platelets were stimulated by thrombin alone. In contrast, the VIII binding ability of platelets developed equally on separate stimulation by collagen and ADP in the experiments of Sewerin and Andersson.[41] These data suggest that the membrane component required for the binding of VIII is not identical with the phospholipids that ensure the binding of factors IXa and X.

3. Endothelial Cells

It is generally held that the intact endothelial cell lining of vascular walls constitutes a nonthrombogenic surface.[43] Recent data suggest, however, that reactions of the clotting process may take place also on the surface of endothelial cells. Zymogen and active factors IX and X can bind to the vascular endothelial cells.[44,45] Factor Xa and prothrombin when added to cell culture gave rise to thrombin.[46] Stern et al.[47] working with bovine aortic endothelial cells have observed the activation of factor X some 60 s after the addition of bovine factors IXa, VIII, and X. The formation of factor Xa was relatively moderate on the endothelial cell monolayer surface, but it was much more pronounced, if the cell culture had been suspended. The combined presence of factors VIII and X induced the appearance of a new, high affinity factor IXa binding site on the bovine aortic endothelial cell surface.[48] When factors XIa, IX, VIII, X, prothrombin, and fibrinogen were added to the bovine endothelial cell monolayer, fibrinopeptide A release was observed and the formation of cell associated fibrin strands was detected.[49] These data led Stern et al.[49] to the conclusion that the endothelial cells can readily propagate coagulation reactions leading to fibrin formation on their surface.

In our experiments with human venous endothelial cells and human factors, the lag phase preceding the formation of factor Xa on the cell monolayer surface was considerably longer than that observed in the bovine system. As seen in Figure 3, in the presence of VIII$_t$, the stabilization of reaction velocity required 6 min, whereas in the presence of nonactivated VIII maximal activity was attained after about a 10-min lag phase.[50]

The formation and function of the IXa-VIII complex play a central role in the coagulation process. As shown in Table 2, the formation of the IXa-VIII complex on human venous

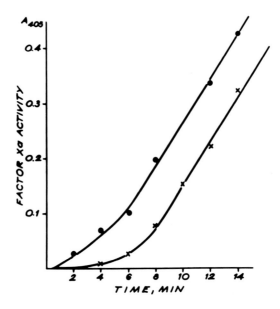

FIGURE 3.   Activation of factor X on the surface of endothelial cells. To the human venous endothelial cell monolayer VIII, IXa, X, calcium, and factor Xa substrate S-2222 were added. Activation of factor X was monitored by the increase of absorbancy of samples taken at intervals. Activation of factor X in the presence of thrombin-activated ●–● and nonactivated ×–× VIII.[50]

Table 2
EFFECT OF BINDING SURFACE AND VIII$_t$ ON THE RATE OF ASSEMBLY OF THE IXa-VIII COMPLEX[4,13,50]

Composition	Lag phase (min)
Factor IXa, Ca^{2+} plus:	
VIII, PL	5
VIII$_t$, PL	3
VIII, plt	3
VIII$_t$, plt	1
VIII, EC	10
VIII$_t$, EC	6

Note: PL — phospholipid, EC — endothelial cell monolayer, plt — thrombin aggregated platelets.

endothelial cells is a relatively slow process as compared to that taking place on either phospholipid or platelet surfaces. The question arises as to whether such a slow reaction could have any appreciable role in physiological coagulation. It is obvious that the platelet membrane ensures more favorable conditions for the binding of the IXa-VIII complex than the surface of endothelial cells. If any inference can be made from experiments in cell culture as to the process occurring *in vivo,* then we may venture the tentative hypothesis that in the slow venous circulation, the factor IXa-VIII complex formed at low rate on the venous endothelial cells may be related to the development of venous thrombosis.

III. ADVANTAGES OF THE SURFACE BINDING OF FACTOR VIII

Surface binding markedly alters the kinetic parameters of factor X activation. Factor IXa is capable of activating factor X also in solution, but the reaction is very slow and the

Table 3
KINETIC PARAMETERS OF FACTOR X ACTIVATION

Composition	Source of proteins	K_m, M	V_{max} (mol Xa/min/mol IXa)	Ref.
IXa	B	3×10^{-4}	0.0022	10
IXa, PL, Ca	B	6×10^{-8}	0.0025	10
IXa, PL, Ca	B	6×10^{-7}	0.007	15
IXa, PL, Ca	H	—	2.0	4
IXa, PL, Ca, VIII	B	6×10^{-8}	500	10
IXa, PL, Ca, VIII	B	5×10^{-7}	2.9	15
IXa, PL, Ca, VIII	H	—	46	4
IXa, plt, Ca, VIII	H	—	54	65

Note: H — human, B — bovine, PL — phospholipid, plt — platelets.

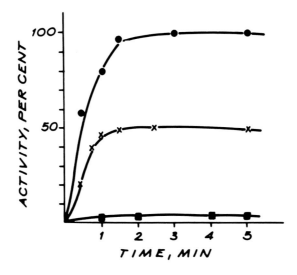

FIGURE 4.   Effect of granulocyte proteases on the assembly of the factor IXa-VIII complex. Formation of the complex in the presence of proteases with nonactivated ■-■ and with thrombin-activated ×-× VIII. Formation of the complex with VIII$_t$ in the absence of proteases ●-●.[54]

Michaelis constant, i.e., the K_m value, indicative of enzyme-substrate affinity, is high. In the presence of phospholipid and calcium the K_m value decreases considerably, the enzyme being saturated at much lower substrate concentrations. As seen from the data shown in Table 3, VIII does not affect the K_m value, while it increases the rate of factor X activation by several orders of magnitude.

It is known that VIII is very susceptible to proteolytic cleavage. The activating/inactivating effect of thrombin has been dealt with previously. Other proteases, e.g., plasmin, trypsin, and chymotrypsin, rapidly inactivate VIII.[51,52] We have shown when studying the effect of granulocyte proteases that even minute amounts of these enzymes inactivate VIII.[53] In contrast, VIII, when incorporated into the IXa-VIII complex, becomes practically resistant to proteolytic inactivation.[54] Analyzing the basis of this resistance we have come to the conclusion that factor IXa is protected by calcium, whereas VIII is protected from proteolysis by the calcium-shielded factor IXa.[54,55] It appears that in the development of proteolytic resistance, an important role is played by the binding rate of VIII. As shown in Figure 4, in the presence of proteases, with native VIII, the activity of the IXa-VIII complex does not develop, presumably owing to the rapid inactivation of VIII. With thrombin-activated

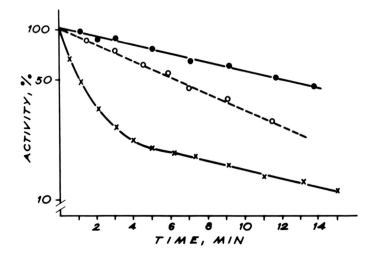

FIGURE 5.   Protection of surface-bound VIII from the effect of specific antibody. Effect of anti-VIII IgG on VIII in solution ×—×, in the presence of aggregated platelets ○—○, and in the platelet surface-bound IXa-VIII complex ●—●. (From Elődi, S., and Váradi, K., *Thromb. Res.*, 33, 557, 1984. With permission.)

VIII, about 50% of the maximal activity of the complex developed even in the presence of proteases, probably because VIII$_t$ binds to the complex rapidly and becomes no longer accessible to proteases.[54] Surface binding also stabilizes the otherwise labile VIII$_t$ activity. According to Lollar et al.[56] the inactivation rate of VIII$_t$ markedly decreases in the presence of phospholipid factor IXa and calcium.

Protection against proteolysis may play a role also in the control of the physiological coagulation process. Activated protein C, which regulates the function of VIII, inactivates VIII through proteolytic degradation.[57,58] However, in the presence of factor IXa, phospholipid, and calcium, VIII becomes protected to a great extent against the attack of activated protein C.[59]

Surface binding protects VIII not only against proteolysis, but also against antibody binding. Studying the effect of specific inhibitors on the IXa-VIII complex, we observed that complex-bound VIII is protected against specific factor VIII antibodies.[60] Figure 5 shows that platelets alone also decrease the inactivation rate of factor VIII, and inactivation caused by the antibody is further decreased by the presence of factor IXa.[61] Factor VIII proved to be protected against factor VIII antibody also in the complex formed on the endothelial cell surface.[50] The effect of factor VIII antibody is decreased by phospholipid preparations as well. On the basis of the foregoing observations, it can be assumed that the protective effect of lipids might be utilized in the case of therapeutic factor VIII preparations. Interestingly, in experiments aimed at the oral administration of factor VIII entrapped in liposomes, the *in vivo* recovery of VIII:C was low both in hemophiliacs and in patients with von Willebrand's disease.[62,63] Obviously, in oral administration, conditions are entirely different from the usual route of i.v. administration. Therefore, the suggested procedure of Barrowcliffe et al.[64] expecting beneficial effects from factor VIII preparations enriched in phospholipids, seems promising in the treatment of hemophilia patients with inhibitors.

IV. SUMMARY

In summary, surface-bound VIII entails several advantages for the coagulation process. It significantly increases the rate of factor X activation and thereby the efficiency of the coagulation cascade. Surface binding stabilizes the activity of VIII$_t$ for prolonged times and renders the otherwise vulnerable protein protected against proteolytic degradation. The resistance also exercised against activated protein C makes it possible that physiological coagulation runs undisturbed even in the presence of the physiological inhibitor of factor VIII. Surface-bound VIII is protected against the inactivation effect of specific antibodies. This phenomenon may open new possibilities in the treatment of hemophilia patients with antibodies.

REFERENCES

1. **Hemker, H. C. and Kahn, M. J. P.,** Reaction sequence of blood coagulation, *Nature,* 215, 1201, 1967.
2. **Hougie, C., Denson, K. W. E., and Biggs, R.,** A study of the reaction product of factor VIII and factor IX by gel filtration, *Thromb. Diath. Haemorrh.,* 18, 211, 1967.
3. **Østerud, B. and Rapaport, S. I.,** Synthesis of intrinsic factor X activator. Inhibition of the function of formed activator by antibodies to factor VIII and to factor IX, *Biochemistry,* 9, 1854, 1970.
4. **Elōdi, S. and Váradi, K.,** Optimization of conditions for the catalytic effect of the factor IXa-factor VIII complex: probable role of the complex in the amplification of blood coagulation, *Thromb. Res.,* 15, 617, 1979.
5. **Hultin, M. B. and Nemerson, Y.,** Activation of factor X by factors IXa and VIII: a specific assay for factor IXa in the presence of thrombin activated factor VIII, *Blood,* 52, 928, 1978.
6. **Enfield, D. L., Ericsson, L. H., Fujikawa, K., Titani, K., Walsh, K. A., and Neurath, H.,** Bovine factor IX (Christmas factor). Further evidence of homology with factor X (Stuart factor) and prothrombin, *FEBS Lett.,* 47, 132, 1974.
7. **Váradi, K. and Elōdi, S.,** Purification and properties of human factor IXa, *Thromb. Haemost.,* 35, 576, 1976.
8. **DiScipio, R. G., Kurachi, K., and Davie, E. W.,** Activation of human factor IX (Christmas factor), *J. Clin. Invest.,* 61, 1528, 1978.
9. **Bucher, D., Nebelin, E., Thomsen, J., and Stenflo, J.,** Identification of γ-carboxyglutamic acid residues in bovine factors IX and X, and in a new vitamin K-dependent protein, *FEBS Lett.,* 68, 293, 1976.
10. **van Dieijen, G., Tans, G., Rosing, J., and Hemker, H. C.,** The role of phospholipid and factor VIIIa in the activation of bovine factor X, *J. Biol. Chem.,* 256, 3433, 1981.
11. **Suomela, H., Blombäck, M., and Blombäck, B.,** The activation of factor X evaluated by using synthetic substrates, *Thromb. Res.,* 10, 267, 1977.
12. **Brown, J. E., Baugh, R. F., and Hougie, C.,** The inhibition of the intrinsic generation of activated factor X by heparin and hirudin, *Thromb. Res.,* 17, 267, 1980.
13. **Elōdi, S., Váradi, K., and Vörös, E.,** Kinetics of formation of factor IXa-factor VIII complex on the surface of platelets, *Thromb. Res.,* 21, 695, 1981.
14. **Østerud, B., Rapaport, S. I., Schiffman, S., and Chong, M. M. Y.,** Formation of intrinsic factor-X-activator activity with special reference to the role of thrombin, *Br. J. Haematol.,* 21, 643, 1971.
15. **Neal, G. G. and Chavin, S. I.,** The role of factor VIII and IX in the activation of bovine blood coagulation factor X, *Thromb. Res.,* 16, 473, 1979.
16. **Neal, G. G. and Esnouf, M. P.,** Kinetic studies of the activation of factor X by factors IXa and VIII:C in the absence of thrombin, *Br. J. Haematol.,* 57, 123, 1984.
17. **Rick, M. E. and Hoyer, L. W.,** Thrombin activation of factor VIII: the effect of inhibitors, *Br. J. Haematol.,* 36, 585, 1977.
18. **Switzer, M. P. and McKee, P. A.,** Reaction of thrombin with human factor VIII/von Willebrand factor protein, *J. Biol. Chem.,* 255, 10606, 1980.
19. **Hoyer, L. W. and Trabold, N. C.,** The effect of thrombin on human factor VIII, *J. Lab. Clin. Med.,* 97, 50, 1981.
20. **Gitschier, L., Wood, W. I., Goralka, T. M., Wion, K. L., Chen, E. Y., Eaton, D. H., Vehar, G. A., Capon, D. J., and Lawn, R. M.,** Characterization of the human factor VIII gene, *Nature,* 312, 326, 1984.
21. **Wood, W. I., Capon, D. J., Simonsen, Ch. C., Eaton, D. L., Gitschier, J., Keyt, B., Seeburg, P. H., Smith, D. H., Hollingshead, P., Wion, K. L., Delwart, E., Tuddenham, E. G. D., Vehar, G. A., and Lawn, R. M.,** Expression of active human factor VIII from recombinant DNA clones, *Nature,* 312, 330, 1984.
22. **Vehar, G. A., Keyt, B., Eaton, D., Rodriguez, H., O'Brien, D. P., Rotblat, F., Oppermann, H., Keck, R., Wood, E. I., Harkins, R. N., Tuddenham, E. G. D., Lawn, R. M., and Capon, D. J.,** Structure of human factor VIII, *Nature,* 312, 337, 1984.

23. **Fulcher, C. A., Roberts, J. R., Holland, L. Z., and Zimmerman, T. S.,** Human factor VIII procoagulant protein. Monoclonal antibodies define precursor-product relationships and functional epitopes, *J. Clin. Invest.*, 76, 117, 1985.

24. **Vehar, G. A. and Davie, E. W.,** Preparation and properties of bovine factor VIII (antihemophilic factor), *Biochemistry*, 19, 401, 1980.

25. **Griffith, M. J., Reisner, H. M., Lundblad, R. L., and Roberts, H. R.,** Measurement of human factor IXa activity in an isolated factor X activation system, *Thromb. Res.*, 27, 289, 1982.

26. **Mertens, K. and Bertina, R. M.,** Activation of human coagulation factor VIII by activated factor X, the common product of the intrinsic and the extrinsic pathway of blood coagulation, *Thromb. Haemost.*, 47, 96, 1982.

27. **Mertens, K., van Wijngaarden, A., and Bertina, R. M.,** The role of factor VIII in the activation of human blood coagulation factor X by activated factor IX, *Thromb. Haemost.*, 54, 654, 1985.

28. **Rick, M. E.,** Activation of factor VIII by factor IXa, *Blood*, 59, 744, 1982.

29. **Rick, M. E. and Hoyer, L. W.,** Thrombin activation of factor VIII. II. A comparison of purified factor VIII and the low molecular weight factor VIII procoagulant, *Br. J. Haematol.*, 38, 107, 1978.

30. **Zwaal, R. F. A.,** Membrane and lipid involvement in blood coagulation, *Biochim. Biophys. Acta*, 515, 163, 1978.

31. **Zwaal, R. F. A. and Hemker, H. C.,** Blood cell membranes and haemostasis, *Haemostasis*, 11, 12, 1982.

32. **Chuang, T. F., Sargeant, R. B., and Hougie, C.,** The intrinsic activation of factor X in blood coagulation, *Biochim. Biophys. Acta*, 273, 287, 1972.

33. **Váradi, K. and Hemker, H. C.,** Kinetics of the formation of the factor X activating enzyme of the blood coagulation system, *Thromb. Res.*, 8, 303, 1976.

34. **Hoyer, L. W.,** The factor VIII complex: structure and function, *Blood*, 58, 1, 1981.

35. **Andersson, L. A. and Brown, J. E.,** Interaction of factor VIII - von Willebrand factor with phospholipid vesicles, *Biochem. J.*, 200, 161, 1981.

36. **Laimanovich, A., Hudry-Clergeon, G., Freyssinet, J. M., and Marguerie, G.,** Human factor VIII procoagulant activity and phospholipid interaction, *Biochim. Biophys. Acta*, 678, 132, 1981.

37. **Brodén, K., Brown, J. E., Carton, C., and Andersson, L.-A.,** Effect of phospholipid on factor VIII coagulant activity and coagulant antigen, *Thromb. Res.*, 30, 651, 1983.

38. **Yoshioka, A., Peake, I. R., Furlong, B. L. Furlong, R. A., Giddings, J. C., and Bloom, A. L.,** The interaction between factor VIII clotting antigen (VIIICAg) and phospholipid, *Br. J. Haematol.*, 55, 27, 1983.

39. **Hultin, M. B.,** Modulation of thrombin-mediated activation of factor VIII: C by calcium ions, phospholipid and platelets, *Blood*, 66, 53, 1985.

40. **Elödi, S.,** Surface oriented enzyme reactions in blood coagulation, in *Recent Advances in Haemotology, Immunology and Blood Transfusion*, Hollán, S. R., Bernát, I., Füst, Gy., Gárdos, Gy., and Sarkadi, B., Eds., John Wiley & Sons, Chichester, 1983, 107.

41. **Sewerin, K. and Andersson, L.-A.,** Binding of native and thrombin activated factor VIII to platelets, *Thromb. Res.*, 31, 695, 1983.

42. **Rosing, J., van Rijn, J. L. M. L., Bevers, E. M., van Dieijen, G., Confurius, P., and Zwaal, R. F. A.,** The role of activated human platelets in prothrombin and factor X activation, *Blood*, 65, 319, 1985.

43. **Wall, R. T. and Harker, L. A.,** The endothelium and thrombosis, *Ann. Rev. Med.*, 31, 361, 1980.

44. **Heimark, R. L. and Schwartz, S. M.,** Binding of coagulation factors IX and X to the endothelial cell surface, *Biochem. Biophys. Res. Commun.*, 111, 723, 1983.

45. **Stern, D. M., Drillings, M., Nossel, H. L., Hurlet-Jensen, A., LaGamma, K. S., and Oven, J.,** Binding of factors IX and IXa to cultured vascular endothelial cells, *Proc. Natl. Acad. Sci. U.S.A.*, 80, 4119, 1983.

46. **Rodgers, G. M. and Shuman, M. A.,** Prothrombin is activated on vascular endothelial cells by factor Xa and calcium, *Proc. Natl. Acad. Sci. U.S.A.*, 80, 7001, 1983.

47. **Stern, D. M., Drillings, M., Kisiel, W., Nawroth, P., Nossel, H. L., and LaGamma, K. S.,** Activation of factor IX bound to cultured bovine aortic endothelial cells, *Proc. Natl. Acad. Sci. U.S.A.*, 81, 913, 1984.

48. **Stern, D. M., Nawroth, P. P., Kisiel, W., Vehar, G., and Esmon, Ch. T.,** The binding of factor IXa to cultured bovine aortic endothelial cells. Induction of a specific site in the presence of factors VIII and X, *J. Biol. Chem.* 260, 6717, 1985.

49. **Stern, D., Nawroth, P., Handley, D., and Kisiel, W.,** An endothelial cell dependent pathway of coagulation, *Proc. Natl. Acad. Sci. U.S.A.*, 82, 2523, 1985.

50. **Elödi, S. and Váradi, K.,** Formation of the factor IXa/factor VIII complex on the surface of endothelial cells, *Blood*, 69, 442, 1987.

51. **McKee, P. A., Andersen, J. C., and Switzer, M. E.,** Molecular structural studies of human factor VIII, *Ann. N.Y. Acad. Sci.*, 240, 8, 1975.

52. **Rick, M. E., Popovsky, M. A., and Krizek, D. M.,** Degradation of factor VIII coagulant antigen by proteolytic enzymes, *Br. J. Haematol.,* 61, 477, 1985.
53. **Váradi, K., Marossy, K., Asbóth, G., Elõdi, P., and Elõdi, S.,** Inactivation of human factor VIII by granulocyte proteases, *Thromb. Haemost.,* 43, 45, 1980.
54. **Váradi, K. and Elõdi, S.,** Increased resistance of factor IXa-factor VIII complex against inactivation by granulocyte proteases, *Thromb. Res.,* 19, 571, 1980.
55. **Kárpáti, J., Váradi, K., and Elõdi, S.,** Effect of granulocyte proteases on human coagulation factors IX and X. The protective effect of calcium, *Hoppe-Seyler's Z. Physiol. Chem.,* 363, 521, 1982.
56. **Lollar, P., Knutson, G. J., and Fass, D. M.,** Stabilization of thrombin-activated porcine factor VIII:C by factor IXa and phospholipid, *Blood,* 63, 1303, 1984.
57. **Marlar, R. A., Kleiss, A. J., and Griffin, J. H.,** Human protein C: inactivation of factors V and VIII in plasma by the activated molecule, *Ann. N.Y. Acad. Sci.,* 370, 303, 1981.
58. **Fulcher, C. A., Gardiner, J. E., Griffin, J. H., and Zimmerman, T. S.,** Proteolytic inactivation of human factor VIII procoagulant protein by activated human protein C and its analogy with factor V, *Blood,* 63, 486, 1984.
59. **Bertina, R. M., Cupers, R., and van Wijngaarden, A.,** Factor IXa protects activated factor VIII against inactivation by activated protein C, *Biochem. Biophys. Res. Commun.,* 125, 177, 1984.
60. **Váradi, K. and Elõdi, S.,** Protection of platelet surface-bound factor IXa and VIII against specific inhibitors, *Thromb. Haemost.,* 47, 32, 1982.
61. **Elõdi, S. and Váradi, K.,** Altered properties of phospholipid-bound factor VIII, *Thromb. Res.,* 33, 557, 1984.
62. **Hemker, H. C., Hermens, W. T., Muller, A. D., and Zwaal, R. F. A.,** Oral treatment of haemophilia A by gastrointestinal absorption of factor VIII entrapped in liposomes, *Lancet,* 1, 8159, 1980.
63. **Sakuragawa, N., Niiya, K., and Kondo, S.,** Oral administration of factor VIII concentrate preparation in von Willebrand's disease, *Thromb. Res.,* 38, 681, 1985.
64. **Barrowcliffe, T. W., Kemball-Cook, G., and Gray, E.,** Binding to phospholipid protects factor VIII from inactivation by human antibodies, *J. Lab. Clin. Med.,* 101, 34, 1983.
65. **Elõdi, S. and Elõdi, P.,** Surface-governed molecular regulation of blood coagulation, *Mol. Aspect. Med.,* 6, 291, 1983.

Chapter 12

INTERACTION OF FACTOR VIII WITH vWf IN MIXED IMMUNORADIOMETRIC ASSAY SYSTEMS

T. Exner and J. Koutts

TABLE OF CONTENTS

I.   Introduction 228

II.   Methodological Details 228
       A.   Solid Phase Immunoradiometric Assays (IRMAs) 228
       B.   Antibodies..228
       C.   Sources of VIII..229

III.   Effect of Various Interacting Components on the Mixed IRMAs 229
       A.   Effect of Various Hemophilic Antibodies 229
       B.   Effect of Various Dissociating Agents...................................229
       C.   Effect of Thrombin in Various Types of VIII IRMAs..................230
       D.   Effects of Various VIII Preparations 230

IV.   Methodological Interpretation 231

V.   Summary 234

References...234

I. INTRODUCTION

The nature of the interaction between factor VIII coagulant activity (VIII:C) and the von Willebrand factor (vWf) in the VIII/vWf complex has been of interest for a long time. It is clear that though these two components are associated in most simple gel filtraton or precipitation procedures, they have different biological characteristics *in vivo* and are under separate genetic control.[1,2] They have been separated by chromatography in high ionic strength buffers[3,4] and also after exposure of the VIII/vWf complex to low concentrations of thrombin.[5,6]

Hemophilic antibodies directed against VIII antigen (VIII:Ag) have been used in immunoradiometric assays (IRMAs) for the detection of antigenic determinants on the procoagulant component.[7,8] Heterologous antibodies to vWf:Ag have been used to assess this more abundant and more antigenic component of the VIII/vWf complex.[9] More recently monoclonal antibodies to both VIII:Ag and vWf:Ag have been developed and used to characterize these individual factors.[10,11]

The aim of this present work was to investigate the association between VIII:Ag and vWf:Ag using one specific antibody to immunoimmobilize the VIII/vWf complex and a second ^{125}I labeled antibody for detecting other aspects of the bound complex. These reagents have been recently applied to a mixed radioimmunoassay.[12] Using this system the effect of various interacting components has been studied.

II. METHODOLOGICAL DETAILS

A. Solid Phase Immunoradiometric Assays (IRMAs)

Immulon "Removawell" (Dynatech Corp.,) 96-well plastic trays were coated with various antibodies at 10^{-2}-g/l concentration in 0.1 M sodium bicarbonate. After blocking with 5% bovine serum albumin (BSA, grade VI, Sigma, St. Louis, U.S.), the wells were washed with 0.2% BSA in 0.12 M sodium chloride, 0.02 M imidazole, 0.005 M sodium citrate, 0.05% sodium azide, and 20 KIU/ml Trasylol (Bayer, Leverkusen, G.D.R.) pH 7.2 buffer (diluent used throughout). (KIU, kallikrein inhibitory units.) Normal plasma or VIII preparations were then incubated in the wells for 16 h at 20°C. The wells were washed three times with the diluent and incubated with various preparations of VIII dissociating agents, such as thrombin or calcium chloride in 0.2% BSA diluent. After 16 h at 20°C, the wells were thoroughly washed and incubated with various ^{125}I labeled antibodies for an equal period. The wells were finally washed, separated, and counted for radioactivity.

B. Antibodies

Monoclonal antibodies to vWf:Ag were prepared by immunizing Balb/C mice with high molecular weight VIII/vWf complex and following now standard hybridization techniques[13] as previously described.[11] The two main monoclonals used were RPA 21-43, kindly donated by Dr. D. Joshua, Royal Prince Alfred Hospital, Sydney, and WM2C9 prepared locally by A. Kabral, Westmead Hospital, Westmead, NSW. Both showed specificity for antigen(s) absent from plasmas of patients with severe von Willebrand's disease but present in both normal plasmas and plasmas from hemophilic patients. These two antibodies showed little cross-reactivity. WM2C9 inhibited ristocetin co-factor activity and showed more reactivity with higher molecular weight forms of vWf:Ag than did RPA21-43. They were isolated from ascites using protein A Sepharose (Pharmacia, Uppsala, Sweden).

Hemophilic antibodies were kindly donated by patients of Dr. R. Herrman, Perth (W); Dr. E. Berry, Auckland, N.Z. (M); Prof. A. Bloom, Cardiff, Wales (D); and Dr. K. A. Rickard, Sydney (DW and KW). The latter (KW) antibody has been previously described[14] and had a titer of approximately 10,000 Bethesda units (BU)/mg protein after isolation using protein A Sepharose.

Antibodies were labeled with ^{125}I using the chloramine T method[15] isolated on a Sephadex G-25 column and applied at a dilution giving 10^5 cpm per well (0.2 ml) for the monoclonals and 5.10^3 cpm per well with the hemophilic antibodies. [125]I labeled antibodies specifically directed at VIII:Ag were isolated by the immunopurification procedure described by Holmberg et al.[16]

C. Sources of VIII

Blood from patients and volunteers was collected by clean venepuncture into one ninth volume of 0.11 *M* sodium citrate (pH 6.5). Plasma was removed after centrifugation at 1200 g for 10 min at 20°C. Normal plasma was pooled from at least five healthy volunteers. VIII of "intermediate" purity, cryoprecipitate, and cryosupernatant plasma were obtained from the Red Cross Blood Transfusion Service, Sydney. The VIII concentrate was gel filtered on a 2.5 × 70-cm column of Sepharose CL-4B (Pharmacia) in 0.15 *M* sodium chloride 0.05*M* tris chloride buffer pH 7.4 The void volume fractions were used at "high purity" VIII/vWf complex.

Calcium dissociated VIII was obtained as low molecular weight VIII:Ag by gel filtration of high purity VIII/vWf complex in 0.1% BSA buffer on Sepharose 4B-CL as recently described.[18]

VIII was assayed by the one-stage method of Margolis[17] utilizing an activated VIII deficient plasma substrate.

High purity human thrombin was obtained from Dr. John Fenton II (New York State Department of Health, Albany). Plasmin was purchased from Kabi AB (Stockholm, Sweden).

III. EFFECT OF VARIOUS INTERACTING COMPONENTS ON THE MIXED IRMA

A. Effect of Various Hemophilic Antibodies

Hemophilic antibodies isolated from several patient plasmas by elution from protein A Sepharose with 0.1 *M* glycine pH 2.5 buffer were used to coat microtiter wells. The various plasmas had anti-VIII titers, KW 10,000 BU/ml, M 1500 BU/ml, D 800 BU/ml, DW 700 BU/ml, and W 400 BU/ml, respectively.

The coated wells were exposed to dilutions of pooled normal plasma as a source of VIII/vWf complex and subsequently to ^{125}I labeled WM2C9 anti-VIII/vWf antibody. Results obtained after washing and counting are shown in Figure 1. It is apparent that only KW and to a lesser extent, DW bound significant amounts of VIII/vWf. Dilution of the normal plasma affected the binding of ^{125}I anti-VIII/vWf to a greater extent than in two-site assays for either VIII:Ag or vWf:Ag.

B. Effect of Various Dissociating Agents

Microtiter wells coated with hemophilic (KW) antibody were exposed to normal plasma as a source of VIII/vWf and subsequently washed thoroughly. The immunoimmobilized VIII was then exposed to serial dilutions of the following agents, calcium chloride initial concentration 1 *M*, sodium chloride initially 2 *M*, sodium EDTA at pH 7.0 initially 0.1 *M*, human thrombin initially 0.8 NIH U/ml, human plasmin initially 0.005 cu/ml, and lysine pH 7.0 initially 0.1 *M* (cu, casein units). After 16 h at 20°C, the wells were washed thoroughly and then exposed to ^{125}I labeled monoclonal antibody WM2C9 against VIII/vWf. After washing, the wells were separated and assessed in a gamma counter for radioactivity. Results obtained are shown in Figure 2. It is apparent that of the agents tested only thrombin significantly reduced ^{125}I activity bound to the wells, suggesting dissociation of the VIII/vWf. This occurred even at surprisingly low thrombin concentrations. The failure of plasmin to promote dissociation could be attributed to the presence of Trasylol in the buffers used. When Trasylol was deleted, plasmin induced dissociation even at low concentrations.

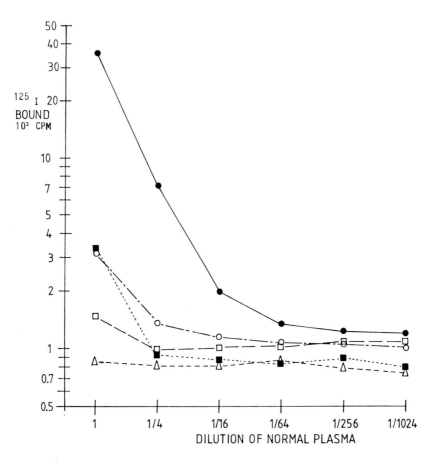

FIGURE 1.   Effect of coating microtiter wells with various antihemophilic antibodies in a mixed IRMA based on ^{125}I WM2C9 anti-VIII/vWf antibody. [125]I cpm plotted against dilution of normal plasma applied to coated wells. DW (○), KW (●), M (□), W (■), D (△).

C. Effect of Thrombin in Various Types of VIII IRMAs

Microtiter wells were coated with various antibodies. Two different monoclonal anti-VIII/ vWfs were used; WM2C9 and RPA 21-43 as well as the hemophilic KW anti VIII:Ag. The wells were then exposed to normal human plasma from which VIII/vWf was bound, presumably by antigenic determinants corresponding to the coating antibody. After exposure to dilutions of high purity human thrombin for 16 h at 20°C, residual associated VIII antigenic determinants were quantitated using various ^{125}I labeled antibodies.

Results obtained are shown in Figure 3. Thrombin failed to affect IRMAs in which antibodies with similar specificities were used for coating and as labeled antibodies. However, thrombin dissociated the VIII/vWf when either the coating antibody was the hemophilic antibody and the labeled antibodies were directed against VIII/vWf or when the coating antibodies were directed against VIII/vWf and the labeled antibody was the hemophilic antibody.

The actual yield of bound ^{125}I in the latter system was much less than in the former.

D. Effect of Various VIII Preparations

The effect of thrombin on VIII/vWf from various sources was investigated. The mixed IRMA based on solid phase hemophilic antibody (KW) and ^{125}I labeled monoclonal anti-vWf RPA 21-43 was used.

Various VIII preparations were applied at dilutions having equal VIII:Ag concentrations

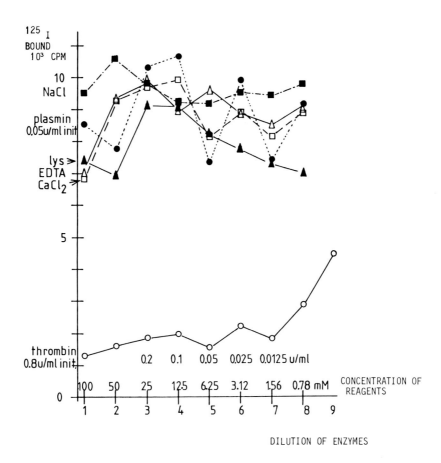

FIGURE 2.   Effect of various agents on VIII complex in the mixed IRMA system. [125]I WM2C9 anti-VIII/vWf antibody binding to VIII complex on KW anti-VIII:Ag coated wells plotted against dilution of $CaCl_2$ (1 *M* initially □), NaCl (2 *M* initially ■), EDTA (0.1 *M* initially △), thrombin (0.8 U/ml initially ○), plasmin (0.05 cu/ml initially ●), lysine (0.1 *M* initially ▲).

(0.5 U/ml in the two-site VIII:Ag IRMA) to KW coated wells. These were successively washed, treated with several dilutions of thrombin for 6 h, and finally exposed to ^{125}I labeled RPA 21-43.

Results obtained are shown in Figure 4.

More purified VIII preparations, for example cryoprecipitate and gel filtered high molecular weight VIII/vWf, showed greater binding of the ^{125}I labeled antibody than VIII from normal plasma, suggesting that VIII:Ag in these preparations was associated with more VIII/vWf than that in normal plasma. However, the VIII/vWf in these more purified preparations was insensitive to thrombin cleavage when immunoimmobilized. VIII/vWf from serum or calcium dissociated VIII:Ag failed to bind significant levels of labeled antibody to the solid phase antihemophilic antibody.

IV. METHODOLOGICAL INTERPRETATION

VIII/vWf bound to certain hemophilic antibodies on microtiter wells was found to contain some vWf:Ag detectable with ^{125}I labeled monoclonal antibodies to vWf:Ag or VIII/vWf.

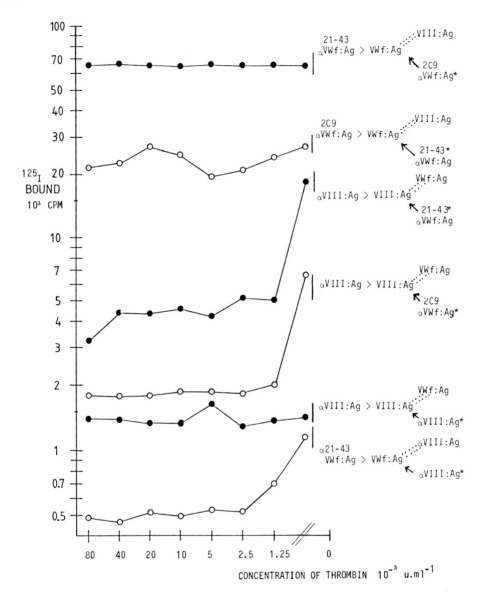

FIGURE 3.   Effect of thrombin on various IRMA methods for VIII complex from normal plasma. ^{125}I cpm bound plotted against thrombin concentration. Code for each assay system shows coating antibody specificity (next to bar) pointing to VIII component bound and labeled antibody (asterisked) binding on right. The bond linking VIII:Ag and vWf moieties in the VIII complex is shown by a double line.

The possibility that the hemophilic antibodies used may have contained components binding vWf:Ag directly was considered unlikely for a number of reasons. Solid phase two-site IRMAs for VIII:Ag using these hemophilic antibodies showed no binding of the vWf:Ag from various severe hemophilic plasmas. Furthermore, no abnormalities in vWf or vWf:Ag were observed in the hemophilic patients who donated their antibodies.

Hemophilic antibodies varied somewhat in their capacity to bind vWf:Ag associated with VIII:Ag, although all of those used in this study performed well in two-site VIII:Ag IRMAs. The reason for this is not clear. It is possible that some antibodies may weaken the association between VIII:Ag and vWf:Ag by binding to particularly sensitive allosteric sites. Conversely, the binding of antibody may interfere with the lability of the VIII/vWf to other agents. Thus, although high calcium and sodium chloride concentrations dissociate the VIII/vWf in free

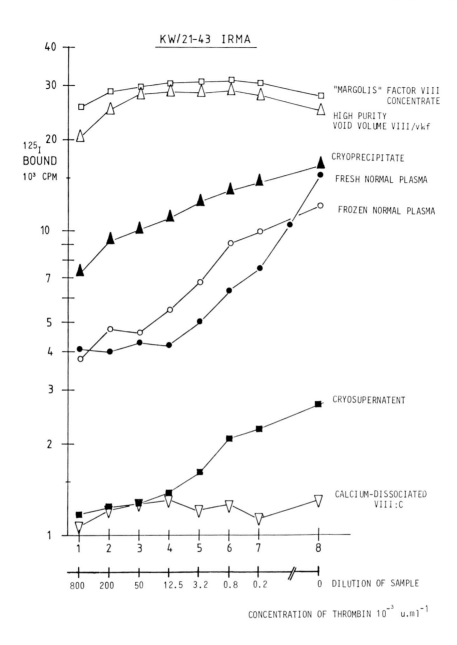

FIGURE 4. Effect of thrombin on VIII complex in various VIII preparations. [125]I RPA21-43 anti-vWf antibody bound to VIII complex on anti-VIII:Ag coated wells plotted against thrombin dilution.

solution,[3,4] they appeared to have little effect on the immunoimmobilized complex detectable by the mixed IRMA.

The results presented here demonstrate that the bond between VIII:Ag and vWf:Ag which is involved in the mixed IRMA is sensitive to dissociation by thrombin. Two-site IRMAs for VIII:Ag and vWf:Ag using the individual antibodies from the mixed IRMA were unaffected by thrombin. These results confirm the observatons of various researchers using other techniques, that thrombin induces the dissociation of VIII:Ag from vWf:Ag.[5,6,19,20]

It is known that thrombin has no apparent effect on vWf:Ag or its functional expression as vWf, but induces several cleavages in the VIII:Ag moiety.[21,22] The cleavages occurring with low concentrations of thrombin result in activation of VIII:C[22] whereas higher thrombin concentrations destroy this activity and result in lower molecular weight fragments such as those seen in serum. These cleavages do not seem to affect most IRMAs for VIII:Ag based on human antibodies.[7,8,16] However, they do affect many of the IRMAs using monoclonal antibodies to VIII:Ag[10,23,24] probably because these bind at individual, more specific epitopes.

The results obtained with the mixed IRMA also suggest some unusual features in the stoichiometry of VIII:Ag and vWf:Ag in the VIII/vWf. Thus, more vWf:Ag is associated with each VIII:Ag in the more purified VIII preparations. These more aggregated forms of VIII appear to be not as sensitive to thrombin cleavage as native VIII/vWf from normal plasma. Complex changes may occur during such VIII isolation procedures.[23] Thus, it is clear that VIII isolated by gel exclusion contains high molecular weight complexes of fibrin(ogen) and probably fibronectin as well as VIII:Ag and vWf:Ag-vWf. This has been suggested by studies in which monoclonal antibodies to fibrin(ogen) were obtained from mice immunized with "void volume" VIII/vWf.[25] It is possible that these other components of the VIII/vWf protect the immunoimmobilized VIII in the mixed IRMA from thrombin cleavage.

Although information on the lability of the VIII/vWf obtained by mixed IRMAs is not completely consistent with results obtained by other methods, this simple technique has considerable potential for investigating interactions between components of this complex.

V. SUMMARY

Microtiter wells coated with a high titer hemophilic antibody to VIII:Ag were found to bind not only directly VIII:Ag from normal human plasma, but also indirectly to vWf:Ag, detectable by the binding of various ^{125}I labeled monoclonal antibodies to vWf:Ag. Such mixed solid phase IRMAs were used to investigate the association between these two components of the factor VIII complex.

High purity thrombin at concentrations down to 10^{-3} U/ml dissociated approximately 70% of the vWf from VIII:Ag as detected by this mixed IRMA. Thrombin did not affect any two-site IRMA for either vWf or VIII:Ag individually. Factor VIII complex immunoimmobilized from normal plasma was much more sensitive to thrombin cleavage than that bound from more purified VIII preparations which were found to contain an increased ratio of VIII vWf per VIII:Ag. EDTA or calcium at concentrations up to 1 M failed to dissociate the components of immuno-immobilized VIII complex.

REFERENCES

1. **Hoyer, L. W.,** The factor VIII complex: structure and function, *Blood,* 58, 1, 1981.
2. **Koutts, J., Howard, M. A., and Firkin, B. G.,** Factor VIII physiology and pathology in man, *Prog. Hematol.,* 9, 115, 1978.
3. **Owen, W. G. and Wagner, R. H.,** Antihemophilic factor: separation of an active fragment following dissociation by salts or detergents, *Thromb. Diath. Haemorrh.,* 27, 502, 1972.
4. **Austen, D. E. G.,** Factor VIII of small molecular weight and its aggregation, *Br. J. Haematol.,* 27, 89, 1974.
5. **Cooper, H. A., Reisner, F. F., Hall, M., and Wagner, R. H.,** Effects of thrombin treatment on preparations of factor VIII and the Ca^{2+}-dissociated small active fragment, *J. Clin. Invest.,* 56, 751, 1975.
6. **Van Mourik, J. A., Lautinga, P. H. G., and Hellings, J. A.,** The effect of coagulation on the association of VIII CAG with VIII RAG, *Thromb. Haemost.,* 46 (Abstr. 793), 254, 1981.
7. **Lazarchick, J. and Hoyer, L. W.,** Immunoradiometric measurement of the factor VIII procoagulant antigen, *J. Clin. Invest.,* 62, 1048, 1978.

8. **Peake, I. R., Bloom, A. L., Giddings, J. C., and Ludlam, C. A.,** An immunoradiometric assay for procoagulant factor VIII antigen, *Br. J. Haematol., 42*, 269, 1979.

9. **Ruggieri, Z. M., Mannucci, P. M., Jeffcote, S. L., and Ingram, G. I. C.,** Immunoradiometric assay of factor VIII-related antigen, with observations in 32 patients with von Willebrand's disease, *Br. J. Haematol., 31,* 129, 1976.

10. **Stel, H. V., Veerman, E. C. T., Huisman, J. G., Janssen, M. C., and Van Mourik, J. A.,** A rapid one step immunoradiometric assay for factor VIII procoagulant antigen utilizing monoclonal antibodies, *Thromb. Haemost., 50,* 860, 1983.

11. **Francis, S. E., Joshua, D. E., Exner, T., and Kronenberg, H.,** Monoclonal antibodies to human FVIII RAG and FVIIIC, *Pathology, 17,* 579, 1985.

12. **Thomas, K. B., Howard, M. A., Koutts, J., and Firkin, B. G.,** Simplified immunoradiometric assay for human factor VIII coagulant antigen, *Br. J. Haematol., 51,* 47, 1982.

13. **Kohler, G. and Milstein, C.,** Continuous cultures of fused cells secreting antibody of predefined specificity, *Nature, 256,* 495, 1975.

14. **Exner, T. and Rickard, K. A.,** Anammestic response to high purity porcine AHF, *Thromb. Haemost., 50,* 623, 1983.

15. **Hunter, W. M. and Greenwood, F. C.,** Preparation of iodine 131-labelled human growth hormone of high specific activity, *Nature, 194,* 495, 1962.

16. **Holmberg, L., Burge, L., Nilsson, R., and Nilsson, I. M.,** Measurement of antihaemophilic factor antigen (VIII:CAG) with a solid phase immunoradiometric method based on homologous non-haemophilic antibodies, *Scand. J. Haematol., 23,* 17, 1979.

17. **Margolis, J.,** An improved procedure for accurate assays of factor VIII, *Pathology, 11,* 149, 1979.

18. **Exner, T., Green, D., and Koutts, J.,** Requirement for carrier protein in the dissociation of antihaemophilic factor from von Willebrand factor, *Thromb. Res.,* in press.

19. **Hoyer, L. W. and Trabold, N. C.,** The effect of thrombin on human factor VIII, *J. Lab. Clin. Med., 97,* 50, 1981.

20. **Muller, H. P., van Tilburg, W. H., Bertina, R. M., and Veltkamp, J. J.,** Immunological studies on the relationship between FVIII related antigen and FVIII procoagulant activity, *Thromb. Res., 20,* 85, 1980.

21. **Weinstein, M., Chute, L., and Deykin, D.,** Analysis of factor VIII coagulant antigen in normal, thrombin treated and haemophilic plasma, *Proc. Natl. Acad. Sci. U. S. A., 78,* 5137, 1981.

22. **Weinstein, M. J., Fulcher, C. A., Chute, L. E., and Zimmerman, T. S.,** Apparent molecular weight of purified human factor VIII procoagulant protein compared with purified and plasma factor VIII procoagulant protein antigen, *Blood, 62,* 114, 1983.

23. **Muller, H. P., van Tilburg, N. H., Derks, J., Klein, E., and Bertina, R. M.,** A monoclonal antibody to FVIIIC produced by a mouse hybridoma, *Blood, 58,* 1000, 1981.

24. **Brown, J., Le Phuc Thuy, Carton, C. L., and Hougie, C.,** Studies on a monoclonal antibody to human factor VIII coagulant activity with a description of a facile two site factor VIII coagulant antigen assay, *J. Lab. Clin. Med., 101,* 793, 1983.

25. **Francis, S., Joshua, D. G., Exner, T., and Kronenberg, H.,** Some studies with a monoclonal antibody directed against human fibrinogen, *Am. J. Hematol., 18,* 111, 1985.

Chapter 13

INTERACTION OF CELL PROTEASES WITH FACTOR VIII AND VON WILLEBRAND FACTOR

Margaret A. Howard

TABLE OF CONTENTS

I. Introduction 238
    A.   Scope of the Chapter 238
    B.   Nature of Factor VIII... 238
    C.   Nature of vWf... 238

II. Interaction with Plasmin 240
    A.   F.VIII 240
    B.   vWf 241
        1.   Structural and Functional Changes 241
        2.   Effect of Plasmin Degradation Products of vWf on
               Platelet Aggregation 242
    C.   *In Vivo* Investigations 242

III. Interaction of Protein C with F.VIII and vWf............................. 242
    A.   F.VIII 242
        1.   F.VIII:C 242
        2.   F.VIII:Ag 243
    B.   vWf 243
    C.   *In Vivo* Considerations 243

IV. Interaction of Leukocyte Proteases with F.VIII and vWf 243
    A.   F.VIII 243
    B.   vWf 244

V. vWf Degradation Products 244
    A.   Identification and Molecular Chemistry 244
    B.   Formation and Enzymes Responsible................................. 244
    C.   Clinical Significance 248

VI. Technical and Clinical Consequences 248
    A.   Purified Material 248
    B.   Infusion Material 249
    C.   Diagnostic Problems... 249

VII. Summary 249

Acknowledgments 250

References... 251

I. INTRODUCTION

A. Scope of the Chapter

Normal hemostasis is achieved by a complex series of interactions between the coagulation factors, blood cells, and the vessel walls. Some of these interactions involve proteolytic cleavage of the coagulation proteins resulting in either augmentation or destruction of functional activity. This chapter is concerned specifically with the effects of cell proteases on the factor VIII/von Willebrand factor (F.VIII/vWf) complex.

F.VIII and vWf are two vital components of the normal hemostatic mechanism. Evidence of their importance is clearly demonstrated by the severity of the bleeding disorders hemophilia and von Willebrand's disease which result from their absence or abnormality. Rapid changes in our understanding of the structure and function of these two proteins have occurred during recent years resulting in some confusion of nomenclature. In an attempt to standardize, the terminology and abbreviations used in this chapter are in agreement with those adopted by the International Committee of Thrombosis and Haemostasis in 1985 and reproduced in Table 1.

Many proteolytic enzymes have been reported to cleave F.VIII and vWf, but the following discussion is restricted to those proteases which are released from cells with which F.VIII/vWf could come into contact during the hemostatic process, i.e., proteases released from the endothelial cells and the circulating blood cells. A listing of these proteases and an overview of their effects on F.VIII and vWf are presented in Table 2.

B. Nature of F.VIII

Other chapters in this series have dealt with structural and functional aspects of the F.VIII molecule so that a brief account is sufficient in this context. F.VIII expresses procoagulant activity (F.VIII:C) *in vivo* acting as a co-factor in the activation of factor X (F.X) by factor IX_a (F.IX) in the presence of calcium ions and phospholipids. This activity is measured *in vitro* either by a clotting assay or by the use of a chromogenic substrate. The antigenic activity of F.VIII (F.VIII:Ag), previously referred to as VIII:CAg, is measured either by an immunoradiometric assay or by an enzyme-linked immunoabsorbant assay (ELISA) using either human or monoclonal antibodies. The circulating concentration of F.VIII has been estimated to be 100 to 200 ng/ml.[1]

Recent cloning and purification has enabled amino acid sequencing and structural analysis.[1-5] These investigators suggest that the size of the F.VIII molecule is consistent with the reported isolation from plasma of a single chain glycoprotein with a molecular weight (MW) of 330 kD.[3,6] During purification, the F.VIII molecule seems to be particularly susceptible to proteolytic degradation, so that most purified preparations demonstrate on sodium-dodecyl sulfate (SDS) polyacrylamide gel electrophoresis (PAGE) a series of polypeptides of MW ranging from 80 to 210 kD. However, highly purified preparations of F.VIII free from proteases are reported to be extremely stable if calcium ions are included in the buffering solution.[3] It has been suggested from experiments investigating the effect of thrombin and protein C on F.VIII:C activity that the active site involved in the conversion of F.X to F.Xa is located on a 90-kD polypeptide.[7]

Recent hybridization experiments using complimentary DNA cloning technology detected mRNA for F.VIII:C in a number of tissues.[8,9] Tissues included liver and spleen hepatocytes, lymph nodes, and kidney. These cells may have the potential for synthesizing F.VIII:C; however, the exact site(s) of synthesis will remain unclear until F.VIII with clotting activity is obtained from a single cell species cultured *in vitro*.

C. Nature of vWf

vWf is intimately involved in the adhesion of platelets to the endothelial cell surface of blood vessels at the site of injury. This interaction involves binding of the vWf molecule

Table 1
NOMENCLATURE AND ABBREVIATIONS FOR
FACTOR VIII AND VON WILLEBRAND FACTOR

Factor VIII	**F.VIII**
Procoagulant activity	F.VIII:C
Antigen	F.VIII:Ag
von Willebrand factor	**vWf**
Ristocetin co-factor activity	RCoF
Botrocetin co-factor activity	BCoF
Antigen	vWf:Ag
Factor VIII/von Willebrand factor complex	F.VIII/vWf

Table 2
EFFECTS OF CELL PROTEASES ON F.VIII AND vWf

	Plasmin	Protein C	ELP/CLP
F.VIII:C	RD	RD	RD
F.VIII:Ag	SD	SD	NK
RCoF	SD	NE	RD
BCoF	NK	NK	NK
vWF:Ag	SD	NE	NK

Note: Table 2 lists the proteases described in this chapter and their known effects on the F.VIII/ vWf complex. RD — rapid decay, SD — slow decay, NE — no effect, and NK — effect not known.

to glycoprotein Ib on the platelet surface,[10-12] but the site on the vWf molecule involved in this interaction is at present unknown. *In vitro* vWf functional activity is measured either by the skin bleeding time,[13] adhesion of platelets to a column of glass beads,[14] or by use of the ristocetin co-factor (RCoF),[15] and botrocetin co-factor (BCoF) assays.[16,17] The antigenic activity of vWf (vWf:Ag) is measured by a number of immunological techniques, including Laurell rocket immunoelectroporesis, immunoradiometric assay, crossed-immunoelectrophoresis (CIE), ELISA assay, and SDS-agarose gel electrophoresis.[18,19] The circulating concentration of vWf has been estimated to be approximately 10 μg/ml.[20]

The molecular structure of circulating vWf remains uncertain; however, *in vitro* heterogeneity is apparent. SDS-agarose gel analysis and CIE indicate that the molecule exists as a series of polymers of MW ranging from 1000 to 20,000 kD.[21,22] Figure 1A and Figure 4, lane A show, respectively, a radio-CIE and a multimeric SDS-agarose analysis of normal vWf. On reduced SDS-PAGE a single polypeptide band with a MW of 220 to 270 kD is present.[20,23,24] This polypeptide has the ability to form intramolecular disulfide bonds and thus aggregates into a series of polymers. It is possible to obtain preparations of vWf which contain limited polymeric forms.[25] From investigations such as these it appears that RCoF activity and skin bleeding time are dependent on the presence of high MW polymers of vWf.[26-31] A function for the lower MW polymers of vWf has yet to be identified.

Both RCoF activity and vWf:Ag activity have been isolated from cultures of endothelial cells and cultures of megakaryocytes and in a cell free system using RNA isolated from endothelial cells.[32-36] The presence of vWf:Ag in tissue sections containing these cell types has been identified using immunological methods.[37,38] Thus, it is reasonable to imply that these cells are the *in vivo* site of synthesis. Endothelial cells also act as a storage site for vWf, releasing it into the circulation in response to exercise and agents such as adrenalin and desamino-D-arginine vasopressin (DDAVP).[39-42]

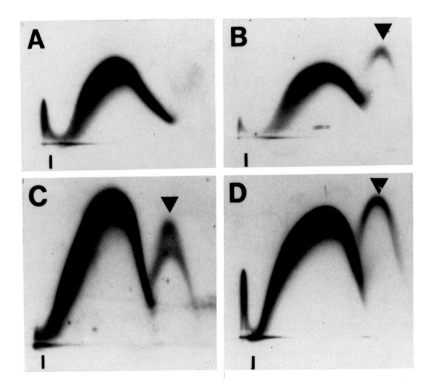

FIGURE 1.   An autoradiograph of a radio-CIE in agarose gel containing ^{125}I rabbit anti-human vWf of (A) normal plasma. (B) normal serum. (C) F.VIII concentrate (Commonwealth Serum Laboratories of Australia), and (D) plasma from a patient with disseminated intravascular coagulation. The solid bars indicate the sample well, and the arrows identify the precipitant peak of vWf:Frag.

II. INTERACTION WITH PLASMIN

Plasmin is the stable activation product of plasminogen which is released from endothelial cells and acts as part of the fibrinolytic system. Substances which activate plasminogen include factor XII (F.XII), kallikrein, streptokinase, urokinase, and tissue plasminogen activator. Although the physiological substrates for plasmin are fibrinogen and fibrin, plasmin will selectively cleave arginyl-X and lysyl-X bonds in many other proteins. Both plasminogen and plasmin are available commercially or can be generated either *in vivo* or *in vitro* by the use of streptokinase and urokinase.

A. F.VIII

Incubation of plasmin with purified F.VIII results in a rapid loss of procoagulant activity.[43-47] This loss is time and concentration dependent.[43-47] Early reports correlated the loss of functional activity with changes in the structure of the F.VIII/vWf complex using SDS-PAGE electrophoresis (PAGE). These experiments were probably demonstrating changes in the structure of the vWf molecule rather than F.VIII since the molecular ratio of vWf to F.VIII is 50:1.[1,20] In one set of experiments, a close correlation was noted between loss of F.VIII:C activity and the destruction of an 85-kD subunit visualized on SDS-agarose electrophoresis.[43]

Changes in F.VIII:Ag levels as a result of interaction with plasmin occur more slowly than the loss of VIII:C activity.[46,48] Direct measurement of F.VIII:Ag levels has confirmed previous observations that the inhibitor neutralizing activity of F.VIII:C was destroyed by plasmin more slowly than procoagulant activity.[49] These results suggest that the first cleavage sites on F.VIII are at or near the site for expression procoagulant activity. Sites on the F.VIII molecule involved in the interaction with antibodies used for measurement of F.VIII:Ag are on that part of the molecule protected from early attack by plasmin.

Loss of F.VIII:C and F.VIII:Ag activities following incubation with plasmin can also be demonstrated in plasma, although the concentration of plasmin required is much greater than for purified material.[48,50] In plasma the F.VIII:Ag levels also decrease more slowly than the clotting activity following incubation with plasmin. The different concentration requirements for plasma may be related to the presence of the plasmin inhibitors, alpha 1 anti-plasmin and alpha 2 macroglobulin, and to the formation of inhibitor-plasmin complexes in plasma. The possiblity that these inhibitor-plasmin complexes retain residual proteolytic activity towards F.VIII has been investigated.[51,52] Some residual activity of the complex has been demonstrated by one group,[51] but it is thought to be insignificant by others.[52]

While the proteolytic products of plasmin digestion of F.VIII have no anticoagulant effect in the F.VIII:C clotting assay,[44] surprisingly, they have been found to augment the apparent F.VIII:C activity when mixed with normal plasma.[44] The mechanism for this effect is at present unknown.

B. vWf
1. Structural and Functional Changes

Structural changes to the vWf molecule have been seen as a change to a more rapidly migrating molecule on CIE, with a concomitant apparent increase in vWf:Ag levels.[50,53] Such changes indicate the presence of a molecule of lower MW which migrates more rapidly in the immunoelectrophoretic assay frequently used for its quantification.[25,53] More frequently SDS-PAGE analysis has been used to assess structural changes in the vWf molecule following plasmin digestion. A progressive cleavage of the basic 220-kD reduced subunit of vWf:Ag to lower MW polypeptides was observed during a 24-h plasmin digestion. At the end of 24 h in a reduced system, protein bands ranging in size from 17.5 to 103 kD have been reported.[49,53-55] These bands stain strongly with periodic acid-Schiffs stain, indicating the presence of carbohydrate.[53,54]

Modification of the carbohydrate structure of the vWf molecule has been achieved by sequential removal of sialic acid, hexoses, and galactose.[56] This carbohydrate modified vWf was more susceptible to proteolytic degradation by plasmin than native vWf rapidly losing its multimeric structure. Possibly carbohydrates serve to protect the molecule from enzymic attack.

This early work has recently been elegantly extended by the use of SDS-agarose electrophoresis which reveals the multimeric structure of vWf.[57] Using this technique a progressive loss of the high MW multimers of vWf following plasmin digestion was observed with release of a 34-kD polypeptide fragment. Interestingly the multimeric structure was preserved while reduced SDS-PAGE demonstrated that no intact 220-kD subunit remained following prolonged plasmin digestion for 60 h. Thus many of the plasmin cleavage sites lie within disulfide loops.[57] These workers were unable to demonstrate proteolysis of vWf:Ag in plasma, fibrin clots, or euglobulin precipitates, suggesting that although purified vWf:Ag acts as a substrate for plasmin it is unlikely that this is the case *in vivo*.

While structural changes of vWf occur under relatively mild proteolytic conditions RCoF activity is more resistant. Even when proteolysis is continued for 24 h, some 20 to 70% of the starting RCoF activity remains.[49,53-55,57] These results indicate that an intact vWf molecule is not essential for expression of RCoF activity. It may be that the activity resides on specific sites which are exposed on the larger multimeric forms of the vWf molecule, concealed in the smaller forms, and again revealed by proteolysis. Such findings have interesting implications for the current interpretation of the molecular abnormalities seen in some variant forms of von Willebrands disease.[18,19]

2. Effect of Plasmin Degradation Products of vWf on Platelet Aggregation

Some controversy surrounds the effect of vWf plasmin cleaved degradation products on platelet aggregation. Reports from the early 1970s showed inhibition of adenosine diphosphate (ADP)-induced platelet aggregation using either platelet rich plasma (PRP) or washed platelets by a dialysable fraction from human vWf plasmin digests.[58-60] That this inhibitory activity was due to vWf cleavage products and not those from contaminating fibrinogen was confirmed by the observation that digested vWd plasma had no effect on ADP-induced aggregation of washed platelets.[60] Similar digests of normal and hemophilic plasma or normal serum are inhibitory. Recently this work has been extended[61] to demonstrate that streptokinase-digested afibrinogenemic plasma inhibits ADP- and collagen-induced aggregation of PRP and collagen-induced release of radiolabeled serotonin from PRP.

This picture is clouded by later reports that plasmin digests of human vWf have no effect on either ADP-induced platelet aggregation or microvascular permeability.[62,63] The differences in these observations may result from the use of vWf of varying purity by different investigators and by the use of different preparations of plasmin. The use of highly purified reagents would help resolve these differences.

C. *In Vivo* Investigations

A limited amount of information is available concerning the effect of plasmin on F.VIII and vWf *in vivo*. It might be expected that competition among the various substrates of plasmin *in vivo* and the presence of its inhibitors may make F.VIII and vWf unlikely candidates for proteolysis. On the other hand, increased concentration of plasmin at sites of vascular injury may occur. One study showing that the F.VIII:C level fell dramatically during the first 30 min of streptokinase therapy[57] suggests that at least under these conditions plasmin cleaves F.VIII.

The appearence of a fast migrating precipitant peak on vWF:Ag CIE (discussed fully in Section V) in patients receiving urokinase therapy implies proteolysis of vWf during this therapy presumably by plasmin.[64] During streptokinase therapy a surprising sequence of changes in vWf:Ag levels and vWf structure occur.[57] During the first 5 to 20 min a decrease in vWf:Ag and RCoF activities and loss of the high MW multimers were noted. However, by 30 to 90 min a dramatic increase in the vWf:Ag and RCoF activities had occurred together with an increase in the high MW multimers. Prolonged streptokinase therapy resulted in a decrease in RCoF activity and a steady loss of the high MW vWf multimers. These observations are consistent with the view that during streptokinse therapy there is degradation of the vWf molecule which may be difficult to observe in some patients due to a simultaneous induction of release of newly formed vWf molecules from storage sites.

III. INTERACTION OF PROTEIN C WITH F.VIII AND vWf

Protein C is an inactive Vitamin K dependent glycoprotein synthesized by endothelial cells and released into the circulation.[65,66] Protein C consists of a heavy and light chain which have a combined MW of 62 kD. It is converted to active protein C (APC) by thrombin which cleaves the heavy chain releasing a short polypeptide of approximately 12 residues. APC has serine amidase activity which can be inhibited by diisopropyl-flurophosphate and acts *in vitro* as an anticoagulant in the presence of phospholipid and calcium ions. This anticoagulant activity may be demonstrated in the presence of phospholipid and calcium ions as a prolonged activated partial thromboplastin time and reduced factor V(F.V) and F.VIII activities.[65,67,68]

A. F.VIII
1. F.VIII:C

The F.VIII:C activity of a purified F.VIII or plasma is rapidly destroyed by APC in the presence of phospholipid and calcium ions.[7,48,68,69] Loss of F.VIII:C activity is paralleled by a corresponding change in the molecular structure. Using a purified preparation of F.VIII, APC has been shown to cleave all fractions of F.VIII with a molecular weight greater than 92 kD producing a polypeptide with a molecular weight of 45 kD, while leaving a doublet at 79 to 80 kD intact.[7] Activation of F.VIII:C by thrombin makes the molecule even more susceptible to cleavage by APC, so that the inactivation process occurs 30 times faster in a sample of activated F.VIII:C than in an unactivated sample.[68]

2. F.VIII:Ag

The levels fo F.VIII:Ag of a highly purified concentrate of F.VIII were only slowly reduced by high concentrations of APC,[48] suggesting that the epitopes for the antibodies used in these assays are carried by the lower MW fragments produced by APC. While F.VIII:C activity is rapidly destroyed by APC in a plasma or purified system, no change in the F.VIII:Ag level was noted in a plasma system.[48]

B. vWf

No effects of APC on either the structure or function of vWf have been reported yet.

C. *In Vivo* Considerations

In 1980 it was suggested that the rare association of F.VIII:C and F.V:C deficiency may be due to an absence of a protein C inhibitor resulting in continuous *in vivo* destruction of these two clotting factors.[70] However, more recent measurements of protein C, its inhibitor, and F.VIII:Ag and F.V antigen levels in patients with a combined F.VIII:C and F.V:C deficiency suggest that a mechanism involving protein C inactivation of F.VIII:C and F.V may not be involved in this bleeding disorder.[71-73]

IV. INTERACTION OF LEUKOCYTE PROTEASES WITH F.VIII AND vWf

Leukocytes contain a number of proteases which are released into the surrounding medium during phagocytosis[74] and coagulation.[75] Two main groups of proteases have been identified and isolated from polymorphonuclear (PMN) cells; these are elastase-like protease (ELP) and chymotrypsin-like protease (CLP).

ELP and CLP while specifically hydrolysing the peptide bond adjacent to the carboxyl group of alanine and phenylalanine, respectively, have been shown to have a broad proteolytic spectrum. Proteins susceptible to attack by these enzymes include fibrinogen,[76,77] complement,[78] fibronectin,[79] coagulation factors,[77,80] plasminogen,[81] and platelet glycoprotein Ib.[82] Since these enzymes have such a broad specificity the suggestion has been made that they may be partly responsible for the coagulation deficiency syndrome seen in cases of disseminated coagulation, acute leukemia, and septicemia.[75,77] Indeed, ELP/antitrypsin complexes have been identified in patients with acute leukemia or disseminated intravascular coagulation,[77,83] but only a few of these patients actually showed reduced levels of coagulation factors.

A. F.VIII

A number of investigators have studied the effect of ELP and CLP on F.VIII:C using either crude leukocyte extracts or enzymes purified from human PMN cells. Under all the experimental procedures used, F.VIII:C was rapidly inactivated by ELP and more slowly by CLP.[76,77,80,84,85] A rapid decrease in F.VIII:C was also noted in a plasma sample exposed to ELP and CLP, indicating proteolysis even in the presence of potent antiproteases.[77]

Cooperation between these two enzymes occurs such that the rate of loss of F.VIII:C activity is greater when both are present than for either alone.[85] Diisopropyl-flurophosphate was an effective inhibitor of this decay.[80] It has also been noted that the formation of a

F.VIII/F.IXa complex in the presence of calcium ions and phospholipid provides protection for both coagulation factors against attack by a crude extract of granulocyte proteases.[84] This protection may be due to the inaccessibility of the susceptible peptide bonds in the F.VIII/IXa complex.

B. vWf

RCoF activity is destroyed by incubation either with purified ELP and CLP or with a crude granulocyte extract, presumably as a result of proteolysis.[76,85] An apparent increase in vWf:Ag level and an increase in the electrophoretic migration of the vWf:Ag precipitant peak on CIE were observed following loss of RCoF activity further suggesting that a proteolytic cleavage of the molecule had taken place.[76]

V. vWf DEGRADATION PRODUCTS

Our current understanding of the molecular changes which occur in the vWf protein following release from the endothelial cell is very limited, and no suggested route for its elimination from the circulation has yet been proposed. Recently a protein has been detected which is thought to be a degradation product of vWf.[64,86,87] It shows partial immunological identity to the vWf molecule and has been identified in circumstances where proteolytic enzymes would expect to be activated. This protein has been variously termed fast moving peak,[64] F.VIII related antigen fragment (VIII:Ag frag),[86] or fast migrating protein.[87] It is possible that a number of degradation products of vWf occur; however, until the relationships between these possible products and vWf are clarified they will be referred to here as vWf:Fragment (vWf:Frag).[88]

A. Identification and Molecular Chemistry

Radio-CIE has been the most common method for identification of vWf:Frag,[64,87-90] although under conditions of increased antigen and antibody concentrations it is possible to visualize the protein by Coomassie blue staining.[86,91,92] VWf:Frag has been observed in normal plasma in trace amounts, in normal serum formed by allowing whole blood to clot but not in recalcified platelet poor plasma or PRP, in F.VIII concentrates, and in the plasma from patients with disseminated intravascular coagulation.

VWf:Frag migrates more rapidly on radio-CIE than vWf:Ag. This suggests that it has a smaller molecular size. As can be seen from Figure 1, vWf:Frag has partial immunochemical identity with the slower moving part of the vWf:Ag precipitant peak. Under other circumstances vWf:Frag shows complete immunological identity with vWf:Ag (Figure 3).[88,92] The exact cause of the different precipitant patterns has yet to be identified.

Partial purification of vWf:Frag has been achieved by using selective ammonium sulfate precipitation and gel filtration.[86,87] An example of clear separation of vWf:Ag from vWf:Frag by differential ammonium sulfate precipitation is shown in Figure 2. The semipurified material migrated on SDS-agarose gel electrophoresis in a similar position to the smallest vWf:Ag multimer and eluted from a Sephacryl 300 gel filtration column in a position suggesting a molecular weight of 900 kD.[86]

A molecular weight of 900 kD and a broad precipitant arc which is seen on radio-CIE suggest that vWf:Frag like its parent molecule is composed of a number of identical subunits noncovalently linked to form a polymeric protein. VWf:Frag has no RCoF activity, but retains some of the antigenic sites involved in the ristocetin interaction by the parent molecule.[91]

B. Formation and Enzymes Responsible

There is good evidence for the concept that vWf:Frag is formed both *in vivo* and *in vitro* as the result of proteolytic degradation of vWf:Ag. VWf:Frag is formed when whole blood

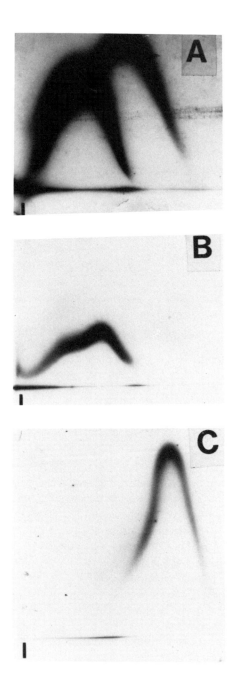

FIGURE 2. An autoradiograph of a radio-CIE in agarose gel containing ^{125}I rabbit anti-human vWf. of (A) starting material containing both vWf and vWf:Frag, (B) precipitate from a 0 to 35% ammonium sulfate cut of the material shown in (A), and (C) precipitate from a 35 to 50% ammonium sulfate cut of the supernate remaining in (B).

is allowed to clot but not when platelet poor plasma or PRP is recalcified. VWf:Frag forms in cryoprecipitate on storage, and this can be prevented by the inclusion of protease inhibitors.[87] All F.VIII concentrates used for patient infusion purified under conditions likely to favor proteases contain significant amounts of vWf:Frag.[64,86,87] Finally, the plasma from all patients investigated with disseminated intravascular coagulation has a distinctive vWf:Frag precipitant peak on CIE.[64,86,87]

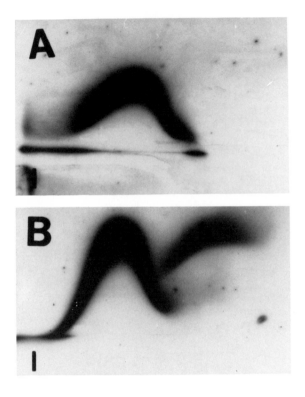

FIGURE 3.   An autoradiograph of a radio-CIE in agarose gel containing
[125]I rabbit anti-human vWf of purified vWf incubated for 60 min at 37°C
with (A) buffer and (B) PMN cells.

Direct confirmation of cellular proteolytic attack on vWf:Ag has recently been obtained. Kunicki et al.[92] have demonstrated that a calcium activated protease (CAP) released from platelets cleaves vWf:Ag to produce a fragment which migrates on CIE to a similar position to the vWf:Frag seen in F.VIII concentrates or in the plasma from patients with disseminated intravascular coagulation. On SDS-PAGE this vWf:Frag has a reduced subunit molecular weight of 206 kD compared to 220 kD for the parent vWf molecule. The platelet protease was inhibited by leupeptin, a specific inhibitor of CAPs, and by a group of calcium chelators but not by a range of chemicals known to inhibit serine proteases and clotting enzymes. It has, therefore, been suggested that a platelet CAP is responsible for the altered vWf:Ag seen under these circumstancs.[92]

An extension of the earlier work from our laboratory trying to identify the protease responsible for formation of vWf:Frag has led to a different conclusion. Platelets, RBCs, monocytes, and PMN cells were separated, washed, lysed, and incubated with purified vWf:Ag. The resultant mixture which was examined by radio-CIE indicated that only PMN cells contained proteases which interacted with vWf:Ag to produce vWf:Frag.[88] The PMN cell protease(s) were inhibited by diisopropyl-flurophosphate, soy bean trypsin inhibitor, and high concentrations of aprotinin, but not by leupeptin, calcium chelators, or inhibitors of coagulation. These experiments suggest that the PMN cell enzyme(s) responsible is a serine protease. The disparity between our results and those of Kunicki et al.[92] may be explained by the presence of ethylene diamine tetra-acetic acid, a powerful calcium chelator in the collecting and wash buffers in our experiments at concentrations sufficient to inhibit any CAPs present in either the platelet or PMN cell preparations.[88]

An example of an autoradiograph of a radio-CIE from an incubation of vWf with PMN cells is shown in Figure 3. It can be seen that vWf:Frag is present following the incubation

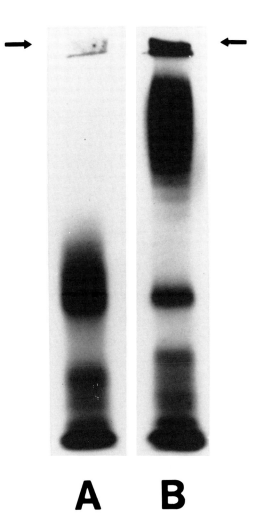

A   B

FIGURE 4.   An autoradiograph of a SDS-agarose gel electrophoresis of [125]I vWf incubated for 60 min at 37°C with (A) PMN cells and (B) buffer.

and that there is a loss of the high MW multimers of vWf. This is further demonstrated on the SDS-agarose gel electrophoresis of this incubation mixture, where there is a clear loss of the large multimeric forms of vWf and an increase in an intermediate sized multimeric form (Figure 4). Attempts to identify the PMN cell protease which cleaves vWf are at an early stage. However, incubation of purified vWf with commercial porcine pancreatic elastase produces a cleavage product which reacts with a rabbit antibody against human vWf:Ag and migrates on radio-CIE in a similar position to vWf:Frag produced by PMN cell cleavage of vWf (Figure 5). A SDS-agarose gel electrophoretic analysis of the incubation product demonstrated a loss of all high MW multimers and a reduction of the smaller forms with formation of an intermediate sized multimer not present in the starting ^{125}I VWf preparation (Figure 6).

The experiments and observations described above indicate that the degradation product(s) of proteolytic cleavage of the vWf molecule retains sufficient of the primary structure of vWf to form into a series of polymers. Part of the molecule lost during the proteolytic process must be necessary for aggregation of the basic vWf subunit into large polymers since after cleavage a variable number of lower MW multimers remain (Figures 4 and 6).

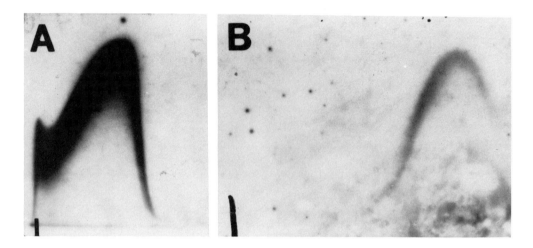

FIGURE 5.   An autoradiograph of a radio-CIE of purified vWf incubated for 30 min at 37° with (A) buffer and (B) elastase 3.0 mg/ml (porcine pancreatic).

A fuller understanding of the structure of those parts of the molecule necessary for the assembling of subunits into polymers should provide a greater insight into the molecular abnormality present in the vWf molecule from patients with type II variant von Willebrand's disease.[18,93]

C. Clinical Significance

Proteins antigenically related to vWf (vWf:Frag) which are presumably the result of proteolytic degradation are present in the plasma from patients with disseminated intravascular coagulation.[64,86,87] A similar protein has been observed in the ascitic fluid from patients with chronic cirrhosis, but without evidence of disseminated intravascular coagulation[89] and in cerebrospinal fluid from one patient.[90] In both chronic cirrhosis and disseminated intravascular coagulation, proteolytic enzymes would be activated, thus the identification of vWf:Frag in body fluids may prove a useful tool for the confirmation of a proteolytic process.

Plasma from patients with severe hemophilia has also been noted to contain increased concentrations of vWf:Frag.[87] No definitive explanation for its presence can be offered; however, it is possible that vWf:Frag represents a normal breakdown product, and the increased amounts seen in the plasma from patients with hemophilia result from delayed clearance. Alternatively, generation of vWf:Frag may be part of the normal process of the reaction of vWf in the hemostatic mechanism, and the increased levels in hemophilia may represent efforts to maintain normal hemostasis. Fragments of vWf are also present in the plasma from patients with hemophilia following transfusion of factor VIII concentrates but not following cryoprecipitate infusion.[86] These results are readily explained by the respective presence and absence of vWf:Frag in the starting material.

VI. TECHNICAL AND CLINICAL CONSEQUENCES

A. Purified Material

A significant loss of F.VIII:C activity occurs during its purification. Some of this loss can be attributed to a natural loss due to methodological inefficiencies, but a number of recent reports have suggested that proteolytic enzymes may also be responsible.[94-97] Thus, attention has been drawn to the need to include either highly specific or, in the absence of detailed information, a battery of proteolytic inhibitors in the blood collection anticoagulant and buffers used for the purification of both F.VIII and vWf.[94-97] Addition of diisopropyl-flurophosphate and heparin to plasma resulted in a significant improvement in the stability of F.VIII:C over 24 h.[95] Maintenance of physiological calcium levels also improves the yield and stability of F.VIII:C[95]

Loss of RCoF activity and change in the structure of the vWf molecule have also been noted in semipurified material during dialysis or storage.[96,97] Some of these changes are prevented by the addition of protease inhibitors.[97] Thus, inclusion of proteolytic inhibitors appears to be essential if an unaltered vWf molecule is to be obtained. Recognition of the effect of proteases in endothelial cell cultures on the vWf and F.VIII molecule is also important.[98,99] The preferred approach is to only include inhibitors of proteases which produce nonphysiological changes to the molecule, otherwise proteolytic cleavages necessary for the normal synthesis of the protein may be retarded.

B. Infusion Material

During the past 20 years F.VIII concentrates have replaced cryoprecipitate as the treatment of choice for bleeding episodes in patients with hemophilia. More recently, they have been used for treatment of patients with von Willebrand's disease. However, despite increased circulating levels of F.VIII:C and RCoF, they have generally been found to be ineffective at controlling the bleeding or reducing the bleeding time.[29,30,100-103]

Alteration in the function/antigen ratio of the F.VIII concentrates compared to cryoprecipitate was noted as well as a structural change to lower MW multimers of the vWf molecule on SDS-PAGE and CIE.[100,103-105] Loss of the high MW multimers of vWf is presumably the cause of loss of *in vivo* function of the concentrates. It has been suggested that proteases present during purification and in the concentrates are responsible for the changes in structure/function.[106] This poses a dilemma. It is not possible to add most proteolytic inhibitors to plasma destined for infusion due to their potential toxicity; therefore, other methods of controlling proteases need to be found. Contamination by cells and their fragments is the most likely route for protease contamination of concentrates.[107,108] Therefore, more efficient removal of cell debris during plasma preparation would be expected to reduce protease contamination.

C. Diagnostic Problems

The normal ratio of functional activity/antigen for both F.VIII:C and vWf is 1.0. Deviations in this ideal ratio have been described in a large number of clinical syndromes.[109-111] Such changes may be the result of proteolytic alteration of the molecule. Thus, whenever abnormal ratios are present clinically one should consider the possibility that proteolytic activation and/or alteration has occurred.

VII. SUMMARY

F.VIII and vWf are both susceptible to cleavage by proteases released from cells with which they would be expected to come into contact during normal hemostatic processing. The proteases which have been discussed in this chapter are plasmin, protein C, an ELP, and a CLP released from leukocytes. To date, no effect of protein C on the vWf molecule has been reported. The functional activity of both proteins is reduced before loss of antigenic activity is evident, following incubation with the proteases suggesting that the first cleavage sites for both proteins are at or near the functionally active sites. Structural changes have been described when the purified proteins are incubated with purified enzymes. Whether these functional and structural changes also occur *in vivo* where the natural inhibitors of the proteases are present remains to be determined. Certainly changes in the levels of F.VIII

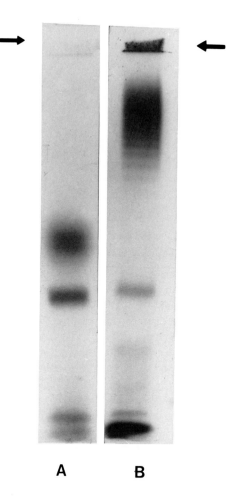

A   B

FIGURE 6. An autoradiograph of a SDS-agarose gel of purified ^{125}I-vWf incubated for 60 min at 37°C with (A) elastase 3.0 mg/ml (porcine pancreatic) and (B) buffer.

and vWf occur in clinical situations where protease may be activated. A proteolytic degradation product of vWf has also been identified in clinical circumstances of proteolytic activation such as disseminated intravascular coagulation; however, definitive identification of the protease(s) responsible has not been made. A clear understanding of the relationship of the proteases described to the physiological functioning of both F.VIII and vWf awaits future research.

ACKNOWLEDGMENTS

I would like to express my gratitude to Professor Barry Firkin and my husband Dr. David Bennett for their help and encouragement in writing this chapter. This work has been carried out with the support of a National Health and Medical Research Council of Australia grant.

REFERENCES

1. **Fay, P. J., Chavin, S. I., Schroeder, D., Young, F. E., and Marder, V. J.,** Purification and characterization of a highly purified human factor VIII consisting of a single type of polypeptide chain, *Proc. Natl. Acad. Sci. U.S.A.*, 79, 7200, 1982.

2. **Toole, J. J., Knopf, J. L., Wozney, J. M., Sultzman, L. A., Buecker, J. L., Pittman, D. D., Kaufman, R. J., Brown, E., Shoemaker, C., Orr, E. C., Amphlett, G. W., Foster, W. B., Coe, M. L., Knutson, G. J., Fass, D. N., and Hewick, R. M.,** Molecular cloning of a cDNA encoding human antihaemophilic factor, *Nature,* 312, 342, 1984.

3. **Vehar, G. A., Keyt, B., Eaton, D., Rodriguez, H., O'Brien, D. P., Rotblat, F., Oppermann, H., Keck, R., Wood, W. I., Harkins, R. N., Tuddenham, E. G. D., Lawn, R. M., and Capon, D. J.,** Structure of human factor VIII, *Nature,* 312, 337, 1984.

4. **Wood, W. I., Capon, D. J., Simonsen, C. C., Eaton, D. L., Gitschier, J., Keyt, B., Seeburg, P. H., Smith, D. H., Hollingshead, P., Wion, K. L., Delwart, E., Tuddenham, E. G. D., Vehar, G. A., and Lawn, R. M.,** Expression of active human factor VIII from recombinant DNA clones, *Nature,* 312, 330, 1984.

5. **Gitschier, J., Wood, W. I., Goralka, T. M., Wion, K. L., Chen, E. Y., Eaton, D. H., Vehar, G. A., Capon, D. J., and Lawn, R. M.,** Characterization of the human factor VIII gene, *Nature,* 312, 326, 1984.

6. **Rotblat, F., O'Brien, D. P., Middleton, S. M., and Tuddenham, E. G. D.,** Purification and characterisation of human factor VIII:C, *Thromb. Haemost.,* 50, 108, 1983.

7. **Fulcher, C. A., Gardiner, J. E., Griffin, J. H., and Zimmerman, T. S.,** Proteolytic inactivation of human factor VIII procoagulant protein by activated human protein C and its analogy with factor V, *Blood,* 63, 486, 1984.

8. **Wion, K. L., Kelly, D., Summerfield, J. A., Tuddenham, E. G. D., and Lawn, R. M.,** Distribution of factor VIII mRNA and antigen in human liver and other tissues, *Nature,* 317, 726, 1985.

9. **Zelechowska, M. G., van Mourik, J. A., and Brodniewicz-Proba, T.,** Ultrastructural localization of factor VIII procoagulant antigen in human liver hepatocytes, *Nature,* 317, 729, 1985.

10. **Jenkins, C. S. P., Phillips, D. R., Clemetson, K. J., Meyer, D., Larrieu, M.-J., and Luscher, E. F.,** Platelet membrane glycoproteins implicated in ristocetin-induced aggregation. Studies of the proteins on platelets from patients with Bernard-Soulier syndrome and von Willebrand's disease, *J. Clin. Invest.,* 57, 112, 1976.

11. **Nachman, R. L., Jaffe, E. A., and Weksler, B. B.,** Immunoinhibition of ristocetin-induced platelet aggregation, *J. Clin. Invest.,* 59, 143, 1977.

12. **Ali-Briggs, E. F., Clemetson, K. J., and Jenkins, C. S. P.,** Antibodies against platelet membrane glycoproteins. I. Crossed immunoelectrophoresis studies with antibodies that inhibit ristocetin-induced platelet aggregation, *Br. J. Haematol.,* 48, 305, 1981.

13. **Ivy, A. C., Nelson, D., and Bucher, G. J.,** The standardisation of certain factors in the cutaneous "venostasis" bleeding time technique, *J. Lab. Clin. Med.,* 26, 1812, 1941.

14. **Salzman, E. W.,** Measurement of platelet adhesiveness: a simple *in vitro* technique demonstrating an abnormality in von Willebrand's disease, *J. Lab. Clin. Med.,* 62, 724, 1963.

15. **Howard, M. A. and Firkin, B. G.,** Ristocetin — a new tool in the investigation of platelet aggregation, *Thromb. Diath. Haemorrh.,* 26, 362, 1971.

16. **Howard, M. A., Perkin, J., Salem, H. H., and Firkin, B. G.,** The agglutination of human platelets by botrocetin: evidence that botrocetin and ristocetin act at different sites on the factor VIII molecule and platelet membrane, *Br. J. Haematol.,* 57, 25, 1984.

17. **Brinkhous, K. M. and Read, M. S.,** Use of venom coagglutinin and lyophilized platelets in testing for platelet-aggregating von Willebrand factor, *Blood,* 55, 517, 1980.

18. **Ruggeri, Z. M. and Zimmerman, T. S.,** Variant von Willebrand's disease. Characterization of two subtypes by analysis of multimeric composition of factor VIII/von Willebrand factor in plasma and platelets, *J. Clin. Invest.,* 65, 1318, 1980.

19. **Meyer, D., Obert, B., Pietu, G., Lavergne, J. M., and Zimmerman, T. S.,** Multimeric structure of factor VIII/von Willebrand factor in von Willebrand's disease, *J. Lab. Clin. Med.,* 95, 590, 1980.

20. **Marchesi, S. L., Shulman, N. R., and Gralnick, H. R.,** Studies on the purification and characterization of human factor VIII, *J. Clin. Invest.,* 51, 2151, 1972.

21. **Hoyer, L. W. and Shainoff, J. R.,** Factor VIII-related protein circulates in normal human plasma as high molecular weight multimers, *Blood,* 55, 1056, 1980.

22. **Pietu, G., Obert, B., Larrieu, M. J., and Meyer, D.,** Structure-function relationship of factor VIII/von Willebrand factor. Application to the study of variant von Willebrand's disease and cryosupernatant prepared from normal plasma, *Thromb. Res.,* 19, 671, 1980.

23. **Lynch, D. C., Zimmerman, T. S., Kirby, E. P., and Livingston, D. M.,** Subunit composition of oligomeric human von Willebrand factor, *J. Biol. Chem.,* 258, 12757, 1983.

24. **Legaz, M. E., Schmer, G., Counts, R. B., and Davie, E. W.,** Isolation and characterization of human factor VIII (antihemophilic factor), *J. Biol. Chem.,* 11, 3946, 1973.

25. **Howard, M. A., Hau, L., Perkin, J., Thomas, K. B., Firkin, B. G., and Koutts, K.,** Causes for the discrepancies in the measurements of factor VIII antigen, *Thromb. Res.,* 19, 63, 1980.

26. **Over, J., Bouma, B. N., van Mourik, J. A., Sixma, J. J., Vlooswijk, R., and Bakker-Woudenberg, I.,** Heterogeneity of human factor VIII. I. Characterization of factor VIII present in the supernate of cryoprecipitate, *J. Lab. Clin. Med.,* 91, 32, 1978.

27. **Martin, S. E., Marder, V. J., Francis, C. W., and Barlow, G. H.,** Structural studies on the functional heterogeneity of von Willebrand protein polymers, *Blood,* 57, 313, 1981.

28. **Hill, F. G. H. and Enayat, M. S.,** Multimeric analysis of eight lyophilized factor VIII concentrates, *Br.. J. Haematol.,* 60, 201, 1985.

29. **Blatt, P. M., Brinkhous, K. M., Culp, H. R., Krauss, J. S., and Roberts, H. R.,** Antihemophilic factor concentrate therapy in von Willebrands disease. Dissociation of bleeding-time factor and ristocetin-cofactor activities, *JAMA,* 24, 2770, 1976.

30. **Green, D. and Potter, E. V.,** Failure of AHF concentrate to control bleeding in von Willebrand's disease, *Am. J. Med.,* 60, 357, 1976.

31. **Doucet-de Bruine, M. H. M., Sixma, J. J., Over, J., and Beeser-Visser, N. H.,** Heterogenity of factor VIII. II. Characterization of forms of human factor VIII binding to platelets in the presence of ristocetin, *J. Lab. Clin. Med.,* 92, 96, 1978.

32. **Chan, V. and Chan, T. K.,** Cell-free synthesis of factor VIII related protein, *Thromb. Haemost.,* 50, 835, 1983.

33. **Tuddenham, E. G. D., Lazarchick, J., and Hoyer, L. W.,** Synthesis and release of factor VIII by cultured human endothelial cells, *Br. J. Haematol.,* 47, 617, 1981.

34. **Nachman, R., Levine, R., and Jaffe, E. A.,** Synthesis of factor VIII antigen by cultured guinea pig megakaryocytes, *J. Clin. Invest.,* 60, 914, 1977.

35. **Edgell, C.-J. S., McDonald, C. C., and Graham, J. B.,** Permanent cell line expressing human factor VIII-related antigen established by hybridization, *Proc. Natl. Acad. Sci. U.S.A.,* 80, 3734, 1983.

36. **Jaffe, E. A., Hoyer, L. W., and Nachman, R. L.,** Synthesis of antihemophilic factor antigen by cultured human endothelial cells, *J. Clin. Invest.,* 52, 2757, 1973.

37. **Rand, J. H., Gordon, R. E., Sussman, I. I., Chu, S. V., and Solomon, V.,** Electron microscopy localization of factor-VIII-related antigen in adult human blood vessels, *Blood,* 60, 627, 1982.

38. **Hoyer, L. W., de los Santos, R. P., and Hoyer, J. R.,** Antihemophilic factor antigen. Localization in endothelial cells by immunofluorescent microscopy, *J. Clin. Invest.,* 52, 2737, 1973.

39. **Prentice, C. R. M., Forbes, C. D., and Smith, S. M.,** Rise of factor VIII after exercise and adrenaline infusion, measured by immunological and biological techniques, *Thromb. Res.,* 1, 493, 1972.

40. **Rizza, C. R. and Eipe, J.,** Exercise, factor VIII and the spleen, *Br. J. Haematol.,* 20, 629, 1971.

41. **Mannucci, P. M., Canciani, M. T., Rota, L., and Donovan, B. S.,** Response of factor VIII/von Willebrand factor to DDAVP in healthy subjects and patients with haemophilia A and von Willebrand's disease, *Br. J. Haematol.,* 47, 283, 1981.

42. **Moffat, E. H., Giddings, J. C., and Bloom, A. L.,** The effect of desamino-D-arginine vasopressin (DDAVP) and naloxone infusions on factor VIII and possible endothelial cell (EC) related activities, *Br. J. Haematol.,* 57, 651, 1984.

43. **Cockburn, C. G., de Beafre-Apps, R. J., Wilson, J., and Hardisty, R. M.,** Parallel destruction of factor VIII procoagulant activivty and an 85,000 dalton protein in highly purified factor VIII/vWf, *Thromb. Res., 21,* 295, 1981.

44. **Pasquini, R. and Hershgold, E. J.,** Effects of plasmin on human factor VIII (AHF), *Blood,* 41, 105, 1973.

45. **Denson, K. W. E. and Redman, C. W. G.,** The destruction of factor VIII clotting activity by thrombin and plasmin, *Thromb. Res.,* 18, 547, 1980.

46. **Rick, M. E., Popovsky, M. A., and Krizek, D. M.,** Degradation of factor VIII coagulant antigen by proteolytic enzymes, *Br. J. Haematol.,* 61, 477, 1985.

47. **McKee, P. A., Anderson, J. C., and Switzer, M. E.,** Molecular structural studies of human factor VIII, *Ann. N. Y. Acad. Sci.,* 240, 8, 1975.

48. **Holmberg, L., Ljung, R., and Nilsson, I. M.,** The effects of plasmin and protein Ca on factor VIII:C and VIII:CAg, *Thromb. Res.,* 31, 41, 1983.

49. **Atichartakarn, V., Marder, V. J., Kirby, E. P., and Budzynski, A. Z.,** Effects of enzymatic degradation on the subunit composition and biologic properties of human factor VIII, *Blood,* 51, 281, 1978.

50. **Lian, E. C.-Y., Nunez, R. L., and Harkness, D. R.,** *In vivo* and *in vitro* effects of thrombin and plasmin on human factor VIII (AHF), *Am. J. Hematol.,* 1, 481, 1976.

51. **Vahtera, E., Varimo, M., and Myllyla, G.,** The effect of 2-macroglobulin-plasmin complex on factor VIII, *Thromb. Res.,* 18, 247, 1980.

52. **Switzer, M. E. P., Gordon, H. J., and McKee, P. A.,** Proteolytic activity of 2-macroglobulin-enzyme complexes toward human factor VIII/von Willebrand factor, *Biochemistry,* 22, 1437, 1983.

53. **Guisasola, J. A., Cockburn, C. G., and Hardisty, R. M.,** Plasmin digestion of factor VIII: characterization of the breakdown products with respect to antigenicity and von Willebrand activity, *Thromb. Haemost.,* 40, 302, 1978.

54. **Andersen, J. C., Switzer, M. E. P., and McKee, P. A.,** Support of ristocetin-induced platelet aggregation by procoagulant-inactive and plasmin cleaved forms of human factor VIII/von Willebrand factor, *Blood,* 55, 101, 1980.

55. **Switzer, M. E. P. and McKee, P. A.,** Immunologic studies of native and modified human factor VIII/ von Willebrand factor, *Blood,* 54, 310, 1979.

56. **Federici, A. B., Elder, J. H., De Marco, L., Ruggeri, Z. M., and Zimmerman, T. S.,** Carbohydrate moiety of von Willebrand factor is not necessary for maintaining multimeric structure and ristocetin cofactor activity but protects from proteolytic degradation, *J. Clin. Invest.,* 74, 2049, 1984.

57. **Hamilton, K. K., Fretto, L. J., Grierson, D. S., and McKee, P. A.,** Effects of plasmin on von Willebrand factor multimers. Degradation *in vitro* and stimulation of release *in vivo, J. Clin. Invest.,* 76, 261, 1985.

58. **Culasso, D. E., Donati, M. B., de Gaetano, G., Vermylen, J., and Verstraete, M.,** Inhibition of human platelet aggregation by plasmin digests of human and bovine fibrinogen preparations: role of contaminating factor VIII-related material, *Blood,* 44, 169, 1974.

59. **Donati, M. B., de Gaetano G., Vermylen, J., and Verstraete, M.,** Inhibition of human platelet aggregation by plasmin digests of human factor VIII, *Blood,* 42, 749, 1973.

60. **Castillo, R., Maragall, S., Martin, E., Guisasola, J. A., and Ordinas, A.,** Inhibition of the platelet function by plasminic effect on human factor VIII, *Thromb. Res.,* 20, 293, 1980.

61. **Castillo, R., Maragall, S., Guisasola, J. A., Casals, F., Profitos, J., and Ordinas, A.,** Inhibition of human platelet aggregation by the proteolytic effect of strepokinase. Role of the human factor VIII-related protein, *Haemostasis,* 5, 306, 1976.

62. **Vermylen, J. and Bottecchia, D.,** Factor VIII and human platelet aggregation. IV. Effect of proteolytic enzymes on platelet aggregation by factor VIII, *Br. J. Haematol.,* 34, 331, 1976.

63. **Stachurska, J., Lopaciuk, S., Gerdin, B., Saldeen, T., Koroscik, A., and Kopec, M.,** Effects of proteolytic degradation products of human fibrinogen and of human factor VIII on platelet aggregation and vascular permeability, *Thromb. Res.,* 15, 663, 1979.

64. **Lombardi, R., Mannucci, P. M., Seghatchian, M. J., Vicente Garcia, V., and Coppola, R.,** Alterations of factor VIII von Willebrand factor in clinical conditions associated with an increase in its plasma concentration, *Br. J. Haematol.,* 49, 61, 1981.

65. **Stenflo, J.,** A new vitamin K-dependent protein. Purification from bovine plasma and preliminary characterization, *J. Biol. Chem.,* 251, 355, 1976.

66. **Esmon, C. T., Stenflo, J., and Suttie, J. W.,** A new vitamin K-dependent protein A phospholipid-binding zymogen of a serine esterase, *J. Biol. Chem.,* 251, 3052, 1976.

67. **Kisiel, W.,** Human plasma protein C isolation, characterization, and mechanism of activation by α-thrombin, *J. Clin. Invest.,* 64, 761, 1979.

68. **Marlar, R. A., Kleiss, A. J., and Griffin, J. H.,** Mechanism of action of human activated protein C, a thrombin-dependent anticoagulant enzyme, *Blood,* 59, 1067, 1982.

69. **Vehar, G. A. and Davie, E. W.,** Preparation and properties of bovine factor VIII (antihemophilic factor), *Am. Chem. Soc.,* 19, 401, 1980.

70. **Marlar, R. A. and Griffin, J. H.,** Deficiency of protein C inhibitor in combined factor V/VIII deficiency disease, *J. Clin. Invest.,* 66, 1186, 1980.

71. **Canfield, W. M. and Kisiel, W.,** Evidence of normal functional levels of activated protein C inhibitor in combined factor V/VIII deficiency disease, *J. Clin. Invest.,* 70, 1260, 1982.

72. **Giddings, J. C., Sugrue, A., and Bloom, A. L.,** Quantitation of coagulant antigens and inhibition of activated protein C in combined factor V/VIII deficiency, *Br. J. Haematol.,* 52, 495, 1982.

73. **Seligsohn, U., Zivelin, A., and Zwang, E.,** Decreased factor VIII clotting antigen levels in the combined factor V and VIII deficiency, *Thromb. Res.,* 33, 95, 1983.

74. **Ohlsson, K. and Olsson, I.,** The extracellular release of granulocyte collagenase and elastase during phagocytosis and inflammatory processes, *Scand. J. Haematol.,* 19, 145, 1977.

75. **Plow, E. F.,** Leukocyte elastase release during blood coagulation. A potential mechanism for activation of the alternative fibrinolytic pathway, *J. Clin. Invest.,* 69, 564, 1982.

76. **Henriksson, P. and Nilsson, I. M.,** Effects of leukocytes, plasmin and thrombin on clotting factors a comparative *in vitro* study, *Thromb. Res.,* 16, 301, 1979.

77. **Egbring, R., Schmidt, W., Fuchs, G., and Havemann, K.,** Demonstration of granulocytic proteases in plasma of patients with acute leukemia and septicemia with coagulation defects, *Blood,* 49, 219, 1977.

78. **Taylor, J. C., Crawford, I. P., and Hugli, T. E.,** Limited degradation of the third component (C3) of human complement by human leukocyte elastase (HLE): partial characterization of C3 fragments, *Biochemistry,* 16, 3390, 1977.

79. **McDonald, J. A. and Kelley, D. G.,** Degradation of fibrinonectin by human leukocyte elastase release of biologically active fragments, *J. Biol. Chem.,* 255, 8848, 1980.

80. **Schmidt, W., Ebring, R., and Havemann, K.,** Effect of elastase-like and chymotrypsin-like neutral proteases from human granulocytes on isolated clotting factors, *Thromb. Res.,* 6, 315, 1975.

81. **Moroz, L. A.,** Mini-plasminogen: a mechanism for leukocyte modulation of plasminogen activation by urokinase, *Blood,* 58, 97, 1981.

82. **Brower, M. S., Levin, R. I., and Garry, K.,** Human neutrophil elastase modulates platelet function by limited proteolysis of membrane glycoproteins, *J. Clin. Invest.,* 75, 657, 1985.

83. **Brower, M. S. and Harpel, P. C.,** Alpha-1-antitrypsin-human leukocyte elastase complexes in blood: quantification by an enzyme-linked differential antibody immunosorbant assay and comparison with alpha-2-plasmin inhibitor-plasmin complexes, *Blood,* 61, 842, 1983.

84. **Varadi, K. and Elodi, S.,** Increased resistance of factor IXa-factor VIII complex against inactivation by granulocyte proteases, *Thromb. Res.,* 19, 571, 1980.

85. **Varadi, K., Marossy, K., Asboth, G., Elodi, P., and Elodi, S.,** Inactivation of human factor VIII by granulocyte proteases, *Thromb. Haemost.,* 43, 45, 1980.

86. **Montogomery, R. R. and Johnson, J.,** Specific factor VIII-related antigen fragmentation: an in vivo and in vitro phenomenon, *Blood,* 60, 930, 1982.

87. **Thomas, K. B., Howard, M. A., Salem, H. H., and Firkin, B. G.,** Fast migrating protein, immunologically related to human factor VIII, studied by crossed immunoelectrophoresis in agarose, *Br. J. Haematol.,* 54, 221, 1983.

88. **Thompson, E. A. and Howard, M. A.,** Proteolytic cleavage of human von Willebrand factor (vWf) induced by enzyme(s) released from polymorphonuclear cells, *Blood,* 67, 128b, 1986.

89. **Vicente, V., Alberca, I., Calles, E., and Lopez Borrasca, A.,** Evidence of degradation of factor VIII-antigen in ascitic fluid, *Br. J. Haematol.,* 55, 555, 1983.

90. **Vicente, V., Alberca, I., Calles, I., Gonzalez, R., and Lopez Borrasca, A.,** Demonstration of FVIII-related antigen in human cerebrospinal fluid, *Haemostasis,* 12, 160, 1982.

91. **Montgomery, R. R. and Corcoran, M.,** Antigenic sites on a fragment of factor VIII (VIIIR:AG fr 1) are important for ristocetin-induced platelet aggregation (RIPA), *Clin. Res.,* 30, 324A, 1982.

92. **Kunicki, T. J., Montgomery, R. R., and Schullek, J.,** Cleavage of human von Willebrand factor by platelet calcium-activated protease, *Blood,* 65, 352, 1985.

93. **Kinoshita, S., Harrison, J., Lazerson, J., and Abildgaard, C. F.,** A new variant of dominant type II von Willebrand's disease with aberrant multimeric pattern of factor VIII-related antigen (type IID), *Blood,* 63, 1369, 1984.

94. **Switzer, M. E. P., Pizzo, S. V., and McKee, P. A.,** Is there a precursive, relatively procoagulant-inactive form of normal antihemophilic factor (factor VIII)?, *Blood,* 54, 916, 1979.

95. **Rock, G. A., Cruickshank, W. H., Tackaberry, E. S., Ganz, P. R., and Palmer, D. S.,** Stability of VIII:C in plasma: the dependence on protease activity and calcium, *Thromb. Res.,* 29, 521, 1983.

96. **Furlan, M. and Beck, E. A.,** Degradation of purified factor VIII by endogenous contaminating enzymes, *Thromb. Res.,* 10, 153, 1977.

97. **Beck, E. A., Bachmann, P., Barbier, P., and Furlan, M.,** Importance of protease inhibition in studies on purified factor VIII (antihaemophilic factor), *Thromb. Haemost.,* 35, 186, 1976.

98. **Booyse, F. M., Quarfoot, A. J., Radek, J., and Feder, S.,** Correction of various abnormalities in cultured porcine von Willebrand endothelial cells by inhibition of plasminogen-dependent protease activity, *Blood,* 58, 573, 1981.

99. **Stead, N. W. and McKee, P. A.,** Destruction of factor VIII procoagulant activity in tissue culture media, *Blood,* 52, 408, 1978.

100. **Jakab, T., Pflugshaupt, R., Furlan, M., and Beck, E. A.,** Variable degradation of factor VIII-related protein in lyophilised concentrates of antihaemophilic factor (AHF), *Vox Sang.,* 35, 36, 1978.

101. **Chediak, J. R., Telfer, M. C., and Green, D.,** Platelet function and immunologic parameters in von Willebrand's disease following cryoprecipitate and factor VIII infusion, *Am. J. Med.,* 62, 369, 1977.

102. **Perkins, H. A.,** Correction of the hemostatic defects in von Willebrand's disease, *Blood,* 30, 375, 1967.

103. **Nilsson, I. M. and Hedner, U.,** Characteristics of various factor VIII concentrates used in treatment of haemophilia A, *Br. J. Haematol.,* 37, 543, 1977.

104. **Weinstein, M. and Deykin, D.,** Comparison of factor VIII-related von Willebrand proteins prepared from human cryoprecipitate and factor VIII concentrate, *Blood,* 53, 1095, 1979.

105. **McCue, M. J., Brossoit, A. D., Marmer, D. J., and Head, D. R.,** Von Willebrand factor (VIII$_{VWF}$) in lyophilized factor VIII concentrates, *Am. J. Hematol.,* 9, 39, 1980.

106. **Orthner, C. L.,** Characterization of proteases in AHF concentrates: effect on factor VIII:von Willebrand protein as assessed by high-pressure gel permeation chromatography, *J. Lab. Clin. Med.,* 104, 816, 1984.

107. **Howard, M. A., Coghlan, M., David, R., and Pfueller, S. L.,** Coagulation activities of platelet microparticles, *Thromb. Res.,* 50, 145, 1988.

108. **George, J. N., Pickett, E. B., and Heinz, R.,** Platelet membrane microparticles in blood bank fresh-frozen plasma and cryoprecipitate, *Blood,* 68, 307, 1986.

109. **Tran, T. H., Lammle, B., and Duckert, F.,** Factor VIII (procoagulant activity VIII:C, and antigen VIII:CAg, related antigen VIIIR:Ag and ristocetin cofactor VIIIR:Cof) in intensive care patients with clinically suspected disseminated intravascular coagulation (DIC), *Am. J. Clin. Pathol.,* 82, 565, 1984.

110. **Holmberg, L. and Nilsson, I. M.,** AHF related protein in clinical praxis, *Scand. J. Haematol.,* 12, 221, 1974.

111. **Howard, M. A., Whitworth, J. A., Hendrix, L. E., Thomas, K. B., and Firkin, B. G.,** Abnormal factor VIII in chronic renal failure, *Med. J. Aust.,* 1, 148, 1979.

Chapter 14

THE INTERACTION OF FACTOR VIII/vWf WITH SOLID MATRICES AND MATRIX-BOUND LIGANDS

R. H. Saundry and P. Harrison

TABLE OF CONTENTS

I.   Introduction...258

II.   General Considerations 258

III. Physiological Interactions of VIII/vWf Related Activities......................259
      A.   Interactions between VIII and vWf....................................259
      B.   Interactions with Phospholipid.......................................259
      C.   Interactions with Factors IX and X...................................260
      D.   Interactions with Fibrinogen and Fibronectin.........................260
      E.   Interactions Necessary for Platelet Adhesion to the
            Subendothelium 260
      F.   Interaction with Immunoglobulins 261
      G.   Interaction with Metal Cations 261

IV.   Conventional Ion Exchange Chromatography 262

V.   Amino Alkane-Derivatized Matrices 263

VI.   Sulfated Matrices 264

VII. Precipitation with Polyvinyl Pyrrolidone...................................268

VIII. Interaction with Polyelectrolytes 268

IX.   Interaction with Lipid Vesicle Matrices....................................268

X.   Interaction with Immobilized Metal Chelate Affinity Matrices................269

XI.   Interactions with Matrix Bound Specific Proteins...........................271
      A.   Immobilized Factor X...271
      B.   Immobilized Fibrin Monomer 271
      C.   Immobilized vWf..271

XII. Interaction with Thiol Matrices 271

XIII. Conclusions and Future Developments.......................................272

References...272

I. INTRODUCTION

The interaction of factor VIII/von Willebrand factor (VIII/vWf) with solid matrices and matrix bound ligands has proved to be a topic of major scientific interest over the last 25 years. Experimental data from such studies have contributed significantly to our perception of possible *in vivo* interactions of VIII/vWf with various physiological components circulating in plasma. Furthermore, the application of the techniques developed for the studies has provided the basis of a number of novel approaches to the purification of one or both of the VIII/vWf components for scientific study and for the production of therapeutic materials.

As much of the earlier studies on VIII/vWf focused on the physicochemical characterization of the VIII moiety alone and/or its interactions with other plasma components, many previous experimental results and conclusions require reevaluation in the light of current knowledge of the interaction of VIII with vWf and in respect to the role of vWf in stabilizing VIII.

In this chapter we review methods that have been used for the purification, isolation, and further study of VIII, vWf, and the VIII/vWf macromolecular complex involving the interaction of VIII/vWf related activities with solid matrices. New approaches for the purification and further study of VIII and vWf will be discussed in detail.

II. GENERAL CONSIDERATIONS

Modern methods for the purification of proteins normally involve affinity chromatography steps.[1,2] This is the method of choice for the purification of macromolecules which are present initially as only minor components of complicated mixtures. Affinity chromatography exploits unique interactions found in biological systems based upon high affinity and specificity of binding with defined ligands. In principle, affinity chromatography can be used for the isolation of either component of a reversible interacting biological system. The basic requirement is the immobilization of one of the components (the ligand) on an insoluble support or matrix such that its specific binding characteristics are retained. The matrix can then be employed for the isolation of that protein from a complex mixture using either batch-wise or column chromatography procedures. Following removal of unbound, noninteracting, undesired components, the specifically bound protein can be reeluted using appropriate conditions, i.e., change in pH, ionic strength, or change in competing ligand concentration. Ultimate success often depends upon how closely the adopted procedures mimic those that pertain in nature since the reeluted component should still be capable of expressing full biological activity. Choice of the inert support is critical in that it should be relatively hydrophilic, stable to chemical reagents, resistant to microbial and enzymic degradation, not impose steric restrictions on the interaction of ligand with the desired component, and display few nonspecific adsorption/absorption sites.

There are two classes of ligands: general and specific. General ligands interact with many different proteins whereas specific ligands interact with only one, or very few families of proteins as in immunopurification. In fact, immunoglobulins have been successfully employed for immunoaffinity chromatographic procedures for the isolation of VIII[3] or vWf[4] as discussed elsewhere. In this chapter the use of general ligands in the purification of VIII/vWf related activities will be presented.

When considering the choice of general ligands a number of factors should be taken into account. The affinity of the matrix bound ligand for the VIII/vWf related active component should ideally be sufficiently high or unique so that the latter is firmly bound. This permits complete separation of the ligand from the unbound contaminants. The affinity for the ligand, however, should not be too great since harsh conditions will be required to effect reelution and may lead to denaturation and loss of biological activity. The number of ligand molecules bound to the matrix should be high such that the matrix will have high capacity and following reelution the VIII/vWf related activity can thus be recovered in a highly concentrated form. The major drawback with the use of generalized ligand affinity matrices is that because of their broad specificities it is most unlikely that a homogeneous product will be obtained using a single matrix procedure. It can be anticipated that sequential combinations of two or more general ligand affinity matrices will have to be used, or one chromatography step in combination with a totally different method of purification, in order to obtain a pure material.

On the basis of current knowledge of the various interactions between the VIII/vWf complex, or either VIII or vWf alone and other components, it is possible to interpret the binding properties of VIII/vWf to various solid matrices. Furthermore, it should be feasible to design even more suitable ligand affinity matrices for the isolation of both VIII and vWf.

III. PHYSIOLOGICAL INTERACTIONS OF VIII/vWf RELATED ACTIVITIES

A. Interactions between VIII and vWf

There is a considerable body of evidence indicating that *in vivo* VIII exists as one component of a macromolecular complex with vWf.[5-9] The VIII moiety is now known to be a comparatively small heterodimeric glycoprotein with an apparent molecular weight variously estimated between 250 and 80 kDa.[10-12] The amino acid sequence has been determined by cDNA gene cloning experiments.[13-15] In contrast, the normal vWf moiety is believed to be a large polymeric glycoprotein with an apparent molecular weight of up to 20×10^6 Da comprised of a minimum of 20 discrete multimeric forms amenable to resolution by sodium-dodecyl sulfate agarose gel electrophoresis analysis.[18-22] Each of the multimeric forms is comprised of integral numbers of the protomeric form which is identical with or very similar to the smallest multimeric form of approximately 10^6 Da. Following complete chemical reduction, subunit structures of approximately 260 kDa are formed suggesting that the basic protomer is comprised of either two or four subunits.[23,24] Mild chemical reduction followed by gel filtration has allowed separation and characterization of both the VIII and vWf moieties.[25-27] Dissociation of VIII from vWf by reduction suggests that these two moieties may be linked together by disulfide bonds. However, there is evidence that other forces may be involved in these interactions. High ionic strength or high concentration of Ca^{2+} ions also results in complete dissociation of VIII from vWf[28-33] as does lowering of the pH value.[31,34] Additionally it has been reported that the multimeric structure of VIII/vWf can be broken down into subunits of approximately 690 kDa by periodate oxidation[35] implying that the carbohydrate side-chains of the subunits may play a part in the subunit interactions. It is possible, however, that periodate oxidation could cleave disulfide bonds.

B. Interactions with Phospholipid

At the present time it is unclear whether or not lipoproteins or phospholipids (PL) are indispensable for the maintenance of the VIII/vWf complex. On the one hand, Hershgold et al.[36,37] reported that highly purified preparations of VIII contained PL, although treatment with phospholipase C variously inactivates VIII[37,38] or has little effect,[39-42] and phospholipase D increases VIII procoagulant (VIII:C) activity.[37] On the other hand, it has been reported that VIII/vWf contains little or no lipid[43,44] and that the PL content may reflect chylomicron content of the starting plasma[45] which is known to affect the size distribution of the VIII/vWf complexes.[39] Indirect evidence that VIII may interact with PL under physiological conditions is derived from observations that PL apparently blocks the antigenic sites on VIII antigen (VIII:Ag)[46-48] and can influence the dissociation of VIII from vWf.[49] Whether or not PL plays a structural role in maintaining the stability of the VIII/vWf complex, it is now widely accepted that PL is an essential component of the ''tenase'' complex wherein IXa, VIII:C, PL, and Ca^{2+} are indispensible for the conversion of factor X to Xa.[48,50,52] It has also been demonstrated that VIII may be protected against proteolysis by granulocyte proteases if the VIII is permitted to form a complex with IXa and PL.[53]

C. Interaction with Factors IX and X

Much of the experimental data on the interaction of VIII/vWf with PL also indicate that in the presence of PL and Ca^{2+}, VIII/vWf interacts with both factors IX or IXa to form the "tenase" complex. In this complex, PL and Ca^{2+} are believed to lower the binding constant of IXa for the substrate moiety factor X, whereas VIII having minimal effect on the binding constant enhances the rate of the reaction of IXa on factor X.[54]

D. Interactions with Fibrinogen and Fibronectin

The starting material for most methods of purification of VIII/vWf is cryoprecipitate,[55] which contains fibrinogen (Fg) and fibronectin (Fn) in addition to VIII/vWf.[55-57] Early work on Fn described it as an insoluble component of Cohn fraction 1.[58,59] Fn is characterized by its ability to form stable complexes with Fg and fibrin, and originally it was believed that it was a special form of Fg. Mosesson and Umfleet,[60] however, demonstrated that it could be resolved from Fg.[60] The "purified" Fn contained appreciable quantities of VIII raising the question of identity of these two plasma constituents. Subsequently, it has been clearly demonstrated that Fn and VIII are complete and separate entities.[61] Furthermore, Mazurier et al.[62,63] have studied cryoprecipitates isolated from Fn-depleted and afibrinogenemic plasmas and have shown that in each case both Fn and Fg are required for cryoprecipitation. Addition of extra Fn to normal plasma induced a higher recovery of VIII in cryoprecipitates. It is believed that at physiological temperatures there is little interaction among the three major components found in cryoprecipitate, but that at lower temperatures such interactions become significant. Possible conformational changes in the structures of the proteins induced by changes in ionic strength during the freezing process may strengthen the protein-protein interactions giving rise to the relatively insoluble cryoprecipitate.

It is believed that Fg and/or fibrin monomer does interact with VIII/vWf to form high molecular weight complexes. Mixtures of radiolabeled VIII/vWf with increasing concentrations of Fg show progressive shift of Fg to higher molecular weightforms.[17] It is believed that low concentrations of Fg are required to ensure the stability, recovery, and normal biological half-life of purified VIII preparations. Although most preparations tend to contain Fg, some reports indicate that its presence is not essential.[3,24] The interaction of VIII and Fg may be relevant for our understanding of the mechanism of platelet aggregation in primary hemostasis since both vWf and Fg bind at, or near to, the same receptor sites (glycoprotein [Gp] IIb/IIIa) on stimulated platelets.[65,68]

E. Interactions Necessary for Platelet Adhesion to the Subendothelium

The vWf moiety of the VIII/vWf complex is known to participate in primary hemostasis and is discussed in detail elsewhere.[69,70] Apart from the interaction of vWf with platelet Gp Ib[70-78] and Gp IIb/IIIa, its binding to collagen is of relevance in the anchorage of the platelet to the subendothelium.[79-85]

There are, however, other components of the subendothelium in addition to collagen which exhibit high affinity for vWf. Human vWf binds specifically and with high affinity to sulfated glycolipids, and the characteristics of binding parallel very closely those required for vWf-induced platelet adhesion or platelet aggregation.[86] Interaction of vWf with sulfated mucopolysaccharides and sulfated glycolipids may play an additional fundamental role, not only in vWf-induced platelet adhesion to endothelium, but also in the processing steps of vWf during biosynthesis and storage in the Weibel-Palade bodies of endothelial cells and in the megakaryocytes.[87] The affinity of VIII/vWf for sulfated polysaccharides can be used as the basis of an affinity chromatographic procedure for the isolation of the VIII/vWf macromolecular complex (see below).

F. Interaction with Immunoglobulins

The correlation of high concentrations of certain paraproteins and abnormal bleeding is well recognized, but the mechanism of the defective hemostasis observed in such cases is uncertain. Disproportionate reduction of VIII:C levels in patients with paraproteinemia raises the question of a possible interaction of VIII with the specific paraproteins present.[88] In cases of IgA and IgM paraproteinemia, the incidence of low levels of plasma VIII:C is common. The bleeding which occurs in these patients resembles that in von Willebrand's disease (vWD), and there would seem to be a direct correlation of incidence of bleeding with paraprotein levels. The evidence is not clear, however, since there is a direct correlation between hemorrhage and raised total plasma protein levels which, in turn, correlates with viscosity and prolongation of the thrombin time, the partial thromboplastin time (PTT), and the thromboplastin generation test. These findings raise the possibility of direct interaction of paraproteins with platelets or inhibition of coagulation factors other than VIII. Addition of paraprotein preparations (at 10 mg/ml) to normal plasma only prolongs the thrombin time. Thus, there is little evidence that, *in vivo*, VIII/vWf interacts with immunoglobulins. On the other hand, indirect evidence for an interaction of VIII/vWf with immunoglobulin can be inferred from the presence of immunoglobulin in VIII/vWf preparations obtained by gel filtration. Since both IgM and IgA tend to polymerize during handling processes, it is most likely that the resulting high molecular weight complexes cochromatograph with VIII/vWf. Such immunoglobulin contaminants in VIII/vWf preparations used to raise heterologous antisera may explain the apparent cross-reactivity of IgM as observed in gels obtained in the vWf multimer sizing technique developed using enzyme linked immunofixation methods.[22]

It would seem likely, therefore, that any interaction between VIII/vWf and immunoglobulins would be nonspecific in character and of insufficient stability to be of use in affinity chromatographic procedures for the isolation of VIII/vWf.

G. Interaction with Metal Cations

The VIII/vWf complex is involved in physiologically important interactions with metal cations. Free Ca^{2+} ions are crucial for both the intrinsic and extrinsic coagulation pathways, and blood may be conveniently anticoagulated by removal of free divalent metal cations by adding chelators such as oxalate, citrate, or EDTA. Calcium ions are indispensable for the formation of the "tenase" complex.[51,52,89] Here the absolute requirement of Ca^{2+} for the stability of this complex is largely explained through the part played by Ca^{2+} binding to the Gla residues of factor IX inducing the conformation changes necessary for full expression.[90] It has, however, been established that free Ca^{2+} ions are necessary for the preservation of VIIIa.[91,92] In citrated plasma, VIII:C has a relatively short half-life making isolation of the active VIII component more difficult when citrate-containing buffers are used.[93,94] Many investigators have found a beneficial effect of adding Ca^{2+} ions to their buffers, and special attention should be paid to the delicate balance between the stabilizing effect of free Ca^{2+} ions and the use of metal chelating anticoagulants in the buffers used for affinity chromatography procedures for isolation of VIII.

Calcium ions are now believed to play a crucial part in maintaining the VIII structure. Interchain metal ion bridges (probably Ca^{2+} bridges) have been identified holding the two chains of the heterodimeric VIII molecules together.[95-97] Addition of EDTA to VIII/vWf causes complete dissociation of the VIII from the vWf,[64,98] and apparently, binding of Ca^{2+} occurs at or near the antigenic determinants of VIII.[98] The presence of Ca^{2+} ions is also obligatory for the binding of vWf to the Gp IIb/IIIa binding sites of metabolically activated platelets,[65,67,68] and here the involvement of Ca^{2+} can be explained in part through the role that it plays in maintaining the necessary Gp interactions within the Gp IIb/IIIa complex itself.[99] Ca^{2+} ions seem to be less essential for the ristocetin-dependent binding of vWf to platelet Gp Ib sites, although it has been reported that removal of Ca^{2+} using 2 mM EGTA results in 86% inhibition of binding of vWf to this receptor.[74] The relevance of Ca^{2+} ions in the function of vWf is still under debate since there is a stoichiometric 1:1 ratio of Ca^{2+} to vWf subunits as assessed by atomic absorbtion.[100] Calcium ions do not seem to be influential in vWf multimer formation.

IV. CONVENTIONAL ION EXCHANGE CHROMATOGRAPHY

VIII and vWf are both acidic proteins. The electrophoretic mobility,[36] amino acid composition,[21,33] and sequence data[13,15,96] indicate that VIII should have a low isoelectric point. Similarly the electrophoretic mobility[101-105] amino acid composition[106,107] and sequence data[108] of purified vWf suggest that this protein should also have an acidic isoelectric point. The isoelectric points of both bovine and human vWf have been determined. A pI for human vWf of 4.61 to 4.80 was determined by isoelectric focusing in small columns, and by isoelectric focusing in agarose gels the pI was estimated to be between 4.91 and 4.96.[109] The acidic nature of vWf was further confirmed by isoelectric focusing in agarose gels in the presence of 7 M urea when it was found that the vW protein could be resolved into three components with pI values between 5.7 and 5.9.[110]

Since both VIII and vWf are most stable at neutral, or near neutral, pH values it is logical that at these pH values both VIII and vWf should carry net negative charges. Thus, they should be amenable to binding and reelution from anion-exchange matrices without employing conditions that would lead to denaturation and low yields. In the earliest application of anion-exchange principles for the isolation of VIII, ECTEOLA-cellulose was used,[111] but soon it was found that better yields could be obtained if either DEAE-Floc or DEAE-Sephadex A25[112] were used. The probable explanation for the better yields is the higher capacity of DEAE matrices, e.g., DEAE-Sephadex A25 contains 3.2 meg. DEAE groups per gram resin. Methodology in the earlier experiments was largely confined to binding on and reelution using the same buffers. Veder[112] was able to obtain a highly concentrated form of VIII, with Cohn fraction 1 as starting material, employing a chromatography step on DEAE-Sephadex A25 and phosphate buffer pH 7.5 in 1.6% NaCl. Michael and Tunnah[113] extended these findings using DEAE-Cellulose (DE50) for the purification of bovine VIII starting with a 2 M sodium phosphate precipitate of $BaSO_4$-absorbed oxalated plasma. In these experiments active material was redissolved in 16% urea, 0.4 M NaCl, 20 mM imidazole buffer pH 7.1 and following the binding step, VIII was recovered through application of a 0.85 M NaCl, 64 mM sodium phosphate buffer pH 6.35. In the light of what we now know of the role that Ca^{2+} ions play in maintaining VIII:C, it is not surprising that the final product was unstable, when Ca^{2+} was not incorporated into the buffer systems. Hynes et al.[114] refined the procedure further by eluting human VIII from phosphate-equilibrated DEAE-Cellulose using a series of step-wise elution buffers combining both increase in phosphate concentration and decrease in pH value: the final product was essentially free of Fg.

The use of DEAE-matrices for the purification of VIII/vWf was extended further when salt gradients were used to reelute the bound activities. McKee et al.[115] showed that VIII bound to DEAE-Cellulose could be reeluted using a 0 to 0.5 M linear NaCl gradient in 50 mM Tris buffer pH 7.35. VIII:C eluted as a single peak of activity in fractions with conductivities between 8 and 15 mmhos. In another series of experiments, DEAE-agarose was used to show that vWf:Ag bound in redissolved cryoprecipitate could be resolved into two components using a linear NaCl gradient in 10 mM Tris buffer pH 7.5.[116] vWf:Ag with the faster electrophoretic mobility was first to elute from the matrix suggesting that charge differences may exist between the two forms of vWf:Ag resolved by this anion-exchange chromatography procedure. Olson et al.[106] showed that all detectable vWf ristocetin cofactor (vWf:RCo) eluted between 0.25 and 0.4 M NaCl with overall yields of 20 to 40% if a linear 50 to 550 m*M* NaCl gradient in 25 m*M* citrate buffer pH 6.15 was used to elute from DEAE-Cellulose. In this particular series of experiments partially purified human vWf:RCo obtained by gel filtration methods was applied to the anion-exchange matrix. No detectable VIII:C was found in any of the fractions, but this may be explained through cumulative losses experienced in the succession of procedural steps performed at 20°C, culminating in the final anion-exchange chromatographic step.

Despite the limitations placed by DEAE matrices for the purification of either VIII or vWf, it has still been of use for the isolation of a low molecular weight chemically reduced form of VIII which was then subsequently used for VIII structural studies. In this manner, Vehar and Davie[11] recovered reduced bovine VIII as a single broad peak from DEAE-Sephadex A50 using a complicated combined linear gradient of 0.15 to 1.5 *M* NaCl, 0 to 0.01 *M* 4-morpholine ethane sulfonic acid (MES), and pH gradient 6.6 to 6.3 in 20 m*M* imidazole.

More recently investigators have favored the quaternary amino ethyl (QAE)-bound matrices as ion exchanges rather than DEAE supports. Baugh et al.[117] were able to reelute both vWf and VIII following binding to QAE Sephadex A25 with a linear 0.15 to 2 *M* NaCl gradient in 20 m*M* imidazole buffer pH 6.0. The vWf eluted first at approximately 0.35 *M* NaCl, followed by the VIII at 0.5 *M* NaCl. In this study it was found that the isolated VIII:C was unstable in that it lost 98% activity at 4°C in 3 d, whereas the initial material, the void peak from a Sepharose 4B chromatography step, was stable for several weeks at 4°C. This is additional evidence for the role that vWf plays in stabilizing VIII:C within the VIII/vWf complex. In a similar procedure[118] QAE cellulose was used for the isolation of porcine VIII using a 0.15 to 0.8 *M* NaCl gradient in a 10 m*M* histidine, 5 m*M* CaCl$_2$ buffer pH 6.0. Here VIII:C was resolved from the vWf which presumably eluted off the matrix at low salt concentrations.

More recently, in an elegant procedure Fay et al.[10] have used Mono Q resin to resolve VIII:C into two active components using a linear 0.05 to 1.0 *M* LiCl gradient in 20 m*M* HEPES, 5 m*M* CaCl$_2$, 10% glycerol buffer pH 7.2. As part of their purification strategy, they concentrated the fraction eluting from a column of aminohexyl sepharose (see below) by first absorbing it onto a small column of trisacryl *M* DEAE using 20 m*M* imidazole, 50 m*M* NaCl, 5 m*M* CaCl$_2$, 1 m*M* sodium citrate buffer pH 7.0, and then quantitatively eluting with a 0.25 *M* CaCl$_2$ salt-step and desalting on a column of Sephacryl S 400 before applying to the Mono Q column. These procedural steps are of considerable relevance in that they illustrate the sequential use of two anion exchange matrices.

V. AMINO ALKANE-DERIVATIZED MATRICES

In the preceeding section the use of matrices with positively charged tertiary (DEAE) or quarternary (QEAE, syn. QAE) amino groups as ligands for anion-exchange chromatography of VIII/vWf was considered. Austen,[119,120] Austen and Smith,[121] and Neal et al.[122] have pioneered procedures for the isolation of VIII from either citrated plasma or redissolved cryoprecipitate as preferred source material through affinity binding to aminohexyl sepharose (AH Sepharose). The presumed site of binding to this matrix was believed to be the primary amino residues of the AH groups. Application of buffers containing 0.1 *M* sodium acetate, 0.1 *M* L-lysine pH 5.5 could be expected to fully protonate the AH groups and thus act as anion-exchange groups. In high-loading semi-batch experiments,[122] VIII:C and vWf could be reeluted using linear 0 to 0.86 *M* NaCl gradients giving a highly concentrated product with an overall yield of approximately 40% VIII:C. This material demonstrated a specific activity of 1.8 U VIII:C per milligram total protein which represented a three- to fourfold purification with respect to the activity of the VIII starting material. In these experiments, apparently the total recovery of vWf:Ag must have been even higher since the ratio vWf:Ag to VIII:C had increased from 3.4 to 6.9. This would indicate that during the purification step some of the VIII:C had lost its biological activity. The encouraging aspect of the use of AH Sepharose is the high capacity of the matrix (7 µmol AH ligand groups per milliliter resin) permitting high loading of VIII/vWf and recommending its use for batch-wise binding procedures. The VIII:C in the eluted material was stable and almost completely devoid of Fg.

The earlier data from experiments with AH Sepharose indicated that under the chosen binding and elution conditions (pH 5.5) there is some degree of dissociation of VIII:C from vWf. When elution was achieved with linear NaCl gradients the vWf normally eluted from the columns before the VIII:C.[124,120] This dissociation has been turned to advantage by Amphlett and Hrinda[125] who bound VIII/vWf to AH Sepharose equilibrated with 20 mM imidazole, 0.1 M L-lysine buffer pH 6.8. The resolution of vWf and the VIII was achieved with two sequential salt steps of 0.4 M NaCl, 10 mM CaCl$_2$, and either 0.3 to 0.5 M CaCl$_2$ or 1.0 M NaCl, 10 mM CaCl$_2$. The VIII:C was obtained in high yield and free of vWf. In these experiments, the higher pH value used would favor preservation of the functinal integrity of the VIII/vWf complex in the initial material throughout the binding step. Additionally, the incorporation of 0.1 M lysine and 10 mM CaCl$_2$ in the eluting buffer favored stabilization of VIII:C.[123]

Morgenthaler[124] has questioned whether or not an anion-exchange mechanism is solely responsible for the binding to AH Sepharose. He studied the binding of both VIII and vWf to a series of diaminoalkyl and aminoalkyl derivatives of Sepharose 4B using similar conditions to those chosen by Austin,[119,120] Austen and Smith,[121] and Neal et al.[122] Increasing amounts of protein as well as VIII were bound to matrices derivatized with ligands of increasing chain length. When coupling different derivatized matrices with ligand groups of the same chain length but with free tertiary amino groups rather than free primary amino groups, the elution profiles were remarkably similar. Furthermore, the effect of the free amino groups was investigated by chromatography of VIII/vWf using matrices where the series of aminoalkyl ligand groups could be directly compared with the homologous series of alkyl chain groups. The results suggested that in these matrices, VIII could bind via additional mechanism(s) other than simple anion exchange, presumably via hydrophobic interaction. It was concluded that the mechanism of binding of both VIII and vWf to AH Sepharose combined elements of both ionic and hydrophobic interactions and that VIII and vWf probably bound independently of each other. The implication from the order of elution that VIII probably has a lower isoelectric point than vWf need not necessarily be true.

It is both relevant and interesting that agmatine-sepharose has been used as one of the steps for the purification of human vWf. The bound vWf could be reeluted ahead of, and resolved from Fn and Fg, using linear NaCl gradients at neutral pH.[107] In this matrix the ligands are alkyl guanidinium groups, and it could be expected that ion-exchange mechanisms similar to those that pertain for AH Sepharose are operative for the binding of vWf.

VI. SULFATED MATRICES

In the light of the foregoing section, it would not be expected that any success could be achieved using sulfated matrices under physiological conditions of pH and ionic strength since here both the VIII/vWf and the matrices should display net negative charges.

Sulfated dextran beads[126] and dextran sulphate (DS) Sepharose[127,128] have been employed with great success for the resolution of human coagulation factors II, IX, and X and protein C[130] isolated by batch-wise adsorption and reelution from BaSO$_4$. Vehar and Davie[11] showed that chemically reduced bovine VIII was bound to sulfated Sepharose CL-4B using 20 mM imidazole, 20 mM glycylethyl ester, 10 mM CaCl$_2$, 0.15 M NaCl buffer pH 6.8 and could then be reeluted with 0.65 M NaCl. In our laboratory it has been possible to isolate both human VIII and vWf from either citrated plasma or cryoprecipitate using sulfated matrices. Cryoprecipitate redissolved in 14 mM citrate, 0.15 NaCl, 2.5 mM CaCl$_2$ buffer pH 6.85 was bound onto sulfated Sepharose CL 4B at 4°C, and VIII/vWf was resolved from most of the bound plasma proteins through use of a linear NaCl gradient. In these experiments the order of elution was Fg, Fn, and VIII/vWf with total vWf and VIII:C recoveries of 80 and 35%, respectively.[129] It would seem that the VIII/vWf complex itself or some other related component interacting with the complex must be binding directly to the highly anionic charge groups.

It has been recognized for some time that the sulfated glycosamino glycans (GAGs) heparin and DS[133] are powerful inhibitors of the ristocetin dependent vWf activity mediating platelet aggregation. This inhibition could not be explained adequately through interaction of the negatively charged heparinoids with the polycationic aminoglycoside antibiotic ristocetin. It has been shown that both VIII and vWf could bind to either heparin or DS immobilized onto agarose beads[132,133] by the CNBr-coupling method of Andersson.[149] Bound VIII:C and VIII:Ag could be recovered through application of linear NaCl gradients. It was further demonstrated that the affinity of binding of VIII/vWf correlated with the degree of sulfation of the matrix ligand. DS preparations with only 5% sulfur content displayed little binding capacity, whereas DS with 17% sulfur displayed high affinity for VIII/vWf. One interesting aspect of these experiments was the apparent co-elution of VIII and vWf:RCo/vWf:Ag such that the potential presence of the vWf moiety could stabilize VIII:C.

The interaction of VIII/vWf with DS-agarose matrices has been developed further in this laboratory[135,136] by studying the interaction of VIII/vWf with high molecular weight DS (500,000 Da 17% sulfur) immobilized onto either 4% agarose or porous glass beads. It was shown that if binding was performed at ambient room temperatures vWf:Ag was detected in both the column wash-through fractions and as a peak of high vWf:RCo/vWf:Ag on the gradient at approximately 0.47 M NaCl. The salt-gradient fraction contained all the vWf:RCo detectable in the applied samples. The observation that only that part of the total vWf that contains the vWF:RCo bound to the matrix correlates well with the observations of Roberts et al.[86] that the high multimeric forms of vWf have the highest affinity for sulfated glycolipids. This could imply that glycolipids could be a possible vWf:RCo binding site on platelets. Indirect evidence that the platelet-binding site(s) of vWf are implicated in binding to DS or sulfated GAGs is the observation that of the two major peptide fragments produced by *Staphylococcus* V8 protease digestion of purified vW protein, only one (fragment 2) could bind to heparin- or DS-agarose. This fragment retained affinity for the Gp Ib platelet-binding site.[87]

We have investigated the pH dependence of binding of vWf:Ag to DS-agarose at ambient room temperature and found that binding was optimal at pH 6.85. At this pH value vWf:Ag could be reeluted with 0.47 M NaCl, whereas at pH values removed from 6.85, lower NaCl was required to effect reelution. Thus, it is possible to use either increasing salt concentration or decreasing pH gradients to effect the reelution of VIII/vWf bound at pH 6.85. We have found that at 4°C where VIII is sufficiently stable, combined increasing linear NaCl and convex decreasing pH gradients permitted almost complete separation of Fg and Fn from VIII/vWf as shown in Figure 1. Yields of 90% vWf:Ag, 90% vWf:RCo, 65% VIII:Ag, and 35% VIII:C were observed. In these experiments the initial material, Al(OH)$_3$-adsorbed cryoprecipitate redissolved in 14 mM citrate, 2.14 mM CaCl$_2$, and 0.15 M NaCl, was applied to the columns of DS-agarose equilibrated at pH 7.3. Using the same buffer with added 1.0 M glycine, elution was performed with a gradient to a final buffer concentration of 1.0 M NaCl at pH 5.5. Under these conditions the VIII/vWf eluted at 0.38 M NaCl, pH 6.5. Furthermore, the overall yields can be improved (100% VIII:Ag, 80% VIII:C) if the initial Al(OH)$_3$-adsorbed cryoprecipitate is also adsorbed against celite to remove the contact factors, and if lysine is incorporated into the eluting buffers. As the stability of VIII:C is

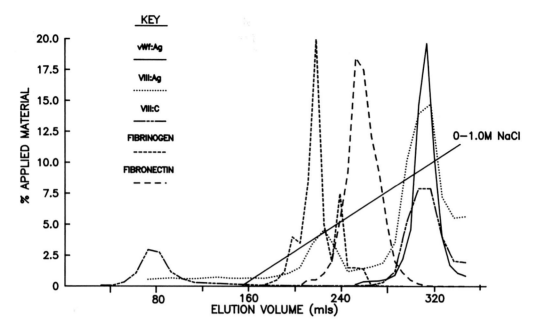

FIGURE 1.   The purification of VIII/vWf on DS Sepharose (combined pH/salt gradient). Both VIII and vWf were completely resolved from Fn and Fg. Albumin and IgG remained unbound. The equilibration buffer was 14 m*M* trisodium citrate, 2.14 m*M* calcium chloride, 0.15 *M* NaCl, 1.0 *M* glycine, pH 7.3. The gradient buffer was 0.15 to 1.0 *M* NaCl in the same buffer at pH 5.5.

dependent upon the presence of free Ca^{2+} ions, we have found it beneficial to incorporate $CaCl_2$ at a final concentration of 2.5 to 10 m*M* into all the buffers. Alternatively, $CaCl_2$ gradients can be used to effect resolution of vWf:Ag from VIII:Ag.[12] Under such elution conditions detectable VIII:C is not entirely coincident with the chromatographic profiles of vWf:Ag or VIII:Ag.

Most of the proteolytic enzyme contaminants as assessed by chromogenic substrate assays (S2222 and S2238) of eluted fractions from DS-agarose columns could be removed by precipitation with 10% PEG 6000, when the bulk of the enzymic activity remains in the supernatant. Alternatively, the use of celite absorbed cryoprecipitate with the incorporation of L-lysine into equilibrating and eluting buffers eradicates such enzymic activity in the eluted fractions. The specific activity of the final products is usually of the order of 1.5 U VIII:C per milligram total protein when assayed by the Lowry method.[137] However, it is conceivable that this value is an underestimate, since SDS-PAGE demonstrated only trace amounts of protein in these fractions. As α and β lipoproteins were detected by enzyme linked immunoabsorbant assay (ELISA) in these fractions, an overestimate of protein concentration is most probable since these substances are known to give falsely high values in conventional protein estimation methods.[138]

At the present time there is no clear evidence for the mechanism of binding of VIII/vWf to DS-agarose. The order of elution is Fg, Fn, and VIII/vWf. In some experiments where there is partial dissociation of the VIII:Ag from vWf:Ag, the VIII:C would appear to have higher affinity for DS than the vWf. This order of elution is precisely the reverse of that observed for reelution of Fg, Fn, and VIII/vWf from agmatine-[107] or AH[122] Sepharose. Since binding to agmatine- or AH Sepharose may be mediated in part through anion-exchange mechanisms, it is logical to assume that binding of VIII/vWf to sulfated matrix could be mediated through cation-exchange mechanisms. Over the pH range investigated, however, both VIII and vWf should bear net negative charges so that to invoke cation-exchange mechanisms it is feasible that whole domains on each of the proteins are positively charged,

Table 1

Salt	Molarity of Elution (pH 6.85) (*M*)
Lithium chloride (LiCl)	0.94
Sodium chloride (NaCl)	0.46
Potassium chloride (KCl)	0.29
Sodium sulfate (Na_2SO_4)	0.35
Potassium sulfate (K_2SO_4)	0.17
Ammonium chloride (NH_4Cl)	0.73
Magnesium chloride ($MgCl_2$)	0.43
Sodium fluoride (NaF)	0.73
Sodium bromide (NaBr)	0.38
Sodium formate ($NaHCO_2$)	0.58
Sodium acetate ($NaCH_3CO_2$)	0.64
Ammonium sulfate ($[NH_4]_2SO_4$)	0.42

a concept that is supported by the observations of vWf binding to heparin.[87] Alternatively, binding may be mediated through metal ion bridges or PLs. In our experience we have not observed any differences in the chromatography elution profiles of dialysed VIII and vWf:Ag on DS-agarose; both equilibrated and eluted on the one hand with buffers comprising EDTA and on the other with buffers comprising 10 m*M* $CaCl_2$. These results indicate that the presence of metal ion bridges between the bound protein and the DS groups is unlikely, but such a mechanism has not been sufficiently well investigated to be completely discounted. It is likely that the mechanism(s) of binding will be complex, and as is believed binding to AH Sepharose will probably incorporate elements of both hydrophilic and hydrophobic interactions. vWf:Ag can be reeluted with a whole range of salts in addition to NaCl at room temperature pH 6.85. For each individual salt the VIII/vWf elutes at a distinct and separate ionic strength. In general, efficacy of elution is found for the series $F^- < Cl^- < Br^- < I^-$, and $Li^+ < Na^+ < K^+$ as shown in Table 1. These findings do not support any theory for the binding of VIII/vWf to immobilized sulfate groups with cation exchange as the sole mechanism of interaction.

It is fortuitous that the use of matrix bound high molecular weight DS allows co-chromatography of VIII and vWf. It is not yet established whether these two components bind concertedly with the bonds between VIII and vWf remaining unbroken, or whether they bind independently of each other. In some experiments, the VIII:Ag eluted close to, but just subsequent to vWf:Ag, indicating that they may bind independently of each other. The true order of affinity would thus be Fg < Fn < vWf:Ag < VIII:Ag. As further support for the view that VIII:Ag may bind to the DS groups independently is the finding that cryoprecipitate obtained from heparinized plasma is rich in vWf, but the bulk of the original VIII:Ag is recovered in the cryosupernatant. Here the inference is that heparin interacts preferentially with the vWf:Ag causing dissociation from VIII:Ag.[125,139,140] One important additional observation is the time course in batch-wise binding experiments performed at 4°C using redissolved cryoprecipitates — all the Fg and Fn bound to the DS-agarose beads within 15 min. The vWf:Ag, however, bound much slower in that after 10 and 18 h of mixing, only 50 and 90%, respectively, of the initial activity vWf was found. Although VIII/vWf has a higher affinity for DS-agarose than Fg and Fn in cryoprecipitate, the overwhelming proportion of the latter proteins can act as effective competitors for the VIII/vWf-binding sites. The binding of VIII/vWf is slow, but when favorable conditions pertain as apparently occur during salt gradient elution column chromatography, the true affinity of VIII/vWf for the DS ligand groups is revealed. This is exemplified by the procedure described by Andersson et al.[141] to remove Fg from cryoprecipitate in the purification of VIII. If the competitive effect of Fg is reduced either by increasing the ionic strength conditions of the applied sample or by using Fg-depleted samples, the kinetics of VIII/vWf binding are dramatically enhanced. These procedures increase the capacity of the matrix to bind cryo-precipitate vWf from 9 vWf U/ml resin to 25 vWf U/ml resin.

VII. PRECIPITATION WITH POLYVINYL PYRROLIDONE

Various chemical methods have been tried to selectively precipitate the VIII:C moiety from whole citrated plasma. Casillas and Simonetti[142] have reported that polyvinyl pyrrol-idone (PVP) at a final concentration of 4% (w/v) can be used to precipitate VIII from either acid citrate dextrose (ACD) or citrate phosphate dextrose (CPD) plasma at 5°. Following resolubilization of the washed precipitates in citrate saline, the product was estimated to have a specific activity of 1.5 VIII:C U/mg total protein at a concentration of 17 VIII:C U/ml. In view of the proven nontoxicity of PVP the procedure for isolation of VIII:C from whole plasma is very attractive, but in a subsequent report it was suggested that the original claims for the effectiveness of PVP as a precipitating agent may not be so dramatic as originally claimed.[143]

VIII. INTERACTION WITH POLYELECTROLYTES

Polycationic matrices[144,145] have been used for the isolation of VIII/vWf. Solid phase cross-linked polyelectrolytes (PEs) synthesized through co-polymerization of ethylene and maleic anhydride have been manufactured with differing charge densities depending upon the proportion of maleic anhydride that has been substituted with dimethyl-amino propylimide (DMAPI) residues. Each dimethyl-amino group has a pKa value of between 8.0 and 8.5. At physiological conditions of pH and ionic strength, these tertiary amino groups will be expected to be fully protonated. These matrices can act as polycationic supports to selectively purify VIII and vWf, and the vitamin K dependent factors from citrated whole plasma. When adsorption is performed at pH 7.8 using E-100 (PE resin in which there is only DMAPI and no maleic anhydride residues), the acidic vitamin K dependent factors are preferentially bound leaving both VIII and vWf in the supernatant. If the pH is lowered to 6.0 and adsorbed against E-5 (copolymer of 5% DMAPI and 95% maleic anhydride) added at 80 mg/ml, only VIII:C binds which can be reeluted with 50 mM citrate, 1.0 M NaCl buffer pH 6.7. The supernatant from the E-5 adsorption step is then treated with an E-100 matrix whereby vWf binds and can subsequently be reeluted by 0.75 M NaCl.

The results obtained with these matrices indicate that their interactions with vWf and VIII are predominantly via cation exchange mechanisms. It was found, however, at pH 8.6 to 9.0 where the resin should be uncharged, that reelution of bound vWf by NaCl was not enhanced. This suggests the possibility that hydrophobic forces in addition to the expected electrostatic forces play a part in the binding process comparable to the mechanism of VIII/vWf binding to AH Sepharose.[124] PEs can be used in an alternative manner for the purification of VIII:C. When citrated whole plasma is subjected to partial chemical reduction with 1 mM DTT for 1 h at pH 7.8 to 8.2, all vWf:RCo is inactivated. Following alkylation of free thiol groups with iodocetamide and partial purification of the resulting VIII:C by gel filtration and PEG precipitation procedures, VIII:C could still be bound onto E-5 resin using 20 mM citrate, 0.15 M NaCl buffer pH 6.0. The matrix is then washed with 0.3 M NaCl to remove nonspecifically bound proteins, and the reduced alkylated VIII:C could be recovered using a 0.4 to 0.5 M linear NaCl gradient.[146]

IX. INTERACTION WITH LIPID VESICLE MATRICES

The important role of PL in stabilizing the ''tenase'' complex has been discussed. One interesting development arising from such studies is that it has been possible to use the interaction of VIII:C with PL to devise a column chromatographic procedure for the isolation of VIII with enriched with respect to vWf content.[147] PL vesicles comprising equal amounts of phosphatidyl serine and phosphatidylethanolamine (PS/PE) were chemically immobilized onto a Biogel A 15 *M* matrix by a two-step CNBr method. Coagulation factors II, IX, and X were bound to the matrix in a Ca^{2+} ion dependent manner. In the presence of 5 m*M* $CaCl_2$, II, IX, and X could be bound as the prothrombin complex in 20 m*M* imidazole, 0.15 *M* NaCl buffer pH 7.3. Following washing procedures, the bound Vitamin K dependent factors could be reeluted by omitting the Ca^{2+} from the buffer. At the same time, VIII/vWf was also observed to bind to the PL matrix, but was Ca^{2+} ion independent. The bound VIII could not be reeluted with 1.0 *M* NaCl, although a significant amount could be recovered through use of chaotropic reagents such as 1 *M* KSCN. The final product demonstrated an VIII:C vWf ratio of 1.82:1. These studies suggest that the primary mechanism underlying the interaction of VIII with PL is predominantly hydrophobic.

X. INTERACTION WITH IMMOBILIZED METAL CHELATE AFFINITY MATRICES

Immobilized metal affinity chromatography (IMAC) is a technique whereby ligands can be separated through differential interaction with metal cations immobilized on inert matrices.[148] When Zn^{2+} or Cu^{2+} ions are immobilized,[151] the ligand groups displaying highest binding affinity contain atoms with lone pairs of electrons. Such potential ligand groups on proteins are the sulfur atoms of free thiol groups, the nitrogen atoms of the ε amino side-chains of lysine residues, and the two nitrogen atoms in the imidazole rings of histidine residues.[150] Binding of proteins will be pH dependent since protonated nitrogens cannot bind to the immobilized metal cations, thus protein binding will be favored at higher pH. Protein binding is independent of ionic strength. Bound proteins can be reeluted from IMAC columns by either lowering pH or through the use of increasing competitor ligand concentrations. Most of the investigations that have been performed on plasma proteins have used serum as the starting material,[149] presumably because the metal chelators used as anticoagulants for plasma have made IMAC methods difficult. It is not surprising that IMAC principles have only been of use for the purification of few coagulation factors. Both Fg[152] and Factor XII[153,154] have been successfully isolated using Zn^{2+} ions coupled to bis-(carboxymethyl amino) agarose beads, probably because both are basic proteins with sufficiently high affinity for the matrix to compete with the anticoagulants.

There is much evidence that VIII/vWf forms stable complexes with Ca^{2+} ions. There are purifications methods for VIII based upon selective binding to tricalcium phosphate,[155,156] calcium citrate-cellulose,[23,157] or $BaSO_4$.[156,158] There is amino acid sequence homology of VIII[115] with the Cu^{2+}-containing protein ceruloplasmin which suggests that metal-binding sites on VIII should exist although no metals other than Ca^{2+} have so far been detected in highly purified VIII.[100] On the other hand, VIII probably interacts only weakly with other cations, since Zn^{2+} can be used to precipitate preferentially Fg and Fn from redissolved cryoprecipitates leaving VIII/vWf in the supernatant.[159] There is even one report that VIII does not bind to Zn^{2+} immobilized chelate affinity matrices.[153]

We have reinvestigated the binding of VIII/vWf from citrated plasma and cryoprecipitate to both Zn^{2+} and Cu^{2+} immobilized onto bio(amino-carboxymethyl) Sepharoses 4B and 6B. Contrary to the earlier reports,[153,159] VIII/vWf displays high affinity for immobilized Zn^{2+} or Cu^{2+}. On the other hand, we found that VIII/vWf would not bind to the same matrices loaded with Ca^{2+}, Mg^{2+}, Cd^{2+}, or Mn^{2+} ions. These observations are of interest in that separation of VIII/vWf from citrated buffers onto either Zn^{2+} or Cu^{2+} columns while maintaining the Ca^{2+} concentrations may be achieved with high recovery. When either $Al(OH)_3$-adsorbed citrated plasma or redissolved cryoprecipitate is applied to either Zn^{2+}

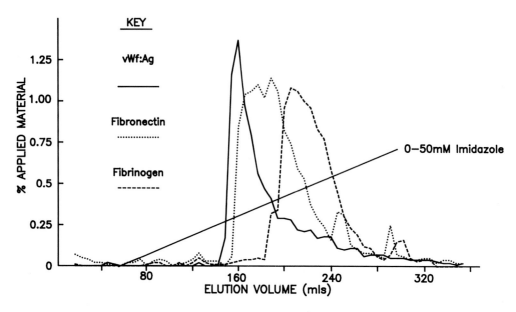

FIGURE 2.   Metal chelate chromatographic separation of VIII/vWf from Fn and Fg (imidazole gradient). Albumin and IgG remained unbound to the matrix.

or Cu^{2+} columns from 14 mM citrate, 0.15 M NaCl, 2.5 mM $CaCl_2$ buffer pH 7.4 at ambient room temperature, the bound VIII/vWf could be reeluted through either application of a decreasing pH gradient (VIII and vWf co-eluted at pH 6.5) or of a linear increasing imidazole gradient (VIII and vWf co-eluted at approximately 9 mM imidazole). When the citrate in the buffers used to create the decreasing pH gradients was replaced with a two-chamber system comprised of 0.1 M Tris HCl pH 7.5 and 0.1 M succinic acid pH 5.5, the VIII/vWf co-eluted at pH 6.05. This observation verifies the competitive nature of citrate for binding to the immobilized metals. At 4°C the apparent affinity of citrate for immobilized metal ions was so high that it precluded all binding of VIII/vWf. In order to perform IMAC studies at 4°C on VIII/vWf, it is necessary to remove the citrate prior to application or to use heparinized plasma.

At ambient room temperatures, the recoveries of VIII/vWf by IMAC methods were good. In binding experiments, step-wise elutions with 25 mM imidazole, 0.15 M NaCl, 14 mM citrate, 2.5 mM $CaCl_2$ pH 7.4 gave yields of VIII:C in excess of 80% with a procedural time of approximately 5 h. When either decreasing pH or increasing imidazole gradients were used for elution, the VIII/vWf was located in fractions eluting just ahead of the Fn and Fg as shown in Figure 2. Although these three proteins were poorly resolved from one another there was complete separation from all the albumin and the immunoglobulin-containing fractions. If bovine serum albumin (BSA) (5 mg/ml) were incorporated into eluting buffers, the VIII/vWf was recovered in the wash-through fractions, completely resolved from bound Fn and Fg. The use of albumin provides a novel method for the separation of the VIII/vWf from contaminating Fg and Fn.

One disadvantage in using IMAC methods for the isolation of VIII/vWf from plasma is the order of elution (VIII/vWf, Fn, Fg immunoglobulins). The VIII/vWf demonstrates lower affinity for the matrix than most of the other major plasma proteins other than albumin. The apparent capacity of the matrix for VIII/vWf from plasma is low. One volume of matrix is required to absorb the total VIII/vWf from an equal volume of citrated cryoprecipitate (3 to 5 U VIII:C per milliliter). IMAC principles, however, may ultimately prove useful for the further purification of VIII/vWf partially purified by other methods.

XI. INTERACTIONS WITH MATRIX BOUND SPECIFIC PROTEINS

A. Immobilized Factor X

Although this review has excluded mention of immunoaffinity chromatography matrices for the purification of VIII/vWf,[3,4] there are, however, a few reports of the application of known VIII/vWf-protein interactions for the design of solid matrices for isolation, purification, and further characterization of VIII/vWf. Vehar and Davie[11] used coagulation factor X immobilized onto Sepharose CL-4B beads for the further purification of reduced bovine VIII:C. Following binding in 20 mM imidazole, 8 mM CaCl$_2$, 17 mM glycylethyl ester buffer pH 6.6, the bound VIII:C protein was reeluted with 0.5 M NaCl.

B. Immobilized Fibrin Monomer

Loscalzo et al.[160] have investigated the use of soluble fibrin monomer (SFM) immobilized onto agarose beads to study the requirements for binding of vWf and glycocalicin, the water soluble proteolytic fragment of platelet Gp Ib. vWf displayed high affinity (Kd 15µg/ml vWf producing half-maximal binding) and stoichiometry (1.3 vWf molecules [monomers] bound per SFM molecule). The data presented indicate that glycocalicin could only bind when the vWf:SFM binary complex had been formed. SFM is believed to be the physiological equivalent of ristocetin and may play an important role in the initiation of vWf-dependent platelet binding to expose subendothelium at sites of vascular injury.[160]

C. Immobilized vWf

Use can be made of the affinity of the VIII moiety for the vWf moiety within the VIII/vWf complex to design matrices for the isolation of VIII:C. When VIII/vWf is immobilized onto agarose beads and allowed to interact with redissolved VIII concentrates, the bound VIII:C can be reeluted after removal of nonspecific proteins by the application of a 1.3 M NaCl, 50 mM Tris buffer pH 7.2. In this report [161] 1.8 U VIII:C were found to bind per milliliter matrix to which 6.7 U VIII/vWf had been covalently immobilized. This method demonstrates the slow kinetics of binding of VIII to affinity matrices. A steady state equilibrium between bound and free VIII:C was only achieved after 2 to 4 h incubation at ambient room temperature.

XII. INTERACTION WITH THIOL MATRICES

Both VIII and vWf are protein moieties of a macromolecular complex which can be separated following reduction of disulfide bonds.[25] Apparently little[25] if any[7] of either moieties *in vivo* have free thiol groups. There are methods for the isolation of VIII in a chemically reduced form but which still retains procoagulant activity. Harris et al.[162] have used both thiol-Sepharose 4B and thiopropyl-Sepharose 4B in the reduced form for the binding of the VIII/vWf-containing fractions obtained by PE E5 fractionation of the protein mixed disulfides formed with pyridyl disulphide. Bound proteins could be reeluted using a 0.1 to 5.0 mM DTT gradient, and the VIII:C was found to elute between 1 and 1.6 mM.

Using a similar strategy Wagner and Marder[163] were able to show that in human umbilical endothelial cells that biosynthetic processing of vW protein involved dimerization of large precursor subunits through disulfide bond formation in the rough endoplasmic reticulum and further multimerization of these protomers in the Golgi apparatus. Immune-purified vWf prepared from cells in which posttranslational processing had been inhibited by the ionophore monensin contained dimers with free thiol groups that could be separated from the fully reduced dimers by chromatography on thiol sepharose.

XIII. CONCLUSIONS AND FUTURE DEVELOPMENTS

The VIII complex is a multifunctional Gp displaying a broad spectrum of binding properties with a large number of plasma, platelet, and vessel wall components. The knowledge of these interactions can be utilized in the design of affinity matrices for the isolation, purification, and further characterization of either VIII, vWf, or the VIII/vWf complex. Knowledge of the charge density of both the VIII and the vWf moieties has been exploited in designing ion-exchange procedural steps, in particular the use of PE matrices of different affinities.

Much attention has been focused in recent times on the possible manufacture of VIII for therapeutic purposes using gene cloning methods. Whereas such methods have yielded VIII in moderately high yields,[13] the product will have to be further purified before clinical use.[164] Whereas immune affinity matrices show great promise for this purpose, they may not prove to be the most cost effective. Furthermore, it is remarkable that ligands known to interact with VIII/vWf, e.g., concanavalin A[165,166] and other lectins,[167] ristocetin, and collagen,[168] have not been exploited for the design of specific matrices.

An affinity resin with a nonimmunological ligand showing high specificity for both components of the VIII complex would be ideal. Because of the nature of VIII/vWf, however, it is unlikely that both components of the complex could bind independently of each other to the same class of matrix bound ligand group with similar binding characteristics allowing subsequent co-elution.

Dual ligand or amphipathic matrices may have to be utilized.[169] Although technically difficult to synthesize, such matrices with two different kinds of ligands immobilized onto the same matrix beads can be envisaged to take advantage of the unique binding properties of VIII and vWf for their ligands. The success of such an approach will largely depend upon finding appropriate conditions where not only will the VIII/vWf be resolved from the undesired components in the source material, but the individually bound VIII and vWf moieties will co-elute. Advantage can then be taken of the stabilizing effect of the vWf on the VIII:C activity providing conditions favor reassociation. If this approach is found to be unsuccessful then attention will have to be focused on the stability of the VIII/vWf complex on binding and elution from new or existing affinity matrices.

REFERENCES

1. **Cuatrecasas, P. and Anfinsen, C. B.,** Affinity chromatography, *Ann. Rev. Biochem.,* 40, 259, 1971.
2. **Lowe, C. R. and Dean, P. D. G.,** *Affinity Chromatography,* John Wiley & Sons, London, 1974.
3. **Tuddenham, E. G. D., Trabold, N. C., Collins, J. A., and Hoyer, L. W.,** The properties of factor VIII coagulant activity prepared by immunoadsorbant chromatography, *J. Lab. Clin. Med.,* 93, 40, 1979.
4. **Jorieux, S., Mazurier, C., de Romeuf, C., and Goudemand, M.,** Properties and interactions of a monoclonal antibody to human von Willebrand factor, presented at Int. Conf. on F VIII/vWF, Bari, June 10 to 15, 1985, 14.
5. **Davie, E. W. and Fujikawa, K.,** Basic mechanisms in blood coagulation, *Ann. Rev. Biochem.,* 44, 799, 1975.
6. **Hoyer, L. W.,** The factor VIII complex: structure and function, *Blood,* 58, 1, 1981.
7. **McKee, P. A.,** Observations on structure-function relationships of human antihemophilic/von Willebrand factor protein, *Ann. N.Y. Acad. Sci.,* 370, 210, 1981.
8. **Hoyer, L. W.,** Biochemistry of factor VIII, in *Hemostasis and Thrombosis: Basic Principles and Clinical Practice,* Coleman, R. W., Hirsh, J., Marder, V.-J., and Salzman, E. W., Eds., Lippincott, Philadelphia, 1982, 39.
9. **Koutts, J., Lavergne, J.-M., and Meyer, D.,** Immunological evidence that human factor VIII is composed of two linked moieties, *Br. J. Haematol.,* 37, 415, 1977.

10. **Fay, P. J., Anderson, M. T., Chavin, S. I., and Marder, V. J.,** The size of human factor VIII heterodimers and the effects produced by thrombin, *Biochim. Biophys. Acta,* 871, 268, 1986.
11. **Vehar, G. A. and Davie, E. W.,** Preparation and properties of bovine factor VIII (antihemophilic factor), *Biochemistry,* 19, 401, 1980.
12. **Hamer, R. J., Koldam, J. A., Beeser-Visser, N. H., and Sixma, J. J.,** Human factor VIII: purification from commercial factor VIII concentrate, characterisation, identification and radiolabeling, *Biochim. Biophys. Acta,* 873, 356, 1986.
13. **Toole, J. J., Knopf, J. L., Wozny, J. M., Sultzman, L. A., Buecker, J. L., Pittman, D. D., Kaufman, R. J., Brown, E., Shoemaker, C., Orr, E. C., Amphlett, G. N., Foster, W. B., Coe, M. L., Knutson, G. S., Fass, D. N., and Hewick, R. M.,** Molecular cloning of a cDNA encoding human antihaemophilic factor, *Nature,* 312, 342, 1984.
14. **Gitschier, J., Wood, W. I., Goralka, T. M., Wion, K. L., Chen, E. Y., Eaton, D. H., Vehar, G. A., Capon, D. J., and Lawn, R. M.,** Characterisation of the human factor VIII gene, *Nature,* 312, 326, 1984.
15. **Wood, W. I., Capon, D. J., Simonsen, C. C., Eaton, D. L., Gitschier, J., Keyt, B., Seeburg, P. H., Smith, D. H., Hollingshead, P., Wion, K. L., Delwart, E., Tuddenham, E. G. D., Vehar, G. A., and Lawn, R. M.,** Expression of active human factor VIII from recombinant DNA clones, *Nature,* 312, 330, 1984.
16. **Van Mourik, J. A., Bouma, B. N., LaBruyere, W. T., de Graf, S., and Mochtar, I. A.,** Factor VIII, a series of homologous oligomers and a complex of two proteins, *Thromb. Res.,* 4, 155, 1974.
17. **Savidge, G. F., Mahmood, N. M., Saundry, R. H., and Seghatchian, M. J.,** Interaction between F VIII/von Willebrand protein and fibrinogen, *Thromb. Haemost.,* 50, 255, 1983.
18. **Fass, D. N., Knutson, G. J., and Bowie, E. J. W.,** Porcine Willebrand factor: a population of multimers, *J. Lab. Clin. Med.,* 91, 307, 1978.
19. **Hoyer, L. W. and Shainoff, J. R.,** Factor VIII-related protein circulates in normal human plasma as high molecular weight multimers, *Blood,* 55, 1056, 1980.
20. **Meyer, D., Obert, B., Pietu, G., Lavergne, J.-M., and Zimmerman, T. S.,** Multimeric structure of factor VIII/von Willebrand factor in von Willebrand's disease, *J. Lab. Clin. Med.,* 95, 590, 1980.
21. **Ruggeri, Z. M. and Zimmerman, T. S.,** Variant von Willebrand's disease: characterisation of two subtypes by analysis of multimeric composition of factor VIII/von Willebrand factor in plasma and platelets, *J. Clin. Invest.,* 65, 1318, 1980.
22. **Chow, R., Harrison, P., and Savidge, G. F.,** Enzyme linked antibody systems for the visualisation of F VIII multimers, *Thromb. Haemost ,* 54, (Abstr. P440), 75, 1985.
23. **Counts, R. B., Paskell, S. L., and Elgee, S. K.,** Disulfide bonds and the quartenary structure of factor VIII/von Willebrand factor, *J. Clin. Invest.,* 62, 702, 1978.
24. **Legaz, M. E., Schmer, G., Counts, R. B., and Davie, E. W.,** Isolation and characterisation of human factor VIII (antihemophilic factor), *J. Biol. Chem.,* 248, 3946, 1973.
25. **Austen, D. E. G.,** Thiol groups in the blood clotting action of factor VIII, *Br. J. Haematol.,* 19, 477, 1970.
26. **Austen, D. E. G., Carey, M., and Howard, M. A.,** Dissociation of factor VIII-related antigen into subunits, *Nature (London),* 253, 55, 1975.
27. **Kirby, E. P. and Mills, D. C. B.,** The interaction of bovine factor VIII with human platelets, *J. Clin. Invest.,* 56, 491, 1975.
28. **Owen, W. G. and Wagner, R. H.,** Antihaemophilic factor: separation of an active fragment following dissociation by salts or detergents, *Thromb. Diath. Haemorrh.,* 27, 502, 1972.
29. **Cooper, H. A., Griggs, T. R., and Wagner, R. H.,** Factor VIII recombination after dissociation by $CaCl_2$, *Proc. Natl. Acad. Sci. U.S.A.,* 70, 2326, 1973.
30. **Weiss, H. J., Philips, L. L., and Rosner, W.,** Separation of subunits of antihemophilic factor (AHF) by agarose gel chromatography, *Thromb. Diath. Haemorrh.,* 27, 212, 1972.
31. **Brockway, W. J. and Fass, D. N.,** The nature of the interaction between ristocetin-Willebrand factor and the factor VIII coagulant activity molecule, *J. Lab. Clin. Med.,* 89, 1295, 1977.
32. **Floyd, K., Burns, W., and Green, D.,** On the interaction between ristocetin and ristocetin cofactor (RCoF), *Thromb. Res.,* 10, 841, 1977.
33. **Vukovich, T., Koller, E., and Doleschel, W.,** Low-molecular weight factor VIII requires a cofactor for its procoagulant activity, *Thromb. Res.,* 19, 503, 1980.
34. **Baugh, R., Brown, J., Sargeant, R., and Hougie, C.,** Separation of human factor VIII activity from the von Willebrand's antigen and ristocetin platelet aggregating activity, *Biochim. Biophys. Acta,* 371, 360, 1974.
35. **Kaelin, A. C.,** Sodium periodate modification of factor VIII procoagulant activity, *Br. J. Haematol.,* 31, 349, 1975.
36. **Hershgold, E. J., Davison, A. M., and Janszen, M. E.,** Isolation and some chemical properties of human factor VIII (antihemophilic factor), *J. Lab. Clin. Med.,* 77, 185, 1971.

37. **Hershgold, E. J., Davison, A. M., and Janszen, M. E.,** Human factor VIII (antihemophilic factor): activation and inactivation by phospholipases, *J. Lab. Clin. Med.,* 77, 206, 1971.

38. **Yoshioka, A., Peake, I. R., Furlong, R. A., Giddings, J. C., and Bloom, A. L.,** The interaction between factor VIII clotting antigen (VIIICAg) and phospholipid, *Br. J. Haematol.,* 55, 27, 1983.

39. **Vukovich, T., Marktl, M., and Nemeth, G.,** Heterogeneity of human factor VIII/vWF in lipaemic plasma, *Thromb. Res.,* 38, 215, 1985.

40. **Fukui, H., Mikami, S., Okuda, T., Murashima, N., Takase, T., and Yoshioka, A.,** Studies of von Willebrand factor: effects of different kinds carbohydrate oxidases, SH-inhibitors and some other chemical reagents, *Br. J. Haematol.,* 36, 259, 1977.

41. **Blecher, T. E., Westry, J. C., and Thompson, M. J.,** Synthesis of prococoagulant antihaemophilic factor in vitro, *Lancet,* i, 1333, 1978.

42. **Giddings, J. C., Shearn, S. A. M., and Bloom, A. L.,** Platelet-associated coagulation factors: immunological detection and the effect of calcium, *Br. J. Haematol.,* 39, 569, 1978.

43. **Green, D.,** A simple method for the purification of factor VIII (antihemophilic factor) employing snake venom, *J. Lab. Clin. Med.,* 77, 153, 1971.

44. **Marchesi, S. L., Shulman, N. R., and Gralnick, H. R.,** Studies on the purification and characterisation of human factor VIII, *J. Clin Invest.,* 51, 2151, 1972.

45. **Ratnoff, O. D., Kass, L., and Lang, P. D.,** Studies on the purification of antihemophilic factor (factor VIII): separation of partially purified antihemophilic factor by gel filtration of plasma, *J. Clin. Invest.,* 48, 957, 1969.

46. **Barrowcliffe, T. W., Gray, E., and Kemball-Cook, G.,** Binding to phospholipid protects factor VIII from inhibition by human antibodies, *Thromb. Haemost.,* 46, 15, 1981.

47. **Broden, K., Brown, J. E., and Andersson, L.-O.,** Effect of phospholipid on factor VIII coagulant activity and coagulant antigen, *Thromb. Res.,* 30, 651, 1983.

48. **Kobayashi, I., Lamme, S., and Nilsson, I. M.,** The interaction between factor VIII clotting antigen and phospholipids in genetic variants of haemophilia and von Willebrand's disease, *Thromb. Res.,* 35, 65, 1984.

49. **Andersson, L.-O. and Brown, J. E.,** Interaction of factor VIII-von Willebrand factor with phospholipid vesicles, *Biochem. J.,* 200, 161, 1981.

50. **Hemker, H. C., Kahn, M. J. P., and Devilee, P. P.,** The adsorption of coagulation factors onto phospholipids. Its role in the reaction mechanism of blood coagulation, *Thromb. Diath. Haemorrh.,* 24, 216, 1970.

51. **Lollar, P., Knutson, G. J., and Fass, D. N.,** Stabilisation of thrombin-activated porcine factor VIII:c by factor IXa and phospholipid, *Blood,* 63, 1303, 1984.

52. **Lollar, P., Knutson, G. J., and Fass, D. N.,** Activation of porcine factor VIII:c by thrombin and factor Xa, *Biochemistry,* 24, 8056, 1985.

53. **Varadi, K. and Eloidi, S.,** Increased resistance of factor IXa-factor VIII complex against inactivation by granulocyte proteases, *Thromb. Res.,* 19, 571, 1980.

54. **Hultin, M. B.,** Role of human factor VIII in factor X activation, *J. Clin. Invest.,* 69, 950, 1982.

55. **Pool, J. G., Hershgold, E. J., and Pappenagen, A. R.,** High-potency anti-haemophilic factor concentrate prepared from cryoglobulin precipitate, *Nature (London),* 203, 312, 1964.

56. **Over, J., Bouma, B. N., and van Mourik, J. A.,** Heterogeneity of human VIII — characterisation of VIII in the supernatant, *J. Lab. Clin. Med.,* 91, 32, 1964.

57. **Weinstein, M. and Deykin, D.,** Comparison of VIII related proteins prepared from cryoprecipitate, *Blood,* 53, 1095, 1979.

58. **Cohn, E. J., Strong, L. E., Hughes, W. L., Jr., Mulford, D. J., Ashworth, J. N., Melin, M., and Taylor, H. L.,** Preparation and properties of serum and plasma proteins. IV. A system for the separation into fractions of the protein and lipoprotein components of biological tissues and fluids, *J. Am. Chem. Soc.,* 68, 459, 1946.

59. **Blomback, B. and Blomback, M.,** Purification of human and bovine fibrinogen, *Ark. Kemi,* 10, 415, 1956/1957.

60. **Mosesson, M. W. and Umfleet, R. A.,** The CIG of human plasma, primary characteristics and relationship to fibrinogen, *J. Biol. Chem.,* 245, 5728, 1970.

61. **Cooper, H. A., Wagner, R. H., and Mosesson, M.,** CIG of human plasma and its relationship to VIII, *J. Lab. Clin. Med.,* 84, 258, 1974.

62. **Mazurier, C., Samor, B., Deromeuf, C., and Goudemand, M.,** The role of fibronectin in factor VIII/von Willebrand factor cryoprecipitation, *Thromb. Res.,* 37, 651, 1985.

63. **Mazurier, C., Samor, B., Lefebvre, A., and Seghatchian, G.,** Influence of fibronectin and fibrinogen in the F VIII/vWF cryoprecipitation process, *Thromb. Haemost.,* 50, 117, 1983.

64. **Mahmood, N., Chakraborty, R., and Savidge, G. F.,** The effect of calcium ions on the sedimentation velocity properties of F.VIII in anticoagulated plasma, *Thromb. Haemost.,* 54, 22, 1985.

65. **Furby, F. H., Berndt, M. C., Castaldi, P. A., and Koutts, J.,** Characterisation of calcium-dependent binding of exogenous factor VIII/von Willebrand factor to surface activated platelets, *Thromb. Res.,* 35, 501, 1984.
66. **Gralnick, H. R., Williams, S. B., and Coller, B. S.,** Fibrinogen competes with VIII for binding to glycoprotein IIb/IIIa when platelets are stimulated with thrombin, *Blood,* 64, 797, 1984.
67. **Lombardo, V. T., Hodson, E., Roberts, J. R., Kunicki, T. J., Zimmerman, T. S., and Ruggeri, Z. M.,** Independent modulation of von Willebrand factor and fibrinogen binding to the platelet membrane glycoprotein IIb/IIIa complex as demonstrated by monoclonal antibody, *J. Clin Invest.,* 76, 1950, 1985.
68. **Ginsberg, M. H., Lightsey, A., Kunicki, T. J., Kaufmann, A., Maguerie, G., and Plow, E. F.,** Divalent cation regulation of the surface orientation of platelet membrane glycoprotein IIb, *J. Clin. Invest.,* 78, 1103, 1986.
69. **Tschopp, T. B., Weiss, H. J., and Baumgartner, H. R.,** Decreased adhesion of platelets to subendothelium in von Willebrand's disease, *J. Lab. Clin. Med.,* 83, 296, 1974.
70. **Meyer, D. and Baumgartner, H. R.,** Role of von Willebrand factor in platelet adhesion to the subendothelium, *Br. J. Haematol.,* 54, 1, 1983.
71. **Weiss, H. J., Baumgartner, H. R., Tschopp, T. B., Tvritto, V. T., and Cohen, D.,** Correction by factor VIII of the impaired platelet adhesion to subendothelium in von Willebrand's disease, *Blood,* 51, 267, 1978.
72. **Doucet-de Bruine, M. H. M., Sixma, J. J., Over, J., and Beeser-Visser, N. H.,** Heterogeneity of human factor VIII. II. Characterisation of forms of factor VIII binding to platelets in the presence of ristocetin, *J. Lab. Clin. Med.,* 92, 96, 1978.
73. **Schneider-Trip, M. D., Jenkins, C. S. P., Kahlé, L. H., Sturk, A., and Ten Cate, J. W.,** Studies on the mechanism of ristocetin-induced platelet aggregation: binding of factor VIII to platelets, *Br. J. Haematol.,* 43, 99, 1979.
74. **Kao, K-J., Pizzo, S. V., and McKee, P. A.,** Demonstration and characterisation of specific binding sites for factor VIII/von Willebrand factor on human platelets, *J. Clin. Invest.,* 63, 656, 1979.
75. **Morisato, D. K. and Gralnick, H. R.,** Selective binding of the factor VIII/von Willebrand factor protein to human platelets, *Blood,* 55, 9, 1980.
76. **Fujimoto, T., Ohara, S., and Hawiger, J.,** Thrombin-induced exposure and prostacyclin inhibition of the receptor for factor VIII/von Willebrand factor on human platelets, *J. Clin. Invest.,* 69, 1212, 1982.
77. **Harrison, R. L. and McKee, P. A.,** Comparison of thrombin and ristocetin in the interaction between von Willebrand factor and platelets, *Blood,* 62, 346, 1983.
78. **Ruggeri, Z. M., de Marco, L., Gatti, L., Bader, R., and Montgomery, R. R.,** Platelets have more than one binding site for von Willebrand factor, *J. Clin. Invest.,* 72, 1, 1983.
79. **Scott, D. M., Griffin, B., Pepper, D. S., and Barnes, M. J.** The binding of purified factor VIII/von Willebrand factor to collagens of differing type and form, *Thromb. Res.,* 24, 467, 1981.
80. **Morton, L. F., Griffin, B., Pepper, D. S., and Barnes, M. J.,** The interaction between collagens and factor VIII/von Willebrand factor: investigation of the structural requirements for interaction, *Thromb. Res.,* 32, 545, 1983.
81. **Santoro, S. A.,** Preferential binding of high molecular weight forms of von Willebrand factor to fibrillar collagen, *Biochim. Biophys. Acta,* 756, 123, 1983.
82. **Kessler, C. M., Floyd, C. M., Rick, M. E., Krizek, D. M., Lee, S. L., and Gralnick, H. R.,** Collagen-factor VIII/von Willebrand factor protein interaction, *Blood,* 63, 1291, 1984.
83. **Bockenstest, P., McDonagh, J., and Handin, R. I.,** Binding and covalent cross-linking of purified von Willebrand factor to native monomeric collagen, *J. Clin Invest.,* 78, 551, 1986.
84. **Perret, B. A., Furlan, M., Jeno, P., and Beck, E. A.,** Von Willebrand factor-dependent agglutination of washed fixed human platelets by insoluble collagen isolated from bovine aorta, *J. Lab. Clin. Med.,* 107, 244, 1986.
85. **Roth, G. S., Titani, K., Hoyer, L. W., and Hickley, M. J.,** Localisation of binding sites within human von Willebrand factor for monomeric type III collagen, *Biochemistry,* 25, 8357, 1986.
86. **Roberts, D. D., Williams, S. B., Gralnick, H. R., and Ginsberg, V.,** von Willebrand factor binds specifically to sulphated glycolipids, *J. Biol. Chem.,* 261, 3306, 1986.
87. **Bockenstedt, P., Greenberg, J. M., and Handin, R. I.,** Structural basis of von Willebrand factor binding to platelet glycoprotein Ib and collagen, *J. Clin. Invest.,* 77, 743, 1986.
88. **Perkins, H. A., MacKenzie, M. R., and Fudenberg, H. H.,** Haemostatic defects in dysproteinaemias, *Blood,* 35, 695, 1970.
89. **Van Dieijen, G., Tans, G., Rosing, J., and Hemker, H. C.,** The role of phospholipid and factor VIIIa in the activation of bovine factor X, *J. Biol. Chem.,* 256, 3433, 1981.
90. **Jones, M. E., Griffith, M. J., Monroe, D. M., Roberts, H. R., and Lentz, B. R.,** Comparison of lipid binding and kinetic properties of normal, variant, and γ-carboxyglutamic acid modified human factor IX and IXa, *Biochemistry,* 24, 8064, 1985.

91. **Weiss, H. J.,** A Study of the cation- and pH-dependent stability of factors V and VIII in plasma, *Thromb. Diath. Haemorrh.,* 14, 32, 1965.

92. **Stibbe, J., Hemker, H. C., and Creveld, S.,** The inactivation of factor VIII in vitro, *Thromb. Diath. Haemorrh.,* 27, 43, 1972.

93. **Foster, P. R., Dickson, I. H., McQuillan, T. A., and Dawes, J.,** Factor VIII stability during the manufacture of a clinical concentrate, *Thromb. Hemostas.,* 50, (Abstr. 0347), 117, 1983.

94. **Foster, P. R., Dickson, I. H., and McQuillan, T. A.,** Stability of factor VIII during the preparation of an intermediate-purity factor VIII concentrate, *Br. J. Haematol.,* 53, 343, 1983.

95. **Fass, D. N., Knutson, G. J., and Katzmann, J. A.,** Monoclonal antibodies to porcine factor VIII coagulant and their use in the isolation of active coagulant protein, *Blood,* 59, 594, 1982.

96. **Truett, M. A., Blacher, R., Burke, R. L., et al.,** Characterisation of the polypeptide composition of human factor VIII:c and the nucleotide sequence and expression of the human kidney cDNA, *DNA (New York),* 4, 333, 1985.

97. **Andersson, L.-O., Forsman, N., Huang, K., Larsen, K., Lundin, A., Pavlu, B., Sandberg, H., Sewerun, K., and Smart, J.,** Internal duplication and sequence homology in factors V and VIII, *Proc. Natl. Acad. Sci. U.S.A.,* 82, 1688, 1985.

98. **Tran, T. H. and Duckert, F.,** Dissociation of factor VIII procoagulant antigen VIII:CAg and factor VIII related antigen VIIIR:Ag by EDTA-influence of divalent cation on the binding of VIII:CAg and VIIIR:Ag, *Thromb. Haemost.,* 50, 547, 1983.

99. **Fujimura, K. and Phillips, D. R.,** Calcium cation regulation of glycoprotein IIb-IIIa complex formation in platelet plasma membranes, *J. Biol. Chem.,* 258, 10247, 1983.

100. **Mikaelsson, M. E., Forsman, N., and Oswaldsson, U. M.,** Human factor VIII: a calcium-linked complex, *Blood,* 62, 1006, 1983.

101. **Legaz, M. E., Schmer, G., Counts, R. B., and Davie, E. W.,** Isolation and characterisation of human factor VIII (antihemophilic factor), *J. Biol. Chem.,* 248, 3946, 1973.

102. **Kernoff, P. B. A., Gruson, R., and Rizza, C. R.,** A variant of factor VIII related antigen, *Br. J. Haematol.,* 26, 435, 1974.

103. **Zimmerman, T. S., Roberts, J., and Edgington, T. S.,** Factor VIII related antigen: multiple molecular forms in human plasma, *Proc. Natl. Acad. Sci. U.S.A.,* 72, 5121, 1975.

104. **Thomas, K. B., Howard, M. A., Salem, H. H., and Firkin, B. G.,** Fast migrating protein, immunologically related to human factor VIII, studied by crossed immunoelectrophoresis in agarose, *Br. J. Haematol.,* 54, 221, 1983.

105. **Seghatchian, M. J.,** Electrophoretic distribution of F VIIIc: measured by chromogenic and clotting methods and comparison with other FVIII-associated activities, *Thromb. Haemost.,* 42, (Abstr. 0254), 111, 1983.

106. **Olson, J. D., Brockway, W. J., Fass, D. N., Bowie, E. J., and Mann, K. G.,** Purification of porcine and human ristocetin-Willebrand factor, *J. Lab. Clin. Med.,* 89, 1278, 1977.

107. **Chopek, M. W., Girma, J.-P., Fujikawa, K., Davie, E. W., and Titani, K.,** Human von Willebrand factor: a multivalent protein composed of identical subunits, *Biochemistry,* 25, 3146, 1986.

108. **Shelton-Inloes, B. B., Titani, K., and Sadler, J. E.,** cDNA sequences for human von Willebrand factor reveal five types of repeated domains and five possible protein sequence polymorphisms, *Biochemistry,* 25, 3164, 1986.

109. **Thay, LeP., Brown, J. E., Baugh, R. F., and Hougie, C.,** Electroisofocusing of bovine and human von Willebrand factor, *Fed. Proc. Fed. Am. Soc. Exp. Biol.,* 40, 777, 1981.

110. **Fulcher, C. A., Ruggeri, Z. M., and Zimmerman, T. S.,** Isoelectric focusing of human von Willebrand factor in urea-agarose gels, *Blood,* 61, 304, 1983.

111. **van Creveld, S., Pascha, C. N., and Veder, H. A.,** The separation of AHF from fibrinogen III, *Thromb. Diath. Haemorrh.,* 6, 282, 1961.

112. **Veder, H. A.,** Further purification of the antihaemophilic factor (AHF), *Thromb. Diath. Haemorrh.,* 16, 738, 1966.

113. **Michael, S. E. and Tunnah, G. W.,** The purification of factor VIII (antihaemophilic globulin). II. Further purification and some properties of factor VIII, *Br. J. Haematol.,* 12, 115, 1966.

114. **Hynes, H. E., Owen, C. A., Bowie, E. J. W., and Thompson, J. H.,** Citrate stabilisation of chromatographically purified factor VIII, *Blood,* 34, 601, 1969.

115. **McKee, P. A., Andersen, J. C., and Switzer, M. E.,** Molecular structural studies of human factor VIII, *Ann. N.Y. Acad. Sci.,* 240, 8, 1975.

116. **Zimmerman, T. S., Roberts, J., and Edgington, T. S.,** Factor VIII-related antigen: multiple molecular forms in human plasma, *Proc. Natl. Acad. Sci. U.S.A.,* 72, 5121, 1975.

117. **Baugh, R., Brown, J., Sargeant, R., and Hougie, C.,** Separation of human factor VIII activity from the von Willebrand's antigen and ristocetin platelet aggregating activity, *Biochim. Biophys. Acta,* 371, 360, 1974.

118. **Knutson, G. J. and Fass, D. N.**, Porcine factor VIII:c prepared by affinity interaction with von Willebrand factor and heterologous antibodies: sodium dodecyl sulphate polyacrylamide gel analysis, *Blood,* 59, 615, 1982.
119. **Austen, D. E. G.**, Separation of factor VIII by ion exchange chromatography, *Thromb. Haemost.,* 42, 111, 1979.
120. **Austen, D. E. G.**, The chromatographic separation of factor VIII on aminohexyl sepharose, *Br. J. Haematol.,* 43, 669, 1979.
121. **Austen, D. E. G. and Smith, J. K.**, Factor VIII fractionation on aminohexyl sepharose with possible reduction in hepatitis B antigen, *Thromb. Haemost.,* 48, 46, 1982.
122. **Neal, G. C., Hersee, D., and Smith, J. K.**, Purification of factor VIII on aminohexyl sepharose, *Thromb. Haemost.,* 54, 78, 1985.
123. **Faure, A., Caron, M., and Tepernier, D.**, Improved buffer for the chromatographic separation of factor VIII coagulant, *J. Chromatogr.,* 257, 387, 1983.
124. **Morgenthaler, J.-J.**, Chromatography of antihemophilic factor on diaminoalkane- and aminoalkane-derivitized sepharose, *Thromb. Haemost.,* 47, 124, 1982.
125. **Amphlett, G. W. and Hrinda, M. E.**, Process for Purifying Factor VIII:c, U.S. Patent 4, 508, 709, 1985.
126. **Miletich, J. P., Broze, G. J., and Majerus, P. W.** The synthesis of sulphated beads for isolation of human coagulation factors II, IX, and X, *Anal. Biochem.,* 105, 304, 1980.
127. **Pepper, D. S. and Prowse, C.**, Chromatography of human prothrombin complex on dextran sulphate agarose, *Thromb. Res.,* 11, 687, 1977.
128. **Modi, G. J., Blajchman, M. A., and Ofusu, F. A.**, The isolation of prothrombin factor IX, and factor X from human factor IX concentrates, *Thromb. Res.,* 36, 537, 1984.
129. **Saundry, R. H., Harrison, P., and Savidge, G. F.**, Isolation of the factor VIII/von Willebrand factor complex by affinity chromatography using sulphate- and dextran sulphate-derivatized agarose, unpublished results.
130. **Marlar, R. A., Kleiss, A. J., and Griffin, J. H.**, Mechanism of action of human protein c, a thrombin-dependent anticoagulant enzyme, *Blood,* 59, 1067, 1982.
131. **Kirby, E. P. and Tang, S. M.**, The binding of bovine factor VIII to human platelets, *Thromb. Haemost.,* 38, 126, 1977.
132. **Maderas, F. and Castaldi, P.A.**, Isolation and insolubilisation of human F VIII by affinity chromatography, *Hemostasis,* 7, 321, 1978.
133. **Suzuki, K., Nishioka, J., and Hashimoto, S.**, Inhibition of factor VIII-associated platelet aggregation by heparin and dextran sulphate, and its mechanism, *Biochim. Biophys. Acta,* 585, 416, 1979.
134. **Andersson, L.-O., Borg, H., and Miller-Anderson, M.**, Purification of human factor IX, *Thromb. Res.,* 7, 451, 1975.
135. **Saundry, R. H. and Savidge, G. F.**, Purification of Factor VIII, British Patent Application 699957, 1985.
136. **Saundry, R. H., Harrison, P., and Savidge, G. F.**, The purification of factor VIII using dextran sulphate-agarose chromatography, *Thromb. Haemost.,* 54, 79, 1985.
137. **Lowry, O. H., Rosebrough, N. J., Farr, A. H., and Randall, R. J.**, Protein measurement with the folin phenol reagent, *J. Biol. Chem.,* 193, 265, 1951.
138. **Kaplan, R. S. and Pederson, P. L.**, Determination of microgram quantities of protein in the presence of milligram levels of lipid and amido black 10B, *Anal. Biochem.,* 150, 97, 1985.
139. **Amrani, D.**, Process for the Separation and Isolation of the AHF Fraction, the Fibronectin Fraction and the von Willebrand's Ristocetin Cofactor Fraction from Blood Plasma, European Patent 0,022,052, 1980.
140. **Amrani, D. L., Mosesson, M. W., and Hoyer, L. W.**, Distribution of plasma fibronectin (cold-insoluble globulin) and components of the factor VIII complex after heparin-induced precipitation of plasma, *Blood,* 59, 657, 1982.
141. **Andersson, L.-O., Borg, H. G., Forsman, N., Hanshoff, G., Lindross, G., Miller-Andersson, M., and Ehrenberg, C.**, Isolation of Coagulation Factors from Biological Material Using Cross Linked Sulphated, Sulphonated Carbohydrates, U.S. Patent 3,920,625, 1975.
142. **Casillas, G. and Simonetti, C.**, Polyvinylpyrrolidone (PVP): a new precipitating agent for human and bovine factor VIII and fibrinogen, *Br. J. Haematol.,* 50, 665, 1982.
143. **Zuber, T. and Morgenthaler, J.-J.**, Polyvinylpyrrolidone as a precipitating agent for factor VIII and fibrinogen, *Br. J. Haematol.,* 52, 517, 1982.
144. **Johnson, A. J., MacDonald, V. E., Semar, M., Fields, J. E., Schuck, J., Lewis, C., and Brind, J.**, Preparation of the major plasma fractions by solid-phase polyelectrolytes, *J. Lab. Clin. Med.,* 92, 194, 1978.
145. **Middleton, S.**, Polyelectrolytes and preparation of factor VIIIc, in *Unresolved Problems in Haemophilia,* Forbes, C. D. and Lowe, G. D. O., Eds., M.T.P. Press, Lancaster, 1982, 109.

146. **Harris, R. B., Newman, J., and Johnson, A. J.,** Partial purification of biologically active, low molecular weight, human antihemophilic factor free of von Willebrand factor. I. Partial characterisation and evidence for disulphide bond(s) susceptible to limited reduction, *Biochim. Biophys. Acta,* 668, 456, 1981.

147. **Andersson, L.-O., Thuy, LeP., and Brown, J. E.,** Affinity chromatography of coagulation factors II, VIII, IX and X on matrix-bound phospholipid vesicles, *Thromb. Res.,* 23, 481, 1981.

148. **Porath, J., Carlsson, J., Olsson, I., and Belfrage, G.,** Metal chelate affinity chromatography, a new approach to protein fractionation, *Nature,* 258, 598, 1975.

149. **Andersson, L.,** Fractionation of human serum proteins by immobilised metal affinity chromatography, *J. Chromatogr.,* 315, 167, 1984.

150. **Hansson, H. and Kagedal, L.,** Adsorption and desorption of proteins in metal chelate affinity chromatography, *J. Chromatogr.,* 215, 333, 1981.

151. **Moroux, Y., Boschetti, E., and Egly, J. M.,** Preparation of metal-chelating trisacryl gels for chromatographic applications, *Sci. Tools,* 32, 1, 1985.

152. **Scully, M. F. and Kakkar, V. V.,** Structural features of fibrinogen associated with binding to chelated zinc, *Biochim. Biophys. Acta,* 700, 130, 1982.

153. **Weerasinghe, K. M., Scully, M. F., and Kakkar, V. V.,** A rapid method for the isolation of coagulation factor XII from human plasma, *Biochim. Biophys. Acta,* 839, 57, 1985.

154. **Pixley, R. A. and Colman, R. W.,** Purification of human factor XII from plasma using zinc chelate affinity chromatography, *Thromb. Res.,* 41, 89, 1986.

155. **Miemetz, J., Weilland, C., and Soulier, J. P.,** Preparation d'une fraction plasmatique humaine riche en facteur VIII (antihemophilique A) et pauvre en fibrinogene, *Nouv. Rev. Fr. Hematol.,* 1, 880, 1961.

156. **Simonetti, C., Casillas, G., and Pavlovsky, A.,** Studies on the adsorption of factor VIII: application to the purification of bovine factor VIII, Br. *J. Haematol.,* 23, 29, 1972.

157. **Legaz, M. E., Schmer, G., Counts, R. B., and Davie, E. W.,** Isolation and characterisation of human factor VIII (antihaemophilic factor), *J. Biol. Chem.,* 248, 3946, 1973.

158. **McCarroll, D., Trent, D., Chen, J., and Lange, R.,** Adsorption of human factor VIII to barium sulphate, *Thromb. Haemost.,* 46, 667, 1981.

159. **Foster, P. R., Dickson, I. H., MacLeod, A. J., and Bier, M.,** Zinc fractionation of cryoprecipitate, *Thromb. Haemost.,* 50, 117, 1983.

160. **Loscalzo, J., Inbal, A., and Handin, R. I.,** von Willebrand protein facilitates platelet incorporation into polymerising fibrin, *J. Clin. Invest.,* 78, 1112, 1986.

161. **Horowitz, B., Lippin, A., and Woods, K. R.,** Purification of low molecular weight factor VIII by affinity chromatography using factor VIII-sepharose, *Thromb. Res.,* 14, 463, 1979.

162. **Harris, R. B., Johnson, A. J., and Hodgins, L. T.,** Partial purification of biologically active, low molecular weight, human antihaemophilic factor free of von Willebrand factor. II. Further purification with thiol-disulphide interchange chromatography and additional evidence for disulphide bonds susceptible to limited reduction, *Biochim. Biophys. Acta,* 668, 471, 1981.

163. **Wagner, D. D. and Marder, V. J.,** Biosynthesis of von Willebrand protein by human endothelial cells: processing steps and their intracellular localisation, *J. Cell Biol.,* 99, 2123, 1984.

164. **Warren, D. C.,** New frontiers in membrane technology and chromatography, applications for biotechnology, *Anal. Chem.,* 56, 1528, 1984.

165. **Kass, L., Ratnoff, O. D., and Leon, M. A.,** Studies on the purification of antihaemophilic factor (factor VIII). I. Precipitation of antihaemophilic factor by concanavalin A, *J. Clin. Invest.,* 48, 351, 1969.

166. **Peake, I. R. and Bloom, A. L.,** Abnormal factor VIII related antigen (FVIIIag) in von Willebrand's disease (vWd): decreased precipitation by concanavalin A, *Thromb. Haemost.,* 37, 361, 1977.

167. **Mikami, S., Ueda, M., Yasui, M., Takahashi, Y., Nishinu, M., and Fukui, H.,** Heterogeneity of sugar composition of factor VIII/von Willebrand factor in von Willebrand's disease: analysis by crossed affinoimmunoelectrophoresis using lectin (Ricinus communis-120), *Thromb. Haemost.,* 49, 87, 1983.

168. **Pareti, F. I., Fujimura, Y., Dent, J. A., Holland, L. Z., Zimmerman, T. S., and Ruggeri, Z. M.,** Isolation and characterisation of a collagen binding domain in human von Willebrand factor, *J. Biol. Chem.,* 261, 15310, 1986.

169. **Levi, Y., Dupechez, T., Rimmele, D., Allary, M., Boschetti, E., and Saint-Blancard, J.,** Nouvelle methode chromatographique pour la purification du facteur VIII:c, *C. R. Acad. Sci. Paris,* 296, 257, 1983.

Chapter 15

FACTOR VIII IN REGIONAL BLOOD BANKING PRACTICE

C. Th. Smit Sibinga

TABLE OF CONTENTS

I.   Introduction 280

II.   Collection of Source Material 280
        A.   System of Collection 281
        B.   Choice of Anticoagulant 281
        C.   Donor Management 281
        D.   Processing of Source Material 281
        E.   Quality Assurance 285

III.   Future Developments in Factor VIII Production 285

References 286

I. INTRODUCTION

Hemophilia treatment has made great advances over the last 2 decades. The principle reason is the discovery of the cryoprecipitation process by Rémigy (1955)[1] and Pool (1959)[2] for harvesting and concentrating factor VIII (VIII) as a cryoglobulin from source plasma. The implementation of this process both in practical blood banking[3,4] and plasma fractionation has led to an increasing availability of concentrated and more purified clotting factor preparations required by hemophiliacs for the control of bleeding.

Clinical demands for antihemophilic VIII products have exceeded the supply in many countries, apparently because of a diversifying process in technical development, and logistic and procedural adaptations among the blood banking, plasma fractionation, and hemophilia treater communities.

This situation presents an interesting and stimulating challenge to those organizations involved in the provision of plasma and plasma products required for hemophilia care. It applies equally to the blood banking organization at national, regional, or local level responsible for the procurement and the production of cryoprecipitate, and to the various organizations at regional, national, or supranational levels involved in the production of plasma fractions on an industrial scale.

However, it is noticeable that the blood banking and blood processing community does not show the necessary unity and cooperation as to allow optimal usage of available resources. In some parts of the world, plasma fractionation is not developed at all, where blood banks do exist. In other areas, competition has created a dualistic system of blood donation and processing. Donors are either motivated in a purely altruistic manner as encouraged by the system or alternatively stimulated to frequently donate plasma on the basis of compensation by attractive bonuses. The processing of the collected blood is either done routinely and orientated for the immediate use of the principal components, or directed to sophisticated fractionation techniques for the optimal recovery of the different protein fractions.

II. COLLECTION OF SOURCE MATERIAL

The collection of source material for blood transfusion is the primary responsibility of blood banks. Not only does this involve the mere collection, but encompasses the organization of a well-motivated blood donor community and a carefully controlled mechanism to avoid malcollection — both under- and over-collection. In this context, where this primary responsibility should be the greatest, the blood banking organization overall has shown the least progress in development. Many situations illustrate the seemingly unreachable ideal of self-sufficiency, a philosophy of intent advocated by those who avow to the principle of discrete independence.

It is now generally accepted that the principle of self-sufficiency may be defined as the ability to collect and process the necessary amounts of source material to provide any quality product for clinical use.[6]

VIII preparations are one such quality product. At the present time, as a result of less than optimal techniques for purification of VIII, a discouraging amount of fresh plasma is needed to meet regional and national demands.

Furthermore, in the collection and immediate processing of blood and plasma, manufacturing conditions are not always maintained at optimal levels. As a consequence of persistent retention of conventional concepts in the face of marginal levels of professional motivation and paucity of commitment to plasma, the progressive utilization of this extremely valuable and important source material has been grossly neglected in routine blood banking. This has ultimately led, in clinical transfusion practice, to the concept that fresh frozen plasma is still a magic commodity. Such practice has significantly contributed to its continual abuse. In the collection of source plasma certain fundamental decisions have to be made.

A. System of Collection

The major system is the collection of whole blood in multiple plastic bloodbags to permit processing in a closed system. This method unavoidably relies upon prior planning as to what component will be made and for what purpose.

Plasmapheresis is a second system for source plasma collection. This can be done either manually or by automated machine apheresis. In both collection systems, processing strategies have to be defined in advance to avoid the implementation of plasma decisions that may be cost ineffective and clinically inappropriate. The type of container used, the destiny of the source material, and the logistics of collection, preparation, and distribution are of great relevance in this context.

B. Choice of Anticoagulant

By tradition, citrate is used as the common anticoagulant in blood/plasma collection systems. Citrate chelates the divalent cations Ca^{2+} and $Mg,^{2+}$ thereby preventing catalysis of the coagulation cascade. However, calcium ions play an important role in stabilizing the complex VIII molecule.[7,8] They noncovalently bridge the VIII coagulant (VIII:C) moiety to the carrier protein von Willebrand factor: antigen (vWf:Ag).[9] Citrate competes by its favorable Ca^{2+} affinity with the intrinsic Ca^{2+} of the VIII/vWf complex, causing disruption of ionic bonds leading to unfolding of the complex molecular structure. This is a time related phenomenon and consequently leads to loss of coagulant activity.

Alternatively, collection of source plasma such that physiological calcium concentrations are rapidly restored either following citrate collection by the addition of heparin and calcium chloride or by the initial collection in heparin has been shown to result in extremely stable VIII:C.[10,11] For practical reasons, cellular components and cryosupernatant plasma are subsequently applied to conventional citrate containing preservative media.

C. Donor Management

Source plasma collection by apheresis permits an increase in volume per donation of up to 600 ml of plasma.[12] Additionally, the principle allows the donor to donate more frequently. Up to 25 600-ml collections seem to be justified and permissible.[13] However, from a moral or ethical point of view, it is debatable as to whether it would not be more acceptable and advisable to have access to a larger number of donors supporting a plasmapheresis program, each donating less frequently, than to load the burden of total plasma collection on the shoulders of a few by encouraging them to donate as frequently as possible.

Another approach is to increase the absolute amount of VIII per volume donated by 1-desaminocysteine-8-D-arginine-vasopressin (DDAVP) stimulation of the donor prior to donation. Intranasal administration of DDAVP 1 h before donation results in a two- to three-fold increase in plasma VIII:C levels.[14] However, a major obstacle in introducing DDAVP stimulation in routine source plasma collection is the ethical question. It is debatable as to whether in a volunteer nonrenumerated blood donor system the introduction of drugs on a repeated basis is permissible and justified. Plasmapheresis as a collection system reflects a more special willingness to endure inconveniences to donate, such as time commitment, the exposure to hazards related to an extracorporeal circuit, the equipment, and the solutions to be used. Awareness of this extra dimension should, therefore, be expressed by full appreciation and efforts to make the donor as comfortable and safe as possible during the procedure, rather than stimulating the donor to feelings of heroism and pride.

D. Processing of Source Material

Once the collection of blood and plasma has been completed, the decision has to be made as to how to process the source material into whatever intermediate or finished products are relevant. In principle, each unit of source material collected, whether whole blood or plasma, should be processed into separate components. Such a policy represents the fundamental approach to self-sufficiency, where the blood bank is the primary contributor.

Apart from optimizing the conditions for the initial processing of plasma involving the time duration between collection and centrifuging, spinning conditions, and temperature and time, much attention needs to be given to the freezing and thawing conditions of source plasma for VIII harvesting.

Fast freezing under conditions of optimal heat exchange has been shown to be significantly better for VIII:C recovery compared to slow freezing.[15,16] An essential criterium is the rate at which the core of the plasma mass is solidly frozen.[17] When the freezing process is slow, water crystallizes from the outer layers inward. The concentration of ions, proteins, and other substances slowly but constantly increases, resulting in dramatic changes in osmolarity and pH.[18] The freezing point then drops and the molecular structure of the VIII/vWf complex is affected. VIII and the variety of other cold insoluble proteins such as fibrinogen and fibronectin co-precipitate during the freezing process. For recovery of the VIII/vWf complex, thawing conditions of the frozen plasma should be determined. Factors, such as heat exchange, rate of heating, temperature control, time, and determination of end points are of critical importance. When thawing is carefully controlled in rate, heat exchange, and timing, the noncold precipitable constituents will resolve leaving the cryoprecipitate in a gel state. Continuous siphoning off of the thawed, watery material significantly influences both the amount of contaminating proteins and the VIII:C yield.[19] Cold insoluble proteins show a temperature range over which solubility changes occur from the gel phase to complete resolution. Although each protein seems to have its own characteristics in this respect, some proteins such as VIII/vWf more likely co-precipitate with other proteins as exemplified by fibronectin and fibrinogen. When conditions for freezing and thawing of citrated plasma are carefully standardized and controlled, VIII:C can be recovered in the cryoprecipitate at levels approximately 40 to 60% of the starting concentration.[16] Cryoprecipitate is a crude material highly contaminated with all other cryoglobulins, immunoglobulins, and a variety of other plasma proteins. Although this procedure increases the specific activity of VIII:C, the material is still bulky. Cryoprecipitate can be frozen and used as a wet preparation or freeze-dried. Freeze-drying results in another relative loss of 15 to 20% of VIII:C without any additional advantage in concentration or purity. Since cryoprecipitation was accepted as a standard technique for VIII:C recovery, large-scale cryoprecipitate extraction from fresh frozen plasma was introduced in plasma fractionation, replacing the original Cohn fraction 1 methodology.[20] Whatever effort is made at blood bank level to optimize the processing and preservation of source plasma, large-scale purification technologies at the present time only result in ultimate recoveries of 10 to 20% VIII:C relative to the starting material. Increased purity and potency are certainly major achievements to be attained in technological advances. However, safety has been shown to be the major concern since large pools of source plasma collected from numerous donors must be processed.[21] The risk of transmitting viral diseases is well established and closely related to the size of the pool.[22] By implementing reduction in pool size, transmission of disease through chronic exposure to concentrates is expected to be reduced.[23] Additional application of physiochemical principles such as heat treatment will further reduce the risk of transmitting infectious agents as exemplified by human immunodeficiency virus (HIV) and non-A, non-B retroviruses.[24] Recent developments have shown the feasibility of application of virus inactivation technology at blood bank level. There is no need to reinvent the wheel, now that the fundamental techniques have been validated extensively and have become accessible to the blood banking profession. Furthermore, introduction at blood bank level of small pool approaches, together with the implementation of high-yield production methods for improved purification of VIII, should be regarded as a major step forward in blood banking technology and significantly contribute to the attainment of self-sufficiency.[10,25]

It has been recognized that the principal loss of VIII:C is in the initial freezing and thawing of plasma.[26] Therefore, the thaw-siphon principle as developed by Mason[19] has been introduced at blood bank level with a number of practical modifications. Fast thawing of the frozen plasma, maintaining a constant temperature of 3 to 5°C, reduces the time during which losses of VIII:C may occur. When the thawed, liquified plasma is siphoned off into a satellite bag, the thawing process is completed in a relatively short time. Reported recoveries average 60% at a specific activity of 0.3 VIII:C U/mg protein. However, the amount of VIII:C per milliliter of the final product does not differ significantly from routine cryoprecipitate.

Based on the same principle of fast-thawing fresh frozen plasma, in 1976 Margolis[27] introduced an improved procedure for preparation of cryoprecipitate by blood banks. The thawing method uses a mechanically rocking waterbath, kept at 4°C. The cryoprecipitate then settles during the thawing process as a compact layer at the bottom of the plastic bag, allowing easy separation without centrifugation. This greatly reduces the handling and preparation time, thereby limiting the losses of VIII:C. Washing this pooled cryoprecipitate material in ice-cold tris citrate saline (TCS) buffer at pH 7.4 results in a small pool of purified concentrate with a yield of 25 to 35% relative to the starting source plasma and a specific activity of 0.3 to 0.5 VIII:C U/mg protein. However, the most important condition for preserving the complex VIII molecular structure is in the maintenance of physiological concentrations of calcium ions.

When changing the anticoagulant from citrate solutions to heparin, the VIII:C level in the plasma increased remarkably. After cryoprecipitation of heparinized plasma, VIII:C is recoverable at levels on the order of 80% of the starting material, while the remainder can be found in the cryosupernatant.[11] Heparin stabilizes VIII:C in plasma. Heparinized plasma stored for 24 h at room temperature does not show any significant decline in VIII:C.[28] This increase in VIII:C levels is not so much a mere heparin effect but a consequence of the presence of normal calcium levels. When citrated plasma is heparinized after 4-h storage at room temperature, there is only a moderate effect noticeable on the VIII:C inactivation process. However, when the citrated plasma is heparinized and recalcified under identical conditions, a remarkable restorative effect is noticeable up to the initial VIII:C levels. When the same experiment is done following longer storage times of citrated plasma, the restorative effect becomes less optimal.[9] Heparin enhances the cryoprecipitability of VIII/vWf and other cold insoluble proteins from plasma.[11] When the principle of fast-thawing plasma is combined with the important effects of heparin and calcium ions on VIII:C preservation, a cryoprecipitate with a remarkably high VIII:C recovery of 70% is obtained. This concentrated material expresses 10 to 15 VIII:C U/ml and a specific activity of up to 0.3 VIII:C U/mg protein. Such a high yield heparin cryoprecipitate is an ideal starting material for further purification with simple technology at blood bank level. Different fractions of the cold insoluble globulin (CIG) material show precipitability at specific temperature ranges, permitting separation and therefore purification from the crude cryoprecipitate. Reprecipitation in a rocking waterbath at 0°C for approximately 2 h results in a second cryoprecipitate which shows intermediate VIII concentrate characteristics (15 to 25 VIII:C U/ml and an average specific activity of 0.7 VIII:C U/mg protein). The recovery following this second cold precipitation step is about 80% relative to the previous step or 45 to 55% relative to the starting material.[29]

Freeze-drying and heat treatment of the dried material in the presence of sucrose or amino acids as protective stabilizers complete the manufacturing process.[30] Clinical studies have shown the efficacy of this small pool, high-yield VIII preparation.[30-32] *In vivo* recovery is 100% with a biological half-life of 8 h (6.5 to 11.6 h). There was no difference in biological behavior of heat treated and nonheat treated freeze-dried preparations as shown in Figure 1. The hemostatic capacity has been studied in hemophilia patients undergoing elective

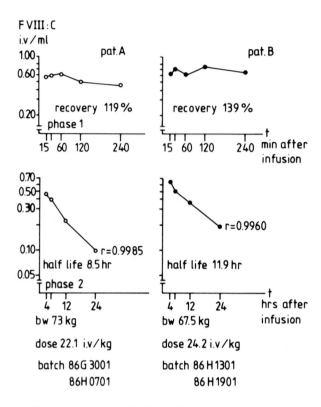

FIGURE 1.   Recovery and half-life of heat treated, small pool, high yield VIII preparation. Four batches were tested in two severe hemophilia A patients.

Table 1
COMPARISON OF VIII CRYOPRECIPITATE
PRODUCTION METHOD

	Potency (U/ml)	Purity (U/mg protein)	Yield (%)
Plasma (fresh)	$\leqq 1$	0.016	100
Cryoprecipitate			
Routine (Judith Pool)	3—6	0.05	44
Fraction 1-0	5	0.2	30
Thaw-siphoning	5—8	0.21	63
Quick thaw, freeze-dried	5—6	0.19	50
Heparin/CIG, freeze-dried	15—25	0.78	55
CPG chromatography	15—25	0.4—0.6	24

orthopedic, GI, or oral surgery.[33] Long-term prophylaxis at a dose of 10 VIII:C U/kg body weight or an average of 1000 VIII:C U/kg body weight per year has shown that the preparation is easy to handle, reliably potent, and safe. The preparation has been in use since 1984, and at this time of writing no clinical or hematological side effects have been reported. Liver function tests remained stable, and no seroconversion for hepatitis B or HIV could be detected.[34]

This supercryoprecipitate compares very favorably with other blood bank produced preparations, as shown in Table 1. The procedure does not require high powered technology, large capital investment, or highly skilled personnel. The method has been shown to be practically feasible and within the reach of most well-equipped, motivated, and dedicated blood banks; it is a natural extension of routine blood banking technology.

E. Quality Assurance

To implement the primary responsibilities in the collection and processing of source material for manufacturing VIII, regional blood banks need to explore the concept of quality assurance. The purpose of quality assurance is to guarantee safe and effective blood bank and transfusion practice. The goal is qualitative rather than quantitative and depends on attitude more than on technical skills. To assure quality in a blood bank, prevention of errors should be the primary goal. Errors can be defined as inadvertent or unauthorized deviations from standard procedures. The first and most important requirement needed for a quality assurance program is, therefore, a standardized and written procedure for every service and every test which the blood bank intends to provide to donors, patients, and physicians. These procedures must be based on a sound philosophy and generally accepted standards. Different procedures entail different kinds of tasks and require different kinds of people. Therefore, it is necessary to define the responsibilities and personnel needs required to fulfill each procedure. Separate job descriptions must be written for each employee group with responsibility for a different type of procedure. In fact, job descriptions are an important tool of quality assurance.

More traditional, although equally important, is the quality assurance of equipment and reagents. In this respect the VIII:C assay illustrates the need for an integral quality assurance program. In order to ensure that the expected performance — reagents, equipment, personnel, or their products — is in fact achieved, a most important element of a quality assurance program is the monitoring of performance. In theory, when we have developed and accepted a policy as, for instance, to achieve self-sufficiency and optimal use of blood and plasma, and have selected appropriate procedures and suitable personnel, equipment, and reagents, we should obtain accurate results and safe and effective products and services. Obviously this does not always happen. An important approach to evaluate the results of a blood bank VIII program, both logistic procedures and end products, is through the recognition and analysis of errors and failures. Although often neglected, continuous awareness of primary responsibilities and the implementation of a quality assurance program including a mechanism to control errors and failures constitute the fundamental role regional blood banks have to play in the manufacture of VIII preparations meeting the standards of safety, purity, potency, and efficacy.[35]

III. FUTURE DEVELOPMENTS IN FACTOR VIII PRODUCTION

Rapid progress in blood banking technology in the last decade converted the first generation transfusion services to high standard second generation organizations. Most second generation services offer advanced technology for implementation and development. These developments not only regard fundamental approaches to blood donors, screening procedures, and optimal collection systems, but do extend into more sophisticated processing technology. This requires specific motivation, training, and expertise, and implementation of pharmaceutical principles and small scale fractionation technology to increase safety. The production of cryoprecipitate should be regarded as the absolute baseline contribution of regional blood banks to hemophilia treatment. With adequate knowledge and expertise, quality cryoprecipitate can be produced routinely. Freeze-drying and heat treatment of these cryoprecipitates, protected by balanced stabilizing buffers (e.g., sucrose or amino acids), should be the first step in the process of technical developments for the immediate future.

Options for increasing both purity and potency of cryoprecipitates at blood bank level are in implementing the combined thaw-siphon/controlled pore glass chromatography (CPG) technology or the heparin double cold precipitation method. Both procedures do not require high powered technology, large capital investment, or highly skilled personnel. The CPG method is currently under development in Australia and New Zealand blood banks, and some fractionation centers are in the process of implementing the principle on a large scale to reduce the losses during purification of cryoprecipitated plasma.

The heparin double cold precipitation technique seems to be more open to routine implementation because of its ease of handling and the flexibility in volume of starting material to be processed. However, this purified, concentrated, high yield VIII preparation still contains a considerable amount of fibrinogen, fibronectin, and heparin. Following this principle, a third cold precipitation step in the presence of additional heparin (25 U/ml) at 4°C for 30 min allows a remarkable further purification with minimal VIII:C losses.[36] In the presence of this increased heparin concentration, fibronectin and fibrinogen co-precipitate, leaving the purified VIII material in the supernatant. This results in a crystal clear, sterile, filterable concentrate with a specific activity of around 1.5 U/mg protein. The recovery is 80 to 90% relative to the previous step at a 20- to 25-u/ml VIII concentration and a final heparin content of 0.2 to 1.0 U/ml.[37-41] Such a technique has major advantages:

1. Simple blood bank technology
2. High yield
3. Small pool principle
4. Increased safety
5. Optimal use of source material

The challenge for the future to the regional blood bank in adequately and sufficiently providing plasma and plasma products required for hemophilia care indeed is interesting and stimulating. However, this statement does not guarantee development of activity and increase in productivity in the field of blood transfusion. More important is the fundamental development of the blood banking profession to a stimulating, dynamic, respected, and fully accepted new discipline in medicine. Blood transfusion medicine should be recognized by the device — *salus donores et aegroti suprema lex.*

REFERENCES

1. **Rémigy, E.,** Essais de Traitement par Plasma Cryoconcentré, academical thesis, University of Nancy, 1955.
2. **Pool, J. G. and Robinson, J.,** Observations on plasma banking and transfusion procedures for haemophilic patients and quantitative assay for antihaemophilic globulin (AHG), *Br. J. Haematol.,* 5, 24, 1959.
3. **Pool, J. G. and Shannon, A. E.,** Simple production of high-potency of antihaemophilic globulin (AHG) concentrates in a closed bag system, *Fed. Proc. Fed. Am. Soc. Exp. Biol.,* 24, 512, 1965.
4. **Pool, J. G. and Shannon, A. E.,** Production of high-potency concentrate of antihaemophilic globulin in a closed bag system, *N. Engl. J. Med.,* 273, 1443, 1965.
5. **Webster, W. P., Roberts, H. R., Thelin, G. M., Wagner, R. H., and Brinkhous, K. M.,** Clinical use of new glycine-precipitated antihemophilic fraction, *Am. J. Med. Sci.,* 250, 643, 1965.
6. Socio-economic aspects of blood transfusion, *Vox Sang.,* 44, 328, 1983.
7. **Rock, G. A., Cruickshank, W. H., Tackaberry, E. S., Ganz, P. R., and Palmer, D. S.,** Stability of VIII:C in plasma: the dependence on protease activity and calcium, *Thromb. Res.,* 29, 521, 1983.
8. **Krachmalnicoff, A. and Thomas, D. P.,** The stability of factor VIII in heparinized plasma, *Thromb. Haemost.,* 49, 224, 1983.
9. **Mikaelsson, M. E., Forsman, N., and Oswaldsson, U. M.,** Human factor VIII: a calcium-linked protein complex, *Blood,* 62, 1006, 1983.
10. **Smit Sibinga, C. Th., Welbergen, H., Das, P. C., and Griffin, B.,** High-yield method of production of freeze-dried factor VIII by blood banks, *Lancet,* ii, 449, 1981.

11. **Rock, G. A., Cruickshank, W. H., Tackaberry, E. S., and Palmer, D. S.,** Improved yields of factor VIII from heparinized plasma, *Vox Sang.,* 36, 294, 1979.
12. WHO Tech. Rep. Ser. 626, Geneva, 1978, 28.
13. **Smit Sibinga, C. Th.,** The apheresis donor: how much and how often?, *Vox Sang.,* 46 (Suppl. 1), 40, 1984.
14. **Mikaelsson, M. E., Nilsson, I. M., Vilhardt, H., and Wiechel, B.,** Factor VIII concentrate prepared from blood donors stimulated by intranasal administration of a vasopressin analogue, *Transfusion,* 22, 229, 1982.
15. **Wensley, R. T. and Snape, T. J.,** Preparation of improved cryoprecipitated factor VIII concentrate. A controlled study of three variables affecting the yield, *Vox Sang.,* 38, 222, 1980.
16. **Slichter, S. J., Counts, R. B., Henderson, R., and Harker, L. A.,** Preparation of cyroprecipitated factor VIII concentrate, *Transfusion,* 16, 616, 1976.
17. **Smith, J.K., Snape, T. J., Haddon, P. M., Gunsson, H. H., and Edwards, R.,** Methods of assessing factor VIII concentrate, *Transfusion,* 18, 530, 1978.
18. **Over, J., Piët, M. P. J., Loos, J. A., Henrichs, H. P. J., Hoek, P. J., von Meyenfeldt, M. A., and Oh, J. I. H.,** Contribution to the optimalization of factor VIII production: improved cryoprecipitation and controlled pore glass adsorption, in *Plasma Fractionation and Blood Transfusion,* Smit Sibinga, C. Th., Das, P. C., and Seidl, S., Eds. Martinus Nijhoff, Boston, 1985, 67.
19. **Mason, E. C.,** Thaw-siphon technique for production of cryoprecipitate concentrate of factor VIII, *Lancet,* ii, 15, 1978.
20. **Watt, J. G.,** Plasma fractionation, in *Clinics in Haematology,* Vol. 5, No. 2, Cash, J. D., Ed., W. B. Saunders, London, 1976, chap. 7.
21. **Seidl, S.,** Needs, quality versus quantity, in *Plasma Fractionation and Blood Transfusion,* Smit Sibinga, C. Th., Das, P. C., and Seidl, S., Eds., Martinus Nijhoff, Boston 1985, 189.
22. What is the importance of the "small pool concept" in the preparation of fraction I and cryoprecipitates for the prevention of post-transfusion hepatitis?, (International forum), *Vox Sang.,* 38, 106, 1980.
23. **Smit Sibinga, C. Th. and Das, P. C.,** Small pool versus large pool in plasma fractionation: reevaluation of a concept, in *Plasma Fractionation and Blood Transfusion,* Smit Sibinga, C. Th., Das, P. C., and Seidl, S., Eds., Martinus Nijhoff, Boston, 1985, 43.
24. **Gerety, R. J.,** Prevention of transmission of virus infections by blood transfusions and removal of virus infectivity from clotting factor concentrates, in *Plasma Fractionation and Blood Transfusion,* Smit Sibinga, C. Th., Das, P. C., and Seidl, S., Eds., Martinus Nijhoff, Boston, 1985, 143.
25. **Margolis, J. and Rhoades, P. H.,** Preparation of high-purity factor VIII by controlled pore glass chromatography, *Lancet,* ii, 446, 1981.
26. **Smith, J. K. and Evans, D. R.,** Processing criteria for recovery of FFP for fractionation, in *Plasma Fractionation and Blood Transfusion,* Smit Sibinga, C. Th., Das, P. C., and Seidl, S., Eds., Martinus Nijhoff, Boston, 1985, 15.
27. **Margolis, J.,** Improvement in production of anti-haemophilic factor (FVIII) concentrates, in *Proc. 11th Int. Cong. World Fed. of Hemophilia,* Academic Press, Tokyo, 1976, 223.
28. **Prowse, C. V.,** Donation procedure: collection lesion, fibrinopeptide A and factor VIII, in *Plasma Fractionation and Blood Transfusion,* Smit Sibinga, C. Th., Das, P. C., and Seidl, S., Eds., Martinus Nijhoff, Boston, 1985, 25.
29. **Smit Sibinga, C. Th. and Das, P. C.,** Heparin and factor VIII, in *New Frontiers in Hemophila Research,* Blombäck, M., Ed.; *Scand. J. Haematol.,* 33 (Suppl. 40), 111, 1984.
30. **Smit Sibinga, C. Th., Schulting, P., Notebomer, J., Das,, P. C., Marrink, J., and v.d. Meer, J.,** Double cryoprecipitated factor VIII concentrate from heparinised plasma and its heat treatment, *Blut,* 56, 111, 1988.
31. **Smit Sibinga, C. Th., Daenen, S. M. G. J., van Imhoff, G. W., Maas, A., and Das, P. C.,** Heparin small pool high-yield purified factor VIII: in vivo recovery and half-life of routinely produced freeze-dried concentrate, *Thromb. Haemost.,* 51, 12, 1984.
32. **Rock, G. A., Smiley, R. K., Titley, P., and Palmer, D. S.,** In vivo effectiveness of a high-yield factor VIII concentrate prepared in a blood bank, *New Engl. J. Med.,* 311, 310, 1984.
33. **Smit Sibinga, C. Th., Waltje, J., McShine, R. L., Maas, A., Das, P. C., Daenen, S. M. G. J., van Imhoff, G. W., and Nieweg, H. O.,** Small pool high-yield factor VIII concentrate: in vitro and in vivo study, *Transfusion,* 24, (Abstr.), 420, 1984.
34. **Smit Sibinga, C. Th., van Loon, J. K., Maas, A., and Das, P. C.,** Long-term efficacy study of heparin high-yield factor VIII in haemophiliacs, *Transfusion,* 26 (Abstr.), 581, 1986.
35. *Quality Assurance in Blood Banking and its Clinical Impact,* Smit Sibinga, C. Th., Das, P. C., and Taswell, H. F., Eds., Martinus Nijhoff, Boston, 1984.
36. **Uithof, J.,** Optimalization of Factor VIII Preparation from Heparinized Plasma, Project Report, Red Cross Blood Bank Groningen-Drenthe, Groningen, 1985.

37. **Smit Sibinga, C. Th., Uithof, J., McShine, R. L., Waltje, J., and Das, P. C.,** Advances in purification of heparin high-yield factor VIII concentrate, *Transfusion,* 25 (Abstr.), 467, 1985.
38. **Wallevik, K., Ingerslev, J., Stenbjerg Bernvil, S., Glavind Kristensen, S., Jørgensen, J., and Kiss-meyer-Nielsen, F.,** Manufacturing in the blood bank of high-purity heat-treated factor VIII concentrate from heparin stabilised blood and its consequences for the red cell and supernate plasma components, in *Future Developments in Blood Banking,* Smit Sibinga, C. Th., Das, P. C., and Greenwalt, T. J., Eds., Martinus Nijhoff, Boston, 1986, 95.
39. **Muntinga, S.,** Introduction of an Improved Production Method (Third Precipitation Step) for Heat Treated Purified Factor VIII Derived from Heparinized Plasma, Project Report, Red Cross Blood Bank Groningen-Drenthe, Groningen, 1986.
40. **teWierik, H.,** Optimalization of the third precipitation step for heat treated factor VIII derived from heparinized plasma. Project Report, Red Cross Blood Bank Groningen-Drenthe, Groningen, 1987.
41. **v. Kan, E., Nieborg, G., Sloot, E., and Vlek, J.,** FVIII Hep/CIG 5: ready to go. Project Report, Red Cross Blood Bank Groningen-Drenthe, Groningen, 1987.

Chapter 16

ADVANCES IN PLASMA FRACTIONATION AND IN THE PRODUCTION OF FACTOR VIII CONCENTRATES

J. K. Smith, T. J. Snape, and R. S. Lane

TABLE OF CONTENTS

I.   Dominance of Freeze-Dried Concentrates in Current Treatment of
        Hemophilia 290

II.   Aims of Plasma Fractionation for Therapeutic Use 291

III.   Current Routes to Therapeutic Concentrates 291
        A.   Large-Scale Cryoprecipitation 291
        B.   Intermediate Purity Concentrates 292
                1.   Washing Bulk Cryoprecipitate 292
                2.   Adsorption of Prothrombin Complex.............................292
                3.   Removal of Fibronectin by "Cold Precipitation" 293
                4.   Partial Removal of Fibrinogen 293
        C.   "High Purity" Concentrates...293
        D.   Chromatographic Purification of Factor VIII 294

IV.   Transmission of Blood-Borne Viruses 296

V.   Possible Developments in Purification of Factor VIII Concentrates.............298

References...298

I. DOMINANCE OF FREEZE-DRIED CONCENTRATES IN CURRENT TREATMENT OF HEMOPHILIA

The treatment of hemophilia A requires above all the reliable supply of a safe, well-characterized factor VIII (VIII) concentrate. Hemophiliacs can now expect a life-span nearly the same as that of unaffected people, and rapid relief from the painful bleeding episodes which formerly limited their choices and opportunities. Should it be necessary to repair the consequences of less effective treatment earlier in life, most surgical procedures can be contemplated under adequate cover with VIII concentrates. The success of this replacement therapy, however imperfect, can be gauged by the depth and volume of dismay expressed when these benefits have been jeopardized, either by doubts about the risks of treatment or by threats to the continued supply of a familiar concentrate.

Every community places an implied finite value on the treatment of hemophilia. Some measures to make safer concentrates may be expensive in terms of processing costs or, less directly, in terms of a limited plasma supply. While more efficient plasmapheresis systems promise to reduce ethical limitations on plasma procurement even outside the overtly commercial sector of the fractionation industry, plasma for VIII recovery will remain relatively expensive if the demand for VIII outstrips that for the equivalent recovered albumin, immunoglobulins, and other therapeutic proteins. Even so, most communities accept both the economic prudence of adequate treatment of hemophilia and the likelihood that, with improved life expectancy, more VIII will have to be provided. Demand may ultimately be limited, not by arbitrary economic factors, but by greater clinical consensus on optimal levels of therapy, especially on prophylactic levels necessary to avert bleeding or rebleeding. The projected demand for VIII concentrate in the U.K. is approximately 2 million U per million population. This demand for VIII dominates calculations of plasma supply, since current fractionation technology, especially with the stages recently introduced to prevent transmission of blood-borne viruses, does not yield more than about 200 U/kg of fresh-frozen plasma (FFP) fractionated. There are, therefore, fresh incentives to improve the yield of VIII:C from plasma processing and to weigh very carefully the losses of activity sacrificed in the pursuit of complete safety.

Even when the quality of single-donor cryoprecipitate has been improved and standardized — and there is a weighty literature of worthy attempts to achieve that goal — local production of frozen cryoprecipitate has never offered a secure basis for treatment of hemophilia in a large population. The main drawbacks have been variability of VIII:C content, difficulty of keeping stable stockpiles, and the maintenance of consistently high quality and yield under a high daily workload. Statistical and procedural variability has led to over-prescribing, nullifying the potential yield advantages of a simple process. Since each unit or pool of a few units constitutes a batch, quality control is inherently inferior to that achieved in the manufacture of concentrates dispensed from a single large batch. The incidence of unpleasant allergic reactions to infusions of cryoprecipitate can be diminished by washing, sometimes as a prelude to freeze-drying, but this is achieved at the expense of further manipulations and losses of activity. Until recently, cryoprecipitate was preferred on grounds of viral safety for mildly deficient patients needing the product of only a few donations per year. However, by 1984 the production of cryoprecipitate in the U.K. had diminished to less than 5% of all factor VIII used, even before heat treated concentrates became available.

It seems likely that cryoprecipitate will follow FFP on the list of superseded therapeutic materials for hemophilia A; however, it may still find uses as a source of unmodified vWf, XIII, or fibrinogen where safer and more effective concentrates are not immediately available.

II. AIMS OF PLASMA FRACTIONATION FOR THERAPEUTIC USE

Plasma fractionation is the eccentric in the pharmaceutical family. The industry is familiar with the refinement of a pure compound from its source in nature, and with the synthesis of compounds from pure materials. Fractionation exploits a unique and limited resource to provide many proteins with a wide and fluctuating range of market values. It is, therefore, hardly surprising that no two companies use the same fractionation scheme. Each must be flexible enough to respond to its particular market and possible changes on the horizon. In particular, national fractionators with a virtual monopoly of the plasma supply of a country must be ready to interpolate new processes, perhaps initially for only a few users, without disturbing the efficient recovery of established proteins.

The fractionator aims first at concentration of a useful protein, not its purification. Factor VIII illustrates all the attractions of increased purification, and their penalties. The *in vivo* half-life, recovery, and therapeutic level (virtually 100% of normal levels, approaching major surgery) dictate that VIII concentrates should be capable of infusion at a potency of about 20 U/ml. Below about 10 U/ml, extensive replacement would mean infusions of inconveniently large volumes; at very high potencies, on the other hand, there is much mechanical wastage during processing and preparation for infusion. Some stages of fractionation are intended to remove contaminants, such as fibronectin and fibrinogen, which would otherwise limit the solubility and potency of VIII. Potency may also be increased by concentration stages, e.g., ultrafiltration or precipitation of VIII without the intention of purification. Other stages may be aimed at separating from crude VIII a contaminant, such as fibrinogen, which may be clinically useful in its own right — although this would not usually justify a large penalty in yield of VIII:C. Finally, there may be a need to remove contaminants, often present at low concentrations, which might threaten the stability or safe use of the concentrate. For such reasons, VIII often undergoes an adsorption stage to remove the proteins of the prothrombin complex. Purification is not pursued further than these considerations dictate, because every extra stage incurs substantial mechanical losses simply by wetting vessels and transfer lines with concentrated VIII. Every stage brings a compromise on discrimination, some VIII being sacrificed into the discarded contaminant fraction. As VIII is purified, its stability may have to be preserved by the readdition of an inert protein such as albumin. This is the context in which the "high purity" designation is accorded to concentrates containing perhaps one part of VIII procoagulant activity (VIII:C) in 5000 parts of other proteins.

III. CURRENT ROUTES TO THERAPEUTIC CONCENTRATES

A. Large-Scale Cryoprecipitation

This is the method universally used in the industry (with only one exception[1]) for the primary recovery of crude VIII from plasma, because it offers acceptable yield and selectivity, does not use precipitating reagents which might complicate the subsequent recovery of other valuable plasma proteins, and demands only close temperature control while FFP is thawed for processing.

A number of hypotheses have been entertained to explain the phenomenon of cryoprecipitation. In the simplest terms, the solubility of certain plasma proteins is very low and changes only slowly as a function of temperature between the solid/liquid transition, near 0°C, and about 5°C; above about 5°C, solubility of these "cryo-proteins" increases rapidly. The key cryo-protein is fibronectin, which appears to associate with VIII and influence its solubility in the plasma medium.

Some VIII:C is always found in the cryosupernatant after removal of cryoprecipitate. Over et al.[2] attributed this to a proportion of circulating VIII with low molecular weight and a different solubility curve from the majority of larger complexes in plasma. Although there may be a small irreducible proportion of plasma VIII which cannot be recovered by cryoprecipitation, losses during large-scale cryoprecipitation are more likely to be due to poor control of heat input to the thawing mass. It is a complex task to ensure that all the heat supplied from the vessel jacket is absorbed by the solid ice to change its physical state, without raising the temperature of the liquid plasma above 0°C and initiating resolution of the particles of cryoprecipitate already formed in it. Although thaw-siphoning[3] cannot be applied directly to large volumes of plasma, some of its lessons can be applied in manufacturing to give worthwhile improvements in efficiency.[4,5] Imperfect control of cryoprecipitate solubility during thawing can be compensated to some extent by adding low concentrations of reagents such as ethanol or polyethylene glycol (PEG), often used in higher concentrations to precipitate VIII from aqueous solution. Indeed, there have been proposals to include such precipitants in the plasma even before freezing. However, these reagents may increase the unwanted precipitation of proteins along with the VIII, or interfere in other ways with further processing of the cryosupernatant.

The selectivity of cryoprecipitation is quite high. Cryoprecipitate contains 50 to 80% of the VIII:C, about half of the fibrinogen, about two thirds of the fibronectin, and about one third of the XIII in plasma. All other plasma proteins are present as supernatant trapped in the cryoprecipitate, which has a solids content of less than 30%, but the overall specific activity is increased some 20-fold over plasma and the precipitate can be redissolved at a concentration of about 10 U VIII:C per milliliter.

During the 1970s, several national fractionators had some success in preparing small-pool (up to 12 donations) or large-pool cryoprecipitate on an industrial scale. Small-pool cryoprecipitate was usually prepared aseptically to avoid difficult terminal sterilization by filtration. Methods were developed for washing the bulk cryoprecipitate, redissolving it in carefully formulated solvents, sterilizing and dispensing as a batch of identical vials, and freeze-drying. This represented the most economical use of scarce plasma resources, but the quality and convenience of freeze-dried cryoprecipitate could not compete with concentrates of higher purity as these became available.

B. Intermediate Purity Concentrates

Some relatively simple improvements can be made to crude cryoprecipitate solutions, without large losses of VIII, yielding freeze-dried "intermediate purity" concentrates. These dissolve readily within 5 to 10 min at a potency of 10 to 20 U VIII:C per milliliter and specific activity of 0.3 to 0.5 U VIII:C per milligram protein, quite adequate for all modes of replacement therapy. Many national fractionators, constrained to make the most of limited plasma sources, have adopted such processes over the last 10 years, in a variety of combinations.

1. Washing Bulk Cryoprecipitate

Washing the precipitate with cold buffer before resolution reduces the burden of trapped plasma proteins, including undesirable and unstable porcoagulants, carried over to subsequent stages. It may also be tailored to reduce the ionic strength of the cryoprecipitate solution, facilitating later removal of fibronectin.

2. Adsorption of Prothrombin Complex

This is usually accomplished by stirring aluminium hydroxide gel with the solution of cryoprecipitate, the duration, temperature, and gel concentration being chosen to minimize adsorption of VIII and maximize removal of prothrombin. The concentration of other unwanted proteins is also diminished, and the solution of factor VIII is more stable during later processing.

Table 1
SOME METHODS IN CURRENT USE FOR THE PARTIAL
SEPARATION OF FIBRINOGEN (AND FIBRONECTIN) FROM FACTOR
VIII CRUDE SOLUTIONS OF CRYOPRECIPITATE

Method	Ref.
Precipitation with 2 *M* glycine	10
Precipitation with 3% PEG	11
Precipitation with Zn^{++} (and heparin)	12
Precipitation with high concentration of heparin	13
Precipitation by brief heating in solution	14
Adsorption on insolubilized heparin	15

3. Removal of Fibronectin by "Cold Precipitation"

If cryoprecipitate is redissolved in a buffer solution of low ionic strength, proteins are progressively precipitated as pH is lowered towards pH 6.3 and the solution cooled. Factor VIII is precipitated less readily than fibrinogen or fibronectin, and a good compromise between yield and purification is usually achieved at pH values between 6.3 and 6.8, with the temperature between 5 and 10°.[6,7] Removal of fibronectin improves the solubility of the factor VIII preparation more dramatically than the modest 1.5- to 2-fold increase in specific activity suggests.

4. Partial Removal of Fibrinogen

Most of the methods discussed below in the corresponding section on high purity concentrates can be adapted to give a higher yield of VIII at the expense of lower specific activity, i.e., less fibrinogen is removed. In particular, it has been found convenient in large-scale fractionation to use controlled pore glass (CPG) in a batch-adsorption mode rather than make full use of its chromatographic potential.[8]

One further approach defies categorization. Rock and Palmer[9] found that replacement of conventional citrate anticoagulants with heparin resulted in a cryoprecipitate with an increased content of VIII activity and fibronectin. After resolution of the cryoprecipitate in a buffer containing heparin, a second cold precipitation separated VIII and fibronectin from many other contaminants. The process has some advantages over conventional cryoprecipitation in small-pool production, but is not readily adapted to large-scale fractionation.

C. "High Purity" Concentrates

The last 5 years have seen a growing demand for concentrates for home therapy and self-administration. Patients prefer a freeze-dried concentrate which dissolves very rapidly, giving a highly potent solution (>20 U VIII:C per milliliter) administered from a small syringe. These features are not readily obtained by the simple processes outlined above, and a two-stage strategy is commonly adopted for concentrates of higher purity (>1 U VIII:C per milligram protein).

The first stage may use one of the simple processes described above, perhaps extended to give more complete removal of fibrinogen, at the expense of VIII yield. Table 1 lists some alternative processes, which in practice are employed only as the first of several purification stages from bulk cryoprecipitate extracts.

After such stages VIII is left in solution but can then be concentrated to a high potency with less interference from troublesome contaminants. Concentration may consist simply of removing water and low molecular weight solutes (ultrafiltration), usually accompanied by a change of buffer salts to those appropriate for freeze-drying (diafiltration). Some manufacturers prefer to reprecipitate the VIII, often gaining further purification by leaving contaminants in solution, and to redissolve the VIII in a small volume of buffer. Excess precipitant remaining in the VIII may have to be removed by an extra desalting or diafiltration stage, but this can be done rapidly on the greatly reduced volume of solution. Some of the precipitation methods used in the second stage are cold ethanol,[16] glycine and sodium chloride,[14] and PEG.[17]

Additional purification stages usually mean increased losses of activity during the handling of concentrated VIII solutions, right up to the point of use by the patient. The gain over good intermediate purity concentrates in terms of rapid resolution and convenience to the patient may be quite small.

However, a new incentive to prepare concentrates of higher purity has arrived — the need to inactivate blood-borne viruses in all coagulation factor concentrates. Manufacturers who elect to heat VIII concentrates, either in protected solution or in the dry state, have found that fibrinogen and fibronectin limit the solubility of the heated product. Removing these proteins before heating permits the more severe regimes of heat treatment which seem to be needed to inactivate hepatitis viruses.

Manufacturers have other encouragements to become adept at purifying VIII still further. Some think it likely that recovery from human plasma will eventually be supplemented or supplanted by human-sequence VIII material from recombinant DNA sources. In this event, the raw material for fractionation will consist largely of nonhuman proteins from the host cell and culture medium. Primary capture of VIII as cryoprecipitate may be impossible because the carrier proteins fibrinogen and fibronectin will be absent. The VIII coagulant activity may be expressed by a protein of low molecular weight, unlike the large complex molecule purified from plasma by most current methods. Above all, it may be necessary to purify VIII almost completely from potentially antigenic or toxic nonhuman proteins in the medium. Intravenous injections in patients several times a week for life will test the safety of any genetically engineered protein much more severely than other current uses of such proteins, e.g., as a single dose in acute illness. In contrast to a plasma-derived concentrate containing one part of VIII:C in 10,000 parts of contaminating protein, nonhuman sources may have to achieve virtually pure VIII:C containing less than 0.1% contaminants.

Precipitation and simple adsorption techniques are seldom better than 90% selective, especially when total yield of one component is a major consideration. Even after hard packing in industrial centrifuges, precipitates typically contain <30% solids and >70% protein from the supernatant. The sheer mass of fibrinogen which has to be removed from cryoprecipitate solutions to achieve VIII of high purity physically entraps a significant proportion of the VIII from the supernatant, and washing is not usually practicable. For all these reasons, purification of VIII in excess of specific activity of 5 U VIII:C per milligram protein calls for the resolving power of chromatography.

D. Chromatographic Purification of Factor VIII

Chromatography or semiselective adsorption methods may be distinguished by the type and degree of selectivity imposed and by the strategic choice to adsorb either VIII or the contaminants to be removed from it. The methods discussed in this section have been used on a preparative scale for therapeutic use or have the requisite potential for high capacity.

On simple molecular exclusion chromatography at low ionic strength on large-pore gels, VIII:C activity remains complexed with von Willebrand factor (vWf) and emerges in the void volume. The degree of separation from smaller contaminants such as fibrinogen and fibronectin depends on column loading and the initial concentrations of these proteins. Viscosity limits the concentration of protein which can be applied to the column, and the dilute eluate must be reconcentrated for most purposes. When the running buffer includes calcium chloride at >20 mmol/l or sodium chloride at >0.8 mol/l, the VIII/vWf dissociates, and VIII:C activity is eluted mainly in the included volume with many other plasma proteins.

Solid phases which strongly adsorb VIII have some advantages over those which adsorb contaminants. It is often possible to achieve concentration rather than dilution of the VIII.There may be opportunities for varied and extensive washing after adsorption, with the intention of removing most other proteins and even reducing viral contamination. The same procedure can be used for many different sources of VIII, the capacity of the adsorbent being determined by the concentration of VIII rather than by the concentrations of contaminants. A disadvantage is that the adsorbent may be more reluctant to release VIII as the selectivity and strength of initial binding are increased. The solutions used to dissociate VIII from the adsorbent may dissociate the VIII/vWf complex, have irreversible effects on VIII:C activity, or complicate further processing towards i.v. use.

Controlled pore glass[8] probably acts both as a molecular exclusion medium and as a semispecific inorganic adsorbent for VIII (cf. bentonite). Immobilized heparin[15] probably acts both as a highly charged ligand and a broadly specific affinity reagent. Either adsorbent may be used to remove most of the fibrinogen and fibronectin from crude or partly processed solutions of cryoprecipitate. Metal chelating adsorbents for fibrinogen[18] and immobilized gelatin as an affinity adsorbent for fibronectin have the potential selectivity for large-scale separations, but their use in fractionation has not been published, possibly because of their limited capacities.

Anion exchangers,[19,20] solid phase polyelectrolytes (PE),[21] immobilized amino-alkanes, and some analogues[22,23] all bind factor VIII at physiological ionic strength and near-neutral pH. Elution under dissociating conditions can result in high purification factors and, at least in the case of amino-hexyl Sepharose (AHS), more than 70% yield of VIII:C activity.[24] The performance of PE and AHS are best attributed to both charge and hydrophobic interactions between the solid phase and VIII, but it is not certain whether the latter binds solely through the procoagulant moiety, VIII:C. vWf is present in the eluates in a reduced proportion. Conditions for all these kinds of chromatography can be manipulated to remove fibrinogen, fibronectin, and much of the vWf from crude solutions, but resolution is inversely related to loading. Ion exchangers tend to have a low capacity for VIII and yield a dilute eluate, whereas PE and AHS have a high capacity (>50 U VIII:C per milliliter bed volume), and conditions can be chosen so that VIII is eluted at a higher concentration than in the loaded sample. In all these applications, there is competition between VIII and contaminating proteins for binding sites, and at present they are used to the best advantage after at least partial processing of cryoprecipitate.

If specificity of binding were the only consideration in the chromatography of VIII, one would expect immunoaffinity separation on immobilized antibodies to be widely used. The most popular variant on a laboratory scale features the binding of VIII/vWf complex to an immobilized polyclonal or monoclonal antibody to VIII/vWf,[25] dissociation of the complex to elute VIII:C under relatively mild increments in sodium chloride or calcium chloride concentration, and chaotropic release of VIII/vWf to recycle the immunoadsorbent. Currently, the capacity and, more surprisingly, the selectivity of the readily available antibodies would limit their industrial application, but these obstacles may be temporary. Applying today's fractionation criteria for adding further purification stages, immunoaffinity chromatography may seem to offer less than, say, AHS in terms of capacity and yield, but the balance might change if the premium on selectivity were raised, e.g., by the need to recover human-sequence VIII:C from a source other than human plasma. It is attractive to avoid binding through VIII/vWf and subsequent dissociation of the complex, by effecting reversible binding to an immobilized antibody against VIII:C. Ideal antibodies would combine a high capacity for VIII:C with the propensity to release it under mild conditions, but conventional strategies for the selection of clones may not be ideally suited to detecting more than one virtue. In another mode, immunoaffinity adsorbents can be used to remove awkward contaminants at a late stage. Currently, all immunoaffinity methods are inhibited by lack of confidence in the complete stability of the matrix-antibody link, and fears of releasing nonhuman protein into the product. This constraint may weigh less heavily as human-sequence VIII:C from cell culture is developed and the tolerable limits for such contaminants are established.

Fractionators have appeared hesitant in applying to very large pools the methods pursued in the isolation of factor VIII for laboratory study. Translation of laboratory chromatographic techniques to columns of over 100 l presents challenges in maintaining processing rates and hygiene, especially when "soft" gels are used as matrices, but these are being answered by growing confidence in column, matrix, and process design. In compensation, chromatography is inherently more amenable to continuous highly automated processing than essentially discontinuous methods based on precipitation or simple adsorption. Coagulation factors can pose unusual problems in the selection of contact materials, especially as purification increases. Another serious obstacle to the large-scale exploitation of some highly resolving methods is their requirement for toxic reagents, e.g., protease inhibitors, which one could scarcely contemplate adding to a protein for ultimate i.v. use.

It is commonly found that, as VIII is purified, losses of coagulant activity through the action of proteases are alleviated, but new sources of loss appear in the form of irreversible adsorption to surfaces and unexplained instabilities on storage, freezing, etc. No single measure to combat these losses seems to be applicable under all circumstances, and we are constantly reminded that increased purification needs economic justification. Since the replacement of the cruder cryoprecipitate preparations by the better intermediate purity and higher purity concentrates, clinicians have not reported a consistent correlation between side effects and either the specific activity or a particular method of manufacture. Hemolysis after high doses of VIII is now rarely seen, since most manufacturers control the concentrations of isoagglutinins and total IgG in their products. However, pressure is mounting to reduce the burden of processed proteins repeatedly infused into hemophiliacs. Although there is no evidence that the development of factor VIII inhibitors is determined by the other proteins in the concentrate, it does seem that protracted treatment with today's relatively impure concentrates may be the source of some immune dysfunction in hemophiliacs, possibly unrelated to lymphotropic viruses.[26] Identification of the offending proteins would signal further changes in processing to remove specific contaminants or increase overall specific activity.

IV. TRANSMISSION OF BLOOD-BORNE VIRUSES

All coagulation factor concentrates share the stigma of transmitting blood-borne viruses, partly because they are recovered by less denaturing techniques than ethanol fractionation, and partly because they have been considered too delicate to survive the kind of heat treatment accorded to albumin preparations. The most serious risk associated with VIII replacement therapy is the transmission of viruses causing hepatitis B, non-A non-B hepatitis (NANBH), and acquired immune deficiency syndrome (AIDS). Although screening of blood donations and increasing vaccination of hemophiliacs have greatly reduced the incidence of hepatitis B, careful prospective clinical trials have shown that until 1985, patients given large pool VIII concentrates for the first time were almost certain to acquire NANBH. No donor screening has been available to exclude NANBH virus from plasma, and the incidence of NANBH has been almost as high in products from unpaid as from paid donors.[27,28] Inactivation of NANBH virus in concentrates was being tackled seriously by most manufacturers when the AIDS "epidemic" struck so harshly at hemophiliacs. Fortunately, the human immunodeficiency virus (HIV) appears to be susceptible to heat treatment of freeze-dried concentrates or to heating in protected solutions of VIII.[29] NANBH has proved to be more resistant to these treatments and continues to present the greater challenge in other important respects.

The absence of even a qualitative test for NANBH virus or its antibody is the most serious obstacle to success. Although chimpanzees are susceptible to the virus which affects humans, results obtained by painstaking and expensive work in chimpanzees do not seem to be wholly applicable to human hemophiliacs.[30] The generally accepted test protocol for detection of NANBH transmission in man is infusion of concentrate into susceptible hemophiliacs with two to four weekly blood samplings for liver function tests. Although many patients who have received VIII on an infrequent basis remain susceptible to NANBH from later infusions, some of the most carefully controlled studies are restricted to patients being treated for the first time. Since the latter are often very young or very mildly affected patients who do not regularly attend hemophilia clinics, regular follow-up is often difficult to achieve. It is always possible that a batch of concentrate used in clinical trials may not contain an infective titer of virus even before the intended inactivation treatment. Any trial of a new inactivation method must, therefore, accumulate 50 patients or more using at least ten batches. By these criteria, none of the trials published to date has yet confirmed that any VIII concentrate is free of transmitting NANBH. In the struggle with NANBH, fractionators have a more limited range of weapons than they had against hepatitis B. Donor screening and immunological approaches, e.g., immunoadsorption of virus, are not available, and they cannot detect partial removal or inactivation of the infective agent during fractionation stages. It has to be assumed that each batch is infective after conventional processing.

It is unfortunate and somewhat surprising that many physical and chemical insults affect the organization of protein molecules more severely than complex viruses. On the assumption that the NANBH virus is lipid envelope, VIII concentrates have been treated with chloroform, but remain infective.[31] Heating at 60° in *n*-heptane, as used by one manufacturer, might also be expected to affect the lipid enveloped, but some batches appear to be infective even after such treatment.[32] A more promising attack on the lipid envelope is now being mounted,[33] in which the "solvent" effect of tri-*n*-butyl phosphate is assisted by a detergent such as sodium cholate. Model virus and chimpanzee studies suggest that NANBH will be inactivated, the loss of VIII activity seems acceptable, and the results of clinical trials are eagerly awaited. Another promising virucidal treatment, using β-propiolactone and UV irradiation,[34] appears to give a high assurance of inactivating NANBH. However, the esterification and acylation of proteins induced by this reagent affect the function of VIII more than many other plasma proteins.

Some workers are investigating gamma irradiation of freeze-dried VIII, at doses similar to those used to sterilize surgical equipment, foods, and drugs.[35] The "window" between inactivation of VIII and inactivation of NANBH may again be rather narrow.

To date, most manufacturers have chosen heat treatment as the means of inactivating NANBH in VIII concentrates. The search for suitable heating regimes has had a considerable impact on the fractionation process itself. If VIII:C activity is to survive heating in solution, it must be protected by the addition of very high concentrations of stabilizers, e.g., amino acids and sugars, which may also protect the virus. Although heating at 60° for 10 h has been chosen by analogy with the pasteurization of albumin, the inclusion of protective agents makes a comparison untenable. Although VIII:C activity survives protected pasteurization, the high concentrations of fibrinogen and fibronectin in cryoprecipitate must be reduced before the solution is heated, if heavy precipitation is to be avoided.

Similarly, the heating regimes tolerated by freeze-dried VIII concentrates are determined less by the stability of VIII:C itself, which proves to be rather robust, than by loss of solubility of accompanying proteins, particularly the usual contaminants fibrinogen and fibronectin. Difficulty in resolution after drying and heating may be alleviated in various ways, e.g., by addition of low concentrations of amino acid mixtures or nonreducing sugars before freeze-drying. Even crude freeze-dried cryoprecipitate, with such modifications, can be heated to 60° with probable inactivation of HIV. However, NANBH is not inactivated after even 72 h at 60°,[30] and model virus studies suggest that higher temperatures may offer a broader window between VIII:C and virus inactivation. In order to heat VIII to 80° for 72 h in the hope of inactivating NANBH as well as HIV, it may prove necessary to improve on the processes used for intermediate purity concentrates. For example, a new concentrate with ten-fold less fibrinogen and fibronectin has had to be developed in England to permit such severe heating without impairment of solubility and unacceptable loss of VIII:C activity.[13] A small penalty in process yield was incurred, balanced by better survival of VIII:C, even under the more severe heating which offers the possibility of a concentrate free of transmitting NANBH.

V. POSSIBLE DEVELOPMENTS IN PURIFICATION OF FACTOR VIII CONCENTRATES

When success in inactivating HIV in finished products is followed by final elimination of NANBH and hepatitis B, it will be difficult to justify the continued use of frozen cryoprecipitate, which had been assumed to be the safest source of VIII until AIDS altered the scene. Manufacturers who have promoted the development of human sequence VIII from nonhuman cell cultures may also regret pressing the viral safety of their projected product so emphatically, particularly if mammalian cells prove to support viruses affecting man. The benefits of today's work on virus inactivation in plasma-source VIII may, therefore, reach far into the future, whether plasma VIII is ultimately supplemented from other sources or plasma fractionation continues to be the best way of supplying a comprehensive range of therapeutic proteins. The likeliest outcome is a protracted co-existence of plasma and recombinant DNA-based VIII concentrates while the latter acquire an acceptable record of safety and efficacy, and the economic comparisons become more reliable than current extrapolations.

Recombinant sources of human sequence VIII for conventional replacement therapy may be overtaken by other approaches. Direct manipulation of a hemophiliac's "faulty" DNA is not yet in sight. It is, however, less fanciful to envisage implantation of exogenous tissue competent to retain a low prophylactic level of VIII:C in the hemophiliac's circulation. Oral administration of VIII would virtually eliminate the fractionator's worries about purification, sterility, and viral transmission. Recovery of VIII in the circulation from oral liposomes[36] has not been satisfactorily confirmed, but the technology of microencapsulation is growing fast and may yet offer new options, in combination with a cheap source of human sequence VIII, for the economical treatment of hemophilia.

REFERENCES

1. **Blombäck, B. and Blombäck, M.,** Purification of human and bovine fibrinogen, *Ark. Kemi,* 10, 415, 1956.
2. **Over, J., Bouma, B. N., Sixma, J. J., Bolhuis, P. A., and Vlooswijk, R. A. A.,** Heterogeneity of human factor VIII. III. Transitions between forms of factor VIII present in cryoprecipitate and in cryosupernatant plasma, *J. Lab. Clin. Med.,* 95, 323, 1980.
3. **Mason, E. C., Pepper, D. S., and Griffin, B.,** Production of cryoprecipitate of intermediate purity in a closed system thaw-siphon process, *Thromb. Haemost.,* 46, 543, 1981.
4. **Foster, P. R., Dickson, A. J., McQuillan, T. A., Dickson, I. H., Keddie, S., and Watt, J. G.,** Control of large-scale plasma thawing for recovery of cryoprecipitate factor VIII, *Vox Sang.,* 42, 180, 1982.
5. **Foster, P. R., Dickson, A. J., and Dickson, I. H.,** Improving yield in the manufacture of factor VIII concentrates, *Scand. J. Haematol.,* 33 (Suppl. 40), 103, 1984.
6. **Smith, J. K., Evans, D. R., Stone, V., and Snape, T. J.,** A factor VIII concentrate of intermediate purity and higher potency, *Transfusion,* 19, 299, 1979.

7. **Horowitz, B., Lippin, A., Chang, M. Y., Shulman, R. W., Vandersande, J., Stryker, M. H., and Woods, K. R.,** Preparation of antihemophilic factor and fibronectin from human plasma cryoprecipitate, *Transfusion,* 24, 357, 1984.

8. **Margolis, J., Gallovich, C. M., and Rhoades, P.,** A process for preparation of "high-purity" factor VIII by controlled pore glass treatment, *Vox Sang.,* 46, 341, 1984.

9. **Rock, G. A. and Palmer, D. S.,** Intermediate purity factor VIII production utilising a cold-insoluble globulin technique, *Thromb. Res.,* 18, 551, 1980.

10. **Thorell, L. and Blombäck, B.,** Purification of the factor VIII complex, *Thromb. Res.,* 35, 431, 1984.

11. **Brinkhous, K. M., Shanbrom, E., Roberts, H. R., Webster, W. P., Fekete, L., and Wagner, R. H.,** A new high-potency glycine-precipitated antihemophilic factor (AHF) concentrate, *JAMA,* 205, 613, 1968.

12. **Bier, M. and Foster, P. R.,** Purification of Antihemophilia Factor VIII by Precipitation with Zinc Ions, U.S. Patent Application 4,406,886, 1983.

13. **Winkelman, L., Owen, N. E., Haddon, M. E., and Smith, J. K.,** A new therapeutic factor VIII concentrate of high specific activity and high yield, *Thromb. Haemost.,* 54, 19, 1985.

14. **Heimburger, V. N., Schwinn, H., Gratz, G., Lüben, G., Kumpe, G., and Herchenhan, B.,** Faktor VIII-Konzantrat, Hochgereinigt und in Lösung Erhitzt, *Arzneim. Forsch./Drug Res.,* 31(4), 619, 1981.

15. **Andersson, L. O., Borg, H. G., Forsman, N., Hanshoff, G., Lindroos, G., Miller-Andersson, M., and Carling, E. C.,** Isolation of Coagulation Factors I and VIII from Biological Material, U.S. Patent 4,022,758, 1977.

16. **Hershgold, E. J., Pool, J. G., and Pappenhage, A. R.,** The potent antihemophilic globulin concentrate derived from a cold insoluble fraction of human plasma; characterisation and further data on preparation and clinical trial, *J. Lab. Clin. Med.,* 67, 23, 1966.

17. **Newman, J., Johnson, A. J., Karpatkin, M. H., and Puszkin, S.,** Methods from the production of clinically effective intermediate- and high-purity factor-VIII concentrates, *Br. J. Haematol.,* 21, 1, 1971.

18. **Scully, M. F. and Kakkar, V. V.,** Structural features of fibrinogen associated with binding to chelated zinc, *Biochim. Biophys. Acta,* 700, 130, 1982.

19. **Fay, P. J., Chavin, S. I., Schroeder, D., Young, F. E., and Marder, V. J.,** Purification and characterization of a highly purified human factor VIII consisting of a single type of polypeptide chain, *Proc. Natl. Acad. Sci. U.S.A.,* 79, 7200, 1982.

20. **Levi, Y., Dupechez, T., Rimmele, D., Allary, M., Boschitti, E., and Saint-Blancard, J.,** Nouvelle methode chromatographique pour la purification du facteur VIII, *C.R. Acad. Sci. Paris,* 296, 257, 1983.

21. **Tuddenham, E. G. D., Lane, R. S., Rotblat, F., Johnson, A. J., Snape, T. J., Middleton, S., and Kernoff, P. B. A.,** Response to infusions of polyelectrolyte fractionated human factor VIII concentrate in human haemophilia A and von Willebrand's disease, *Br. J. Haematol.,* 52, 259, 1982.

22. **Austen, D. E. G. and Smith, J. K.,** Factor VIII fractionation on amino-hexyl Sepharose with possible reduction in hepatitis B antigen, *Thromb. Haemost.,* 48, 1, 1982.

23. **Morgenthaler, J.-J.,** Chromatography of antihemophilic factor on diaminoalkane- and aminoalkane-derivatized Sepharose, *Thromb. Haemost.,* 47, 124, 1982.

24. **Neal, G. G., Hersee, D., and Smith, J. K.,** Purification of factor VIII on aminohexyl-Sepharose, *Thromb. Haemost.,* 54, 78, 1985.

25. **Fulcher, C. A. and Zimmerman, T. S.,** Characterization of the human factor VIII procoagulant protein with a heterologous precipitating antibody, *Proc. Natl. Acad. Sci. U.S.A.,* 79, 1648, 1982.

26. **Lee, C. A., Bofill, M., Janossy, G., Thomas, H. C., Rizza, C. R., and Kernoff, P. B. A.,** Relationships between blood product exposure and immunological abnormalities in English haemophiliacs, *Br. J. Haematol.,* 60, 161, 1985.

27. **Fletcher, M. L., Trowell, J. M., Craske, J., Pavier, K., and Rizza, C. R.,** Non-A non-B hepatitis after transfusion of factor VIII in infrequently treated patients, *Br. Med. J.,* 287, 1754, 1983.

28. **Kernoff, P. B. A., Lee, C. A., Karayiannis, P., and Thomas, H. C.,** High risk of non-A non-B hepatitis after a first exposure to volunteer or commercial clotting factor concentrates: effects of prophylactic immune serum globulin, *Br. J. Haematol.,* 60, 469, 1985.

29. **McDougal, J. S., Martin, L. S., Cort, S. P., Mozen, M., Heldebrant, C. M., and Evatt, B. L.,** Thermal inactivation of the acquired immunodeficiency syndrome virus, human T lymphotropic virus-III/lymphadenopathy-associated, with special reference to antihemophilic factor, *J. Clin. Invest.,* 76, 1, 1985.

30. **Colombo, M., Carnelli, V., Gazengel, C., Mannucci, P. M., Savidge, G. F., Schimpf, K., and the European Study Group,** Transmission of non-A, non-B hepatitis by heat-treated factor VIII concentrate, *Lancet,* 2, 1, 1985.

31. **Mannucci, P. M., Colombo, M., and Rodeghiero, F.,** Non-A, non-B hepatitis after factor VIII concentrate treated by heating and chloroform, *Lancet,* 2, 1013, 1985.

32. **Kernoff, P. B. A., Miller, E. J., Savidge, G. F., Machin, S. J., Dewar, M. S., and Preston, F. E.,** Wet heating for safer factor VIII concentrate?, *Lancet,* 2, 721, 1985.

33. **Horowitz, B., Wiebe, M. E., Lippin, A., and Stryker, M. H.,** Inactivation of viruses in labile blood derivatives. I. Disruption of lipid-enveloped viruses by tri(n-butyl)phosphate detergent combinations, *Transfusion,* 25, 516, 1985.

34. **Prince, A. M., Stephan, W., and Brotman, B.,** β-propiolactone/ultraviolet irradiation: a review of its effectiveness for inactivation of viruses in blood derivatives, *Rev. Infect. Dis.,* 5, 92, 1983.

35. **Horowitz, B., Wiebe, M. E., Lippin, A., Vandersande, J., and Stryker, M. H.,** Inactivation of viruses in labile blood derivatives. II. Physical methods, *Transfusion,* 25, 523, 1985.

36. **Hemker, H. C., Muller, A. D., Hermens, W. Th., and Zwaal, R. F. A.,** Oral treatment of haemophilia A by gastrointestinal absorption of factor VIII entrapped in liposomes, *Lancet,* 1, 70, 1980.

Chapter 17

VIRUS TRANSMISSION BY FACTOR VIII PRODUCTS

D. L. Aronson

TABLE OF CONTENTS

I.   Introduction 302

II.   Viruses Transmitted by Plasma Coagulation Products...........................302
        A.   Hepatitis B and Non-A, Non-B Hepatitis...............................303
        B.   Retroviruses: Human Immunodeficiency Virus 304
        C.   Parvovirus 305
        D.   Miscellaneous 305

III.   Determinants of Viral Transmission by Plasma Products......................305
        A.   Transient Viremic State in the Donor 306
        B.   Instability of the Extracellular Virus...............................306
        C.   Low Virus Titer in the Plasma 306
        D.   Neutralizing Antibody Present in the Pooled Plasma 306
        E.   Inactivation of the Virus by the Processing Steps 307
        F.   Host Defense Mechanisms 307
        G.   Inability to Detect Infection in the Recipients 308

IV.   The Impact of Infectious Agents on the Hemophiliac........................308

V.   Viral Inactivation Methodologies 312
        A.   Donor Screening 312
        B.   Viral Inactivation Procedures..313

VI.   Strategies for Patient Treatment..316

VII.   Summary 316

References...317

I. INTRODUCTION

The development of plasma concentrates for the treatment of hemophilia has resulted in profound improvement in the length and quality of life for the hemophiliac.[1-3] This advance has not been made without increasing risks for these patients. As expected, the leading adverse effect of repeated transfusion of plasma products from large numbers of donors is transmission of infectious (viral) disease and infection. In the era prior to the availability of fractionated antihemophilic factor (factor VIII), the sole replacement therapy available to the hemophiliacs was plasma, and the intensity of treatment was considerably less than now. For example, prior to 1965, an intensively treated hemophiliac may have been exposed at the most to 100 blood donors a year and several thousand in his lifetime. In contrast, current treatment even with a single donor product such as cryoprecipitate results in the exposure to 500 donors per year while treatment with concentrate results in exposure to products derived from 10,000 donors for each lot and millions of donors during a lifetime.

While for viral infections with a high carrier rate, such as hepatitis B or non-A, non-B hepatitis, the exposure to more donors makes little difference, it can be argued that we are exposing patients to rare and exotic viruses from the one donor in a million who is a carrier. Of perhaps more concern is the probability of infecting a patient with two viruses which operate in concert to produce disease. If, for example, a virus and a "helper virus" coexist in 1/1000 donors, the probability of infection with both agents using single donor products is 1/1 million whereas using a pool of 1000 donors this probability increases to more than 50%. This is apparently the case with the interaction of the hepatitis B virus and the "delta" agent.[4] On the other hand, it may also be argued that the dilution of a few contaminated donations in large pools might be beneficial in reducing the morbidity associated with any given virus.

II. VIRUSES TRANSMITTED BY PLASMA COAGULATION PRODUCTS

The number of viruses known to be transmitted by blood products is extremely limited, and that known to be transmitted by plasma products is even less. The first known of the blood-borne viral diseases was hepatitis. As blood and plasma therapy developed during World War II, it became clear that the transmission of hepatitis was a not uncommon event.[5-7] Despite the fact that the follow-up of blood and plasma recipients and the diagnosis of hepatitis were based on clinical presentation and limited tests of liver function such as thymol turbidity, cephalin flocculation, and bilirubin, the incidence of hepatitis was considered sufficiently high so that programs were developed to reduce or remove this risk.[8,9] The most commonly used plasma fraction at the time was albumin. However, other products, derived from pooled human plasma, such as thrombin and fibrinogen, were both associated with a high incidence of hepatitis.

On the basis of epidemiologic characteristics and the incubation period, two clinical forms of hepatitis were defined: "serum" hepatitis and "infectious" hepatitis. The former was associated with the use of blood products, while the latter with a shorter incubation period was associated with the classic fecal-oral type of transmission.

In the 1950s, the introduction of the current tests for the diagnosis of liver disease, i.e., the serum glutamic oxaloacetic transaminase (SGOT) and the alanine amino transferase (ALT), indicated that blood transfusion was commonly associated with an elevation of transaminase values within 6 months of receiving blood products. In some reports as many as 15% of those receiving blood transfusions developed ALT elevations consistent with some form of hepatitis.[10]

This is the status of transfusion associated viral diseases as of 1970. At this time hepatitis included either a single clinical entity associated with jaundice, which, on epidemiologic grounds, was felt to be due to multiple causes, or, as in the case of a larger fraction of patients, an anicteric condition, but in which the measurement of transaminase elevation indicated the presence of liver disease.

A. Hepatitis B and Non-A, Non-B Hepatitis

With the advent of serologic tests for hepatitis B,[11-13] strides were made not only in the substantial reduction of the transmission of at least one form of hepatitis, but also in the unravelling of a still tangled story concerning the origins of posttransfusion hepatitis and "transaminitis".[14] The former, serum hepatitis, has been shown to be in part caused by what is now referred to as hepatitis B. Other forms comprising the rest are due to "non-A, non-B hepatitis(s)", while little if any infection is due to hepatitis A. Hepatitis B is a virus, endemic around the world, and associated with a chronic carrier state in 5 to 10% of those with evidence of infection. Depending on the given population the carrier state for hepatitis B is between 1/100 and 1/1000. Since the advent of screening for hepatitis B antigen the incidence of carriers in the blood donor populations has been reduced to well under 1/1000. The chronic carrier state is associated with a high titer of infectious virus in the plasma. From both human and chimpanzee transmission experiments the level of infectious virus can be 10^8 particles per milliliter.[15,16]

The hepatitis B virus is now known to be a lipid coated virus with an outside "class" antigen referred to as the surface antigen (HBsAg). In the carrier state, the circulating level of this antigen is as high as 100 µg/ml. The interior is a DNA core surrounded by another membrane containing a different antigen, the "core antigen" (HBcAg).[17,18] Infection with hepatitis B results in the production of antibodies to both the core and the surface antigen.

Under certain circumstances, infection with hepatitis B virus results in the production of three antibodies. The time course of infection usually shows the appearance of the core antibody first. If the hepatitis becomes chronic the level of the core antibody remains relatively high. Following the viremic antigen positive stage and the production of the core antibody, there is the development of the antibody against the surface protein: the anti-HB sometimes appears as another antigen which is referred to as the e-antigen.[19] This antigen is not, as yet, identified with any viral structure and may arise from liver necrosis. The e-antigen disappears and the antibody to the e-antigen appears when the viral DNA is integrated into the hepatocyte genome.[20] There is continued secretion of the surface antigen but no further viral replication. With the development of the e-antibody the liver disease picture changes from chronic active hepatitis to an inactive stage.

A recent addition to the transmissible agents is that referred to as the delta agent which was originally identified by serologic measurement.[4,21-23] The delta agent is a 34-nm particle without an envelope and which, in contrast to the hepatitis B virus, contains only RNA. The number of infectious particles in plasma is as high as 10^{11} per milliliter, and there is a chronic carrier state. The estimated frequency of the carrier state is not known, although the antibody occurs in several percent of most populations, and the plasma containing the antibody can be infectious. No production lots of either factor VIII or factor IX complex products were found to contain detectable delta antigen despite strong epidemiologic evidence of transmission by factor VIII. Infection with the delta agent after infection with hepatitis B results in a new hepatitis with release of a virus made up of the RNA from the delta agent and the surface antigen of the hepatitis B.

The ubiquitous non-A, non-B hepatitis virus is a conundrum.[24,25] This infection is defined by the appearance of an elevated ALT which persists. Epidemiologic studies indicate that the carrier rate in all populations of blood donors is probably greater than 1%.[26] Along with the persistent elevation of the ALT, there is also evidence of histologic changes in the liver ultimately leading to some degree of cirrhosis.

Clinical studies in blood product recipients, however, give inconsistent results for the incubation period after exposure to blood products. For example, the ALT rise seen in recipients of blood and single donor plasma occurs at 35 d. In contrast, in pooled plasma product recipients, such as hemophiliacs, the ALT rise is seen in some cases much earlier (8 to 20 d).[27,28]

The only animal model other than humans currently available for the study of non-A, non-B hepatitis, is the chimpanzee.[29,30] The incubation time in chimpanzees seems to be 5 to 12 weeks. In contrast to hepatitis B, it is reported that there is no apparent relationship between the incubation time and the dose of infective material administered. The infective level found in plasma after chimpanzee inoculation is about 10^2 infectious U/ml, although one inoculum has been found to contain as high as 10^6 infectious U/ml. Chimpanzee transmission has been accomplished with plasma samples taken years after the acute infection when the donor plasma had only minimal elevation of the ALT.[31] Evidence of the heterogeneity of the agent causing non-A, non-B hepatitis is derived from chimpanzee cross-challenge experiments.[29] Chimpanzees exposed to non-A, non-B hepatitis inoculum are refractory to reinfection with the same inoculum. However, there are other inocula which will cause a subsequent rise in the ALT. No virus has been isolated, although some electron microscope pictures of putative agents have been published.[32-36] Recently there have been reports suggesting that at least one form of non-A, non-B hepatitis is a retrovirus.[36,37] These reports are based on the occurrence of particle bound reverse transcriptase in the plasma of patients or chimpanzees with acute non-A, non-B hepatitis. Electron microscopy also reveals budding particles similar to that seen with retrovirus infections of other types.

A variety of immunologic test systems have been proposed for the diagnosis of non-A, non-B hepatitis infection. As of this time of writing none of these have been verified.[38,39]

B. Retro Viruses: Human Immunodeficiency Virus

In the last few years a new syndrome, acquired immune deficiency syndrome (AIDS) has been described in association with transfusion of blood and blood products. Early reports associated AIDS in hemophiliacs with the presence of antibodies to a retrovirus, human T-cell leukemia virus-I (HTLV-I). In 1983 to 1984 another retrovirus, variously referred to as human T-cell lymphotropic retrovirus #3 (HTLV-III), lymphadenopathy associated virus (LAV), AIDS related virus (ARV), or human immunodeficiency virus (HIV), was found to be the causative agent of AIDS.[40-43] The early implication of HTLV-I in this disease[44,45] was probably due to the presence of related antigens in these two viruses. More recent data indicate a low frequency of HTLV-I antibody in a variety of hemophilia populations.[46,47] The prevalence of the antibody to HTLV-I in the hemophilia population is similar to that in the general population. This would indicate that HTLV-I virus is probably not transmitted by factor VIII or factor IX concentrates. A single report has been published on the presence of the genome of HTLV-II (another retrovirus related to HTLV-I and HTLV-III) in the lymphocytes of a hemophiliac with chronic pancytopenia.[48] HIV selectively infects the helper lymphocytes and blunts the cellular immune system. After infection with the virus, there may be an acute disease characterized by, among other symptoms, an acute glandular fever-like disorder occurring within 6 weeks. The more usual pattern is for the severe clinical illness to show up months to years following the initial infection following a stage characterized by generalized lymphadenopathy. The net result in a certain as yet undefined number of infected patients is death caused by secondary opportunistic infections. The virus has been isolated from all body fluids.

Although HIV is the most recent of the transmissible plasma agents to be identified, in many ways there is more known about it than there is of the other transmissible plasma agents. It is a coated virus, which can be cultured in either peripheral lymphocytes or in a transformed cell line. The genome has been characterized from various isolates derived from AIDS patients. Immunologic characterization shows both similarities and differences with

HTLV-I and HTLV-II viruses. Unequivocal identification of the agent by electron microscopy has been accomplished.

The occurrence of a prolonged carrier state has been established by culture studies from patients with AIDS related complex, i.e., generalized lymphadenopathy. While virus isolation from the cells can be done consistently, only rarely has there been isolation from plasma, and never from a blood product. At the same time as the virus can be isolated from the cells by an infected patient, the plasma has antibody to viral proteins specific for the HIV virus. Antibody screening would indicate that about 1/5000 blood donors have antibodies to HIV that can be confirmed by immunoblotting methods (the so-called Western blot). Many of these donors, although not all, are associated with high risk activities including homosexuality and the use of i.v. narcotics.

C. Parvovirus

Another recent addition to the viruses transmitted by blood and blood products is human parvovirus (HPV) which is identical to the serum parvo-like virus (SPLV). This virus may be identical to that responsible for the "fifth" disease of childhood, an acute febrile illness associated with a rash. The carrier rate in blood donors has been estimated to be between 1/4000 and 1/40,000, and the viremic stage lasts approximately 3 weeks in duration.[49,50] The number of particles in the blood during the viremic stage is large and has been estimated to be as high as 10^{12} infection particles per milliliter. While a relatively low frequency of antibody has been found in nontransfused populations, there is an almost universal occurrence of antibody to this virus in hemophiliacs.[51]

While little is known about this particular parvovirus, the parvoviruses as a class are nonenveloped, single stranded DNA viruses without either lipid or glycoprotein. While some are associated by themselves with acute infectious disease, others are in the class of "helper" viruses that can multiply only in the presence of helper adenovirus.

D. Miscellaneous

Efforts have been made to establish whether other common viruses might be transmitted by factor VIII preparations. These studies do not indicate that there is an excessive proportion of treated hemophiliacs with exposure to viruses including measles, mumps, and rubella.[52] While the proportion of hemophiliacs showing evidence of infection with cytomegalovirus (CMV) and Epstein-Barr virus (EB virus) is not unusual, the type of antibody indicates more "reactivation" in hemophiliacs.[53] Specific studies show no excess antibody to hepatitis A in hemophiliacs compared to aged matched controls from the same geographic area.[54]

While it is heartening to realize that there is evidence for only a few viruses being transmitted to plasma products, this must be tempered by the knowledge that of the five viruses mentioned above, four have been implicated only in the last few years. It would seem likely that there may be other viruses transmitted by factor VIII products that are as yet undiscovered. However, there seems to be little in the way of serious infectious disease in the hemophiliac that cannot be explained by the viruses listed above — AS OF TODAY. The one lesson from AIDS is that new viruses can be introduced into the blood supply with dire consequences. A second concern is the interaction of multiple virus infections. As noted above, co-infection with hepatitis B and the delta agent results in a disease different from infection with the individual agents. One report indicates that co-infection with CMV and HIV leads to more T-helper cell suppression. Table 1 lists the viruses known to be transmitted by plasma products and gives estimates of the carrier rate in blood donors.

III. DETERMINANTS OF VIRAL TRANSMISSION BY PLASMA PRODUCTS

Possible reasons for the limited number of viruses transmitted by plasma products are varied and numerous.

Table 1
VIRUSES TRANSMITTED BY PLASMA PRODUCTS AND THEIR
ESTIMATED CARRIER FREQUENCY

Virus	Carrier rate
Hepatitis B	2—5/1000
Non-A, non-B hepatitis	10/1000
Delta agent	?10/1000
HIV	0.2/1000
Parvovirus	0.1/1000

A. Transient Viremic State in the Donor

Most viral infections are characterized by a viremic stage of only a few days, so that there is little probability of a viremic donor giving blood during this phase. A further limitation is that the viremic donor may not feel well enough to donate or is deferred as a donor at the blood bank. There are, however, many viruses (and more are being discovered all the time) with a persistent carrier state in the face of apparently good health. It is interesting to note that all of the viruses mentioned above, with the exception of the parvovirus, are characterized by a carrier state of months to years.

B. Instability of the Extracellular Virus

Many viruses are so unstable that they cannot maintain infectivity outside the cell and are transmitted directly from cell to cell. Salient examples of this type virus are CMV, EB virus, and HTLV-I. All three of these viruses are easily transmitted by the cellular components of the blood. Plasma and plasma products have never been implicated in transmission of these viruses despite intensive investigation.[55] Preliminary reports of increased prevalence of antibody to HTLV-I in the serum of hemophiliacs have not been confirmed with more specific tests.

C. Low Virus Titer in the Plasma

Many viruses, while present in the blood, are present at such a low titer that transmission is unlikely when pooled into a large volume of noninfective plasma. Again, it is to be noted that any of the transmissible agents such as hepatitis B virus, the delta agent, and parvovirus are present in high concentration. In contrast, low titers of non-A, non-B hepatitis virus, such as 100 to 1000 infectious U/ml, have been reported in carriers as assessed in chimpanzees.[29] No data are available as of this writing on the concentration of HIV in the plasma of infectious donors.

D. Neutralizing Antibody Present in the Pooled Plasma

Pools derived from several thousand different donors are used for the commercial production of plasma products. These pools presumably contain protective antibody to many endemic viruses, and thus the occasional viremic plasma may well be neutralized prior to fractionation. This phenomenon probably explains the decrease in hepatitis B transmission by pooled plasma products after the removal of the detectably HBsAg positive donors, despite the presence of one unit per several thousand which can transmit hepatitis. The increase in the amount of free antibody to hepatitis B surface antigen found in immunoglobulin preparations after the advent of screening and excluding donations positive for the hepatitis B antigen has been reported.[56] This large excess antibody can neutralize the residual infectious virus. Indeed, it has been proposed that the addition of small amounts of antibody to pooled plasma products would ensure more satisfactorily that hepatitis B would not be transmitted.[57,58]

E. Inactivation of the Virus by the Processing Steps

The process of fractionation can reduce the infectivity of viruses by two different mechanisms. The first is by inactivating the viruses which are present. While the methods used for fractionation of therapeutic plasma proteins are ''gentle'', the methods used involving shifts of pH and high concentrations of alcohol, along with drying, are sufficient to inactivate many viruses. Furthermore, the distribution of the residual virus may be predominantly into fractions not used for therapeutic preparations. Unfortunately, factor VIII is made under the most gentle of conditions with little or no alcohol being used, and residual viruses of all types are found in the cryoprecipitate as well as the final factor VIII material.[59-62] In general, about 10% of the virus is precipitated with the cryoprecipitate, and there is a further one log reduction in virus content during freeze drying.

There are few precise data on the effect of alcohol on the specific viruses transmitted by plasma fractions. However, in most studies of the effect of fractionation on added viruses, only a fraction of the added virus is recovered. Pennell[59] recovered only 10% of virus added to plasma prior to fractionation. More recently there are contradictory reports on the effect of alcohol on HIV. The report of Martin et al.[63] indicates that the conditions used for the fractionation of the immune globulins rapidly kill HIV, while other reports[64,65] find little inactivation under these conditions. It is well established that exposure to even 40% alcohol does not prevent the transmission of hepatitis B, and that immune globulin preparations exposed to 25% alcohol transmit non-A, non-B hepatitis.

During the fractionation of plasma by the cold ethanol technique there is a general pattern of viral fractionation. Most of the recoverable virus is found in either fraction 1, the fraction containing fibrinogen, the cryoprecipitate, the starting fraction for the production of factor VIII or in Cohn fraction 3, a waste fraction containing a mixture of alpha and beta globulins. The act of fractionation seems to separate the viruses from the fraction 2, the fraction from which therapeutic immune globulin preparations are derived. Hepatitis B virus is found more in fraction 3 than in other fractions used for therapy, as assessed both by measuring the hepatitis DNA and the presence of the RNA polymerase.[60,61] The retroviruses seem to have a similar distribution during ethanol fractionation of plasma.[62,65] This is in no way to say that these procedures make a product incapable of transmitting viral diseases. All Cohn plasma fractions including albumin and immunoglobulin preparations have been indicated in the transmission of viral diseases. However, in many cases these fractionation procedures may prevent a marginally infected pool from transmitting infection.

F. Host Defense Mechanisms

Host defense mechanisms have been, by default, an explanation for the wide spectrum of sequelae seen after exposure of a population to a given infectious agent. For many years, it has been well established that age was an important determination for both morbidity and mortality after exposure to infectious agents.[66] The age relationship is almost independent of the virus involved with a high mortality during the first few years of life followed by a minimum mortality during early adolescence. This is followed by increased case fatality with further increase in age.

Inherent and acquired differences in the immunologic status of patients may also explain some of the differences in morbidity and mortality from the same infection. The heavily treated hemophiliac has measurable abnormalities of the immune system independent of and preceding exposure to HIV.[67-70] These include increased circulating immune complexes, increased immunoglobulin level, increased T-suppressor cells, and relative anergy to skin test antigens. It is possible that the increased immunoglobulin level is associated with the chronic liver disease seen in hemophiliacs. The presence of increased levels of circulating immune complexes is associated with the use of factor VIII concentrates rather than with single donor cryoprecipitate, and one can speculate that the origin is the infusion of allogeneic

Table 2
DEATHS FROM INFECTIOUS
DISEASES IN U.S. HEMOPHILIACS
(1968—1979)

Hepatitis (8)	Food poisoning (1)
Septicemia (3)	Tuberculosis (1)
Candidiasis (2)	Measles (1)
Unspecified virus (1)	Infectious mononucleosis (1)
Syphilis (1)	Encephalitis (1)

proteins. Similarly, there is no mechanism to explain the increased T-suppressor cells although the concept of "antigen overload" is evoked. The same concept of antigen overload is invoked to explain the blunted response to skin test antigens. These phenomena can be explained by viral infection as well as by the "antigen overload" thesis.

The prior immunologic state has been found to affect the reaction of the hemophiliac to infusion of factor VIII concentrates contaminated with HIV.[70] Those hemophiliacs with an aberrant T-cell ratio were more likely to develop antibodies to HIV after exposure to a lot of infected factor VIII, while those with a normal ratio infused with the same factor VIII preparation were less likely to develop antibody.

G. Inability to Detect Infection in the Recipients

Along with all of the above limitations on viral disease transmission, one must add our inability to detect the pathologic changes produced by infection. With the classic transmissible disease of hepatitis, there is a clear clinical end point, i.e., jaundice, that can easily be associated with blood products. Following the development of the more accurate tests for liver function, such as the ALT, it has become routine to screen blood product recipients or others at risk for the occurrence of increased ALT as an indicator of liver pathology. Similar clinical or laboratory end points are not available for diseases of other organ systems, and therefore we may be missing other types of pathologies induced by viral agents in plasma products, and in particular factor VIII concentrates.

IV. THE IMPACT OF INFECTIOUS AGENTS ON THE HEMOPHILIAC

The classic virus disease was an acute infection from which one either recovered or died. Any long-term sequelae, such as cirrhosis following hepatitis, were considered as residual damage of the acute infection. However, more and more viruses are being discovered which are by nature persistent and with long-term sequelae, as a result of the persistence of the viral genome. These long-term sequelae include organ specific inflammatory changes, such as in liver disease, ultimately resulting in cirrhosis and immunologic paralysis resulting in opportunistic infection. Even malignant diseases including leukemias, lymphomas, hepatocellular carcinoma, and CNS tumors are associated with the presence of persistent viral infection.

Review of 949 hemophiliac deaths in the U.S. from 1968 to 1979 showed that there were a variety of infectious disease deaths listed, as shown in Table 2. The overall occurrence of death from infectious disease was somewhat higher than that for the normal population. The individual infectious diseases noted were not in themselves unusual. Death from acute hepatitis was the leading infectious disease death noted. The other infectious disease deaths listed were unremarkable except for the presence of two deaths stated to be due to candidiasis and one death with a secondary diagnosis of cryptococcosis. While these deaths currently would be considered to be secondary to AIDS, they occurred well before there was any evidence of HIV infection of the U.S. hemophilic population. No deaths were listed under the category of opportunistic infection prior to 1980.

Deaths from pneumonia are surprisingly high. This is listed as the primary cause of death in several patients per year, and as an associated cause in another 5% of patients. In the recent experience in the U.K., the same trend is seen with a substantial number of deaths caused by pneumonia.[1] In most cases no organism is identified.

The malignancies attributed to viral infection include primary hepatocellular carcinoma, T-cell leukemias, lymphomas, and CNS tumors. The death caused by malignancies in the hemophilic population show no unusual frequency of these particular tumors. While no case of Burkitts lymphoma was identified between 1965 and 1979 in the U.S., there has been a published report of one after 1980 in the U.S. and a second report from Japan.

Thus, up until 1979, there was no evidence of unusual or unsuspected infectious diseases in the intensively treated hemophilic populations. However, the era of intensive treatment only commenced in 1970, and long-term outcomes must still be watched. Currently, there is serologic evidence of hepatitis B infection in 90% of heavily treated hemophiliacs, 35% have antibody to the delta agent, and about 80% have HIV antibodies. In one study there was universal evidence of infection with serum parvolike virus.[51] While there is no serologic test for non-A, non-B hepatitis, epidemiologic studies show 100% transmission in carefully studied hemophiliac populations.

Essentially all hemophiliacs heavily treated with any product prepared prior to screening for HBsAg have serologic evidence of infection with hepatitis B.[71] Approximately 5% are chronic HBsAg carriers, and it is the chronic carriers who are at risk for late sequelae of hepatitis B infection including cirrhosis and hepatocellular carcinoma. Many hemophiliacs (30%), also have antibody against the delta agent indicating that at least at one point their infection with hepatitis B could have been exacerbated by this co-infection.[72] However, since 1975, the time when hepatitis B antigen screening was instituted on donor plasma, only one acute hepatitis death has been reported in the U.S. In the U.K., acute hepatitis was listed as the cause of death in 5% of the hemophiliacs dying between 1976 and 1980.[1] The reported deaths were presumably due to either acute fulminant hepatitis or chronic active hepatitis. If one also includes the deaths from cirrhosis, most of which may be a sequelae infection in this group of patients, about 8% have liver disease as either the primary or an associated cause of death. It is probable that the acute hepatitis deaths were caused by hepatitis B, but it is not determined at this time what role the non-A, non-B hepatitis agent would have in chronic liver disease. Some reports have concluded that, in general, chronic hepatitis and liver disease are numerically a negligible cause of death in hemophiliacs.[73]

With the advent of hepatitis B antigen screening of plasma donations, the frequency of contaminated lots was reduced. However, there was still serologic conversion of young hemophiliacs.[74] As of today, all antigen negative patients and those younger patients receiving the hepatitis B vaccine should have no evidence of liver disease as a result of hepatitis B.

While the consequences of infection with hepatitis B virus are well understood, the consequences of infection with non-A, non-B hepatitis are less well understood. Acute non-A, non-B hepatitis infection is characterized by nausea, vomiting, and jaundice in about 15% of infected patients. The case fatality rate has been reported to be as high as 1% in some patient populations. Hemophiliacs around the world have chronically increased levels of ALT, and when liver biopsy is performed there is a high frequency of inflammatory disease in the liver.[75-77] By default, these abnormalities are considered to be due to chronic infection with non-A, non-B hepatitis. It may be that the young hemophiliacs exposed to non-A, non-B hepatitis have less morbidity and mortality over the short term.

The long-term consequences of non-A, non-B hepatitis are under intense study. Hay et al.[75] found that 38% of hemophiliacs who were biopsied because of chronically elevated ALT had signs of chronic active hepatitis or cirrhosis. Another study, while finding a high incidence of histological changes on repeat biopsy, felt there was no progression.[73,76] In recipients of single donor products, Alter[78] found an inconsistent pattern of progression of

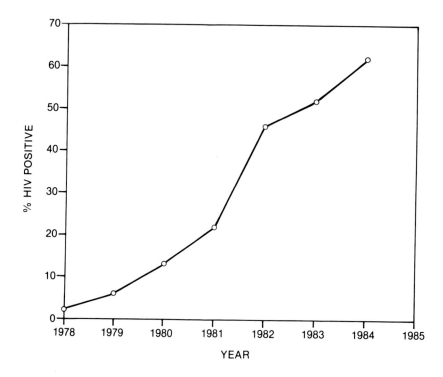

FIGURE 1.   Reported prevalence of antibody (1978—1985) to HIV in hemophiliacs. Data from the U.S. and Europe.

biopsy changes in some patients and regression in others. However, it has also been estimated from these same data that 10% of those infected with non-A, non-B hepatitis will develop cirrhosis. However, the cirrhosis may be milder than that associated with alcoholism, but with a case fatality rate estimated at about 1%.[78]

The new scourge of blood products is infection with HIV. From serologic surveys the first appearance of this virus in the hemophilic population was in 1978.[79] Most of the hemophiliacs developed evidence of exposure to HIV between 1980 and 1983,[80-89] as demonstrated in Figure 1.

The early spread of the virus in the hemophiliac population has been traced to contamination of the source plasma drawn in the U.S. and used as the source of most of the world's supply of factor VIII concentrates. However, even in countries with isolated blood supplies, such as Australia and Scotland, the hemophiliac population was exposed to HIV at almost the same time.[90,91] In January 1982, the first hemophiliac death attributed to AIDS was reported. After almost 2 years of little increase in the reported cases of AIDS in hemophiliacs, there was a dramatic rise of reported cases of AIDS in hemophiliacs in the first half of 1984,[92] as shown in Figure 2. With rare exceptions, the terminal event was infection with pneumocystis carinii. While almost all of the early patients with AIDS were older, severely affected, and intensively treated hemophiliacs, approximately half of the new cases of AIDS in hemophiliacs since the middle of 1984 have occurred in moderately affected and infrequently treated hemophiliacs or in factor V deficient and von Willebrand disease patients.[92] Some of these latter cases have only been treated with single-donor products. In patients treated only with single-donor cryoprecipitate the annual serologic conversion rate to HIV was 18%/year.[86]

The retrospective serologic studies, noted above, indicate that the onset of exposure of the hemophiliacs to HIV began in 1978.[88] By the time the serologic test became available the majority of hemophiliacs throughout the world treated with factor VIII concentrates, as

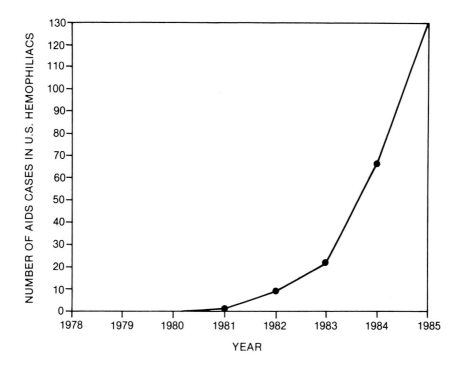

FIGURE 2.   AIDS cases by CDC definition (Centers for Disease Control) in the U.S. hemophiliac population by year.

opposed to single-donor products, were positive for antibody to HIV (60 to 80%). Currently there is no evidence that any of the serologic conversions have been due to passive immunization with infused inactivated virus. Virus can be cultured from the peripheral lymphocytes of approximately 30% of the antibody positive hemophiliacs. Surprisingly even those treated solely with single-donor cryoprecipitate showed an unexpectedly high rate of conversion to seropositivity.[85,86] Patients receiving 2000 factor VIII U/year of cryoprecipitate had an annual seroconversion rate of 20%. This is to be compared with the experience in Scotland where all recipients of material derived solely from Scottish plasma remained seronegative until a single lot was apparently contaminated with HIV.[93]

The long-term consequences of infection with HIV are unknown.[94] Many hemophiliacs have laboratory evidence of abnormal immune function as characterized by high immunoglobulin, low T4/T8 ratios, increased suppressor cells, decreased T-helper lymphocytes, depressed reactivity to cutaneous antigens, etc.[95-102] The general patterns, prior to infection with HIV, is an increased serum immunoglobulin level and increased number of T-suppressor cells. After infection with HIV, i.e., in those patients with antibody to HIV, there is a decrease in the number of T-helper cells. There is some evidence of slow progression of these immunologic changes in some of the hemophiliacs.[95,100]

Some of the antibody positive hemophiliacs progress to the "lymphadenopathy syndrome".[102-107] The frequency of LAD/PGL varies from 5 to 40% in reports from different hemophilia centers. In the report of deShazo et al.,[102] it is the younger hemophiliacs who exhibit the lymphadenopathy syndrome. From the current experience, the attack rate for AIDS in hemophiliacs as of this writing is about 1%. It has been reported that the appearance of the lymphadenopathy syndrome occurs about 10 months after evidence of infection with HIV, but that the appearance of AIDS occurs after 4 years. This is to be contrasted to the incubation period of 2 to 3 years in the documented cases of AIDS transmitted by blood transfusion in adults, and the incubation period of less than a year associated with neonatal transfusion. There are several patients with documented positive serology for more than 6 years with no evidence of clinical disease.[107]

Not only do plasma transmitted diseases impact on the hemophiliac but as with other transmissible diseases it involves the family members. Several reports indicate that the spouses and other household contacts of HIV antibody positive hemophiliacs develop antibodies to HIV.[107,108] One case of vertical transmission of HIV infection has been reported.[109] Similarly hepatitis B is transmitted within households and transmitted vertically to children. While the data on non-A, non-B hepatitis are incomplete, in at least one epidemic in nonhemophiliacs, there was transmission from infected mothers to their infants.[110]

V. VIRAL INACTIVATION METHODOLOGIES

Viral contamination of plasma products was an anticipated adverse effect of production procedures, and methods to limit viral transmission have been investigated since the mid-1940s. There were three traditional approaches. The first was to only accept ''healthy'' donors. This assumed that one could tell which donors were healthy by physical and laboratory examination. The only laboratory test used to detect infectious disease in plasma donors was the serologic test series for syphilis. The second approach was withdrawal of the product from clinical use. This was used when it was discovered that human thrombin transmitted hepatitis. The same approach was used to remove fibrinogen from the market. This approach can only be used if there are other satisfactory options available. Human thrombin was replaced with bovine thrombin, and fibrinogen from pooled plasma was replaced by single-donor cryoprecipitate.[111] The third approach was to use a viral inactivation step: traditionally, heating. Heating albumin solutions at 60°C for 10 h has been used for 40 years to prevent viral transmission. However, most proteins cannot be heated to the degree that albumin can tolerate without adverse effects. Similarly, pooled plasma was stored at room temperature and irradiated with UV light to prevent hepatitis transmission.[112] The introduction of products such as factor VIII and factor IX was done with full knowledge that virus transmission would be a problem, and over the years a variety of methods have been tried to reduce this risk.

A. Donor Screening

The first step to reduce viral transmission by blood and blood products is donor screening. This screening starts with the history and physical examination of the donor. All blood donors with a history of hepatitis, of taking street drugs, more recently of homosexual activity, or any other illness that would indicate a transmissible disease or indeed a negative impact on the donor have been excluded. Unfortunately, self-exclusion of high risk donors such as homosexuals and drug users is of limited success, both in volunteer as well as in commercial blood banks. Both specific and global blood screening tests have been proposed for the removal of potentially infectious plasma units. In general, the global tests lack specificity and sensitivity, i.e., they will screen out some safe donors and allow a number of unsafe donors to be bled. Recent data on screening with the ALT indicate that with very carefully standardized ALT testing about two thirds of the donations transmitting non-A, non-B hepatitis would be excluded.[26] However, the majority of donors who would be excluded would not necessarily have a transmissible disease. While this is a significant advantage to the single blood recipient it is doubtful that it would have much impact on a product from thousands of donors.

In contrast, specific sensitive tests can be of great value. The development of the specific test for hepatitis B has had a major impact on the transmission of hepatitis B in both blood and plasma products.[14] The impact on the pooled products was not expected and probably represents the neutralization of residual virus by excess antibody. The hepatitis B viral load in the current plasma pools is probably 1/10,000 that of pools prior to screening. Fortuitously, this screening procedure also removes those donors who are carriers of the delta agent. The impact of screening plasma for the presence of HIV antibody will not be appreciated for some time. However, with all of its imperfections it will be better than the surrogate tests that have been proposed such as hepatitis core antibody or beta microglobulin. The most urgent need is the development of accurate tests for non-A, non-B hepatitis.

There is a limit to the number of screening tests that can be done on blood donors. At some point the cost effectiveness and yield of positive results and exclusion of healthy donors make this a limited approach. While the standard syphilis test is relatively cheap it can be estimated that tests such as those for hepatitis B and HIV cost $5 U.S. each. If, or when, a test for non-A, non-B hepatitis is developed, this will add further to the cost of blood and plasma therapy.

B. Viral Inactivation Procedures

The next approach is to inactivate the virus contaminants from the individual donations, the plasma pool, or the final product. No satisfactory approach has, as yet, been developed for the removal or inactivation of all types of viruses in the plasma pool, but a variety of approaches have been and are being used on the final products. These methods include the use of fractionation procedures and physical and chemical inactivation methods.

The major difficulties in the development of improved viral inactivation procedures are appropriate test systems with which to validate the viral inactivation methodologies and the development of inactivation procedures which do not denature the plasma proteins. While hepatitis has been and is one of the major problems with plasma products, the test systems are limited to chimpanzee testing. In retrospect, this model is insufficient to evaluate inactivation procedures for non-A, non-B hepatitis. All procedures currently being used for the inactivation of viruses in factor VIII have been shown to prevent transmission to chimpanzees of non-A, non-B hepatitis. However, the clinical data in human subjects do not correlate with the chimpanzee data. No other direct approach is available for the study of hepatitis inactivation except such clinical studies. HIV inactivation has been studied in tissue culture systems utilizing measurements of the products of HIV replication in either peripheral lymphocytes or lymphocyte cell lines. In the absence of adequate test systems for the viruses known to be transmitted, another approach to the study of viral inactivation in plasma products is the use of a panel of ''marker'' viruses of different structure. The desirable properties of a marker virus are stability, ease of measurement, nonpathogenic characterization, and the absence of inhibiting antibodies in human plasma. This method has been used to develop many of the viral inactivation procedures currently used. As clinical data are developed, it will be possible to correlate marker virus kill with clinical outcome.

The removal of infectious agents by fractionation has been discussed previously. In general, the procedures currently in practice for the production of factor VIII result in the elimination of 99% of all viruses studied. Specific steps have been proposed for the elimination of infectious virus. Precipitation with polyethylene glycol has been proposed for the elimination of hepatitis B virus from certain plasma fractions.[113] Unfortunately, this approach would have little impact on the production of factor VIII since the conditions under which hepatitis B and probably other viruses are precipitated are the same conditions which precipitate factor VIII enriched fractions. This procedure has been used for the removal of hepatitis from factor IX concentrates. A novel approach is the use of hydrophobic column chromatography as proposed by Einarsson et al.[114] This technique uses an octanoic hydrazine linked to sepharose to remove viruses. Adsorption and elution conditions for the removal of hepatitis B antigen were elevated first on factor IX concentrates. However, current clinical trials indicate that such material submitted to this procedure has transmitted hepatitis.

A second approach to the physical removal of viruses is the use of immunoadsorbents

Table 3
**VIRAL INACTIVATION PROCEDURES FOR FACTOR VIII CONCENTRATES
AS USED BY DIFFERENT MANUFACTURERS**

Armour
  60°C for 30 h lyophilized
Alpha
  (A) 60°C for 10 h suspended in heptane
  (B) 60°C for 24 h in lyophilized state
Behringwerke
  60°C for 10 h heated in sugar-glycine solution
Cutter
  (A) 68°C for 72 h in lyophilized state
  (B) 60°C for 10 h heated in sugar-glycine solution
Hyland
  60°C for 72 h in lyophilized state
New York Blood Center
  Extraction with *N*-butyl phosphate and Tween®

such as antibody to hepatitis B surface antigen for the selective adsorbtion of a given infectious agent. This procedure has been tested under extreme conditions and seems able to remove some, if not all, of the contaminating hepatitis B virus. In the absence of known antibody for a given virus, this approach has limited feasibility.[115] While there has been substantial development in the field of filtration technology, there are no techniques proposed to use filtration for the removal of viruses.

Physical inactivation of viruses has been the approach commonly used or attempted. For heat inactivation to be successful, some constituent of the virus must be more sensitive than the plasma protein being treated. The heating of albumin is done in the presence of a specific ligand, either caprylate or tryptophanate, which does not stabilize viruses, but substantially increases the temperature of denaturation of the protein. After 10 h at 60°C invariably albumin is almost free of detectable transmissible agents. Recently Shikata et al.[116] demonstrated that this procedure inactivates approximately 10^4 hepatitis B virus. However, the fractionation procedure also removes much of the virus in the starting plasma pool, and essentially it is a combination of the fractionation methodology and heat treatment that contributes to the safety of the final product.

In the last decade, several new approaches to the "pasteurization" of factor VIII have been developed. Recent reports show that factor VIII can be heated for 10 h at 60°C when the protein is stabilized by the addition of high concentrations of sucrose and glycine.[117] Chimpanzee experiments indicate that this procedure kills some hepatitis B virus although the degree of viral kill by the heating process as opposed to the fractionation procedure is unclear. Unfortunately, stabilizers of protein stabilize viruses at the same time and decrease the effectiveness of heat inactivation.[118] Stabilization of virus has been shown by the addition of high citrate concentrations used to prevent heat denaturation of the factor IX complex.[119] The use of high concentration of citrate to stabilize the factor IX also resulted in the stabilization of hepatitis B virus, as shown by both chimpanzee and "marker" virus studies. Another approach to viral inactivation is the heat treatment of dried protein preparations. Lyophilization is a well-established method to stabilize dry proteins, but it also stabilizes viruses. As of this time, most factor VIII is heated by this method. The dry heat methods have been developed utilizing both "marker" viruses and chimpanzee experiments for validation. As of this writing, all methods have been shown to inactivate HIV.[118,120-122]

Table 3 lists the methods currently used to heat treat factor VIII. These methods are variable in their effectiveness in inactivating non-A, non-B hepatitis.[123-127] Colombo et al.[124] reported that Hyland factor VIII heated in the dry state for 72 h at 60°C infused into 13 "virgin" hemophiliacs resulted in evidence of non-A, non-B hepatitis infection in 11 recipients. Two patients who received factor VIII heated in the dry state at 60°C for 30 h developed clinical hepatitis within 3 weeks. No patients developed HIV antibody. However, it now seems that several processes have the capacity to inactivate non-A, non-B hepatitis in most lots of factor VIII.[132-134] Another product heated at 68°C for 72 h has no reported clinical follow-up. The sucrose-glycine method has been reported to be effective in preventing the transmission of non-A, non-B hepatitis. Kernoff et al.[125] reported on the effectiveness of the Alpha heating method for the inactivation of viruses. Multiple lots of this factor VIII concentrate, heated in the presence of heptane, showed that one out of five lots infused transmitted non-A, non-B hepatitis. The one lot transmitting non-A, non-B hepatitis was derived from a pool which was unwittingly derived from a plasma pool with increased ALT levels.

As of this writing, the clinical follow-up of patients receiving viral inactivated factor VIII products has been encouraging in that no patient has been reported to have seroconverted to HIV antibody. None of eight virgin hemophiliacs developed HIV antibodies after receiving Hemofil-T. In contrast, 8 of 29 patients treated with the same quantity of nonactivated product developed antibody to HIV.[135,136] Felding et al.[129] have reported on 46 patients treated with a heated factor VIII without HIV antibody seroconversion. Similarly, Mosseler et al.[131] have reported on 30 patients treated with heat inactivated products, and Kernoff et al.[125] have reported on 18 patients treated with another product without serologic conversion. The number of lots involved is limited in these studies as is the time of follow-up.

The heating procedures currently used are effective to prevent the transmission of HIV, but have variable impact on the transmission of non-A, non-B hepatitis. In none of the reported studies has follow-up reported any cases of hepatitis B infection. No *in vitro* or *in vivo* studies have been conducted to investigate the inactivation of delta agent or the serum parvovirus. While the current procedures are marginally effective against non-A, non-B hepatitis, one can anticipate that in the next few years all products will have improved safety.

Other physical methods are available for viral inactivation in blood products. Early attempts at viral inactivation used UV irradiation.[139] It was only after sufficient irradiation to do substantial damage to the protein that there was evidence of inactivation of hepatitis B. More recently that has been coupled with chemical treatment to inactivate viruses in factor IX. Ionizing radiation such as X-rays kill viruses, but also can damage the protein. No published data exist to establish the usefulness of ionizing radiation to inactivate viruses in plasma products.

There are several chemical agents used for the sterilization of virus vaccines that have been proposed for the sterilization of blood products. The most studies of these is the alkylating agent, beta propiolactone (BPL).[140] More recently it has been proposed to sterilize factor IX complex with BPL in conjunction with UV irradiation[141] and to apply this principle for the sterilization of factor VIII.[142] While no data are available concerning the sterilization of factor VIII, there are substantial data that the factor IX so treated does not transmit hepatitis. *In vitro* studies indicate that it is also effective in inactivating HIV. The production of antigenic derivatives is of concern when using BPL with protein solutions. While much attention has been given to the carcinogenicity of BPL, this material is rapidly hydrolyzed, and there should be no residual BPL in the final product. Naturally, if used without adequate safeguards, BPL would be a hazard within the fractionation plant. The strategy of pretreating the plasma before purifying the factor IX complex seems to be effective in removing neoantigens. Whether this can be a useful procedure for improving the safety of factor VIII is unproven.

A second chemical approach recently developed is the use of lipid solvents to inactivate the viruses in plasma products.[143] With the exception of the parvovirus all pathogenic viruses in plasma thus far described are lipid coated. Classically, inactivation of viruses by ether has been utilized to define the presence of essential lipid. Substantial investigation of mixtures of lipid solvents and detergents is ongoing, and at this time seems to have great promise. The data available thus far are either *in vitro* or chimpanzee studies of hepatitis transmission. In all cases all lipid coated viruses have been inactivated. These include hepatitis B; non-A, non-B hepatitis; and HIV. In the next few years clinical data should be available to verify the effectiveness of this approach. The clinical and laboratory data on viral inactivation are focused on hepatitis B; hepatitis non-A, non-B; and HIV, and no information is available on the effectiveness of currently applied procedures on the delta agent or parvovirus.

The information on viral inactivation of blood products is being rapidly expanded, and the state of the art at this time of writing may change considerably in the near future. The ultimate solution to this very serious problem will likely be a combination of the above strategies, i.e., donor screening, removal, and inactivation of viruses. For a variety of reasons including donor and recipient safety, the screening methods should be improved where possible. As products such as factor VIII become more purified there will be a further reduction in the viral bioburden in the final product. This will, in turn, render the inactivation procedures more effective.

While there are great expectations in the safety of proposed products made by recombinant DNA technology, it must be remembered that many of the cell substrates that will be used will have their own, as yet unidentified, viruses. However, on the more optimistic side, these will be highly purified and current technology and guidelines will control through strict constraints the content of total DNA at a level which will not be infectious.

VI. STRATEGIES FOR PATIENT TREATMENT

There are various strategies available for the treatment of the hemophiliac. Some propose that cryoprecipitate is the safest product to use and that all patients should be treated with single-donor products when possible. The success of this approach ultimately depends on the carrier rate for a given virus. For example, the carrier rate for non-A, non-B hepatitis is so high in the general population that a severe hemophiliac would be exposed to this virus after only a short period of treatment with a single-donor product. Furthermore, if a single-donor plasma product is contaminated, it will contain several hundreds or thousands more viral particles than the pooled product and will not be exposed to inactivating antibodies that may exist in a plasma pool. A contrasting treatment strategy would be the exclusive use of virally inactivated products for the treatment of all hemophiliacs. Since almost all products contain non-A, non-B hepatitis, this implies the exposure of the hemophiliac patients to non-A, non-B hepatitis at every infusion. The neonate immune system and other defense mechanisms are not fully developed, and the impact of infectious diseases under the age of 3 years is associated with greater morbidity and mortality. Since the very young hemophiliac can be treated with small amounts of factor VIII, a rational approach may be to use single-donor cryoprecipitate until the age of 5 years and then to change therapy to the pooled viral inactivated products. This would imply that non-A, non-B hepatitis exposure would take place in a host with a mature defense mechanism.

Not only are the hemophiliacs themselves at risk for viral diseases, but so also are the family contacts. It is well established that there can be spread within a household of hepatitis B and non-A, non-B hepatitis, and possibly HIV. Therefore, it would seem appropriate that the household members are vaccinated against hepatitis B and trained in the appropriate handling of factor VIII concentrates including the disposal of the used infusion equipment.

VII. SUMMARY

The transmission of viruses by plasma products, and in particular factor VIII, has been a long-standing problem. While it would seem that only a limited number and type of viruses are transmitted by factor VIII (hepatitis B; non-A, non-B hepatitis; HIV; delta agent; and parvovirus) there may be others as yet undescribed transmitted by this blood product. The important lesson gained since the emergence of HIV is that new viruses can appear in the blood supply of the world at any time. Of further concern in the transmission of viruses by factor VIII is the state of the host immune system which may have been depressed previously by the presence of circulating immune complexes or by other mechanisms of immune suppression.

In the last 15 years great progress has been made in reducing the risk of hepatitis B to the hemophiliac. The two major changes have been the screening of the plasma for the presence of hepatitis B antigen and the introduction of the vaccine to protect the newly diagnosed and untreated hemophiliac. The impact of the viral inactivating procedures on the transmission of hepatitis B may be a third approach, although by itself the heating steps would probably have little impact on heavily hepatitis B contaminated factor VIII.

The most common disease associated with the infusion of blood products is non-A, non-B hepatitis, as measured by the elevation of the ALT several weeks after infusion into "virgin" patients. It is clear that with nonactivated factor VIII and with most of the viral inactivated products currently on the market, there is still a very substantial risk of non-A, non-B hepatitis. There is strong evidence that there are multiple agents involved, none of which has thus far been identified or characterized. Whether screening of plasma by global nonspecific tests would have an impact on the transmission of this/these agent(s) has not been established.

The impact of AIDS on the hemophiliac population of the world has been large both pathologically and psychologically. The majority of heavily treated hemophiliacs around the world have developed antibodies to HIV. The long-term impact on the majority of the hemophiliacs is yet to be ascertained. Viral inactivation studies *in vitro* indicate that the current inactivation procedures should prevent transmission of the HIV by factor VIII and other plasma products.

The smaller "helper viruses", the delta agent, and the serum parvovirus most probably will not be inactivated by the current procedures. Hopefully, as hepatitis B disappears from the scene, the impact of the delta agent will also wane. As far as is known the serum parvovirus has little long-term impact, although the effect of i.v. exposure could be different than that of household transmission.

In the near future it can be expected that there will be the elimination of the transmission of the viruses associated with known transmission of disease to hemophiliacs. The specter of other unknown viruses will always be present even with products derived from nonhuman cell lines.

REFERENCES

1. **Rizza, C. R. and Spooner, R. J. D.,** Treatment of haemophilia and related disorders in Britain and Northern Ireland during 1976—1980: report on behalf of the directors of haemophilia centres in the United Kingdom, *Br. Med. J.*, 286, 929, 1983.
2. **National Center for Health Statistics,** Vital statistics data 1965—1979.
3. **Levine, P. H.,** Efficacy of self-therapy in hemophilia: a study of 72 patients with hemophilia A and B, *N. Engl. J. Med.*, 291, 1381, 1974.
4. **Rizzeto, M., Purcell, R. H., and Gerin, J.,** Epidemiology of HBV-associated delta agent: geographical distribution of anti-delta and prevalence in polytransfused HBsAg carriers, *Lancet*, 1, 1215, 1980.
5. **Beeson, P. B.,** Jaundice occurring one to four months after transfusion of blood or plasma, *JAMA*, 121, 1332, 1943.
6. **Oliphant, J. W.,** Jaundice following administration of human serum, *Harvey Lecture, N.Y. Acad. Sci.*, 20, 429, 1944.

7. **MacCallum, F. O.,** Homologous serum hepatitis, *Lancet,* 2, 691, 1947.

8. **Oliphant, J. W. and Hollaender, A.,** Homologous serum jaundice: experimental inactivation of etiologic agent in serum by ultraviolet irradiation, *Public Health Rep.,* 61, 598, 1946.

9. **Murray, R., Oliphant, J. W., Tripp, J. T., Hampil, B., Ratner, R., and Diefenbach, W. C. L.,** Effect of ultraviolet radiation on infectivity of icterogenic plasma, *JAMA,* 157, 8, 1955.

10. **Walsh, P. H., Purcell, R. H., Morrow, A., Chancock, C., and Schmidt, P.,** Post transfusion hepatitis after open-heart surgery, *JAMA,* 211, 261, 1970.

11. **Blumberg, B. S., Alter, H. J., and Visnich, S.,** A ''new'' antigen in leukemia sera, *JAMA,* 191, 541, 1965.

12. **Prince, A.,** An antigen detected in the blood during the incubation period of serum hepatitis, *Proc. Natl. Acad. Sci., U.S.A.,* 60, 814, 1968.

13. **Okochi, K., Murakami, S., Ninomiya, K., and Kaneko, M.,** Australia antigen, transfusion and hepatitis, *Vox Sang.,* 18, 289, 1970.

14. **Goldfield, M., Black, H. C., Bill, J., Srihongse, S., and Pizzuti, W.,** The consequences of administering blood pretested for HBsAg by third generation techniques: a progress report, *Am. J. Med. Sci.,* 270, 335, 1975.

15. **Barker, L. F., Chisari, F. F., McGrath, P. P., Dalgard, D. W., Kirschstein, R. L., Almeida, J. D., Edgington, T. S., Sharp, D. G., and Peterson, M. R.,** Transmission of type B hepatitis to chimpanzees, *J. Infect. Dis.,* 127, 648, 1973.

16. **Barker, L. F., Maynard, J. E., Purcell, R. H., Hoofnagle, J. H., Berquist, K. R., London, W. T., Gerety, R. J., and Krushak, D. H.,** Hepatitis B virus infection in chimpanzees: titration of subtypes, *J. Infect. Dis.,* 132, 451, 1975.

17. **Dane, D. S., Cameron, C. H., and Briggs, M.,** Virus-like particles in serum of patients with Australia antigen-associated hepatitis, *Lancet,* 1, 695, 1970.

18. **Hoofnagle, J. H., Gerety, R. J., and Barker, L. F.,** Antibody to hepatitis B core in man, *Lancet,* ii, 869, 1973.

19. **Magnius, L. O. and Espmark, J. A.,** New specificities in Australia antigen positive sera distinct from the LeBouvier specificities, *J. Immunol.,* 109, 1017, 1972.

20. **Sherlock, S. and Thomas, H.,** Treatment of chronic hepatitis due to hepatitis B virus, *Lancet,* ii, 1343, 1985.

21. **Purcell, R. H., Rizzetto, M., and Gerin, J. L.,** Hepatitis delta virus infection of the liver, *Semin. Liver Dis.,* 4, 340, 1984.

22. **Purcell, R. H. and Gerin, J. L.** Experimental transmission of the delta agent to chimpanzees, in *Viral Hepatitis and Delta Infection,* Verme, G., Bonino, F., and Rizzeto, M., Eds., Alan R. Liss, New York, 1983, 79.

23. **Rizzetto, M., Canese, M. G., Arico, S., Crevelli, O., Trepo, C., Bonino, F., and Verme, G.,** Immunofluorescence detection of a new antigen-antibody system (delta/anti-delta/0) associated with hepatitis B virus in liver and serum of HBsAg carriers, *Gut,* 18, 997, 1977.

24. **Prince, A. M., Brotman, B., Grady, G. F., Kuhns, W. J., Hazzi, C., Levine, R. W., and Millian, S. J.,** Long incubation post-transfusion hepatitis without evidence of exposure to hepatitis B virus, *Lancet,* 2, 241, 1974.

25. **Alter, H. J., Holland, P. V., Morrow, A. G., Purcell, R. H., Feinstone, F. M., and Moritsugu, Y.,** Clinical and serologic analysis of transfusion-associated hepatitis, *Lancet,* 2, 838, 1975.

26. **Aach, R. D., Szmuness, W., Moseley, J. W., Hollinger, F. B., Kahn, R. A., Stevens, C., Edwards, V. M., and Werch, J.,** Serum alanine aminotransferase of donors in relation to the risk of non-A, non-B hepatitis in recipients: the transfusion transmitted virus study, *N. Engl. J. Med.,* 304, 989, 1981.

27. **Craske, J., Dilling, N., and Stern, D.,** An outbreak of hepatitis associated with intravenous injection of factor VIII concentrate, *Lancet,* ii, 221, 1975.

28. **Craske, J., Spooner, R. J. D., and Vandervelde, E. M.,** Evidence for existence of at least two types of factor-VIII-associated non-B transfusion hepatitis, *Lancet,* 2, 1051, 1978.

29. **Tabor, E.,** Development and application of the chimpanzee animal model for human non-A, non-B hepatitis, in *Non-A, Non-B Hepatitis,* Gerety, R. J., Ed., Academic Press, New York, 1981, 186.

30. **Tabor, E., Gerety, R. J., Drucker, J. A., Seeff, L. B., Hoofnagle, J. H., Jackson, D. J., April, M., Barker, L. F., and Pineda-Tamondong, G.,** Transmission of non-A, non-B hepatitis from man to chimpanzee, *Lancet,* 1, 463, 1978.

31. **Tabor, E., April, M., Seeff, L., and Gerety, R. J.** Acute non-A, non-B hepatitis: prolonged presence of the infectious agent in the blood, *Gastroenterology,* 76, 680, 1979.

32. **Gerety, R. J.,** Particles and antigen-antibody systems associated with non-A, non-B hepatitis and non-specific tests to detect virus carriers, in *Non-A, Non-B Hepatitis,* Gerety, R. J., Ed., Academic Press, New York, 1981, 207.

33. **Bradley, D. W., Cook, E. H., Maynard, J. E., McCaustland, J. A., Ebert, J. W., Dolana, G. H., Petzel, R. A., Kantor, R. J., Heilbrun, A., Fields, H. A., and Murphy, B. L.,** Experimental infection of chimpanzees with antihemophilic factor (factor VIII) materials: recovery of virus-like particles associated with non-A, non-B hepatitis, *J. Med. Virol.,* 3, 253, 1979.

34. **Jackson, D. J., Tabor, E., and Gerety, R. J.,** Acute non-A, non-B hepatitis: specific ultrastructural alterations in endoplasmic reticulum of infected hepatocytes, *Lancet,* 1, 1249, 1979.

35. **Shimizu, Y. K., Feinstone, S. M., and Purcell, R. H.,** Non-A, non-B hepatitis: ultrastructural evidence for two agents in experimentally infected chimpanzees, *Science,* 205, 197, 1979.

36. **Iwarson, S., Schaff, Z., Norkeans, G., and Gerety, R. J.,** Retrovirus-like particles in hepatocytes of patients with transfusion-acquired non-A, non-B hepatitis, *J. Med. Virol.,* 16, 37, 1985.

37. **Seto, B., Coleman, W. G., Iwarson, S., and Gerety, R. J.,** Detection of reverse transcriptase activity in association with the non-A, non-B hepatitis agent(s), *Lancet,* 2, 941, 1984.

38. **Shirachi, R., Shiraishi, H., Tateda, A., Kikuchi, K., and Ishida, N.,** Hepatitis "C" antigen in non-A, non-B post transfusion hepatitis, *Lancet,* 2, 853, 1978.

39. **Seto, B., and Gerety, R. J.,** A glycoprotein associated with the non-A, non-B hepatitis agent(s): isolation and immunoreactivity, *Proc. Natl. Acad. Sci. U.S.A.,* 82, 4934, 1985.

40. **Melief, C. M. J. and Goudsmit, J.,** Transmission of lymphotropic retroviruses (HTLV-I and LAV/HTLV-III) by blood transfusion and blood products, *Vox Sang.,* 50, 1, 1986.

41. **Vilmer, E., Barre-Sinoussi, F., Rouzioux, C., Gazengel, C., Vezinet-Brun, F., Danguet, C., Fischer, A., Manigne, P., Cherrmann, J. C., Griscelli, C., and Montagnier, L.,** Isolation of a new lymphotropic retrovirus from two siblings with hemophilia B, one with AIDS, *Lancet,* 1, 753, 1984.

42. **Gallo, R. C., and Wong-Staal, F.,** A human T-lymphotropic virus (HTLV-III) as the cause of the acquired immunodeficiency syndrome, *Ann. Int. Med.,* 103, 679, 1985.

43. **Markham, P. D., Salahuddin, S. Z., Popovic, M., Sarngadharan, M. G., and Gallo, R. C.,** Retrovirus infections in man: human T-cell leukemia (lymphotropic) viruses, in *Viral Mechanisms of Immunosuppression,* Gilmore, G. and Wainberg, M. A., Eds., Alan R. Liss, New York, 1985, 49.

44. **Evatt, B. L., Stein, S. F., Francis, D. P., Lawrence, D. N., McLane, M. F., McDougal, J. S., Lee, T. H., Spira, T. J., Cabradilla, C., Mullens, J. I., and Essex, M.,** Antibodies to human T cell leukemia virus-associated membrane antigens in haemophiliacs: evidence for infection before 1980, *Lancet,* ii, 698, 1983.

45. **Kloster, B. E., Tomar, R. H., Stockman, J. A., Lamberson, H. V., Merl, S. A., John, P. A., Groth, D. M., and Poiesz, B. J.,** Antibodies to human T-cell lymphotropic virus-I membrane antigens and inverted T4/T8 ratios in hemophiliacs, *Am. J. Clin. Pathol.,* 83, 450, 1985.

46. **Chorba, T. L., Jason, J. M., Ramsey, R. B., et al.,** HTLV-I antibody status in hemophilia patients treated with factor concentrates prepared from U.S. plasma sources and in hemophilia patients with AIDS, *Thromb. Haemost.,* 53, 180, 1985.

47. **Goudsmit, J., Miedma, F., Breederveld, C., Terpstra, F., Roos, M., Schellekens, P., and Melief, C.,** Antibodies to the human T-cell lymphoma/leukemia virus type-I in Dutch haemophiliacs, *Vox Sang.,* 50, 12, 1986.

48. **Kalyanaraman, V. S., Narayanan, R., Feorino, P., et al.,** Isolation and characterization of a human T-cell leukemia virus type II from a hemophilia A patient with pancytopenia, *EMBO J.,* 4, 1455, 1985.

49. **Anderson, M.,** The emerging story of a human parvo-virus like agent, *J. Hyg. (London),* 89, 1, 1980.

50. **Anderson, M. J., Davis, L. R., Hodgson, J., Jones, S. E., Murtaza, L., Pattison, J. R., Stroud, C. E., and White, J. M.,** Occurrence of infection with a parvovirus-like agent in children with sickle cell anemia during a two-year period, *J. Clin. Pathol.,* 35, 744, 1982.

51. **Mortimer, P. P., Luban, N. L. C., Kelleher, J. F., and Cohen, B. J.,** Transmission of serum parvolike virus by clotting factor concentrates, *Lancet,* 2, 482, 1983.

52. **McVerry, B. A., Ross, M. G. R., Knowles, W. A., and Voke, J.,** Viral exposure and abnormal liver function in haemophilia, *J. Clin. Pathol.,* 32, 377, 1979.

53. **Cheeseman, S. H., Sullivan, J. L., Brettler, D. B., and Levine, P. H.,** Analysis of cytomegalovirus and Epstein-Barr virus antibody responses in treated hemophiliacs: implications for the study of acquired immune deficiency syndrome, *JAMA,* 252, 83, 1984.

54. **Gerety, R. J., Eyster, M. E., Tabor, E., Drucker, J. A., Lusch, C. J., Prager, D., Rice, S. A., and Bowman, H. S.,** Hepatitis B virus, hepatitis A virus and persistently elevated aminotransferases in hemophiliacs, *J. Med. Virol.,* 6, 111, 1980.

55. **Okochi, K., Sato, H., and Hinuma, Y.,** A retrospective study on transmission of adult T-cell leukemia virus by blood transfusions: seroconversion in recipients, *Vox Sang.,* 46, 245, 1984.

56. **Smallwood, L. and Gerety, R. J.,** Hepatitis B immune globulin and immune serum globulin antibody levels, *N. Engl. J. Med.,* 303, 5290, 1980.

57. **Tabor, E., Aronson, D. L., and Gerety, R. J.,** Removal of hepatitis B infectivity from factor IX complex by hepatitis B immune globulin, *Lancet,* 2, 68, 1980.

58. **Brummelhuis, H. G. J., Over, J., Duivis-Vorst, C. C., Wilson-deSturler, L. A., Ates, G., Hoek, P. J., and Reerink-Brongers, E. E.,** Contribution to the optimal use of blood. IX. Elimination of hepatitis B transmission by (potentially) infectious plasma derivatives, *Vox Sang.,* 45, 205, 1983.

59. **Pennell, R. B.,** The distribution of certain viruses in the fractionation of plasma, in *Hepatitis Frontiers,* Hartmann, F. W., LoGrippo, G., Mateer, J. G., and Barron, J., Eds., Little, Brown, Boston, 1957, 297.

60. **Trepo, C., Hantz, O., Jacquier, M. F., Nemoz, G., Cappel, R., and Trepo, D.,** Different fates of hepatitis B markers during plasma fractionation. A clue to the infectivity of blood derivatives, *Vox Sang.,* 35, 143, 1978.

61. **Shih, J., Cheung, H. N., Holland, P. V., and Gerety, R. J.,** Distribution of hepatitis B surface antigen (HBsAg) and/or specific hepatitis B virus (HBV) DNA in fractions derived from HBsAg positive plasma, *Gastroenterology,* 84, 1397, 1983.

62. **Levy, J. A., Mitra, G., and Mozen, M.,** Recovery and inactivation of infectious retroviruses from factor VIII concentrate, *Lancet,* ii, 722, 1984.

63. **Martin, L. S., McDougal, J. S., and Loskoski, S. L.,** Disinfection and inactivation of the human T-lymphotropic virus type III/lymphadenopathy associated virus, *J. Infect. Dis.,* 152, 400, 1985.

64. **Prince, A. M., Piet, M. P. J., and Horowitz, B.,** Effect of Cohn fractionation conditions on infectivity of the AIDS virus, *N. Engl. J. Med.,* 314, 386, 1986.

65. **Wells, M. A., Wittek, A. E., Epstein, J. S., Marcus-Sekura, C., Daniel, S., Tankersley, D. L., Preston, M. S., and Quinnan, G. V.,** Inactivation and partitioning of human T-lymphotropic virus, type III, during ethanol fractionation of plasma, *Transfusion,* in press.

66. **Burnet, F. M.,** The pattern of disease in childhood, *Australas. Ann. Med.,* 1, 93, 1952.

67. **Tsoukas, C., Gervais, F., Shuster, J., Gold, P., O'Shaugnessy, M., and Robert-Guroff, M.,** Association of HTLV-III antibodies and cellular immune status of hemophiliacs, *N. Engl. J. Med.,* 311, 1514, 1984.

68. **Kaplan, J., Sarnaik, S., and Levy, J.,** Transfusion induced immunologic abnormalities not related to AIDS virus, *N. Engl. J. Med.,* 313, 1227, 1985.

69. **Gjerset, G. F., Martin, P. J., Counts, R. B., Fost, L. D., and Hansen, J. A.,** Immunologic status of hemophilia patients treated with cryoprecipitate or lyophilized concentrate, *Blood,* 64, 715, 1984.

70. **Ludlam, C. A., Carr, R., Veitch, S. E., and Steel, C. M.,** Disordered immune function in haemophiliacs not exposed to commercial factor VIII, *Lancet,* 1, 1226, 1983.

71. **Gerety, R. J. and Eyster, M. E.,** Hepatitis among hemophiliacs, in *Non-A, Non-B Hepatitis,* Gerety, R. J., Ed., Academic Press, New York, 1981, 97.

72. **Rosina, F., Saracco, G., and Rizzetto, M.,** Risk of post-transfusion infection with the hepatitis delta virus. A multicenter study, *N. Engl. J. Med.,* 312, 1488, 1985.

73. **Mannucci, P. M. and Colombo, M.,** Liver Disease in hemophilia, *Lancet,* 2, 774, 1985.

74. **Gomperts, E. D., Lazerson, J., Berg, D., Lockhart, D., and Sergis-Deavenport, E.,** Hepatocellular enzyme patterns and hepatitis B virus exposure in multitransfused young and very young hemophilia patients, *Am. J. Hematol.,* 11, 55, 1981.

75. **Hay, C. R. M., Preston, F. E., Triger, D. R., and Underwood, J. C.,** Progressive liver disease in haemophiliac: an understated problem?, *Lancet,* 1, 1495, 1985.

76. **Mannucci, P. M., Colombo, M., and Rizzetto, M.,** Non-progressive course of non-A, non-B chronic hepatitis in multitransfused hemophiliacs, *Blood,* 60, 655, 1982.

77. **Preston, F. E., Triger, D. R., Underwood, J. C. E., Bardhan, G., Mitchell, V. E., Stewart, R. M., and Blackburn, E. K.,** Percutaneous liver biopsy and chronic liver disease in haemophiliacs, *Lancet,* ii, 592, 1978.

78. **Alter, H. J.,** Posttransfusion hepatitis: clinical features, risk and donor testing in *Infection, Immunity and Blood Transfusion,* Dodd, R. Y. and Barker, L. F., Eds., Alan R. Liss, New York, 1985, 47.

79. **Evatt, B. L., Gomperts, E. D., McDougal, J. S., and Ramsey, R. B.,** Coincidental appearance of LAV/HTLV-III antibodies in hemophiliacs and the onset of the AIDS epidemic, *N. Engl. J. Med.,* 312, 483, 1985.

80. **Eyster, M. E., Goedert, J. J., Sarngadharan, M. G., Weiss, S. H., Gallo, R. C., and Blattner, W. A.,** Development and early natural history of HTLV-III antibodies in persons with hemophilia, *JAMA,* 253, 2219, 1985.

81. **Hall, S. E., Hows, J. M., Wosley, A. M., and Luzzatto, L., Chu, A. C., Meachan, R., Morris, J., Cheinsong-Popov, R., Weiss, R. A., and Tedder, R.,** Seroconversion of human T-cell lymphotropic virus III (HTLV-III) in patients with haemophilia: a longitudinal study, *Br. Med. J.,* 290, 1705, 1985.

82. **Madhok, R., Melbye, M., Lowe, G. D. O., Forbes, C. D., Froebel, K. S., Bodner, A. J., and Biggar, R. J.,** HTLV-III antibody in sequential plasma samples from haemophiliacs 1974—1984, *Lancet,* i, 524, 1985.

83. **Machin, S. J., McVerry, B. A., Cheinsong-Popov, R., and Tedder, R. S.,** Seroconversion for HTLV-III since 1980 in British haemophiliacs, *Lancet,* i, 336, 1985.

84. **Gurtler, L. G., Wernicke, D., Eberle, J., Zoulek, G., Deinhardt, F., and Schramm, W.,** Increase in prevalence of anti-HTLV-III in haemophiliacs, *Lancet,* ii, 1275, 1984.

85. **Kerper, M. A., Kaminsky, L. S., and Levy, J. A.,** Differential prevalence of antibody to AIDS-associated retrovirus in haemophiliacs treated with factor VIII concentrate versus cryoprecipitate: recovery of infectious virus, *Lancet,* i, 275, 1985.

86. **Gjerset, G. F., McGrady, G., Counts, R. B., Martin, P. J., Jason, J., Kennedy, S., Evatt, B., and Hansen, J. A.,** Human lymphadenopathy-associated virus antibodies and T-cells in hemophiliacs treated with cryoprecipitate or concentrate, *Blood,* 66, 718, 1985.

87. **Moffat, E. H., Bloom, A. L., and Mortimer, P. P.,** HTLV-III antibody status and immunological abnormalities in haemophilic patients, *Lancet,* 1, 935, 1985.

88. **Gomperts, E. D., Feorino, P., Evatt, B. L., Warfield, D., Miller, R., and McDougal, J. S.,** LAV/ HTLV-III presence in peripheral blood lymphocytes of seropositive young hemophiliacs, *Blood,* 65, 1549, 1985.

89. **Mathez, D., Leibovitch, J., Sultan, Y., and Maisonneuve, P.,** LAV/HTLV-III seroconversion and disease in hemophiliacs treated in France, *Lancet,* i, 118, 1986.

90. **Rickard, K. A., Joshua, D. E., Campbell, J., Wearne, A., Hodgson, J., and Kroninberg, H.,** Absence of AIDS in hemophiliacs in Australia treated from an entirely voluntary blood system, *Lancet,* 2, 50, 1983.

91. **McGrath, K. M., Thomas, K. B., Herrington, R. W., Turner, P. J., Taylor, L., Ekert, H., Schiff, P., and Gust, I. D.,** Use of heat-treated concentrates in patients with haemophilia and a high exposure of HTLV-III, *Med. J. Aust.,* 143, 11, 1985.

92. Changing patterns of acquired immunodeficiency syndrome in hemophilia patients—United States, *Morbidity Mortality Weekly Rep.,* 34, 241, 1985.

93. **Ludlam, C. A., Tucker, J., Steel, C. M., Tedder, R. S., Cheingsong-Popov, R., Weiss, R. A., McClelland, D. B., Phillip, I., and Prescott, R. J.,** Human T-lymphotropic virus type III (HTLV-III) infection in seronegative haemophiliacs after transfusion of factor VIII, *Lancet,* ii, 233, 1985.

94. **Francis, D. P., Jaffe, H. W., Fultz, P. N., Getchell, J. P., McDougal, J. S., and Feprino, P. M.,** The natural history of infection with the lympadenopathy-associated virus/human T-lymphotropic virus type III, *Ann. Int. Med.,* 103, 719, 1985.

95. **Jason, J., Hilgartner, M., Holman, R. C., Dixon, G., Spira, T. J., Aledort, L., and Evatt, B.,** Immune status of blood product recipients, *JAMA,* 253, 1140, 1985.

96. **Ceuppens, J., Vermylen, J., Colaert, J., Desmyter, J., Gautama, K., Stevens, E. A. L., Vanham, G., Vermylen, C., and Verstraete, M.,** Immunological alterations in haemophiliacs treated with lyophilized factor VIII cryoprecipitate from volunteer blood donors, *Thromb. Haemost.,* 51, 207, 1984.

97. **Counts, R. B. and Hansen, J. A.,** T-cell subsets in hemophilia, *N. Engl. J. Med.,* 308, 1292, 1983.

98. **Jason, J., McDougal, J. S., Holman, R. C., Stein, S. F., Lawrence, D. N., Nicholson, J. K., Dixon, G., Doxey, M., and Evatt, B. L.,** Human T-lymphotropic retrovirus type III/lymphadenopathy-associated virus antibody. Association with hemophiliacs' immune status and blood component usage, *JAMA,* 253, 3409, 1985.

99. **Gill, J. C., Wheeler, D., Menitove, J. E., Aster, R. H., and Montgomery, R. R.,** Persistence and progression of immunologic abnormalities in haemophilia, *Thromb. Haemost.,* 53, 328, 1985.

100. **Brettler, D. B., Forsberg, A. D., Brewster, F., Sullivan, J. L., and Levine, P. H.,** Delayed cutaneous hypersensitivity reactions in hemophiliacs treated with factor concentrate, *Am. J. Med.,* in press.

101. AIDS-Hemophilia French Study Group, Immunologic and virologic status of multitransfused patients: role of type and origin of blood products, *Blood,* 66, 896, 1985.

102. **deShazo, R. D., Daul, C. B., Andes, W. A., and Bozelka, B. E.,** A longitudinal immunologic evaluation of hemophiliac patients, *Blood,* 66, 993, 1985.

103. **Jones, P., Hamilton, P. G., Bird, G., Fearns, M., Oxley, A., Tedder, R., Cheingsong-Popov, R., and Codd, A.,** AIDS and haemophilia: morbidity and mortality in a well defined population, *Br. Med. J.,* 291, 695, 1985.

104. **Johnson, R. E., Lawrence, D. N. A., Evatt, B. L., Bregman, D. J., Zyla, L. D., Curran, J. W., Aledort, L. M., Eyster, M. E., Brownstein, P., and Carman, C. J.,** Acquired immunodeficiency syndrome among patients attending haemophilia treatment centers and mortality experience of hemophiliacs in the United States, *Am. J. Epidemiol.,* 121, 797, 1985.

105. **Bloom, A. L., Forbes, C. D., and Rizza, C. R.,** HTLV-III, haemophilia and blood transfusion, *Br. Med. J.,* 290, 1901, 1985.

106. **Lawrence, D. N., Jason, J. M., Bouhasin, J. D., McDougal, J. S., Knutsen, A. P., Evatt, B. L., and Joist, J. H.,** HTLV-III antibody status of spouses and household contacts assisting in home infusion of hemophilia patients, *Blood,* 66, 703, 1985.

107. **Ragni, M. V., Tegtmeier, G. E., Levy, J. A., Kaminsky, L. S., Lewis, J. H., Spero, J. A., Bontempo, F. A., Handwerk-Leber, C., Bayer, W. L., Zimmerman, D. H., and Britz, J. A.,** AIDS retrovirus antibodies in hemophiliacs treated with factor VIII or factor IX concentrates, cryoprecipitate or fresh frozen plasma: prevalence, seroconversion rate and clinical correlation, *Blood,* 67, 592, 1986.

108. **Kreiss, J. K., Kitchen, L. W., Prince, H. E., Kasper, C. K., and Essex, M.,** Antibody to human t-lymphotropis virus type III in wives of hemophiliacs. Evidence for heterosexual transmission, *Ann. Int. Med.,* 102, 623, 1985.

109. **Ragni, M. V., Urbach, A. H., Kiernan, S., Stambouli, J., Cohen, B., Rabin, B. S., Winkelstein, A., Gartner, J. C. et al.,** Acquired immunodeficiency syndrome in the child of a hemophiliac, *Lancet,* i, 133, 1985.

110. **Renger, F., Porst, H., Frank, K. H., Kunze, D., and Hinkel, G. K.,** Ergebnisse zur Epidemiologie, Klinic, Immunologie und Morphologie der non-A/non-B Hepatitis, *Z. Aerztl. Forbild.,* 75, 894, 1981.

111. **Bove, J. R.,** Fibrinogen—is the risk worth the benefit?, *Transfusion,* 18, 129, 1978.

112. **Aach, R. and Aronson, D. L.,** Association of serum hepatitis with one lot of dried irradiated pooled plasma, *JAMA,* 193, 17, 1965.

113. **Johnson, A. J. and Newman, J.,** Removal or concentration of hepatitis-associated antigen (HAA) from human plasma fractions, *Fed. Proc. Fed. Am. Soc. Exp. Biol.,* 31, 654, 1972.

114. **Einarsson, M., Kaplan, L., Nordenfelt, E., and Miller, E.,** Removal of hepatitis B virus from a concentrate of coagulation factors II, VII, IX and X by hydrophobic chromatography, *J. Virol. Methods,* 3, 213, 1981.

115. **Charm, S. and Wong, B. L.,** An immunoadsorbent process for removing hepatitis antigen from blood and plasma, *Biotechnol. Bioeng.,* 16, 593, 1974.

116. **Shikata, T., Karasawa, T., Abe, K., Takahashi, T., Mayumi, M., and Oda, T.,** Incomplete inactivation of hepatitis B virus after heat treatment at 60 C for 10 hours, *J. Infect. Dis.,* 138, 242, 1978.

117. **Heimburger, N., Schwinn, H., Gratz, P., Luben, G., Kumpe, G., and Herchenhan, B.,** Faktor VIII-Konzentrat, Hochgereinigt und in Losung Erhitzt, *Arzneim. Forsch: Drug Res.,* 31, 619, 1981.

118. **Menache, D. and Aronson, D. L.,** Measures to inactivate viral contaminants of pooled plasma products, in *Infection, Immunity and Blood Transfusion,* Dodds, R., and Barker, L., Eds., Alan R. Liss, New York, 1985, 407.

119. **Horowitz, B., Wiebe, M. E., Lippin, A., van der Sande, J., and Stryker, M. H.,** Inactivation of viruses in labile blood derivatives. II. Physical methods, *Transfusion,* 25, 523, 1986.

120. **Levy, J. A., Mitra, G. A., Wong, M. F., and Mozem, M. M.,** Inactivation by wet and dry heat of AIDS-associated retroviruses during factor VIII purification from plasma, *Lancet,* i, 1985, 1456.

121. **McDougal, J. S., Martin, L. S., Cort, S. P., Mozen, M. M., Heldebrant, C. M., and Evatt, B. L.,** Thermal inactivation of the acquired immunodeficiency syndrome virus, human T-lymphotropic virus-III/lymphadenopathy-associated virus, with special reference to antihemophilic factor, *J. Clin. Inv.,* 76, 875, 1985.

122. **Heldebrant, C. M., Gomperts, E. D., Kasper, C. K., McDougal, J. S., Friedman, A. E., Huang, D. S., et al.,** Evaluation of two viral inactivation methods in the preparation of safer factor VIII and factor IX concentrates, *Transfusion,* 25, 510, 1985.

123. **Mannucci, P. M., Colombo, M., and Rodeghiero, F.,** Non-A, non-B hepatitis after factor VIII concentrate treated by heating and chloroform, *Lancet,* ii, 1013, 1985.

124. **Colombo, M., Mannucci, P. M., and Carnelli, V.,** Transmission of non-A, non-B hepatitis by a heat treated factor VIII concentrate, *Lancet,* ii, 1, 1985.

125. **Kernoff, P. B. A., Miller, E. J., Savidge, G. F., Machin, S. J., Dewar, M. S., and Preston, F. E.,** Wet heating for safer factor VIII concentrate?, *Lancet,* ii, 721, 1985.

126. **Preston, F. E., Hay, C. R. M., Dewar, M. S., Greaves, M., and Triger, D. R.,** Non-A, non-B hepatitis and heat-treated factor VIII concentrates, *Lancet,* ii, 213, 1985.

127. **Mannucci, P. M., Gringeri, A., and Ammassari, M.,** Antibodies to AIDS and heated factor VIII, *Lancet,* i, 1505, 1985.

128. **Rouzioux, C., Charamet, S., Montagnier, L., Carnelli, V., Rolland, G., and Mannucci, P. M.,** Absence of antibodies to AIDS virus in hemophiliacs treated with heat treated factor VIII concentrate, *Lancet,* ii, 271, 1985.

129. **Felding, P., Nilsson, I. M., Hansson, B. G., and Biberfeld, G.,** Absence of antibodies to LAV/HTLV-III in hemophiliacs treated with heat-treated factor VIII concentrate of American origin, *Lancet,* 2, 832, 1985.

130. **Mosseler, J., Schimpf, K., Auerswald, G., Bayer, H., Schneider, J., and Hunsman, G.,** Inability of pasteurised factor VIII preparations to induce antibodies to HTLV-III after long-term treatment, *Lancet,* i, 1111, 1985.

131. **Oliphant, J. W. and Hollaender, A.,** Homologous serum jaundice: experimental inactivation of the etiologic agent in serum by ultraviolet irradiation, *Public Health Rep.,* 61, 598, 1946.

132. **LoGrippo, G. A. and Hayashi, H.,** Efficacy of betaprone with ultraviolet irradiation of hepatitis B antigen in human plasma pools, *Henry Ford Hosp. Med.,* 21, 181, 1973.

133. **Stephan, W. and Prince, A. M.,** Efficacy of combined treatment of factor IX complex (PPSB) with beta-propiolactone and ultraviolet (UV) irradiation, *Hemostasis,* 10, 67, 1981.

134. **Stephan, W., Prince, A. M., and Kotitscheke, R.,** Factor VIII concentrate from cold sterilized human plasma, *Dev. Biol. Stand.,* 54, 491, 1981.
135. **Prince, A. M., Horowitz, B., Brotman, B., Huima, T., Richardson, L., and van den Ende, M. C.,** Inactivation of hepatitis B and Hutchinson strain of non-A, non-B hepatitis viruses by exposure to Tween 80 and ether, *Vox Sang.,* 46, 36, 1984.
136. **Horowitz, B., Wiebe, M. E., Lippin, A., and Stryker, M. H.,** Inactivation of viruses in labile blood derivatives. I. Disruption of lipid-enveloped viruses by tri (n-butyl) phosphate detergent combinations, *Transfusion,* 25, 516, 1986.

APPENDIX

NOMENCLATURE AND ABBREVIATIONS

Factor VIII/von Willebrand Factor:
  (Bimolecular complex) — VIII/vWf
Factor VIII:
  (Native protein) — VIII
  (Recombinant protein) — rVIII
Factor VIII:
  (Procoagulant activity) — VIII:C
  One-stage clotting method — $VIII:C_1$
  Two-stage clotting method — $VIII:C_2$
  Amidolytic methods (one and two stages) — $VIII:Am_1$ and $VIII:Am_2$
Factor VIII:
  (Antigen) — VIII:Ag
von Willebrand Factor:
  (Protein) — vWf
von Willebrand factor:
  (Functional activity)
  Ristocetin cofactor — vWf:RCo
  Botrocetin activity — vWf botrocetin activity
von Willebrand factor:
  (Antigen) — vWf:Ag
von Willebrand's Disease — vWD
  Subtypes of vWD expressed by Roman numerals with alphabetical subclassification

Amino acids — aa
Complementary DNA — cDNA
Fibrinogen — Fg
Fibronectin — Fn
Kilo basepairs — (K)bp
Molecular weight (kilodaltons) — kDa
Nucleotides — ntd
Thymidine kinase — TK
Vaccinia virus — vv
Wild type — WT

INDEX

A

A1-domain, 8, 89—90
A2-domain, 8, 89—90
A23187 ionophore, 175, 179, 180
A3-domain, 89—90
Acetic acid, 100, 137
N-Acetyl galactosamine (GalNAc), 45, 48, 56
N-Acetyl glucosamine (GlcNAc), 48, 52, 56, 69, 71, 191
N-Acetyl neuraminic acid, 48
Acquired autoimmune deficiency syndrome (AIDS), 296, 298, 304—305, 311—312, 317
Acrylamide gels, 50
Activation, see also specific activators
　II, 112
　VII, 112
　VIII, 2, 4, 6—7, 11—19, 102, 109—112, 118, 202, 216—220
　VIII:C, 15, 242—243
　IX, 112
　IXa, 100
　X, 98—99, 102, 112, 219—221
　cold/surface, 99, 117, 119
　prothrombin, 18
Acutin, 116
Adenine, 34, 85
Adenosine
　deaminase (ADA) gene, 28
　diphosphate (ADP), 149—151, 157, 187, 189, 192—194, 218, 241
Adenylate cyclase, 188
Adhesion, platelet, to damaged subendothelium, 28, 41, 61—65, 68, 72, 78, 84, 129—130, 132, 148—155, 158, 163, 174, 182, 187, 192, 237, 257, 260
A-domains, 8—10, 28—29
Adrenaline, 239
Adsorption chromatography
　aluminum hydroxide, 4, 43, 97, 99, 102, 104—108, 110, 119
　aminohexyl sepharose, 4
　on gold granules, 62
Adsorption index, 104
Affinity chromatography, 1, 4, 43—44, 55, 258—260, 271—272
Afibrinogenemia, 192
Agarose electrophoresis systems, 16, 45, 50, 57—59, 115, 136—137, 158—160, 238—239, 244—247, 250, 262, 265—267
Agglutination, platelet, ristocetin-induced, 41, 61—63, 67—68, 189—191
Aggregation, platelet, 63, 130—133, 141, 147, 150—154, 157—159, 161—165, 187, 189, 191—194, 202—206, 220, 237, 242, 260
Agmatine-Sepharose, 44, 266
Agonists, vWf interaction with platelet membrane and, 187—194, see also specific agonists

AIDS, see Acquired autoimmune deficiency syndrome
AL-7 T-cell hybridoma cell line, 28
Alanine, 13, 43, 46—47, 51, 86, 91, 242, 302—304, 308—309, 312, 317
Albumin, 26, 49, 131, 218, 270, 297, 302, 307, 312, 314
Alcohol, 307
Alcoholism, 310
Aldehyde groups, 69
Alditols, oligosaccharide, 55
Alkaline borohydride, 51
Alkane-derivatized Sepharose, 44
Alkylation, 10, 53, 63, 65, 136, 156—157
Alkyl-guanidinium groups, 264
Alloantibodies, human, 147
Allosteric sites, 232
Aluminum hydroxide adsorption, 4, 43, 97, 99, 102, 104—108, 110, 119, 265, 269, 292
Alpha heating method, for viral inactivation, 315
Amidolytic assays, 97—124, 325, see also specific assays
Amino acids, 5, 7—13, 27, 32, 34, 45—47, 50, 53, 56—57, 60—61, 65—66, 72, 84—88, 90—91, 147—148, 154, 157, 158, 179, 262, 283, 297, 325, see also specific amino acids
Amino alkane-derived matrices, 257, 263—264, 295
Amino ethyl-Sepharose chromatography, 44
Aminohexyl (AH) sepharose adsorption chromatography, 4, 44, 263—264, 266—268, 295
Aminoglycoside antibiotics, 265
Ammonium sulfate precipitation, 4, 43, 152, 243—244, 267
Amphipathic matrices, 272
Anergy, relative, to skin test antigens, 307
Anhydrous hydrazine, 51
Anicteric conditions, 303
Animal VIII, 1, 6
Anion exchangers, 262—263, 266, 295
Antagonists, Vitamin K, 115
Antibiotics, 265, see also specific antibiotics
Antibodies
　"anti-", 85
　anti-VIII, 1, 4, 34, 221—222
　anti-VIII/vWf, 173, 228
　anti-hepatitis B, 303, 313
　anti-HIV, 305, 309, 311—313, 315, 317
　anti-light chain, 35
　anti-vWf, 1, 3, 43, 57—59, 135—138, 140—141
　biotinylated, 138, 140
　hemophilic, 227—231
　monoclonal, 147, 191, 201
　　4Fg, 161
　　9, 152, 161
　　21-42, 161
　　202 D3, 152, 161
　　203, 155
　　211-A6, 64

anti-VIII, 4, 17—18, 28, 31, 35, 227—229
anti-VIII:Ag, 227, 232—233
anti-VIII/vWf, 230, 295
anti-IX, 17—18
anti-GPIb, 63—64, 70
anti-GpIIb/IIIa, 63, 66, 70, 192
anti-vWf, 3—4, 44, 61—62, 64—65, 68, 84, 134,
    136, 147—148, 150—154, 156, 160—161,
    163—164, 203—204
anti-vWf:AgII, 91
assays of, 129, 136
B2A, 160
B7, 160
B23, 151, 153, 160
B200, 67
B205, 67
CAG-1 175A7, 29
CLB-RAg 1, 160
CLB-RAg 7, 160
CLB-RAg 20, 160
CLB RAg 21, 67, 160
CLB RAg 34, 68
CLB RAg 35, 64—65, 68, 150—152, 155—156,
    160
CLB-RAg 36, 160
CLB-RAg 201, 151—153, 155, 160
D7, 160
ESvWF 1, 160
ESvWF 5, 151, 160
F4, 160
H9, 65—66, 151, 169
RFF VIII:R1, 64, 136, 150—152, 160—161
RFF-VIII:R2, 64, 136, 160—161, 164
RG21, 65
RPA 21-43, 227, 229, 231—232
in vWd diagnosis, 147, 161—165
W1-2, 153
W1-8, 153
WM2C9, 227—229, 231
neutralizing, present in pooled plasma, 301, 306
polyclonal, 27, 201
    anti-VIII, 17
    anti-VIII/vWf, 295
    anti-IX, 17
    anti-vWf, 3, 84—85, 134, 136
primary unlabeled, 138
quinine/quinidine-dependent, 190
vWf function unaffected by, 147, 154—155
Anticoagulants, oral, 97, 99, 109, 115—118, 241,
    261, 269, 279, 281, see also specific
    anticoagulants
Antigenic determinants, 115, 134, 201, 227, 261
Antigenicity tests, 34
Antigenic sites, 32, 34
Antigen overload, 308
Antihemophilic factor, VIII, 2, 28, 42, 302
α1-Antiplasmin, 241
Antiproteases, 243
Antithrombin III, 100, 114
α1-Antitrypsin, 112, 242
Aorta, 174, 219

Apheresis, 281
APTT assay, 29, 97, 100—102, 106, 124
Arabinogalactan, 131
Arachidonic acid, 189
Arginine, 12—13, 17, 32, 46, 51, 54, 66, 85—87, 90,
    93, 155, 157, 191, 193
Arginyl bonds, 51, 115, 240
Arterial thrombosis, 202
Arteries, 174, 203
Aryl-sulfatase, 202
Ascites, 228
Asialoglycoproteins, 70—71
Asialo-vWf, 69—71, 187, 190—191, 193—194
Asparagine, 7, 13, 28, 46, 51, 66, 158, 192, 194
Aspartic acid, 86, 90
Aspirin, 131
Assays
    amidolytic, 97—124
    APTT, 29, 97, 101—102, 106
    chromogenic substrate, 98—99, 101—102, 107,
        111, 117, 122, 136, 138, 237
    clotting, 98, 100, 119, 121—124
    collagen binding, 129, 134
    ELISA, 129, 134, 136, 141, 162, 237, 266
    immunoradiometric (IRMAs), 122, 129, 134, 158,
        161—165, 177
    mixed, 227—234
    like with like, 112, 117
    monoclonal antibody, 129, 136
    multiple point, 123
    photometric, 100
    quantitative, 129, 134—136
    single site fluid phase, 135
    three-points dose response, 101
    transient expression, 27
    tritiated peptide, 115
    two site solid phase, 135
Asymmetry, vWf, 59
ATIII, 104
ATG codon, 34
Atherosclerosis, 201
Atomic absorption spectroscopy, 9, 262
Autocatalysis, 115
Autologous, 36, 131—132
Automated rate analyzers, 98
Autoprothrombin, 116
Autoradiography, 58, 137—139, 141, 244—247, 249
Autosomal inheritance, 130, 159—160
Avidin-biotin-peroxidase complex, 138, 140

B

B1-domain, 89—90
B2-domain, 89—90
Back-translation, 26
Bacteria, gene expression in, 27
Bacterial, 27, 99, 116
Bacteriophages, vWf:cDNA inserts and, 84—85
Balb/C mice, immunization of with VIII/vWf
    complex, 228
Ball of yarn structures, 59—60

Bank, cDNA, 27

Barbazole, 138

Barium sulfate, 262, 269

Batch-wise binding experiments, 267, 293

BclI, 34

B-domain, 8, 11, 28—29, 32—34, 88

Bentonite, 43, 295

Bernard-Soulier syndrome, 70, 132, 149, 188—190, 192

BgIII, 91

BHK 21 cell line, 29—31, 34—35

Bile salts, 105

Bilirubin, 302

Bimolecular complex, between VIII and IXa, 17

Biocentrifugal analyzers, 102

Biochemical characterization, of VIII, 1—2, 5—11

Biogel A15M gel filtration, 4, 45

Biotechnology
  basic principles of, 25
  of VIII, 25—36

Bleeding
  diathesis, autosomally inherited, 130
  time, 62, 129—141, 147, 153, 261, 280, 290

Blood
  banking practice, regional, VIII in, 279—286
  -borne viruses, transmission of, 289—290, 296—298, 302
  cells, 237
  clotting, 1, 12, 17—19, 215
  donors, 280—281, 285, 296—297, 302, 304—305
  perfusion systems, 191—192
  product contamination, 26
  transfusion, collection of source material for, 44, 279—286, 302, 304—305
  whole, 281

Bloodbags, plastic, 281, 283

Bonds, see specific bonds

Bone marrow, 36, 201, 207—208

Botrocetin, 133—134, 190, 239, 325

Bovine
  VIII, 6, 14, 262—263
  VIII/vWf, 10
  IXa, 98, 117
  X, 98, 116—117, 119
  Xa, 215
  aortic endothelial cell surface, 218
  papilloma virus (BPV), 28
  plasma, 4
  serum albumin (BSA), 31, 35, 227, 270
  vWf, 190, 193

BPV, see Bovine, papilloma virus

5-Bromodeoxyuridine, 29

Burkitt's lymphoma, 309

Burns, severe, 123

N-Butyl phosphate, 314

C

C1-domain, 89—90

C2-domain, 89—90

Cadmium, 269

Calcium, 2, 9, 19, 100—101, 114, 183, 201, 215, 217, 219—221, 228, 231—233, 281
  -activated protease CAP, 245
  bridges, 19
  chelators, 245
  chloride, 31, 35, 43—44, 227—228, 230, 263—271, 281, 294—295
  cytoplasmic, 175
  ion, 3, 7—8, 16, 33, 101—104, 131, 190, 192—193, 215, 237, 241—243, 259—262, 266, 269, 281, 283
  as variable in amidolytic assay of VIII, 97, 102—104

Calibration curves, amidolytic assay, 121

Cancer, widespread, 123

Candidiasis, 308

Capillaries, 173, 202

Caprylate, 314

Carbohydrate, 179, 189, 240, 259, 297
  VIII and, 1, 5, 7, 10—11
  moiety, vWf, 41—42, 45, 48, 62, 68—72, 115
  processing, 181

Carbon, platinum, 49

γ-Carboxy glutamic acid, 216

γ-Carboxylation, 27

Carboxymethylation, vWf, 50

bis-(Carboxymethyl amino) agarose beads, 269

Carcinogens, 315, see also specific agents

Carcinoma, hepatocellular, 308—309

Carrier states, viral, 303, 306

Cascade, clotting, 14—15, 61, 84, 98, 119, 221, 281

Casein, 229

Catalase, 179, 202

Catalysis, 101, 117, 119

Catalytic efficiency, 18

Cations
  divalent, 3, 8—9, 33, 188—190, 261
  exchange, 266—267
  metal, VIII/vWf interaction with, 257, 261—262, 269

C-domains, 7—8, 10, 28, 88

Celite, 265

Cell lines, 28, 31, 34—35, 313, see also specific cell lines

Cell(s), 306, see also specific cell lines
  attachment sites, 90, 157
  proteases, interaction of with VIII and vWf, 237—250
  transfected, 36

Central nervous system (CNS) tumors, 308—309

Central twofold symmetry axis, 58

Centrifugation, 42, 124, 228, 282, 294
  density gradient, 175, 177—178
  discontinuous albumin gradient, 218
  sucrose density gradient, 6, 10

Cephalin flocculation, 302

Ceruloplasmin, 1, 9—10, 28, 269

Chaotropic reagents, 44, 269

Chelate affinity matrices, 269—270

Chelation, 7, 9, 245, 261, 295

Chemical composition, of vWf, 45

Chimpanzees, non-A-non-B hepatitis in, 297, 303—304, 313—314, 316
Chinese hamster ovary (CHO) cells, 182
Chloramine T method, 229
p-Chloromercuribenzoic acid, 10
Chloronaphthol, 138
CHO, see Chinese hamster ovary cells
CHO DHFR⁻ cells, 28
Chromatography, 228, 262, 296
   adsorption, 4, 43, 62, 97, 99, 102, 104—108, 110, 119
   affinity, 1, 4, 43—44, 55, 258—260, 271—272
   aminohexyl-Sepharose, 4, 44, 263—264, 266—268, 295
   controlled pore glass (CPG), 284—286, 293, 295
   discontinous, 296
   gas-liquid, 51
   high performance liquid (HPLC), 1, 4, 6, 8, 43
   hydrophobic column, 313
   ion exchange, 43, 257, 262—263, 272
   salt gradient elution column, 267
   size exclusion, 44
Chromogenic Factor VIII Kit, 119
Chromogenic substrate assays, 98—99, 101—102, 107, 111, 117, 122, 136, 138, 237
Chromosomal vWf gene, 83, 91—92, 174
Chromosome 5, 91
α-Chromotrypsin, 116
Chromozyn-TH, 101
Chylomicrons, 43, 45, 259
Chymotrypsin, 64, 220, 242—243, 248
CIE, see Crossed immunoelectrophoresis
CIG, see Cold insoluble globulin
Circulating immune complexes, 307, 317
Circulation, 241, 243
Cirrhosis, of liver, 303, 308—310
Cisternae, Golgi, 180, 207
Citrate, 42, 101, 131, 261, 263, 265—266, 268—270, 281—283
Citric acid, 100—101
Clean venipuncture, 228
Clearance, delayed, 247
Cleavage, proteolytic, 5—8, 12—17, 28, 32—34, 50, 54, 59—61, 65—66, 86, 92—93, 100—102, 131, 147—148, 154—157, 174, 179—180, 190—191, 220—221, 233, 237, 241—243, 246—248
Cloning, 25—26, 28—30, 83—85, 147, 295, see also specific clones
Clostridium perfringens, neuraminidase from, 70
Clot-end-point method, 98
Clotting
   assays, 1, 10, 16—19, 98, 116, 119, 121—124
   cascade, 14—15, 61, 84, 98, 119, 221, 281
   factors, 17, 215—223, 237, 242—243, 261, 264, 269
   intravascular, 123
   proteases, 15
   proteins, 4—5
CMV, see Cytomegalovirus
CNBr-coupling method, 265
CNS, see Central nervous system tumors

Coagglutinin, 133
Coagulation venom, 190
Coatest factor VIII kit, 97, 99—100, 102, 104—105, 107—108, 117—123
Cochromatography, 261
Codons, 27, 34, 85, see also specific codons
Cohn fractions, 260, 262, 282, 307
Coil regions, 55, 57
Cold ethanol technique, 307
Cold insoluble globulin (CIG), 283—284
Cold precipitation, fibronectin removal by, 289, 293
Cold/surface activation, 99, 117, 119
Collagen, 149, 173—174, 188—189, 192—193, 218, 272
   binding, 41, 63—64, 67—68, 72, 129, 130, 134, 150—151, 154—157, 160, 194, 260
   site, 147, 154—156
   fibrillar, 71, 134
   type I, 67, 70, 84, 134, 148, 150, 153
   type II, 84, 150
   type III, 148, 153
Columns
   anti-VII monoclonal antibody, 4
   anti-vWf monoclonal antibody, 4
   gel filtration, 3
   glass bead, 147, 238
   hydrophobic, 313
   IMAC, 269—270
   lectin insolubilized, 11
   molecular sieving, 49
   Mono-Q, 8
   Sephacryl 300, 243
   Sephadex, 4, 45, 228
   Sepharose, 44—45, 55, 59, 228, 263—264, 271, 313
Competition binding studies, with anti-vWf MAbs, 152
ConA, see Concanavalin A
Concanavalin A (ConA), 43, 45, 55, 69, 272
Conception, 114
Congenitally deficient patients, clotting in, 102
Contamination
   blood product, 25—26
   fibrinogen, 4
   HIV, 35
   Ig, 261
   protease, 248
   viral, 291, 293, 295—296
   vWf, 4, 45
Contraceptives, oral, 108
Controlled pore glass (CPG) chromatography, 285—286, 293, 295
Coomassie blue stain, 49—50, 68—69, 244
Coordination complexes, copper, 9
Copolymerization, 268
Copper, 1, 8—9, 270
Core antigen, 303
COS-7 cells, 29, 34
CPG, see Controlled pore glass chromatography
Crossed immunoelectrophoresis (CIE), 49, 129, 134, 136—137, 238—240, 243—245, 247—248
Cross-linkage, 49

Cryoglobulins, 280, 282
Cryoprecipitation, 1—4, 42—44, 61—62, 69, 124,
    134—135, 228, 230, 232, 247—248, 260,
    262, 265—267, 269—270, 280, 282—286,
    290, 295—298, 302, 307
  large-scale, 289, 291—292
  single-donor, 310—312, 316
  washing bulk, 289, 292
Cryoproteins, 291
Cryptococcosis, 308
Crystallization, water, 282
C-terminal region
  VIII/vWf, 202
  IXa, 18
  X, 116
  B-domain, 10
  vWf, 5, 51—52, 54, 57, 65, 68, 80, 84—85, 90,
      147—149, 155, 157, 190—191, 193
  vWf:AgII, 91
Cutaneous antigens, 311
Cycloheximide, 174—175
Cysteine, 7, 10, 13, 45—47, 51—52, 54, 56—57, 60,
    85, 87, 89—90, 148—149
Cytomegalovirus (CMV), 305—306
Cytoplasmic, 176, 207, 210
Cytosol, 179

D

D1-domain, 90
D2-domain, 90
D3-domain, 90
D4-domain, 90
o-Dansidine, 138
Dansyl, 16, 69
DDAVP, see 1-Desamino-8-D-arginine-vasopressin
DEAE, 262—263
Decarboxylation, 99
Decay reaction, first-order, 16
Default pathways, 173
Deletions, specific, 32
Delipidation, VIII/vWf, 55
Delta agent, 302—303, 305—306, 309, 315, 317
Demarcation membrane, megakaryocyte, 207
Denaturation, 44, 49, 258
Dense bodies, 201
Density gradient centrifugation, 174, 177—178
Depolymerization, vWf, 71
1-Desamino-8-D-arginine-vasopressin (DDAVP), 90,
    120, 123—124, 139, 141, 239, 281
des-Gla proteins, 115—118
Desialylation, 70
Determinants
  antigenic, 134, 201, 227, 261
  of viral transmission by plasma products, 301,
      306—308
Dextran sulfate, 4, 44, 264—267
DFP, see Diisopropylfluorophosphate
DHFR, see Dihydrofolate reductase
Diafiltration, 293
Dialysis, 241
Diaminobenzidine, 138, 140
Dianoalkane, derivatized, 44

Diathesis, autosomally inherited bleeding, 130
Diazotation reaction, 98, 101
Dictyostelium sp., 8
Digitonin, 204
Dihydrofolate reductase (DHFR) gene, for Chinese
    hamster ovary, 28
Diisopropyl-fluorophosphate (DFP), 16, 242—243,
    245, 249
Dimers, vWf, 66, 84—85, 92, 147—150, 155, 179—
    180, 271
Dimethylaminopropylamide (DMAPI), 3, 268
Direct transformation absorbance, 102
Discontinuous albumin gradient centrifugation, 218,
    296
Disseminated intravascular coagulation, 243—245,
    246, 248
Dissociation, see also specific dissociating agents
  VIII, 1, 3, 41, 44, 217, 227, 229
  VIII/vWf, 228, 295
  constant (K_D), of IXa for phospholipid, 18
  vWf, 217
Disulfide bonds, 1, 4—5, 7, 10, 54, 60, 85, 147, 181,
    190, 201—202, 259, 271
Dithiothreitol (DTT), 10, 49, 63, 271
Divalent cations, 3, 8—9, 33, 188—190, 261
DMAPI, see Dimethylaminopropylamide
DNA
  blotted chromosomal, 91
  complementary (cDNA), 29, 181, 237, 325
    VIII, 5, 10, 25—26, 28—29, 34, 72, 121, 215
    bacterial fusion protein, 27
    bank, 27
    B-region, 33
    Escherichia coli, 27
    human kidney library, 28
    isolation, 26
    library, construction of, 26
    rVIII, 29—30, 121
    recombinant technology, 32, 294, 298, 307
    sequencing, 52
    single-stranded (ss), 305
    viral, 303, 316
    vWf, 60—61, 83, 85—88, 91, 179
  exons, 8
Domains, see also specific domains
  globular, 148—149, 157
  homologies among, 88—89
  vWf organization in, 41, 54—57, 64—68
Donor(s)
  screening, 281, 285, 296—297, 301—305, 312—
      313, 316—317
  transient viremic state in, 301, 306
Double reciprocal recombination, 30
Drug users, 312
DTT, see Dithiothreitol
Duplication, of precursor vWf protein, 93
Dye front, low relative molecular weight peptides in,
    17

E

E5 low charge polyelectrolyte, 3
E100 high charge polyelectrolyte, 3

e-antigen, 303
Ear lobe, bleeding time measured following incision
    made in, 130
EB, see Epstein-Barr virus
ECTEOLA-cellulose, 262
Edman degradation, 50, 87, 91
EGTA, 262
EIA, see Electroimmunoassay
Elastase, 64, 190, 242—243, 246—249
Electroblotting, 138, 140—141
Electroimmunoassay (EIA), 129, 134—135
Electron
    dense markers, 203
    inactivation, 10
    microscopy, 45, 57—59, 71, 148—149, 157, 175,
        201—211, 304
Electrophoresis, 49, 68, 122, 134—136, 138, 262
    crossed, 129, 136—137
    disc, 49—50
    flat-bed system, 137
    high voltage, 51, 55
    SDS-agarose, 69, 259
    SDS-PAGE, 5—7, 9—11, 14—15, 31, 57—59, 85,
        92, 147, 155, 160—161, 179—180, 237—
        240, 243, 245—246, 248—249
    two-dimensional, 129, 136—137
Electrophoretic mobility, 49—50, 262
Electrostatic interactions, 147, 217, 268
β-Elimination, 51, 55
ELISA, see Enzyme-linked immunoadsorbent assays
Ellagic acid, 101
Elution gradients, lithium chloride, 8—9
Encephalitis, 308
Endocardium, 202
Endocytosis, 181
Endoglycosidases, 11, 42, 71
Endonucleases, restriction, 84
Endoperoxide analogue, 189
Endoplasmic reticulum, 92, 174, 178, 179, 271
Endothelial cells
    VIII surface-binding, 219—220
    IX binding to, 99
    X binding to, 99
    ds cDNA synthesized from, 84—85
    protein C synthesis in, 241
    vWf synthesis in, 42, 59—60, 62, 71, 115, 130—
        131, 147—149, 156, 173—179, 181, 183,
        188, 192, 201—204, 209, 215, 219, 221,
        237—238, 243, 248, 260, 271
    Weibel-Palade bodies in, 204
Endothelium, rabbit aortic, platelet adhesion to, 68
End-point technique, 100—101
Enzyme-linked immunoadsorbent assays (ELISA),
    129, 134, 136, 141, 162, 238, 266
Enzymes, 84, 115—116, 178, 215, 237, 244—248,
    see also specific enzymes
Epitope(s), 136, 150, 157, 161—162, 191
    VIII, 242
    anti-vWF monoclonal antibody, 61, 66, 147, 155—
        157, 161
    mapping studies, 17, 32, 34

Epstein-Barr (EB) virus, 305—306
Escherichia coli, cDNA, 27
Esters, phorbol, 174—177
Ethanol, 3, 42—43, 292, 294, 307
Ether, 3
Ethylene, 3, 4, 7, 131, 228, 230, 233, 245, 261, 268
N-Ethylmaleimide, 10, 65
Euglobin, 240
Exocytosis, 175
Exoglycosidases, 11
Exons, 8, 29, 84
Expression, gene, basic principles of, 25—30
Extracellular virus, instability of, 301, 306

F

F 1-0 therapeutic fraction, 42
Fab, 136, 153, 191
Factor II, 99, 102, 104, 112, 264, 269
Factor IIa, 101—102, 104, 111, 117, 124
Factor V, 14, 16—17, 28, 241
Factor VII, 99, 102, 104—105, 112, 114, 117, 119
Factor VIII, 1—2, 5, 11, 15, 18—19, 41—44, 89, 98,
        101—102, 106, 111, 114, 119—120, 160,
        181, 227, 229, 237, 240—241, 290, 293—
        296, 304—305, 307—308, 312, 314—317,
        325
    activated, 1, 4, 7—8, 11—19, 102, 109—110, 112,
        118, 215—219
    amidolytic method, 97—124
        one stage (VIII:AM$_1$), 103, 106—109, 113—114,
            116—118, 120—122, 124
        two stage (VIII:AM$_2$), 106—109, 112—114,
            116—121, 124
    antigen (VIII:Ag), 227—233, 237—240, 242—
        247, 266—267, 325
    biotechnology of, 25—36
    cell protease interaction with, 237—250
    clotting method, 116, 325
    concentrates
        advances in production of, 289—298
        freeze-dried, 289—290
        high purity, 289, 293—294
        intermediate purity, 289, 292—293
        future developments in production of, 279, 285—
            286
    deficiency states, 120
    gene, 26, 29—30, 147
    genetically defective, 18
    heat-treated, 121
    inactivated, 1, 11, 16—17, 33, 122, 220—221, 313
    inhibition, 97, 99, 121—122, 296
    native, 1, 10
    leukocyte protease interaction with, 237, 243—244
    native, 109, 112, 216, 220
    nonactivated, 1, 16, 18, 123, 219
    plasma, 35, 42, 173, 217
    procoagulant (VIII:C), 2, 10—19, 29, 31—32, 34,
        62, 97—101, 104—105, 108—110, 112, 115,
        117—118, 120—121, 123—124, 141, 149—
        150, 153, 158, 216, 237—240, 242, 248, 259,

261, 263—264, 266, 268—272, 281—286, 290—298, 325
products, virus transmission by, 301—317
protein C interaction with, 237, 242—243
purification, 1—5, 10, 228, 280, 289, 291, 294, 296
recombinant (rVIII), 25—26, 28—32, 35, 99, 121, 325
in regional blood banking practice, 279—286
structure and biochemical characterization of, 1—2, 5—11
surface-bound, 215—223
Factor VIII/IXa complex, 243
Factor VIII/vWF complex, 41—45, 49, 55, 72, 84, 121, 201—202, 227—234, 238, 282, 294—295, 325
Factor-VIII$_t$, 215—216, 218—219, 221
Factor IX, 4, 18, 27, 100, 102, 264, 269, 304, 312—315
Factor IXa, 1, 9, 14—19, 98, 100, 103—105, 114
Factor IXa/VIII complex, 215—218, 220—221
Factor X, 4, 9, 18, 29, 100, 103, 105, 114, 116—117, 119, 218—221, 237, 259, 264, 269
VIII/vWf interaction with, 257, 260
activated, 98—99, 102, 112, 221
immobilized, 257, 271
native, 115
Factor Xa, 1, 13—14, 16—18, 31—33, 97—124, 150, 215—219, 237, 259, see also specific topics
Factor XIa, 100
Factor XII, 269
Fast migrating protein, 243
Fast-thawing, 283
Fecal-oral transmission, of hepatitis, 302
Fetuses, hemophilic plasma from, 121
Fever, 305
FFP, see Fresh-frozen plasma
Fibrin, 100, 218, 239—240, 257, 271
Fibrinogen, 1—4, 42—43, 45, 66, 70, 98, 101, 117, 119, 149, 158, 183, 190—194, 202—206, 208, 240, 242—243, 257, 260, 264—267, 269—270, 282, 286, 289—295, 297—298, 302, 312, 325
Fibrinolytic system, 17, 114
Fibrinopeptide A (FPA), 111, 218
Fibroblast binding protein, 157
Fibronectin, 2—3, 43, 66, 158, 175, 179, 183, 191, 194, 203, 234, 243, 257, 260, 264—267, 270, 282, 286, 289, 291—295, 297—298, 325
Fifth disease, 305
Filaments, folding of, 60
First-order decay reaction, 16
FITC, see Fluorescein isothiocyanate
Flat-bed electrophoretic system, 137
Flocculation, cephalin, 302
Fluorescein isothiocyanate (FITC), 69, 177
Food poisoning, 308
Forearm, volar surface of, 130
Formalin, 62, 133
FPA, see Fibrinopeptide A
Fractionation, plasma, 3, 41—43, 115, 123, 201—

202, 271, 280, 285—286, 289—298, 307, 313
Frameshift, 34
Freeze-drying, 282—285, 290, 292, 296—297, 307
Freeze-thawing, 131, 174
Fresh-frozen plasma (FFP), 290—291
Frictional ratio, 45
Fucose, 48, 55—56
Fusion proteins, bacterial, 27

G

G418 resistance gene, 28
GAGs, see Glycosaminoglycans
Galactose, 11, 48, 55, 69—71, 190
oxidase, 11, 42, 69—70
penultimate, 189
removal of, 10, 60, 70
β-Galactosidase, 11, 27, 42, 70—71, 138
Gamma counting, 228
Gas-liquid chromatography, 51
G-domain, globular, 57—58, 60
Gelatin-Sepharose, 44
Gel filtration, 3—4, 6, 43—45, 49, 55, 59—62, 138, 223, 227—228, 314
Genetic code, degeneracy of, 27
Gene(s), 173, 272
VIII, 2, 5, 147
defective, 36
expression, basic principles of, 25, 27—28
heterologous in mammalian cells, 27
marker, 27—28
promoter, 29—30
therapy, 36
vWf, chromosomal, 83—93, 179
Glandular fever-like disorders, 304
Glanzmann's thrombasthenia, 70, 149, 189
Gla peptide, 99, 116
Glass bead columns, 147, 238
Global amidolytic assays, of VIII based on APPT principles, 97, 101—102
Globulins, 307
Glutamine, 13, 32, 46, 51, 54, 67—68, 85, 91
Glutaraldehyde, 203
Glycans, 41, 45, 51—53, 55—57, 70—72
Glycerol buffer, 131, 263
Glycine, 4, 13, 42—43, 45—47, 51, 66—68, 86, 90—91, 115, 158, 192, 194, 229, 265—266, 293—294, 314—315
Glycocalicin, 153, 191, 194, 271
Glycolipids, sulfated, 45, 260, 265
N-Glycopeptides, 55
Glycoprotein Ib (GP Ib) complex, 63—67, 84, 89, 130, 132—133, 147, 151, 153—156, 192, 260, 262, 265, 271
Glycoprotein IIb/IIIa (GP IIb/IIIa) complex, 41, 66—68, 84, 89—90, 130, 147, 149, 153—157, 160, 181, 188—193, 205, 260—261
Glycoprotein V (GP V) complex, 191
Glycoproteins, 11, 28, 53, 61, 68, 72, 91—92, 130—131, see also specific glycoproteins
Glycosaminoglycans (GAGs), 265

N-Glycosyl peptide, 55
Glycosylation, 84, 92, 147, 174, 179
 N-, 45, 51—52, 56, 61, 71
 O-, 45, 51—52, 72
 sites, 5—6, 8, 11, 27—28, 54, 86—87
Glycoxyl-agarose, 49
Glycylethyl ester, 264, 271
Goat, 140, 177
Gold, colloidal, 62, 203—205
Golgi apparatus, 93, 175—176, 179—181, 184, 188,
 203, 206—208, 271
GP Ib, see Glycoprotein Ib complex
GP IIb/IIIa, see Glycoprotein IIb/IIIa complex
GP V, see Glycoprotein V complex
Granulocyte proteases, 244, 260
Gray platelet syndrome, 201, 208—211
GRnRG protomeric basic units, vWf, 60
Guanidine HCl, 49
Guanidinium, 264
Guanine, 34, 85
Guinea pig megakaryocytes, 187
Gyration, 62

H

Half-cystinyl residues, 51
Half-life, 16, 33, 70, 150, 284
H-chain, X factor, 116
Head-to-tail triplication of domain, 88
Heat treatment, 121, 282—285, 294
HeLa cells, 29, 31
α-Helices, 53—54, 56
Helper viruses, 302, 305, 317
Hemolysis, 105
Hemolytic uremic syndrome, 123
Hemophilia, 280, 283, 285, 296—298, 302, 304—
 307, 309—311, 314—317
 A, 26, 29, 31, 34—36, 42—44, 117, 120—121,
  150, 173, 221—222, 227—231, 237, 241,
  247—248, 284, 289—290
 treater communities, 280
Hemophiliacs, impact of infectious agents on, 301,
 308—312
Hemorrhagic symptoms, 62, 261
Hemostasis
 local, 182
 normal, 237, 247—248
 primary, 61—62, 84, 98, 130—133, 141, 147,
  149—151, 201, 260
Hemostatic plug, 156, 192
Heparin, 43, 65, 102, 104, 249, 265, 267, 281, 283—
 284, 286, 293, 295
Heparinoids, 265
Hepatitis
 B, 27, 284, 294, 296—298, 301—306, 307, 309,
  312—317
 non-A, non-B (NANBH), 296—298, 301—304,
  306—307, 310, 312—317
HepG2 (human hepatoma G2) cells, 29, 31
Hepatocellular carcinoma, 308—309
Hepes buffer, 263
n-Heptane, 297

Heterodimers, 6—7, 15, 17, 180, 182, 259, 261
Heterogeneity, vWf, 59, 71
β-Hexosaminidase, 178
Hexoses, 48, 71
HGT(P) (FMC) agarose, 137, 139
High molecular weight (HMW), 62, 64, 70—71, 131,
 133—138, 231, 239, 246, 247
High performance liquid chromatography (HPLC), 1,
 4, 6, 8, 43
High resolution epitope mapping, 32
High voltage electrophoresis, 51, 55
Hirudin, 15—16, 46, 51
Histidine, 13, 263
HIV, see Human immunodeficiency virus
HMW, see High molecular weight
Homodimers, vWf, 180
Homology, internal, 28, 85, 88—89
Homosexual activity, 305, 312
Homozygous vWD patients, 158
Horizontal incision, 131
Host defense mechanisms, 301, 307—308
HPLC, see High performance liquid chromatography
HPV, see Human parvovirus
HTLV viruses, see specific human T-cell leukemia
 viruses
Human II, 264
Human VIII, 1, 5—6, 10—11, 13—14, 17, 28, 33,
 52, 55—56, 58, 63
Human VIII/vWf, 45
Human IX, 264
Human IXa, 98
Human X, 98, 116, 264
Human Xa, 215
Human alloantibodies, 147
Human arterial subendothelium, 132
Human asialo-vWf, 190, 193
Human cryoprecipitate, 4
Human endothelial cells, 84
Human hepatitis, 303
Human immunodeficiency virus (HIV), 35, 282, 284,
 296—298, 301, 304—317
Human lymphocytes, 157
Human osteosarcoma cells, 157
Human parvovirus (HPV), 305—306
Human plasma, 26, 57, 117, 295, 302
Human plasmin, 241
Human platelets, 4, 11, 193, 201, 203—204
Human polymorphonuclear leukocytes, 242
Human T-cell leukemia virus, 304—306
Human thrombin, 228—229
Human umbilical endothelial cells, 271
Human vWf, 260
Hybridization techniques, 26, 91
Hybridomas, T-cell, 28
Hydrazine, anhydrous, 51
Hydrazinolysis, 51, 55
Hydrogen, 53, 140
Hydrolases, 201
Hydrophilic interactions, 267
Hydrophobic interactions, 60, 147, 264, 267—269,
 295
p-Hydroxymercuribenzene sulfonic acid, 10

C-6 Hydroxymethyl groups, 69
Hypercoagulable states, elevated VIII in, 97, 99, 104, 108—117
Hypotonic glycerol lysis, 131

I

I-2581, 116—117
IEP, see Immunoelectrophoresis
Ig, 201, 257—258, 261—262, 270, 306—307, 311
IgA, 261
IgG, 31, 135, 153, 176, 190, 221, 296
IgM, 261
IMAC columns, 269—270
Imidazole, 227, 263—264, 269—271
Immobilized amino-alkanes, 295
Immobilized fibrin monomer, 257, 271
Immobilized metal chelate affinity matrices, 257, 269—270
Immobilized vWf, 257, 271
Immobilized X, 257, 271
Immulon plastic trays, 227
Immune complex, electrophoresis of unreduced in presence of SDS, 10
Immunizations, deliberate, with vWf, 150
Immunoadsorption, 43, 155, 295, 297, 313—314
Immunochemical aspects, of vWD, 147—165
Immunoelectrophoresis (IEP), 49, 134, 137, 141, 158, 163—165, 238—240, 243—245, 247—248
Immunofluorescence microscopy, 173—174, 176, 181, 202—203, 206, 210
Immunogold staining, 201—205
Immunoimmobilization, 230, 233
Immunoisolation, 44
Immunolocalization, 207
Immunologic paralysis, 308
Immunoprecipitation, 44, 65, 67, 190
Immunoradiometric assays (IRMAs), 122, 135—136, 159, 162—165, 177, 227—234
Inactivation
  V, 16
  VIII, 1, 11, 16—17, 33, 122, 220—221, 313
  VIII:C, 242
  electron, 10
  hepatitis virus, 294
  HIV, 314
  irradiation, 7
  viral, 301, 307, 312—316
Incubation time, 100, 150
Inhibition, 11
  VIII, 97, 99, 121—122, 296
  hemophilia A, 31, 34
  irreversible, 16
  plasmatic, 114
  plasmin, 240
  plasminogen activator, 114
  protease, 59, 71, 104, 296
  protein C, 242
  proteolytic, 16, 100, 248
  thrombin, 100, 119

INR values, 99, 115, 117—118
Insulin, 27, 180
Integrin, 157
Intensifying screens, for autoradiography, 138
Interchain metal ion bridges, 19, 261
Interleukin-1, 99
Intrachain bridges, 10
Intravascular coagulation, disseminated, 123, 243—245, 247, 249
In vitro bleeding time, 129, 131—141
In vivo bleeding time, 129—131
Iodine isotope (^{125}I), 50, 78, 133, 135, 137—138, 148, 227—233, 239, 244—246, 249
Iodoacetate, 10
Ion-exchange chromatography, 43, 257, 262—263, 272
Ionic interactions, 147, 264
Ionizing radiation, 315
IRMAs, see Immunoradiometric assays
Irradiation inactivation, 7
Irreversible inhibitors, 16
Isoagglutinins, 296
Isoelectric focusing, 59, 262
Isolation, cDNA, 26, 46—47, 51
Isoleucine, 13
Isopropanol, 137

J

Jaundice, 302, 308—309

K

Kallikrein, 112, 115
Kidney, 238
Kill, marker virus, 313—314
K_m (kinetic constant), 18, 102, 220
KSCN, 269

L

Lability, VIII, 26
Lactate dehydrogenase, 178
LAD/PGL, see Lymphadenopathy syndrome
Lag phase, 102—104, 111—113, 117, 119, 215—216, 218—219
Lambda HvWf 3 cDNA clone, 51
Lancets, 131
Large pore gels, 57, 137, 294
LCA, see *Lens culinaris* agglutinin-Sepharose
L-chain, factor X, 116
Lectins, 8, 11, 42, 69, 70, 272
Lens culinaris agglutinin (LCA)-Sepharose, 55
Leucine, 13, 46—47, 51, 54, 87
Leukemia, 123, 243, 308—309
Leukocyte(s), 191, 237, 243—244, 249
Leupeptin, 245
Libraries, cDNA, 28
Ligands, 150, 257—272
Light microscopy, 201
Like with like assays, 112, 117

Lipid(s), 45, 49, 105
-coated viruses, 303, 315—316
envelope, 297
transfer, 45
vesicle matrices, VIII/vWf interaction with, 257, 268—269
Lipopolysaccharides, bacterial, 99
Lipoproteins, very low density (VDL), 45
Liposomes, 221
Lithium chloride elution gradient, 8—9, 267
Liver
VIII synthesis in, 147
disease, chronic, 123, 303, 307—309
function tests, 284, 302
hepatocytes, 237
mRNA in, 28
lectin, 70
Longitudinal incision, 130
Low molecular weight (LMW), 135, 137—138, 246, 248, 294
Low resolution gels, electrophoretic, 138
Lowry method, 266
Lymphadenopathy syndrome (LAD/PGL), 304, 311
Lymph nodes, 237
Lymphocytes, 105, 157, 304, 311, 313
Lymphomas, 308—309
Lysine, 13, 46, 51, 67, 85—86, 155, 231, 263—264, 269
Lysosomes, 178, 201, 207
Lysyl bonds, 51, 240

M

α2-Macroglobulin, 240
Macroglobulinemia, 123
Magnesium, 267, 269, 281
Malate dehydrogenase, 178
Maleic anhydride, 3, 268
Malignancies, attributable to viral infection, 308—309
Manganese, 269
Mammalian cells, cDNA ability to express specific biological function in, 27
Manchester Comparative Reagent, 108, 110
Mannose, 45, 48, 55—56, 69, 179
Mannosidase, 11
Marker(s), 27—28, 178, 203, 313—314
Mass spectrometry, 51
Matrices
amino alkane-derivatized, 257, 263—264
immobilized metal chelate affinity, 257, 269—270
lipid vesicle, 257, 268—269
solid, VIII/vWf interaction with, 257—272
sulfated, 257, 264—268
thiol, 257, 271
Matrix-bound ligands, VIII/vWf interaction with, 257—272
MDCK canine kidney cells, 29, 31
Measles, 305, 308
Megakaryocytes, vWf synthesis in, 42, 60, 181, 192, 201—203, 206—209, 260
Membrane bilayer, 105

2-Mercaptoethanol, 4, 10, 49
Mercurials, 10
MES, see 4-Morpholine ethane sulfonic acid
Metal, 257, 261—262, 269—270, 295
Methionine, 13, 27, 32, 45—47, 51, 54, 177, 180
Methionyl fragments, 51
α-Methyl-D-mannoside, 69
Mice, 36, 157, see also individual species
Micelles, 105, 217
Microscopy
electron, 45, 57—59, 71, 149—150, 158, 175, 201—206, 208—209, 304
immunoelectron, 181
immunofluorescence, 173—174, 176, 202
light, 202
Microsomes, 178
Microtiter procedures, 98, 100—101, 124, 228—230
Microtubules, cytoplasmic, 204, 206, 210
Microvascular permeability, 241
Migration, electrophoretic, 60, 63, 122, 134—137, 243
Mitochondria, 179, 205, 207
Modified one stage amidolytic assay, 97, 100
Molecular
cloning
of VIII gene, 2, 5
of vWf, 83—93
of vWf:cDNA, 83—85
sieving columns, 49, 69
weights
of native human VIII activity devoid of vWf, 10
oligomeric, of purified VIII, 6—7
of vWf, 41, 45, 49, 57, 59, 62—64, 70—71
Monensin, 271
Monocytes, peripheral blood, 105
Monomers, 65, 155, 179, 257, 271
Mononucleosis, infectious, 308
Mono-Q column, 8
Monosaccharides, vWf, 52, 72
4-Morpholine ethane sulfonic acid (MES), 263
MRC, 117
Mucopolysaccharides, sulfated, 260
Multimeric sizing techniques, 41, 44, 58—60, 62—64, 70—72, 84, 92, 129, 131, 134, 136—141, 147—148, 155, 157—163, 179, 188—192, 201—202, 207, 240—241, 243, 246, 259, 262, 265, 271
Multiple dose response bioassays, 109, 123
Mumps, 305
Mutagenesis, site-directed, 84
Mutations, single base, 32
Myelomatosis, 123
Myocardial infarction, 123

N

NADPH, 62, 178
NANBH, see Non-A, non-B hepatitis
Narcotics use, 305
Native
VIII, 1, 10, 109, 112, 216, 220
vWf, 49, 50, 63—65, 67, 70, 109, 189, 240

X, 115
Nausea, 309
NBRF Protein Sequence Database, 51
Neoantigens, 315
Neonatal blood transfusion, 311—312
Nephrotic syndrome, 123
Neuraminic acid, 48
Neuraminidase, 11, 42, 56, 69—71, 132
Neutralization inhibitors, 122
para-Nitroaniline (pNA), 98—101, 103, 116—117,
    119
Nitrocellulose membrane, 138—140
NMR, see Nuclear magnetic resonance spectroscopy
Nonactivated VIII, 1, 16, 18, 219
Non-A, non-B hepatitis (NANBH), 296—298, 301—
    304, 306—307, 309—310, 313—317
Noncovalent bonds, 7
Nonlinearity, 101
Nonparallel dose response, 135—136
Nonplasmatic environments, 98
Nonsense codon, 85
Nonthrombogenic surface, 218
Normal cells, electron microscopic studies of vWf
    distribution in, 201
Northern blotting analysis, 173
N-terminal region, 5—6
    VIII/vWf, 202
    -linked carbohydrate sites, 11
    vWf, 50, 53, 57, 60—61, 67—68, 85—87, 147—
        149, 155, 157, 190—191, 193
    vWf:AgII, 91
Nuclear magnetic resonance (NMR) spectroscopy,
    51
Nucleoids, 203—205
Nucleophilic side chains, 10
5′-Nucleotidase, 178
Nucleotides, 29, 33, 83, 85—88, 91, 325, see also
    specific nucleotides

O

Oligomeric molecular weights, of purified VIII, 6—7
Oligomers, plasma vWf, 58
Oligonucleotide probes, 26—28, 84, 91
Oligosaccharides, 51, 54—55, 72, 190
One-stage VIII amidolytic assay (VIIIAm$_1$), 97, 99—
    101, 106—110, 113—114, 116—118, 120—
    122, 123, 163, 229, 325
Open reading frame, 91
Optical densities, amidolytic assay, 121
Oral anticoagulant therapy, VIII amidolytic activity
    in, 97, 99, 115—117
Oral contraceptives, 108
Organelles, 202, see also specific structures
Osamines, 48
Osteosarcoma cells, human, 157
Oxalate, 261
Oxidases, galactose, 11, 69
Oxidation, 11

P

Pancreatic elastase, porcine, 246—247, 249

Pancytopenia, 304
Papilloma virus, bovine (BPV), 28
Paraformaldehyde, 133
Paralysis, immunologic, 308
Parallelism, 101, 109
Paraproteinemia, 261
Partial specific volume, vWf, 45
Partition cells, 59
Parvoviruses, 301, 305—306, 315—317
PAS, see Periodic acid Schiff staining
Pasteurization, VIII, 314
PEG, see Polyethylene glycol
PE matrices, 271—272, 295
Penultimate galactose, 10, 60, 70, 190
Peptidases, signal, 86—87, 90, 92
Peptides, see also specific peptides
    VIII/IXa, 243
    degradation, 115—116
    N-glycosyl, 55
    inactive VIII, 5
    mapping, 187
    RGD-containing, 66
    signal, 34, 61, 174
    vWf, 41, 50—52, 71—72
Perfusion systems, 63, 191—192
Periodic acid Schiff (PAS) staining, 45, 68, 240
Permeability, microvascular, 241
Peroxidase, 85, 136, 138
Peroxisomes, 178, 201, 207
pH, 3, 43—44, 60, 227, 258, 262—264, 266, 268—
    270, 282, 293
Phagocytosis, 242
Phenylalanine, 13, 46—47, 51, 242
Phenyl-methyl-sulfonyl fluoride (PMSF), 93
Phenylthiodantoins, 52
Phorbol myristate acetate (PMA), 174—177
Phosphate, 262
Phosphatidylcholine, 105, 218
Phosphatidylethanolamine, 105, 218, 269
Phosphatidyl inositol, 105
Phosphatidyl serine, 105, 217, 269
Phospholipase C, 112, 259
Phospholipid(s), 45, 98—101, 102—106, 108—109,
    115, 215—221, 237, 242—244
    VIII interaction with, 9, 16, 18—19, 97, 102—108,
        257, 259—260
    negatively charged, 17, 217
    porcine brain, 104, 107, 111
    surface-bound VIII, 215, 218
    tenase complex stabilization and, 268—269
Photometric assays, 100
Placenta phospholipid/factor VIII complex, 112
Plasma
    VII:C, 119, 281—282
    VIII, 1, 3, 6—8, 10—11, 31, 35, 42, 173, 217
    VIII:C, 149—150
    afibrinogenemic, 241, 260
    autologous citrated PRP, 131—132
    bovine, 4
    citrated, 2, 101
    clotting factors, 17
    coagulation products, viruses transmitted by, 301,
        303—305

fibrinogen, 42—43
fibronectin, 3, 43
fractionation, 3, 280, 289—298
fresh-frozen, 280, 282
glycoproteins, 61
hemophilic, 49, 119, 121
human, 26, 57
lipids, 105
low virus titer in, 301, 306
membrane, 178, 182—183, 188, 203—204, 206
platelet-poor (PPP), 243
platelet-rich (PRP), 122, 241, 243—244
pooled, 301, 306, 312—313
porcine, 4
products, determinants of viral transmission by,
    301, 306—308
proteins, 2—3, 5, 84, 90, 100, 130, 282, 297—298,
    302, 305—307, 313, 315—317
thrombin-like activity in, 112, 114
viremic, 306
vWD, 69—70, 134, 136, 147, 161
vWf, 42—45, 50, 58—62, 72, 131, 133, 135, 137,
    147, 157, 161, 163—164, 192, 201, 217
Plasmapheresis, 124, 281
Plasmatic inhibitors, 114
Plasmids, 27—28, 30, 34, 84—85, see also specific
    plasmids
Plasmin, 50, 57, 60, 67, 71, 158, 220, 228, 230, 237,
    239—242, 248
Plasminogen, 84, 114, 240, 243
Platelet(s)
    activation, 201
    adhesion, to damaged subendothelium, 28, 41,
        60—64, 68, 72, 84, 129—130, 132, 147—
        154, 157, 162, 173, 182, 187, 192, 237, 257,
        260
    agglutination, ristocetin-induced, 41, 62—63, 67—
        68, 71, 188—190
    aggregation, 63, 130—133, 141, 147, 150—154,
        156—158, 160—164, 187, 189, 191—194,
        201—206, 221, 237, 241—242, 260
    -derived growth factor, 201
    factor 3, 105
    factor 4, 201
    α-granules, 42, 181, 188, 192, 201—210
    human washed, 11
    membrane, 188—189, 191, 193, 215, 217—219
    plug, 189
    -poor plasma (PPP), 243
    protease, 245
    receptors, 193
    -rich plasma (PRP), 122, 241, 243—244
    segregation, 163—164
    spreading, 148
    thrombasthenic, 70, 147
    washed concentrate, 111, 153
Platinum carbon, 49
Plot transforms, 135
Plug, 156, 189, 192
PMA, see Phorbol myristate acetate
PMN, see Polymorphonuclear leukocytes

PMSF, see Phenyl-methyl-sulfonyl-fluoride
pNA, see *para*-Nitroaniline
Pneumonia, 309
Polyacrylamide gels, 49
Polyadenylation, 84—85
Polybrene, 188—189
Polycations, 133, 188, 268
Polydispersity, vWf, 49—50, 71
Polyelectrolytes, 1, 3, 257, 268, 295, see also specific
    electrolytes
Polyethylene glycol (PEG), 3—4, 43, 135, 266,
    292—294, 313
Polylysine, 188
Polymerization, 174, 180—181, 183, 189, 202
Polymers, vWf, 41, 58—60, 63, 147, 182, 246—247
Polymorphisms, 29, 91
RFLPs, 91—92
Polymorphonuclear (PMN) leukocytes, 242, 245—
    246
Polypeptide(s)
    VIII, 1, 3, 5—9, 14, 19
    VIII:C, 25, 32—35
    heavy chains, 5—6, 8, 10—15, 17, 32—34, 115,
        215, 241
    light chains, 5—6, 8—15, 32—35, 99, 115, 153,
        215, 241
    vWf, 50, 53—56, 60—61, 72, 90, 92, 174, 179
    vWf:AgII, 91
Polysaccharides, sulfated, 260
Polyvinyl pyrrolidone (PVP), 257, 268
Porcine
    VIII, 6, 14, 28, 33, 122
    brain phospholipid, 98, 101, 104, 107, 111
    pancreatic elastase, 246—247, 249
    plasma, 4
    platelets, 201, 204—206, 208—210
    vWD, 210
    vWf, 153
Porters, 30
Posttranslational modifications, 27, 59, 87, 187, see
    also specific modifications
Potassium, 69—70, 267
Pottering, 177
Precipitation, 1, 3, 43—44, 91, 134, 268, 291, 294,
    296—297
    ammonium sulfate, 4, 43, 152, 244—245, 267
    cold, 289, 293
    glycine, 4
    heparin double cold technique, 286
    polyethylene glycol, 4, 257, 268, 313
Precursor proteins, 1, 5, 83, 88—90, 93, see also
    specific proteins
Pregnancy, VIII amidolytic activity in, 97, 99, 108—
    115, 118
Prenatal diagnosis, of hemophilic plasma, 121
Primary structure, of vWf, 41, 50—53
Probes, 26—28, 36, 91
Processing sites, 32
Procoagulants, 2, 25—26, 32—35, 98, 109, 115—
    116, 147, 187, 216—217, 237—238, 240, see
    also specific coagulants

Proline, 13, 46, 51, 85, 87
Promegakaryoblasts, 188
Promoter genes, 27, 29—30, 58—59, 62
β-Propiolactone, 297, 315
Pro-sequences, vWf, 83, 90—91, 147, 149, 179, 182, 187
Protamine sulfate, 188
Protease(s), 29, 115, 157—158, 160, 220, 244, 249
  calcium ion-activated (CAP), 131, 190, 245
  clotting, 15
  contamination, 248
  granulocyte, 243, 260
  inhibition, 59, 71, 104, 296
  platelet, 245
  serine, 93, 215, 245
  Staphylcoccus aureus V8, 51—52, 63—66, 154—155, 190, 265
Proteinases, 92—93
Protein A, 227—228
Protein C
  activated (APC), 1, 13—14, 16—17, 31—33, 104, 112, 114—115, 221—222, 237, 241—243
  HepG2 cell production of, 29
  /protein S complex, 17
  vWf interaction with, 237, 242
Protein M, 102
Protein S, 17
Protein(s), 4—5, 19, 42, 45, 49, 53, 62, 84, 178, 282, see also specific proteins
  copper-binding, 1, 8—9
  denatured, 27
  fast migrating, 243
  fibroblast-binding, 157
  fusion, 27
  hemostatic, 201
  matrix-bound specific, 257, 271
  nucleophilic side chains in, 10
  plasma, 2—3, 5, 84, 90, 100, 130, 282, 297—298, 302, 305—307, 313, 315, 316—317
  precursor, vWf, 83, 88—90, 93
  viral, 305
  vitamin K-dependent, 110, 115, 117, 217, 241, 268
Proteoglycans, 203
Proteolysis, 5—8, 12—17, 26, 28—29, 32—34, 44, 50, 52, 54—55, 59—61, 64—67, 84, 86, 92—93, 100—102, 123, 134, 147—148, 154—157, 174, 179—181, 187, 189—191, 202, 220—222, 237, 240—243, 246—249, 260
Prothrombin, 18, 141, 218, 260, 269, 289, 291—292
Prothrombinase complex, 13—14, 104, 114
Protomers, vWf, 41, 57—60, 148, 154, 157, 202, 271
PRP(RIPA), ristocetin-induced platelet aggregation in, 129, 132, 141, 147, 150, 153, 156, 158, 160, 162
Pseudo-vWD, 132
Pst I, 91
pTG1016, 34
pTG1021, 34
pTG1025, 34
pUC9, 28
Purification

VIII, 1—5, 280, 291
VIII/vWf, 43—44, 72
vWf, 41—44, 50, 57, 62, 68
PVP, see Polyvinyl pyrrolidone
Pyridyl disulphide, 271

Q

QAE, 4, 263
Quadruplication, of precursor vWf protein, 93
Quasi-elastic light scattering, 60, 62
Quaternary amino ethyl-Sepharose, 44
Quick thaw, 284
Quinidine, 190
Quinine, 190

R

Rabbit(s)
  anti-vWf antibodies, 136, 140, 147, 158, 160, 244—246
  arterial endothelium, 68, 132
  half-life of human asialo-vWf in, 70
  liver lectin, 70
  polyclonal human vWf antibodies, 85
Radioimmunoassay (RIA), 129, 135—136, 227
Radioligands, 138
Rapid decay, 238
Rate of heating, 282
R-domain, 57
N-Reacetylation, 55
Rebleeding, 153, 290
Receptors
  fibrinogen, 205
  fibronectin, 157
  GP Ib, 149—150, 153—154, 156, 161—162, 192
  GP IIb/IIIa, 154, 156—157
  platelet, 187, 191—194
  RGD sequence, 182
  surface, 130
  vWf, 65, 187—188, 191—192, 194, 205
Recipients of plasma, inability to detect infection in, 301, 308
Recombinant
  VIII (rVIII), 25—26, 28—32, 35, 99
  IX (rIX), 29
  vaccinia virus, 27, 29—35
Recombination, double reciprocal, 30
Red blood cells, 245
Reduction, 50, 52—53, 60, 63, 65, 68—69, 155—156, see also specific reducing agents
Regional blood banking practice, VIII in, 279—286
Religation, 34
Remixing, of protein chains in presences of Ca^{++}, 8
Renal disease, 123
Repeated freeze-thawing, 131
Replication, viral, 303
Resin thrombin-agarose, 16
Restriction, 84, 91—92
Retraction, vascular endothelial cell, 156
Retroviruses, 282, 301, 304—305, 307, see also

specific viruses
Reverse transcriptase, 29
RGD sequence, 66, 68, 90, 158, 182
RGDS sequence, 90
RGP sequence, 86
RIA, see Radioimmunoassay
Ricinis communis lectin, 69
Ristocetin, 149, 151, 161, 192—193, 265, 271—272
   co-factor (vWf:RCo), 62—63, 67—71, 129, 132—
     134, 162—164, 188—189, 227, 238, 240—
     241, 243, 248, 262, 265, 325
   -dependent tests, 129—133
   -induced
     binding to platelets, 41, 64—66, 129, 133, 187,
       191, 261—262
     platelet agglutination, 41, 61—63, 67—68
     platelet aggregation in PRP(RIPA), 129, 132,
       141, 147, 150, 153, 156, 158, 160, 162
   /vWf interaction with platelet membrane and, 187,
     189—190, 194
RNA
   hepatitis B, 303
   messenger (mRNA)
     VIII:C, 237
     VIII gene, 2
     albumin-encoding, 26
     library of DNA sequences complementary to, 26
     liver, 28
     poly$^+$, 84—85
     processing, 179
     vWf, 85, 91—92, 179
   polymerase, 307
Romanowsky stain, 207
Rubella, 305
RVV, 116

S

S2222, 100, 103, 115, 219
S2238, 112
Saccharose gradients, 45
Saline, 138, 268
Salt gradient elution column chromatography, 267
Scarring, 131
SCCS, see Surface-connected canalicular system
Screening, donor, 301, 312—313, 316—317
SDS-agarose electrophoresis, 69, 259
SDS-PAGE electrophoresis, 5—7, 9—11, 14—15,
   31, 57—59, 85, 92, 147, 155, 160—161,
   179—180, 237—240, 243, 245—246, 248—
   249
Secondary cleavage bond, 115
Secondary opportunistic infections, 304
Secondary structure, of vWf, 41, 53—56
Secretion, vWf, 173—183
Sedimentation, 3, 6—7, 45, 49, 59, 61
Sephacryl 300 column, 243
Sephacryl S400 column, 4, 263
Sephadex G-25 column, 228
Sephadex G200 column, 4, 45
Sepharose columns, 44, 45, 55, 59, 227—228, 263—
   264, 271, 313

Septicemia, 242, 308
Sequanator analyses, 51
Serine, 12—13, 16—17, 32, 46, 51—52, 54, 85—87,
   90—91, 93, 116, 215, 245
Seroconversion, of HIV antibody, 311, 315
Serotonin, 201, 241
Serum, 302—303, 305, 315, 317
Seryl residues, 52
Shear-induced platelet aggregation, 63, 130, 148,
   150, 161, 192
β-Sheets, 53—54, 56
Sialic acid, 10, 69—71, 189—190
Side chains, nucleophilic, 10
Sieving, molecular, 69
Signal peptides, 28, 34, 61, 86—87, 90, 92, 174
Silica, colloidal, 177
Silver stain technique, 31, 34—35, 137
Simplate II, 130
Single site fluid phase assay, 135
Sinusoidal cells, 181
Site-directed mutagenesis, 84
Size exclusion chromatography, 44
Skin test antigens, relative anergy to, 307
Slime molds, 8
Slow decay, 238
Snake venom, 133
Sodium
   acetate, 267
   azide, 227
   bicarbonate, 227
   bromide, 267
   carbohydride, 137
   carbonate, 137
   chloride, 3, 44, 227—228, 230—231, 262—271,
     294—295
   citrate, 227—228, 266
   dodecyl sulfate (SDS), 44, 49, 60, 137
   fluoride, 267
   formate, 267
   periodate, 11
   phosphate, 262
   sulfate, 267
Soft gels, 296
Solid matrices, VIII/vWf interaction with, 257—272
Solid-phase immunoradiometric assays, 161, 227—
   228, 295
Soluble fibrin monomer (SFM), 271
Sonication, 60, 62
Soy bean trypsin inhibitor, 245
SpI, 54, 67
SpII, 51—52, 54, 57, 64, 66—68, 155
SpIII, 51—52, 54, 57, 63—66, 68, 154—155
Spectrophotometry, 98, 102
Spectroscopy, atomic absorption, 9, 55
SphI, 34
Spleen, hepatocytes in, 237
Spreading, platelet, 148
Stabilization, viral, 314
Staphylococcus aureus, V8 protease, 51—52, 57,
   63—66, 154—155, 190, 265
Start codons, 34, 85
Sterilization, terminal, 292

Stokes radii, 6—7, 9, 45, 59—60, 62
Stop codons, 34, 85
Streptavidin-biotinylated peroxidase complex, 140
Streptokinase, 239, 241
Stringency, low, sequence hybridization in
    conditions of, 27
Structure of VIII, 1, 5—11
Structure/function-relationships, of vWf, 41, 61—71
Subcellular fractionation, 201—202
Subcloning, 27
Subendothelium/vWf interaction, 41, 61, 63, 68, 84,
    130—132, 134, 147—151, 153—154, 157,
    162, 173, 183, 187, 192—193, 201, 257, 260,
    271
Subtilisin, 67, 154—155, 190
Succinic acid, 270
Sucrose, 6, 10, 283, 314—315
Sulfated, 257, 260, 264—268
Sulfate, 4, 267
Sulfation, 84, 87, 92
Sulfhydryl groups, 1, 10, 45, 65
Sulfur, 54, 177, 265, 269
Suppressor cells, 307—308, 311
Surface-bound VIII, interaction of with other
    coagulation factors, 215—223
Surface-connected canalicular system (SCCS), 203—
    204, 207—208
Surgery, 284, 291
Syphilis, 308, 312—313

T

T4/T8 ratios, 311
Tannic acid, 42
T-cell(s), 28, 307—309, 311
Temperature control, 100, 282
Template method, bleeding time and, 130
Tenase complexes, 19, 97, 99—100, 102—109,
    112—114, 121, 259—261, 268
Terminal sterilization, 292
Tetramers, vWf, 57, 147
TGA codon, 34
Thaw-siphoning, 282—285, 292
Therapy, gene, 36
Thermolability, 29
Thermolysin, 64, 154—155, 191
Thiol groups, 10, 257, 269, 271
Thioredoxin, 10, 62
Three-dimensional structure of vWf, 41, 53—57
Three-points dose response assay, 101
Threonine, 13, 46, 51—52, 91
Threonyl residues, 52
Thrombasthenia, Glanzmann's, 70, 149, 188—189,
    192
Thrombin, 1, 7, 11—18, 31—32, 63—64, 70, 98—
    99, 102, 106—107, 110, 112, 114, 116—118,
    123—124, 149—151, 153, 157, 173, 175,
    182, 187—188, 190, 192—194, 204, 215—
    220, 227—233, 242, 302, 312
 -agarose resin, 16
 cleavage, 33, 61, 67
 inhibition, 100, 119

-like activity (TLA), 112, 114, 116, 123
Thrombocythemia, 218
Thrombocytopenia, 141, 149
β-Thromboglobulin, 201
Thrombomodulin, 17
Thromboplastin, 100, 105, 141, 241, 261
Thromboquant-APPT, 101
Thrombosis, 26, 160, 201
Thrombospondin, 174—175, 191, 201, 203, 206
Thrombotic thrombocytopenic purpura, 123
Thrombus formation, 147, 150, 192
Thymidine kinase, 30, 325
Thymine, 34
Thymol turbidity, 302
Tissue
    VII/VIIa complexes, 99
    factor (TF), as variable in amidolytic assay of VIII,
        97, 102, 104—109, 117, 119
    grafts, in gene therapy, 36
    -induced Xa generation, 110—111
    -type plasminogen activator (t-PA), 84, 239
Tourniquets, 130
Toxicity, proteolytic inhibitor, 248
Transfection, 27, 36
Transfer lines, 291
Transfusion, blood, 280, 286, 302—305, 311
Trans-Golgi network, 180
Transient, 27, 301, 306
Translation, 179
Trasylol, 228
Tri-*n*-butyl phosphate, 297
Triplets, vWf, 88, 93, 157—158
Tris, 228, 262, 270—271, 283
Trisodium citrate, 266
Tritiated peptide assay, 115
Triton X-100 detergent, 137—138
Trypsin, 57, 60, 62, 64—65, 67, 116, 155—156, 177,
    190, 220
Tryptophan, 13, 27, 45—47, 51
Tryptophanate, 314
Tuberculosis, 308
Tubular structures, 203, 205—206, 208
Turbidity, thymol, 302
Tween, 314
Two-allele polymorphism, 91
Two-chain complexes, 34
Two-dimensional immunoelectrophoresis, 49, 129,
    136—137
Two-site solid phase assay, 135, 160—163, 228,
    231—232
Two-stage VIII amidolytic assay (VIII:Am$_2$), 97,
    100—102, 105—110, 112—114, 116—121,
    123, 325
Tyrosine, 13, 45—47, 51, 57

U

U46619 endoperoxide analogue, 189
UDP-galactosyltransferase, 178
Ultracentrifugation, 45, 49, 59, 62
Ultrafiltration, 291, 293
Ultrastructural analysis, 201

Ultraviolet (UV) radiation, 297, 315
Umbilical veins, endothelial cell, 84—85, 174
Urea, 49, 59, 161, 262
Uremia, 123
Urokinase, 239, 241
UV, see Ultraviolet radiation

V

Vaccination, 296, 309
Vaccinia virus, 27, 29—32, 34—35, 325
Vacuoles, 209
Valine, 13, 46—47, 51, 57, 67, 193
Vancomycin, 132—133, 189, 193
Variables, affecting amidolytic assay of VIII, 97, 102—108
Vascular
  endothelial cells, 148, 156, 189, 218
  injury, 173, 215, 237, 271
VDL, see Lipoproteins, very low density
Vectors, 29, 34, see also specific vectors
Veins, 173—174, 202
Venipuncture, clean, 228
Venom coagglutinin, 189
Venous pressure, 130
Vero monkey kidney cells, 29, 31, 181
Vertebrates, 203
Very low density lipoproteins (VDL), 45
Vesicles, secretory, 174—175, 177, 179, 183, 205, 207, 209
Vessel wall, 148, 156, 173—184, 201, 237, 272
Vibrio cholerae, neuraminidase from, 70
Viral
  carrier states, 306
  contamination, 295
  diseases, blood-borne, 302
  DNA, 303
  immunadsorption, 297
  inactivation, 307, 315—316
  infections, 306
  promoter/enhancer sequences, 27, 29
  proteins, 305
  replication, 303
  stabilization, 314
Viremic state, transient in donor, 301, 303, 306
Virgin hemophiliacs, 314—315, 317
Virus(es)
  blood-borne, transmission of, 289—290, 296—298
  extracellular, instability of, 301, 306
  helper, 302, 305, 317
  inactivation, 301, 307, 312—316
  transmission by VIII products, 301—317
Vitamin K-dependent protein, 16—17, 104, 106, 110, 115, 117, 217, 241, 268
Vitronectin, 66, 157
V_{max}, for activation of factor X, 18
Void volume, 233, 294

Volar surface, of forearm, 130
Vomiting, 309
von Willebrand's disease (vWD), 42, 45, 61, 69, 71, 92, 120, 147, 158—161, 163—165, 192, 201, 203, 209—210, 221, 237, 240, 248, 261, 325
  diagnosis and classification of, 131, 141, 147, 159—161
  electron microscopic studies of, 201, 209—210
  immunochemical aspects of, 147—165
  mild, 131, 133
  plasma, 134, 147, 161
  platelet-type, 132
  pseudo-, 132
  reliability of diagnosis of carriers for, 92
  severe, 133—134, 136, 148—149, 157, 161—162, 187, 203, 227
  type I, 68, 131, 139, 159, 161—164
  type IA, 159
  type IB, 159
  type IC, 159
  type II, 136—137, 163—164, 247
  type IIA, 68, 70—71, 131, 139, 158—159, 161
  type IIB, 139, 158—161
  type IIC, 159—160
  type IID, 159—161
  type III, 159
  type INY, 159
vWf methodology and, 42, 68, 129—141

W

Washed human platelets, 11, 120, 153
Washing bulk cryoprecipitate, 289, 292
Wash-through fractions, 270
Water, 138, 282
Waterbath, mechanically rocking, 283
Weibel-Palade bodies, 84, 90—91, 93, 174—175, 179—181, 183, 188, 202—204, 260
Western blot analysis, 27
Wetting vessels, 291
Working reagents, 97, 101

X

Xanthine-guanine phosphoribosyltransferase (XGPRT) gene, 28
X chromosome, 29
X-ray, 53, 138, 315

Y

Yeasts, gene expression in, 27

Z

Zymogen, 115, 218
Zinc, 269, 293